D1348782

Biology of the
Mouse Histocompatibility-2 Complex

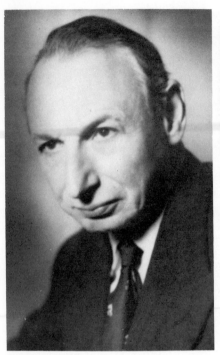

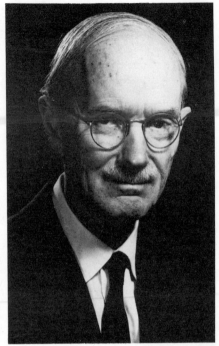

Peter A. Gorer
(Courtesy of Mrs. P. A. Gorer)

George D. Snell
(Courtesy of Dr. G. D. Snell)

Biology of the
Mouse Histocompatibility-2 Complex

Principles of Immunogenetics
Applied to a Single System

Jan Klein

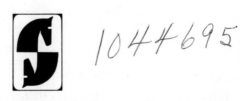

Springer-Verlag   New York · Heidelberg · Berlin   1975

Jan Klein
Department of Microbiology
The University of Texas
Southwestern Medical School
5323 Harry Hines Boulevard
Dallas, Texas 75235

Library of Congress Cataloging in Publication Data

Klein, Jan, 1936–
    Biology of the mouse histocompatibility-2 complex; *principles* ...
    Bibliography: p. 541
    1. H-2 locus. I. Title. [DNLM: 1. Chromosomes.
2. Histocompatibility. 3. Immunogenetics. QH600
K64b].
QR184.3.K54   599′.3233   74–14843
ISBN 0–387–06733–7.

ISBN 0–387–06733–7   Springer-Verlag   New York · Heidelberg · Berlin
ISBN 3–540–06733–7   Springer-Verlag   Berlin · Heidelberg · New York

With love to my mother,
and with apologies to Dagmar, Norman, and Daniel.

"Ach, wenn man doch wissend werden könnte!" rief Knecht.
"Wenn es doch eine Lehre gäbe, etwas, woran man glauben
kann! Alles widerspricht einander, alles läuft aneinander vorbei,
nirgends ist Gewißheit. Alles läßt sich so deuten und läßt sich
auch wieder umgekehrt deuten . . . Gibt es denn keine Wahrheit?
Gibt es keine echte und gültige Lehre?"

Hermann Hesse, *Das Glasperlenspiel*

Preface

Somewhere I heard a story of a bridge and a painter. The bridge was enormous and was made all of metal, and the painter's job was to keep it from rusting. He would start at one end and slowly proceed, day by day, month by month, toward the other end, painting the bridge. But no sooner would he finish with the painting than the bridge would begin to rust again. The rust, too, would start at one end and slowly proceed toward the other end, systematically destroying the painter's endeavor. And so the painter would return to where he had started, and begin painting again, slowly proceeding toward the other end of the bridge, always just one step ahead of the rust. And if the story is true, the painter might still be painting that bridge—a modern Sisyphus!

During the writing of this book, the story of the painter and his bridge kept coming to mind. The field the book covers has been developing so rapidly that, like the painter, I too had to return to where I had started and fight the rust of obsolescence. But unlike the painter, I had a deadline to meet, which constituted a point of no return. And so, sending off this manuscript, I have no choice but to watch the fruits of my endeavor be overtaken by the rust.

In recent years, the *H-2* system has become not only the prototype of similar systems in other species, but also one of the focusing points of modern biology. It forms a bridge between immunology and genetics, between biochemistry and immunology, between virology and genetics, and it carries the potential of broad biological implications. I have tried to cover all these different facets of the system and to present as complete a picture as was in my power.

The breadth of this book's scope forced me to plunge into areas in which I am not an expert and thus increase the risk of having errors slip into the text. Although I tried to minimize such risk through consultations with many of my colleagues, I probably have not avoided it completely. For any errors remaining, I sincerely apologize.

Anticipating that the book might be read by geneticists who know little about immunology, immunologists who know little about genetics, and others who are neither immunologically nor genetically oriented, I have placed at the beginning of each section an introductory chapter summarizing the basic knowledge necessary for understanding the particular section.

Because of the broad area covered and because of the limited space available, I could not document fully by references many important observations mentioned in this monograph. This is particularly true for the introductory chapters. As a rule I have deliberately avoided references to work done in species other than the mouse. This too was motivated only by space limitations.

I am indebted to many individuals who, in different ways, assisted me during the work on this monograph: to Dr. Donald C. Shreffler, with whom I spent my *Lehrjahre;* to Drs. James Forman, Dietrich Götze, Margaret C. Green, Frank Lilly, Eva Lotzová, Hugh O. McDevitt, George D. Snell, and Ellen S. Vitetta who read portions of the book and made invaluable comments and suggestions; to all those quoted in the text who provided me with unpublished data and important documentary material; to Messrs. Jong M. Park and Suresh Savariryan, whose outstanding technical expertise allowed me to continue my research while working on this book, and to Springer-Verlag for having the courage to undertake this venture. But above all, I thank Ms. Pamela Erbe Wiener, who so patiently struggled with my distortions of her native tongue.

Jan Klein

Contents

Part Three: Central Regions of the *H-2* Complex

Section Five: *I*-region associated traits

Section Six: *S* and *X* region-associated traits

Part Four: Conclusion

Part One

Introduction

Chapter One

History

I. Prehistory

The history of the *H-2* system (see Appendix) begins with the advent of tumor transplantation at the turn of the century. By that time, tumor biologists had realized that cancer was a complex disease, with each tumor displaying a certain individuality and uniqueness. Because this individuality limited the length of time a particular tumor would be available, experimenters sought to prolong the observation period by transplanting the neoplastic tissue from one animal to another. However, most attempts at tumor transplantation gave unsatisfactory results because even the few tumors that actually grew in the new host survived only a short time. Only occasionally was a prolonged survival observed, but the conditions under which this occurred were not known. The turning point in the investigation came through the use of inbred stocks of mice by Carl O. Jensen at the Agriculture and Veterinary Institute in Copenhagen, Denmark, and Leo Loeb at the University of Pennsylvania in Philadelphia, Pennsylvania.

Jensen (1903), using a stock of "white mice," successfully propagated a spontaneous alveolar carcinoma through 19 generations. Transplantations of the same tumor to various other stocks of mice failed. The "white mice" apparently achieved a relatively high degree of inbreeding by being maintained in a closed colony in which only matings among relatives were possible.

Loeb used Japanese waltzing mice, which had been bred for centuries in the Far East for their peculiar behavioral characteristics. These mice display extreme nervousness, excitability, and hyperactivity. When excited, they run in circles until exhausted; they whirl, twist, toss their heads, and jerk. These behaviors are caused by an inner ear defect controlled by a single recessive gene. The recessivity of the trait was known to mouse fanciers, who purposely maintained the stock by inbreeding, and thus unknowingly gradually increased its genetic homogeneity. The mice were imported to Europe and to the United States from the Far East at the end of the nineteenth century, and achieved

notoriety among biologists when Loeb (1908) demonstrated their high susceptibility to a tumor of Japanese waltzing mouse origin.

Through Jensen's and Loeb's work, the importance of "race" in susceptibility to tumor transplants was realized and a genetic control of tumor trans-
plantability suggested. The genetics of tumor transplantation was studied by
E. E. Tyzzer (1909), who confirmed Loeb's observation that a tumor of Japanese
waltzing mouse origin (carcinoma JwA) grew in practically all mice of that stock
and not in mice of unrelated stocks. He also observed that F_1 hybrids between
Japanese waltzing and common mice were nearly all killed by the JwA tumor.
Interestingly, the tumor did not grow in the 54 inoculated F_2 hybrids or the 16
inoculated F_3 hybrids, a situation seemingly contradicting simple Mendelian
genetics: in one generation (F_1) a character (susceptibility to a tumor) behaved
as if dominant, but in the following generations (F_2 and F_3) the dominance
vanished. The paradox was explained in 1914 by C. C. Little, who proposed a
genetic theory of tumor transplantation by which he postulated that the susceptibility to a tumor transplant is determined by several dominant genes. The
exact numbers of genes involved can be estimated from the formula $f = (\frac{3}{4})^n$,
where f is the fraction of F_2 mice dying from a tumor and n is the number of
susceptibility genes. A similar formula for the backcross generation is $f = (\frac{1}{2})^n$.
As shown in Table 1-1, the value of f decreases rapidly with the increasing
number of susceptibility genes. With $n = 15$, only about 1 percent of the F_2
and 0.002 percent of the backcross mice are expected to die from the tumor. The

Table 1-1. Relationship between number of genes responsible for susceptibility to a
transplanted tumor and percentage of susceptible mice

Number of genes	Percent susceptible in	
	F_2	backcross to resistant parent
1	75.0	50.0
2	56.2	25.0
3	42.2	12.5
4	31.6	6.2
5	23.7	3.1
6	17.8	1.6
7	13.3	0.8
8	10.0	0.4
9	7.5	0.2
10	5.6	0.1
11	4.2	0.05
12	3.2	0.02
13	2.4	0.01
14	1.8	0.006
15	1.3	0.003

absence of susceptible F_2 and F_3 animals in Tyzzer's experiment can be explained by insufficient sample size.

This theory was experimentally verified by Little and Tyzzer (1916) on a larger sample of mice. Of the 183 F_2 mice inoculated with the JwA tumor, three mice (or 1.6 percent) succumbed to the tumor, leading Little and Tyzzer to conclude that susceptibility to the JwA tumor depended on 14–15 dominant susceptibility genes.

The genetic theory of tumor transplantation was significant not only because it defined the conditions necessary for successful propagation of neoplastic tissue, but also because it stimulated the development of inbred strains—which in turn became an indispensible tool in many areas of biological and medical research. "The introduction of inbred strains into biology is probably comparable in importance with that of the analytical balance into chemistry" (Grüneberg 1952).

The genetic theory of transplantation, however, failed to define the nature of the hypothetical susceptibility genes. Many believed that regression of a tumor in a resistant animal was caused by an active defense mechanism in the host rather than a failure of the tumor tissue to grow. Because inoculation of tumor tissue into a healthy recipient in some ways resembled an invasion of the body by pathogens, it was speculated that the body may respond to foreign tumor cells by production of antibodies, just as occurs during bacterial infections. Although considerable effort was expended searching for the hypothetical antitumor antibodies, none were discovered. Occasionally, reports appeared claiming a demonstration of immunity against cancer cells (Lumsden 1932, Shinoi 1932, and others), but these were lost in the immensity of the negative results. It was generally believed that neoplastic cells differed from normal cells and that the postulated immune reaction was directed against this difference. This hypothesis, however, could not explain why the tumors were not rejected when transplanted within an inbred strain. Haldane (1933) postulated an alternative explanation that the immunity was directed against alloantigens rather than tumor-specific antigens. He predicted that antigenic differences similar to blood-group differences exist in other tissues, and that a tumor arising in a given tissue preserves the alloantigenic characteristics of the donor. He further speculated that the alloantigens induce an immune response in a host lacking them. Transplantation within an inbred strain does not induce such a response, because the donor of the tumor and the host share the same antigens. The mouse, with all its inbred strains and great variety of transplantable tumors, seemed the best experimental animal for testing Haldane's hypothesis. Unfortunately, there was no evidence that alloantigenic or blood-group differences existed in this species. Several investigators tried to find blood groups among the different inbred strains of the mouse, but failed.

II. Early Work

Among those looking for blood-group antigens in the mouse was Peter A. Gorer, then at the Lister Institute in London. Gorer had more luck than his predecessors. Using first normal human group A and later immune rabbit antimouse sera, he was able to detect four blood-group antigens, which he designated I, II, III, and IV (Gorer 1936a, b, 1937a). Antigen II was identified with a rabbit antimouse (strain A) antiserum (Gorer 1936b). The unabsorbed antiserum reacted indiscriminately with red cells of all three inbred strains used by Gorer (A, C57BL, and CBA), apparently due to the presence of a species-specific antibody. After removal of this antibody by absorption with CBA red cells, the antiserum failed to react with CBA and C57BL erythrocytes, although it did react with A erythrocytes. Repeated absorptions with CBA cells lowered the titer against the A cells significantly, but never completely removed the anti-A activity. Absorptions with C57BL cells removed the species-specific antibody, but failed to remove or even decrease the anti-A activity. From these experiments Gorer concluded that the antiserum defined an antigen (antigen II) absent on C57BL and present on both A and CBA cells. Strain A seemed to have a much higher level of antigen II than strain CBA. With this knowledge, Gorer (1937b) proceeded to test the relationship between the blood-group genes and the hypothetical genes for tumor susceptibility. The test involved two inbred strains, A and C57BL, and their hybrids (F_1, F_2, and both backcrosses). The parental strains and the hybrids were inoculated with an A strain carcinoma and at the same time tested serologically with the rabbit antimouse serum for the presence of antigen II. As expected, the A strain, F_1 hybrids, and A backcross were completely susceptible, and the C57BL strain completely resistant to the tumor. In the F_2 generation, of the 65 inoculated mice, 35 were susceptible and 30 were resistant; all the susceptible and 17 of the 61 resistant mice carried antigen II. These results were interpreted by Gorer as an indication that susceptibility to this particular tumor was determined by two or possibly three genes, one of which was identical with the gene for antigen II. The correlation between the presence of an antigen and tumor growth strongly suggested that an immunological mechanism was involved in the regression of the tumor in the resistant animals. The immunological hypothesis of tumor regression was further strengthened by the finding that sera of the C57BL mice that rejected the tumor contained hemagglutinating antibodies directed against A strain erythrocytes. Testing of the F_2 generation (Gorer 1938) revealed that the allo-antibody in the C57BL anti-A antiserum was directed against the same antigen as the rabbit anti-II serum. Of the 24 (A × C57BL)F_2 mice tested, 16 reacted with both the alloantisera and xenoantisera while the remaining 8 reacted with neither, hence establishing antigen II as an alloantigen.

The C57BL anti-A serum reacted strongly with A and weakly with CBA red cells. Absorption with CBA cells removed the anti-CBA but not the anti-A activity. Apparently the antiserum contained at least two antibodies, one specific for A and the other reacting with an antigen shared by A and CBA erythrocytes.

The appearance of anti-II antibodies following tumor regression suggested that the neoplastic tissue shared antigen II with normal tissues. This was confirmed by an absorption experiment in which an A strain tumor absorbed both the anti-A and the anti-CBA alloantibodies from the alloanti-serum.

Gorer's early work established two important facts. First, it demonstrated that the genes for susceptibility to tumor transplants were identical with the genes coding for alloantigens. Second, it provided firm evidence for the immunological nature of resistance to tumor transplants by showing that rejection of a tumor is accompanied by production of alloantibodies. These two discoveries led Gorer to formulate the concept of tissue transplantation. According to Gorer, "normal and neoplastic tissues contain iso-antigenic factors which are genetically determined. Iso-antigenic factors present in the grafted tissue and absent in the host are capable of eliciting a response which results in the destruction of the graft" (Gorer 1938). This immunological theory of transplantation represented one of the major advances in biological sciences of the twentieth century and marked the beginning of the era of transplantation immunology. Curiously, this fact was never formally recognized by prize-awarding committees, which often hailed discoveries of far less significance.

The immunological theory of tissue transplantation was supported by experimentation with normal tissue grafts. Several investigators (e.g. Little and Johnson 1922, Bittner 1936, and others) demonstrated that, for instance, pieces of spleen, when inoculated subcutaneously into individuals of the same strain, survived indefinitely, whereas those transplanted into mice of a different strain were destroyed. Parental spleen transplanted into F_2 hybrids survived in only 1-2 percent of the recipients, indicating involvement of some 12-15 susceptibility genes. Transplanted tissue, whether normal or neoplastic, apparently followed the same laws, the *laws of transplantation*.

The immunological basis of rejection of normal tissue transplants by allogeneic hosts was demonstrated by Medawar and his colleagues at the University of Oxford (Gibson and Medawar 1943, Medawar 1944). Medawar worked with outbred rabbits rather than mice, and used skin rather than splenic tissue as grafts.[1] His experiments were based on the comparison of autografts (grafts on the same animal) to allografts (grafts between genetically different animals of the same species). He demonstrated that in the first week after transplantation auto- and allografts behave in exactly the same way: they heal in and establish a normal blood supply. In the second posttransplantation week, however, differences between the two types of grafts begin to emerge. While the autografts gradually return to the condition of normal skin, the allografts begin to show signs of degeneration. They become inflamed and edematous, and their dermis is infiltrated by mononuclear cells. The inflammatory phase is followed by obliteration of the graft's vascular system and disintegration of the epidermis and dermis. The necrotic graft is then replaced by ingrowth of host epidermis. The destruction (rejection) of the graft is usually completed two to

---

[1] Although skin grafting had been used previously, Medawar's group made it one of the basic techniques of immunological experimentation. The method of skin grafting described by Billingham and Medawar (1951) is still in wide use in numerous modifications in many laboratories around the world.

three weeks after transplantation. A second graft from the same donor placed on the same recipient is rejected much more rapidly than the first one, usually within the first week after transplantation. This *second-set reaction* is sometimes so rapid that the second graft does not have time to heal in. Apparently, the first graft sensitizes the host, which then responds to the second graft in an accelerated fashion. The sensitization is specific: only second-set grafts from the same donor as the first-set grafts are rejected by an accelerated reaction; second grafts from unrelated allogeneic donors are rejected by a typical *first-set* (unaccelerated) reaction. The sensitization is systemic, with the second graft provoking a second-set reaction in almost any part of the body, regardless of the location of the first graft. These three characteristics of the rejection process (accelerated response to second grafts, specificity, and systemic character of sensitization) were considered by Medawar to be evidence that the *allograft reaction* was immunological by nature.

It was assumed that the allograft reaction, like many other immunological phenomena, was mediated by antibodies. Humoral antibodies were indeed frequently found in recipients that rejected tumor (Gorer 1937b) or normal tissue (Amos *et al.* 1954) allografts. Gradually, however, evidence was gathered indicating that the humoral antibody response was not the full explanation of graft rejection. As early as 1910, some investigators noticed that the destruction of the transplants was regularly accompanied by infiltration of the graft by round cells, primarily small lymphocytes. An experimental proof that allograft reaction was not mediated by humoral antibodies was provided in 1954 by Mitchison. In his classical *adoptive transfer* experiment, Mitchison demonstrated that the sensitized state of the recipient rejecting a tumor graft can be transferred to a new recipient with lymphoid cells but not with serum. From this he concluded that the allograft reaction, although frequently accompanied by humoral antibody formation, was basically a cell-mediated type of immunity similar to delayed hypersensitivity. This was later confirmed by many other investigators. By that time, however, immunologists were so used to the idea of antibodies being responsible for specificity of all immunological reactions that they found it difficult to accept a system in which antibodies were not involved. They immediately postulated that the lymphocytes mediating graft destruction carried antibodies firmly bound to their cell surfaces. To this day, the existence of these *cell-bound antibodies* has been neither proved nor disproved. Although it is generally accepted that the lymphocytes involved in cell-mediated immunity carry some kind of recognition structures on their cell membranes, the nature of these structures is still highly controversial.

III. Classical Era

By the middle of the twentieth century, both the genetic theory of transplantation and the immunological explanation of graft rejection were generally accepted. It was clear that a class of genes coded for alloantigens, and that these alloantigens were responsible for rejection of incompatible neoplastic and normal tissue grafts. The antigens responsible for tissue compatibility were summarily designated by Snell (1948) as *histocompatibility antigens*, and the genes coding for these structures as *histocompatibility genes* (*H genes*).

The only known effect of *H* genes[2] is their involvement in graft rejection and the only method available for their detection is transplantation. Because any two inbred strains differ in many *H* loci and because a difference at any single *H* locus can cause graft rejection, in conventional inbred strains the role of individual *H* loci in transplantation cannot be assessed. The analysis of such loci requires specialized genetic methods, the development of which was undertaken by George D. Snell at the Jackson Laboratory in Bar Harbor, Maine.

Snell realized that the first step in genetic analysis of histocompatibility was the separation and identification of individual *H* loci through lines carrying only one *H* difference (Snell 1948). Such lines were first designated *coisogenic*, but this was later changed to *congenic*. Because in any pair of congenic lines one line resisted grafts from the other line, the pairs were also called *congenic resistant* (isogenic resistant, coisogenic resistant). In 1946, Snell began production of several dozen congenic lines, but these were later destroyed by fire. He then began a new set of lines on a scale even more imposing than in the first attempt. This time the program was successful, and its result was a collection of strains that made the mouse the prototype animal in transplantation genetics and immunology. The development of the congenic lines by Snell was the most significant event in transplantation biology since the introduction of inbred strains. Without the lines, progress in many areas of research would have been impossible or considerably hindered.

With a few exceptions, the congenic lines were strikingly similar to the strains from which they were derived. One of the exceptions was strain A.CA, which carried on the A background both the *H* gene for resistance to an A strain tumor and the gene for *Fused tail* (*Fu*). That the *Fu* was introduced along with an *H* gene at once suggested the two were linked, a supposition later confirmed by a linkage test. Furthermore, because Gorer had previously shown that one of the genes for the resistance to A strain tumors was identical with the gene coding for antigen II, Snell set up tests for linkage between genes for antigen II and *Fused tail*. In a joint study with Gorer (Gorer *et al.* 1948), Snell confirmed the identity of the tumor-resistance gene with the gene for antigen II and demonstrated a close linkage between the latter and *Fused tail*. The *H* gene coding for antigen II was designated H_2, later changed to *H-2*.[3] Because the *Fu* gene was previously assigned to linkage group IX (abbreviated LGIX), the *H-2* locus was given the same assignation.

---

[2] According to the genetic convention, gene symbols are italicized, whereas symbols for gene products are printed in a roman type. In this monograph, *H-2* is printed in italics whenever it refers to the genotype (e.g., *H-2* gene, *H-2* complex, *H-2* haplotype, *H-2* recombinant, etc.) and in roman type whenever it refers to the phenotype (e.g., H-2 antigen, H-2 molecule, H-2 chart, etc.). To avoid lengthy expressions such as "antigen controlled by the *H-2ᵃ* haplotype" shorthand expressions are often used such as "*H-2ᵃ* antigens."

[3] Actually, the gene should have been designated *H-1*, because it was the first *H* gene identified.

During the development of the congenic lines, Snell noted that some lines displayed stronger resistance to tumor grafts than others, as though the *H* genes (antigens) differed in strength. After the lines were established, this possibility was tested by Counce and co-workers (1956), who discovered that the *H-2* difference was much more effective in causing rejection of skin or tumor allografts than *non-H-2* differences. Skin grafts exchanged between mice differing at the *H-2* locus were rejected in less than two weeks after grafting, whereas grafts across *non-H-2* barriers were rejected later (sometimes much later) than three weeks after grafting. Tumor grafts quite often overrode a single *non-H-2* barrier, but could not surpass the *H-2* barrier. These experiments led Snell to conclude that there were two types of *H* genes, *major* (strong) and *minor* (weak). Subsequent work by several investigators confirmed this conclusion. The *H-2* gene has remained the sole representative of the strong category, whereas all other known *H* loci (the *non-H-2* loci) are of the weak category. Because the *H-2* locus was later discovered to consist of more than one gene, it also became known as the *major histocompatibility complex* of the mouse.

In 1951, Snell described special genetic methods for the study of tissue compatibility (*histogenetic methods*). Application of these methods to the available congenic lines and inbred strains led to discovery of an astonishing array of alleles at the *H-2* locus. In the original study, Snell and his co-workers described more than a dozen different *H-2* alleles (Snell and Higgins 1951, Snell 1951, Snell *et al.* 1953a). The number of alleles has continued to increase, making it apparent that the *H-2* locus is much more *polymorphic* than any other known locus in the mouse.

About the same time that Snell in Bar Harbor was developing and applying his histogenetic methods, Gorer in England renewed his effort to characterize the *H-2* locus serologically. This effort demonstrated that antigen II was not the only antigen controlled by the *H-2* locus, because antibodies other than anti-II were obtained in several strain combinations (Gorer 1947, Gorer *et al.* 1948, Gorer 1950). However, these were difficult to work with, because they reacted poorly and inconsistently in the saline hemagglutination technique originally used for the detection of antigen II. It was a frustrating experience; it was clear that additional antibodies were present in some antisera, and yet the antisera were unanalyzable because of technical difficulties. Gorer therefore spent much effort developing new serological techniques for the detection of these weak antibodies. After many trials, he evolved two reliable methods, which then became a standard armamentarium not only of *H-2* serologists but of serologists working with other systems as well. The two techniques were the human serum-dextran hemagglutination test[4] (Gorer and Mikulska 1954) and the dye-exclusion cytotoxic test (Gorer and O'Gorman 1956).

With the refined techniques, serological analysis of the *H-2* system progressed rapidly. The work was begun at Guy's Hospital Medical School in London, where Gorer was joined by Z. B. Mikulska and Bernard D. Amos. Amos later

---

[4] This test was later replaced by its modification, the PVP-hemagglutination method of Stimpfling (1961).

continued the work in the United States, first at Roswell Park Memorial Institute in Buffalo, New York, and later at Duke University Medical Center in Durham, North Carolina. In 1952, Gorer was visited by Gustavo Hoecker, who then established another center for *H-2* serology at the Universidad de Chile in Santiago, Chile. The picture that emerged from the early serological analysis of the *H-2* system was one of enormous complexity (Amos *et al.* 1955, Gorer and Mikulska 1959, Hoecker *et al.* 1954, 1959; Amos 1959). It became apparent that the different *H-2* alleles each controlled an array of antigens, some of which seemed to be limited to a single allele while others were shared by two or more alleles. The alleles were designated by small superscript letters ($H-2^a$, $H-2^b$, $H-2^c$, etc.), and the antigens first by capital letters (A, B, C, etc.) and later by Arabic numerals (1, 2, 3, etc.).

The discovery of *serological* complexity was soon followed by the discovery of *genetic* complexity. The first indication that the *H-2* locus was not genetically simple came from a chance observation by Snell (1953) that $H-2^d/H-2^k$ heterozygotes accepted $H-2^a$ tumor grafts. This phenomenon, which later became known as the *dk effect*, was explained by the assumption that the *H-2* locus consisted of two components, *d* and *k*, and that the $H-2^a$ allele was derived by genetic recombination between the components. (For some time $H-2^a$ was written as $H-2^{dk}$). Histogenetic evidence for the occurrence of recombination within the *H-2* locus was provided by Sally L. Allen (1955a), then at the Jackson laboratory in Bar Harbor. She observed among the offspring of an $H-2^a/H-2^f$ heterozygote one exceptional animal which, when crossed to an $H-2^k/H-2^k$ homozygote, produced progeny resistant to an $H-2^a$ tumor. The same animal, when crossed to an $H-2^d/H-2^d$ homozygote, produced progeny that were 50 percent resistant to the same tumor. One explanation offered by Allen for this behavior was that the exceptional animal lost the *d* component of the $H-2^a$ allele by an intra-*H-2* crossing-over. In the outcross to $H-2^d$, the recombinant type was complemented by the $H-2^d$ allele, and the animals carrying the recominant type were therefore susceptible to the $H-2^a$ tumor. In the outcross to $H-2^k$, no such complementation occurred, and the animals were therefore all resistant.

The first intra-*H-2* recombinant detected by serological methods was described by Gorer and co-workers (Amos *et al.* 1955, Gorer and Mikulska 1959). The recombinant was obtained in a cross $H-2^b/H-2^d \times H-2^d/H-2^d$. The progeny of this cross were tested with antisera against antigens 2 and 5 of the $H-2^b$ allele. Of the 32 animals tested, 18 reacted with both antibodies, 13 reacted with neither, and one reacted with anti-2 but not with anti-5. A progeny test with the exceptional animal then confirmed that a genetic change from $+2+5$ to $+2-5$ types occurred. Gorer explained the change as a crossing-over between the genetic determinants for antigens 2 and 5. This interpretation was supported by the finding that the recombinant *H-2* allele gained the H-2.31 antigen of $H-2^d$. Gorer and Mikulska (1959) also described two more recombinants that arose from a heterozygote $H-2^a/H-2^b$. A number of additional *H-2* recombinants were later described by several other investigators.

Serological analysis of individual *H-2* recombinants revealed the *H-2* locus to be a complex consisting of several regions separable by genetic crossing-over. The regions were designated by capital letters (*D*, *C*, *V*, *E*, *A*, *K*), and each region was believed to consist of one locus (or gene cluster) coding for one or more H-2 antigens. An unexpected evidence supporting the multilocus model of the *H-2* system was furnished by Shreffler and Owen (1963), who discovered a genetically controlled quantitative variant in the serum of normal mice, the serum substance (Ss). Shreffler later showed that the locus coding for the Ss antigen was located within the *H-2* complex (Shreffler 1965), with genes for H-2 antigens on both sides of the locus. It was clear that the *H-2* was not a single gene. Under these circumstances, it was no longer appropriate to call the *H-2* a "locus" and the alternative *H-2* forms, "alleles"; consequently, the former was more appropriately termed *H-2 system* or *H-2 complex* and the latter *H-2 haplotype* or *H-2 chromosome*.

By the late 1960s, the *H-2* system consisted of approximately 24 different *H-2* haplotypes, over 30 antigens, and six histocompatibility regions. Because of this system's forbidding complexity, the H-2 workers soon found themselves relatively isolated, and although they continued to probe deeply into the system, they found little outside interest in their accomplishments. The *H-2* system was often considered an exotic curiosity completely detached from reality.

IV. Renaissance of the *H-2* System

The first development of three to revive interest in the *H-2* system was the realization that other mammals besides the mouse also possessed one major histocompatibility complex (MHC) and that these MHC's were remarkable similar to the *H-2* system. A genetic system able so stubbornly to withstand the test of evolution was clearly not just an exotic curiosity. Much renewed interest in the *H-2* system came from those working with the human *HL-A* system; they soon discovered that some of the methodology and many of the conceptual advances developed by the *H-2* workers were also applicable to *HL-A* studies.

The second major development that renewed interest in the *H-2* system was a series of discoveries linking the system to such biologically important functions as susceptibility and resistance to certain viruses and the genetic control of the immune response to certain antigens. In 1964, Lilly and his co-workers demonstrated that the difference in the susceptibility of different strains of mice to the infection with Gross virus was controlled by one major gene closely linked to *H-2*. Subsequent work by Lilly (1970) showed that the gene was probably located within the *H-2* complex. Genetic control of susceptibility to other leukemia viruses was also found to be associated with the *H-2* system.

In 1965, McDevitt and Sela discovered that the level of the humoral antibody response to certain synthetic polypeptides was under strict control by a major gene (*Ir-1*) located within the *H-2* system (McDevitt *et al.* 1972). This discovery was followed by a number of reports indicating that genetic control of the immune response to a variety of other antigens was also linked to the *H-2* system. At present, the response to some 30 different antigens has been in one way or another associated with the *H-2* complex, suggesting that the complex has an important biological function and that elucidation of this function might prove crucial for understanding the genetics and immunology of host suscepti- bility to infectious diseases.

The third development leading to the renaissance of the *H-2* studies was brought about by these studies themselves. In a perfect example of a Hegelian dialectic evolution, at the point when the *H-2* became hopelessly complex, the trend reversed itself and produced a considerably simplified picture of the system. The reversal was triggered by a discovery that similar H-2 antigens might be controlled by different loci of the complex (Shreffler *et al.* 1966). This discovery led to a reinterpretation of serological and genetic data and to a new model of the *H-2* system (J. Klein and Shreffler 1971, Stimpfling 1971, Snell *et al.* 1973a), which viewed the system as consisting of only two histocompatibility genes (or gene clusters), *H-2K* and *H-2D* (*two locus model*). The two-locus model is supported by a number of observations, a most important being that certain H-2 antigens can be arranged into two mutually exclusive series, apparently controlled by alleles at two genetic loci (Snell *et al.* 1971b). The attractiveness of the two-locus model is its simplicity. In this model, the *H-2* system has left its highly specialized realm and has become, once again, public property.

However, if Hegel's dialectic can be trusted, the two-locus model should not be the last word in H-2 genetics. After thesis and antithesis, the synthesis is yet due. There are already signs indicating that the two-gene model is an over- simplification. Evidence has recently been gathered (J. Klein *et al.* 1974b) support- ing the existence of a third histocompatibility locus, *H-2I*, in the vicinity of the *H-2K* locus. The chromosomal segment between *H-2K* and *Ss* has been shown to code for antigens detectable by serological methods, but apparently different from the classic H-2 antigens (David *et al.* 1973a, Hauptfeld *et al.* 1973a), the so-called *Ir region associated* or *Ia antigens*. And the loci responsible for activa- tion of lymphocytes in mixed lymphocyte culture and in graft-versus-host reaction seem to be spread throughout the *H-2* complex (Bach *et al.* 1972a, b, Meo *et al.* 1973a, J. Klein and Park 1973, Oppltová and Démant 1973). There- fore, it is likely that the true picture of the *H-2* system is somewhere between the original multilocus and the simplistic two-locus model.

The interpretation and the nomenclature of the *H-2* complex to be adopted here is depicted diagrammatically in Table 1–2. (See J. Klein *et al.* 1974a.) The complex is divided by the *Ss* locus into two ends, the *K end* between *H-2K* and *Ss*, and the *D end* between *Ss* and *H-2D*. The term "end" will also be used to indicate direction; thus, the *K end* will mean a direction from the *Ss* locus toward the centromere, and the *D end* the direction from the *Ss* locus toward the telomere. The *H-2* complex is composed of regions, subregions, and loci. An *H-2* region is a segment of the *H-2* complex consisting of a marker gene and an indeterminate number of neighboring loci. At present, there are five regions in the *H-2* complex, *K*, *I*, *S*, *X*, and *D*. The *I* region consists of two (or possibly

Table 1-2. Genetic nomenclature of the *H-2* complex*

Complex	*H-2*						
Ends	*K*					*D*	
Regions	*K*	*I*			*S*	"*X*"	*D*
Subregions		*IA*	*IB*	*IC*			
Loci	*H-2K*	*Ir-1A*	*Ir-1B*	*Ia*	*Ss*	*Lad*	*H-2D*
	Lad	*Ir-(T, G)-A--L***	*Ir-LDH*$_B$	*Lad*	*Slp*	*H-2G*	*Lad*
		*Ir-IgA***	*Ir-Nase*	*Ir-GLT?*			
		*Ir-RE***	*Lad?*				
		Ir-OA	*Ia*				
		Ir-OM					
		Ir-BGG					
		H-2I					
		Lad					
		Ia					

* The genetic relationship of the individual loci in each region or subregion is not known.
** The location of this gene into the *IA* subregion is only tentative.

three) subregions, *IA* and *IB* (formerly termed *Ir-1* and *Ir-IgG*, respectively). Each region or subregion contains at least one *locus*, defined as a segment of the genetic material coding for a single polypeptide chain. The loci in the regions or subregions *K*, *IA*, *IB*, *S* and *D* are denoted *H-2K*, *Ir-1A*, *Ir-1B*, *Ss*, and *H-2D*, respectively; no clearly defined locus has as yet been assigned to the region *X*. Loci responsible for graft rejection are designated *H-2* followed by a capital letter (i.e., *H-2K*, *H-2I*, and *H-2D*); loci responsible for genetic control of immune response to antigens are designated *Ir-1* followed also by a capital letter (i.e., *Ir-1A* and *Ir-1B*); loci responsible for lymphocyte activation in mixed lymphocyte culture and in graft-versus-host reaction are denoted *Lad* (lymphocyte-activating determinants) followed by an Arabic numeral (i.e., *Lad-1*, *Lad-2*, *Lad-3*, etc.) and finally, loci controlling *I*-region-associated antigens are designated *Ia.1*, *Ia.2*, *Ia.3*, and so on. For the sake of convenience, the *H-2* regions will be divided here into *peripheral* (*K* and *D*) and *central* (*I*, *S*, and *X*). The first half of this book will deal with the peripheral regions, and the second half with the central regions.

The alternative forms of genes at a single locus, or of subregions and regions, are called *alleles* and are designated by small superscript letters (and numbers) indicating their genetic origin (e.g., $H\text{-}2K^b$, $H\text{-}2D^d$, Ss^k, etc.). The alternative forms of the whole *H-2* complex are called haplotypes and are also designated by small letter (and number) superscripts.

V. The Beginning of the Golden Age?

At the present time, the picture of the *H-2* system resembles a partially assembled puzzle with the main outline rapidly emerging and many pieces still missing. One of the missing pieces is *H-2* biochemistry. Although the first attempt to isolate H-2 antigens was made almost two decades ago (Billingham *et al.* 1956), the biochemists are still struggling with the most basic problems and technical difficulties. Development of methods for isolation and purification of H-2 antigens will undoubtedly lead to progress in the elucidation of the structural basis of H-2 serology, determination of the relationship between H-2 and other biologically important molecules (for example, immunoglobulins), determination of the structural relationship between the products of the different *H-2* regions and subregions, and in other areas of H-2 research.

Another blank in the puzzle is the genetic variability of the *H-2* system. Nothing is yet known about the actual extent of the *H-2* polymorphism, about the forces maintaining it in natural populations, and about its evolutionary significance.

However, the most difficult problem is the function and functional inter-relationship of the different *H-2* regions. Do the regions operate independently of each other, or do they collaborate in performance of their functions? If they collaborate, what is the nature of the collaboration? And even more generally, what is the biological function of the individual *H-2* regions and of the *H-2* complex as a whole?

It appears that at least one region of the *H-2* complex might be involved in the antigen recognition by thymus-derived lymphocytes (T cells). It has been speculated (Benacerraf and McDevitt 1972) that the *I* region codes for the hypothetical recognition structure of the T cells, the T cell receptor, and that the receptor is distinct from conventional immunoglobulin molecules. Should the concept of the *H-2*-associated recognition molecules prove to be correct, it would revolutionize modern immunology. However, even if the hypothesis of the *H-2*-controlled T cell receptors proves to be incorrect, it is already clear from the knowledge available that an in-depth study of the *H-2* complex will change some presently maintained immunological dogmas.

Clearly, the most exciting era of the *H-2* studies is yet to come!

Chapter Two

The Mouse and Its Forms

An understanding of the different aspects of the *H-2* system requires some knowledge of the animal inherent to the system, the mouse. This chapter summarizes the essential information on the various forms of wild and domesticated mice.

I. Taxonomy

The house mouse, *Mus musculus* Linnaeus, is in the order *Rodentia* (Table 2–1), the suborder *Myomorpha*, the superfamily *Muroidea*, the family *Muridae*, and the subfamily *Murinae* (Simpson 1945). In the same subfamily are 75 other genera, only three of which are found in Europe and/or North America: the harvest mouse (*Micromys*), the field mouse (*Apodemus*), and the rat (*Rattus*). In the genus *Mus*, Ellerman (1941) lists 130 different forms. There is no agreement among the taxonomists as to which of these forms are distinct species and which are subspecies, races, and local varieties. One extreme view, held, for instance, by Schwarz and Schwarz (1943) and Schwarz (1945), is that all the forms belong to *one* species, *Mus musculus*. Classification proposed by these latter authors will be adopted here.

Table 2-1. Taxonomical classification of the order *Rodentia**

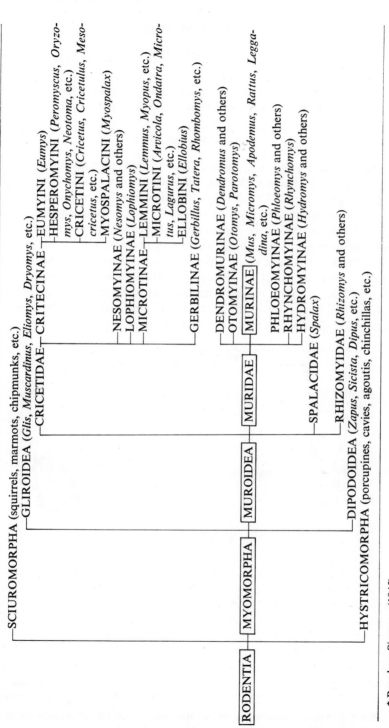

* Based on Simpson (1945).

II. Wild Mice

"Wild mice are unconfined animals over whose reproduction man does not have any control" (Bruell 1970). They are distinguished from domesticated mice, whose breeding in captivity is controlled by man. The term wild mice refers to three different categories of animals: aboriginal, commensal, and feral.

A. Aboriginal Mice

"Aboriginal *M. musculus* are mice that to our best knowledge have never lived in close association with man. They are genuinely wild in the sense this word is usually used" (Bruell 1970). Aboriginal mice are found only on the Eurasian continent, except for one subspecies that is indigenous to Northwest Africa, north of the Atlas Mountains. They are typical dry-area animals, inhabiting steppes and savannahs, where they make burrows in the ground and live on grass, seeds, and grain. Schwarz and Schwarz (1943) distinguish four aboriginal subspecies of *M. musculus*: *M.m. wagneri* Eversmann, *M.m. spicilegus* Petenyi, *M.m. manchu* Thomas, and *M.m. spretus* Lataste. The subspecies differ in body size, head size, tail length, and coat color. The approximate geographical distribution of these subspecies is shown in Fig. 2–1.

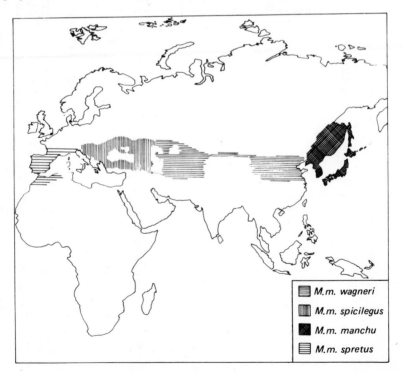

Fig. 2-1. Approximate geographical distribution of four aboriginal subspecies of *Mus musculus*. (Based on Schwarz and Schwarz 1943.)

B. Commensal Mice

Commensal *M. musculus* are mice that live in close association with man in human-built shelters: houses, granaries, corn cribs, stables, chicken coops, tool sheds, barns, and so on. They feed on scraps of food or on man's food supplies. They are derived from three of the four aboriginal subspecies; the fourth subspecies, *M.m. spretus*, has not produced any known commensal form. Schwarz and Schwarz (1943) distinguish 11 commensal subspecies of *M. musculus*, nine derived from *M.m. wagneri* and one each derived from *M.m. spicilegus* and *M.m. manchu*. The origin of the commensal forms is shown in Table 2-2, their geographical distribution in Fig. 2-2. The commensal mice

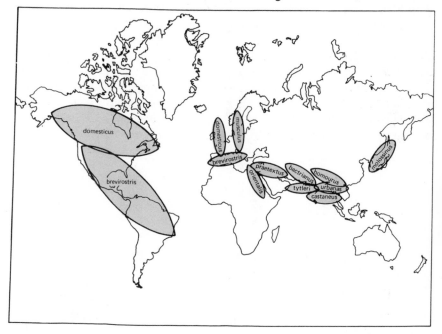

Fig. 2-2. Areas inhabited by commensal subspecies of *Mus musculus*. (Based on Schwarz and Schwarz 1943.)

are true cosmopolitans, remarkably adapted to different climatic conditions. Together with the house rat, they are the most successful mammals. Because of the diversity of conditions in which they live, the commensal forms show much greater variability than the aboriginal subspecies. In general, the commensal mice tend to be larger and to have darker fur and longer tails than the aboriginal mice. The tail of the aboriginal mice is always shorter than the head and the body, whereas the tail of the commensal forms is either as long as the head and the body or longer.

The house mouse was imported to the Americas in the post-Columbian era, apparently on the ships of the first settlers. There were two lines of invasion of

Table 2-2. Origin and dispersal of the commensal subspecies of *Mus musculus**

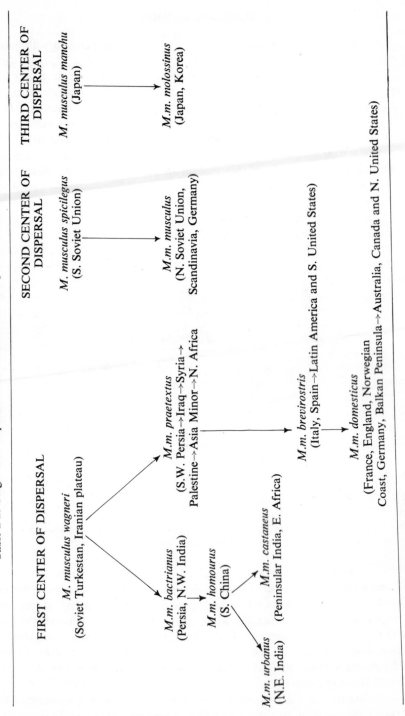

FIRST CENTER OF DISPERSAL

SECOND CENTER OF DISPERSAL

THIRD CENTER OF DISPERSAL

M. musculus wagneri
(Soviet Turkestan, Iranian plateau)

M. musculus spicilegus
(S. Soviet Union)

M. musculus manchu
(Japan)

M.m. praetextus
(S.W. Persia→Iraq→Syria→
Palestine→Asia Minor→N. Africa

M.m. bactrianus
(Persia, N.W. India)

M.m. homourus
(S. China)

M.m. castaneus
(Peninsular India, E. Africa)

M.m. urbanus
(N.E. India)

M.m. brevirostris
(Italy, Spain→Latin America and S. United States)

M.m. domesticus
(France, England, Norwegian
Coast, Germany, Balkan Peninsula→Australia, Canada and N. United States)

M.m. musculus
(N. Soviet Union,
Scandinavia, Germany)

M.m. molossinus
(Japan, Korea)

* Based on Schwarz and Schwarz (1943).

the American continent by the mouse: one along the shipping lanes from Spain and Portugal, the other from northern Europe, primarily from England, France, and Germany. The Spaniards introduced the Mediterranean subspecies, *M.m. brevirostris*, to the Latin American countries and to the southern part of the United States, formerly under Spanish rule. The English, French, and German settlers introduced the North European subspecies, *M.m. domesticus*, to the northern parts of the United States, Canada and Alaska.

C. Feral Mice

Feral mice "are mice that once were commensals of man but reverted to a more feral existence" (Bruell 1970). They are found in areas such as agricultural fields, open grasslands, marshes, sandhills, and coastal islands. Like the aboriginal mice, field mice also live in burrows and feed on grass and grain. Many commensal mice live temporarily as field mice, moving into the fields when the weather is warm and dry and returning to man's shelters when the weather becomes cold and wet. The reversion to field life is more frequent among the less specialized commensals, namely those with shorter tails and lighter fur. Permanent reversion to feral habits usually occurs only in the dry climatic zone.

III. Domesticated Mice

Domesticated *M. musculus* are mice that have been deliberately adapted to life in captivity. The earliest domesticated mice were bred for fancy, particularly in ancient China and Japan, where pet fanciers collected rare variants of mice and kept them for entertainment. The hobby of breeding fancy mice was brought by British traders to Europe, and from there eventually spread to the United States. In the second half of the nineteenth century, domesticated mice found their way into the laboratories and became favorite experimental animals in many areas of research. Originally, mice used for experimentation were provided by pet shops, pet dealers, or mouse fanciers, but later scientists preferred to raise their own animals.

A. Inbred Strains

1. Theory

Random-bred mice, that is, mice mated without regard to their relationship, are usually genetically heterogeneous. In many experiments this heterogeneity is undesirable, because it introduces additional variables into the experimental conditions. Since the cause of genetic heterogeneity is segregation of alleles at heterozygous loci,[1] genetic homogeneity can be achieved by restricting segregation and heterozygosity. The process used to restrict heterozygosity and to increase homozygosity is inbreeding or mating of individuals more closely

---

[1] For explanations of genetic terms, see Chapter Nine.

related to each other than individuals chosen at random from a population. Inbreeding can take different forms, depending on the degree of kinship between the mated individuals. The form most commonly used in the mouse is the full-sib, or brother-sister mating, consisting of breeding individuals that have both parents in common.

The genetic consequences of repeated brother-sister mating can be explained using as an example a single locus with two alleles, A and a. There can be three genotypes with regard to this locus: AA, Aa, and aa. Assume that from a random sample of mice carrying the A locus, two have been selected for mating and that both happen to be Aa heterozygotes. The mating, which can be written genetically as $Aa \times Aa$, produces three types of progeny: AA, Aa, and aa in the ratios $\frac{1}{4}:\frac{1}{2}:\frac{1}{4}$. From these progeny, two mice (littermates) are selected for further mating. Theoretically, the three genotypes can be arranged into six combinations and four types of matings called incrosses, crosses, backcrosses, and intercrosses (E. Green and Doolittle 1963):

Incrosses: $\begin{pmatrix} AA \times AA \\ aa \times aa \end{pmatrix}$

Crosses: $(AA \times aa)$

Backcrosses: $\begin{pmatrix} AA \times Aa \\ aa \times Aa \end{pmatrix}$

Intercrosses: $(Aa \times Aa)$

Because the number of Aa mice is twice as great as the number of either AA or aa mice, the Aa individuals have a better chance to be selected for mating than the AA or aa individuals. The exact probability of selecting a particular combination for mating can be calculated by multiplying the relative frequencies with which the individual genotypes occur. This is best achieved in the form of a checkerboard, as shown in Table 2–3. The probability (P) of the various types of mating in the first generation of inbreeding (F_1) are

$$P \begin{pmatrix} AA \times AA \\ aa \times aa \end{pmatrix} = \tfrac{2}{16} = \tfrac{1}{8}$$

$$P(AA \times aa) = \tfrac{2}{16} = \tfrac{1}{8}$$

$$P \begin{pmatrix} AA \times Aa \\ aa \times Aa \end{pmatrix} = \tfrac{4}{8} = \tfrac{1}{2}$$

$$P(Aa \times Aa) = \tfrac{1}{4}$$

In the next generation (F_2), the following situation ensues. The progeny of the F_1 incrosses, because of the brother-sister mating system, yield only incrosses, with the same probability as in the F_1 generation ($\frac{1}{8}$). The progeny of the F_1 crosses yield only intercrosses (probability $\frac{1}{8}$). The F_2 backcrosses ($AA \times Aa$ or $aa \times Aa$) each produce two types of progeny, AA and Aa or aa and Aa, with probability $\frac{1}{2}$ of each type. These yield three types of mating with probabilities

Table 2-3. Possible mating types and their probabilities in a segregating population consisting of $\frac{1}{4}AA$, $\frac{1}{2}Aa$ and $\frac{1}{4}aa$ genotypes

Parent A	Parent B		
	$\frac{1}{4}\,AA$	$\frac{1}{2}\,Aa$	$\frac{1}{4}\,aa$
$\frac{1}{4}\,AA$	$\frac{1}{16}\,(AA \times AA)$	$\frac{1}{8}\,(AA \times Aa)$	$\frac{1}{16}\,(AA \times aa)$
$\frac{1}{2}\,Aa$	$\frac{1}{8}\,(AA \times Aa)$	$\frac{1}{4}\,(Aa \times Aa)$	$\frac{1}{8}\,(aa \times Aa)$
$\frac{1}{4}\,aa$	$\frac{1}{16}\,(AA \times aa)$	$\frac{1}{8}\,(aa \times Aa)$	$\frac{1}{16}\,(aa \times aa)$

$$P\left(\begin{matrix} AA \times AA \\ aa \times aa \end{matrix}\right) = \tfrac{2}{16} = \tfrac{1}{8}$$

$$P\left(\begin{matrix} AA \times Aa \\ aa \times Aa \end{matrix}\right) = \tfrac{4}{16} = \tfrac{1}{4}$$

$$P(Aa \times Aa) = \tfrac{2}{16} = \tfrac{1}{8}$$

And finally, the F_1 intercrosses, occurring with a probability of $\frac{1}{4}$, produce in F_2 four types of matings with probabilities

Incrosses: $\quad \tfrac{2}{64} = \tfrac{1}{32} = 0.031$

Crosses: $\quad \tfrac{2}{64} = \tfrac{1}{32} = 0.31$

Backcrosses: $\quad \tfrac{4}{32} = \tfrac{1}{8} \ = 0.125$

Intercrosses: $\quad \tfrac{1}{16} = 0.062$

The probability of different crosses in the F_3 and all following generations can be arrived at in a similar way, always using the values from the previous generation. The relationship between frequencies of the four mating types in two successive generations of brother-sister mating is shown in Table 2–4. The relationship can be expressed mathematically in the form of four equations:

$$p_{n+1} = p_n + \tfrac{1}{4}r_n + \tfrac{1}{8}v_n$$
$$q_{n+1} = \qquad\qquad \tfrac{1}{8}v_n$$
$$r_{n+1} = \qquad \tfrac{1}{2}r_n + \tfrac{1}{2}v_n$$
$$v_{n+1} = q_n + \tfrac{1}{4}r_n + \tfrac{1}{4}v_n$$

where p, q, r, and v are the probabilities of incrosses, crosses, backcrosses, and intercrosses, respectively, and n is the generation. The actual values of p, q, r, and v for the first 20 generations of brother-sister mating are given in Table 2–5 which, in addition, also shows the total probability of heterozygotes (h) calculated from the formula

$$h_n = \tfrac{1}{2}r_n + v_n$$

It is apparent from Table 2–5 that in the successive generations of the full-sib mating the probability of incrosses (p), and thus the probability of homozygosity, gradually increases, whereas the probability of heterozygosity (h) decreases.

Table 2-4. Relationship between frequencies of various types of matings in two successive generations of brother-sister mating*

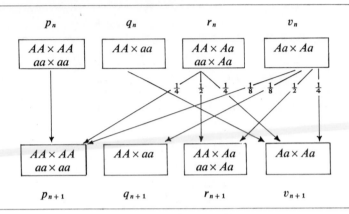

Table 2-5. The probability of incrosses (p_n), crosses (q_n) backcrosses (r_n), intercrosses (v_n), and heterozygosity (h_n) in the first 20 generations (F_n) of brother-sister mating when $v_0 = 1$

F_n	p_n	q_n	r_n	v_n	h_n	h_{n+1}/h_n
F_0	0.000	0.000	0.000	1.000	1.000	—
F_1	0.125	0.125	0.500	0.250	0.500	0.500
F_2	0.281	0.031	0.375	0.312	0.500	1.000
F_3	0.414	0.039	0.344	0.203	0.375	0.750
F_4	0.525	0.025	0.273	0.176	0.312	0.833
F_5	0.616	0.022	0.225	0.138	0.250	0.800
F_6	0.689	0.017	0.181	0.113	0.203	0.812
F_7	0.748	0.014	0.147	0.091	0.164	0.808
F_8	0.797	0.013	0.119	0.073	0.133	0.809
F_9	0.836	0.009	0.097	0.057	0.107	0.809
F_{10}	0.867	0.007	0.078	0.047	0.087	0.809
F_{11}	0.893	0.006	0.062	0.039	0.070	0.809
F_{12}	0.913	0.005	0.051	0.031	0.057	0.809
F_{13}	0.930	0.004	0.041	0.025	0.046	0.809
F_{14}	0.943	0.003	0.033	0.020	0.037	0.809
F_{15}	0.954	0.003	0.026	0.016	0.030	0.809
F_{16}	0.963	0.002	0.021	0.014	0.024	0.809
F_{17}	0.970	0.002	0.018	0.010	0.019	0.809
F_{18}	0.976	0.001	0.014	0.009	0.015	0.809
F_{19}	0.981	0.001	0.011	0.007	0.012	0.809
F_{20}	0.985	0.000	0.009	0.006	0.010	0.809

This is depicted graphically in Fig. 2-3, which shows that the increase of p is at first very rapid, but in later generations levels off. As the ratios h_{n+1}/h_n (i.e., the ratios of the probability of heterozygosity in one generation to the probability of heterozygosity in the preceeding generation) indicate, after the first few generations the heterozygosity is decreasing at a constant rate of 19.1 percent per generation. At 20 generations of brother-sister mating, the p reaches a value close to 100 percent (in principle, it never quite reaches 100 percent). A line that has undergone 20 or more consecutive generations of brother-sister mating is called *inbred*.

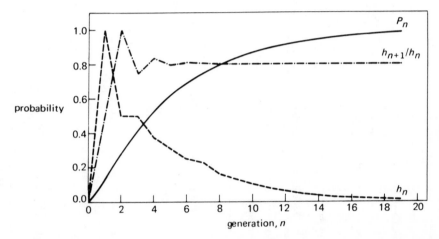

Fig. 2-3. The probability of incrosses (p_n) and of heterozygosity (h_n) in 20 successive generations of brother-sister mating when $v_0 = 1$, and the ratios of successive values of h_{n+1}/h_n. (Reproduced with permission from E. L. Green and D. P. Doolittle: "Systems of mating used in mammalian genetics." In *Methodology in Mammalian Genetics*, W. J. Burdette (ed.) pp. 3–55. Copyright © 1963 by Holden-Day. All rights reserved.)

If in the first generation one would by chance select an incross combination ($AA \times AA$ or $aa \times aa$), there would be no further segregation and all the animals in the subsequent generations would be homozygous at the A locus. However, this still would not make the line inbred. The founders of an inbred line are heterozygous not at one but at a number of different loci, and it is homozygosity at more than 98 percent of these loci that is required for certification of a line as inbred. The probability of selecting in the first generation two animals homozygous at 98 percent of the originally heterozygous loci is negligible.

2. Nomenclature

The symbols designating the individual inbred strains of the mouse consist of letters (capital or small) and/or numerals (Arabic or Roman). The reasons for choosing a particular symbol are often peculiar. For example, in the BALB/c symbol, the BALB stands for *B*agg's *alb*ino, and the c is the gene for albinism;

Table 2-6a. Genealogy of the more commonly used inbred strains (*H-2* haplotypes in parentheses)*

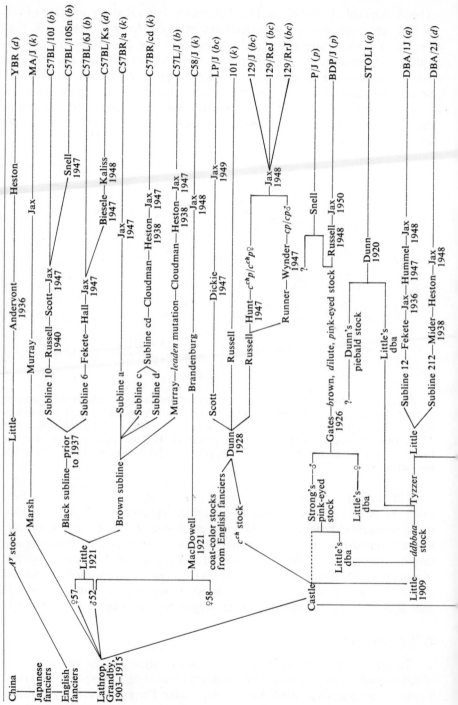

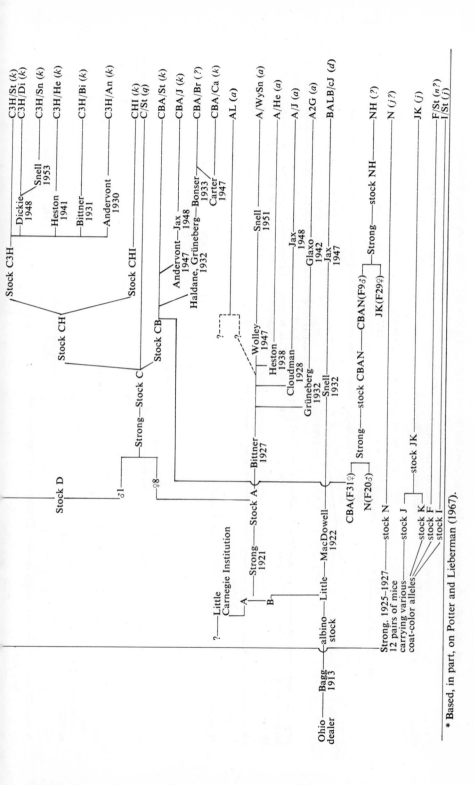

* Based, in part, on Potter and Lieberman (1967).

Table 2-6b. Genealogy of the more commonly used inbred strains (*H-2* haplotypes in parentheses)*

Princeton dealer —— Rockefeller Institute in Princeton, N.J., 1922 —— Stock used in experiments with *pneumonia*-like organisms —— Lynch —— Rockefeller Institute in New York —— Jax 1952 —— PL/J (*u*)

—— BSVS (*t5*)

Rockefeller Institute in New York heterogeneous stock —— albino line —— Webster 1929 —— *bacteria-susceptible-virus-susceptible* stock

—— *bacteria-resistant-virus-susceptible* stock —— BRVS (?)

—— Furth 1928 —— Oak Ridge (Upton) —— Jax 1954 —— RF/J (*k*)

Pennsylvania breeder, supplier to Du Pont, 1928 —— Furth 1928 —— Rockefeller Institute, N.Y. —— Rhoades 1936 —— Lynch 1940 —— F27 —— Law 1948 —— AKR/Lw (*k*)

F32 —— Jax 1948 —— AKR/J (*k*)

—— Oak Ridge (Furth) 1949 —— Upton 1959 —— Cumberland Farms 1960 —— AKR/Cum (?)

—— CIBA (1953) —— AKR/FuA (?)

Swiss stock Lausanne —— de Coulon —— Lynch —— Parker —— Jax 1947 —— SWR/J (*q*)

Denmark —— Street —— Egelbreth —— Holm —— strain ST at > F8 —— subline b —— Heston 1947 —— Jax 1948 —— ST/bJ (*k*)

subline a —— Simonsen —— ST/a (*b*)

inbreeding began circa 1945 —— stock A —— BUA (?)

Brown *University* —— albino stock BU —— stock B —— Jax 1968 —— BUB (*q*)

Wild mutant trapped in Illinois by Knight in 1920 —— Detlefsen —— *ce* stock —— Eaton —— Woolley —— Jax 1948 —— CE/J (*k*)

—— Eaton 1940 —— Woolley 1948 —— Dickie 1949 —— Jax 1954 —— DE/J (*k ?*)

? —— Ohio State University —— Erwin strain —— Eaton —— E strain

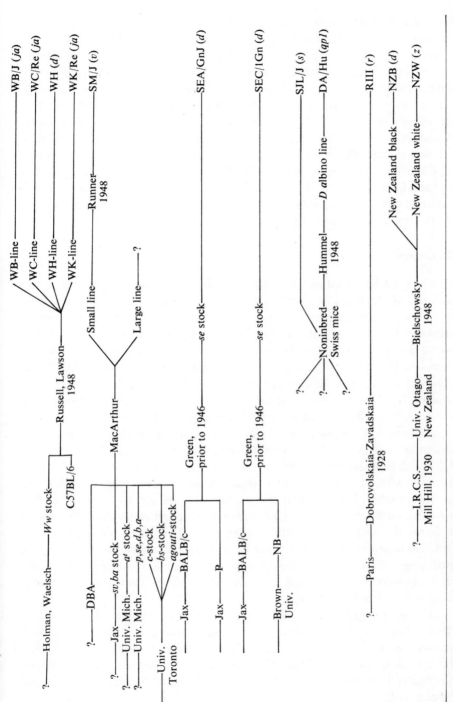

* Based, in part, on Potter and Lieberman (1967).

DBA means *d*ilute, *b*rown non-*a*gouti, three coat-color genes present in the founder stock; C57BL and C57BR got their names from the fact that their founder happened to have number 57 and her descendants were *bl*ack or *br*own, and so on. Different substrains of the same strain are distinguished by an abbreviation, separated from the strain symbol by a slanted line, and indicating the name of the person (or laboratory) who maintains them. For example, C3H/St is a substrain of C3H maintained by L. C. Strong; A/J is a substrain of A maintained by the Jackson Laboratory, and so on. Two or more substrain symbols indicate that the strain changed owners. Thus, C3H/HeJ is a subline of C3H, originally maintained by W. E. Heston and later acquired by the Jackson Laboratory. According to nomenclature rules (Snell *et al.* 1960), a new substrain symbol is assigned to a strain that has been separated from its founder strain for a minimum of five generations of brother-sister mating.

3. Origin

The most recent list of inbred strains (Staats 1972) contains 244 entries, the majority of which can be traced to a few founder stocks derived from domesticated mice of pet dealers and mouse fanciers. One major source of the founder stocks was the mouse farm of A. E. C. Lathrop in Brandby, Massachusetts, where a large collection of fancy mice, mainly coat-color variants imported from England or Germany or obtained from dealers in the United States (Massachusetts, Ohio, New Jersey), was housed. The stocks were probably kept isolated from one another, but no strict inbreeding system was deliberately followed. In the first two decades of this century, Ms. Lathrop supplied mice to several investigators, some of whom used them for development of inbred strains. Lines C57L, C57BR, C58, C57BL, MA, BDP, N, F, JK, NH, C3H, CBA, and probably several others, can all be traced directly or indirectly to the Lathrop collection. Other sources of inbred strain founders included unidentified dealers in Ohio, Pennsylvania, Illinois, and New Jersey. Most of the dealers were in contact with each other, constantly trading and exchanging their stocks, a factor that led to considerable intermixing of the gene pools among the different mouse colonies. Additional intermixing probably occurred during the early stages of inbred strain development, because in many instances the developing lines were not maintained by strict brother-sister mating, and sometimes were not even pedigreed.

The genealogy of the more important inbred strains is summarized in Tables 2–6a and 2–6b. It must be emphasized that in addition to the interconnections shown in these tables, there were probably many more, of which there is no record. For additional information on the inbred strain genealogy, the reader is referred to articles by Staats (1966, 1972), Heston (1949), and Strong (1942).

B. Congenic Lines

1. Theory

Two lines that are genetically identical (*isogenic*) except for a difference at a single (*differential*) locus are referred to as *coisogenic*. True coisogenicity occurs as a result of a point mutation within an inbred strain; partial coisogenicity can be attained by a series of crosses reconstituting the genetic background of one strain and retaining one gene from a second strain. Partially coisogenic lines, that is, lines that differ not only at the desired locus but most likely also at a chromosomal segment of indeterminate length adjacent to this locus, are called *congenic*. Congenic lines that differ at an *H* locus and therefore resist each other's grafts are called *congenic resistant* (*CR*).

Any series of genetic crosses leading to a production of a congenic line always begins with two strains; one provides the genetic background (*background strain, inbred partner*) and the other donates the differential locus (*donor strain*). The background strain must be, and the donor strain may or may not be, inbred.

2. Methods of Production

CR lines differing at the *H-2* complex can be produced by several different mating systems (Snell 1948, E. Green and Doolittle 1963, Snell and Bunker 1965, E. Green 1966), the simplest of which is the NX *backcross system*. The principle of the NX system is explained in Fig. 2–4, using as an example strains B10 (background strain) and A (donor strain). The production of the B10.A congenic line begins with a crossing of the two strains and backcrossing of the (B10 × A)F$_1$(= N1) hybrid to the background strain.

The resulting N2 generation is typed with B10 anti-A (*H–2^b* anti-*H–2^a*) antiserum, the negative animals (*H-2^b/H-2^b*) are discarded, and the positive animals (*H-2^a/H-2^a*) are backcrossed again to the background strain. The N3 generation is then typed with the same reagent and the positive animals again backcrossed. This procedure is repeated for a minimum of 12 generations (N12), after which the *H-2^a/H-2^b* heterozygotes are intercrossed, and the donor-type *H-2^a/H-2^b* homozygotes are selected and maintained by brother-sister (F) matings. The N1 hybrid inherits one-half of its genetic material from the A strain and the other half from the B10 strain; the repeated backcrossing gradually replaces the A strain material with the material of the B10 strain while the selection retains one specific gene complex derived from the A strain (*H-2^a*).

The probability (*P$_n$*) that any locus achieves homozygosity after *n* generations of backcrossing can be calculated from a formula

$$p_n = 1 - (1 - c)^{n-1}$$

where *c* is the frequency of recombination between the locus in question and the differential locus (E. Green and Doolittle 1963). The probabilities for five

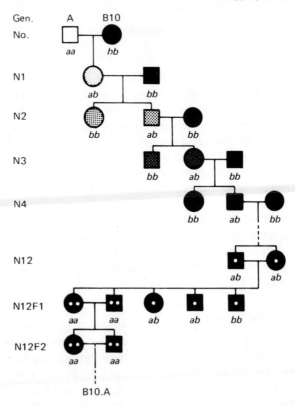

Fig. 2-4. The backcross or NX system of producing congenic lines of mice. Explanation in text. Gen. = generation of backcrossing; A = donor strain; B10 = background strain (inbred partner); $a = H\text{-}2^a$; $b = H\text{-}2^b$. Selection of $H\text{-}2^a/H\text{-}2^b$ heterozygotes is carried out with $H\text{-}2^b$ anti-$H\text{-}2^a$ serum.

different values of c in the first 12 generations of backcrossing are listed in Table 2–7. For any locus unlinked with the differential locus ($c = 0.5$), the probability of homozygosity in the twelfth generation of backcrossing is close to the maximal value of 1.0 ($p_{12} = 0.999$). For this reason, a strain that has been backcrossed for 12 or more generations is regarded as congenic. However, for any locus that is ten map units distant from the differential locus ($c = 0.1$), the probability of homozygosity in the twelfth generation of backcrossing is only 0.68. Evidently, even after 12 generations of backcrossing, the congenic line still carries a long chromosomal segment derived from the donor strain, in addition to the differential locus.

Because only three or four backcross generations can be obtained in the mouse in one year, the development of a CR line takes three to four years, even under ideal conditions. If more complicated mating systems are used, the time is even longer. However, the development can be hastened by a combination of serological typing and skin grafting (Egorov and Zvereva 1967). In this case, the positive animals in each backcross generation are grafted with skin derived

Table 2-7. The probability of homozygosity (p) at a locus X after n generations of back crossing to an inbred strain, calculated for five selected values of the recombination frequency (c) between locus X and the differential locus

c	$n =$	1	2	3	4	5	6	7	8	9	10	11	12
0.5	$p(\%) =$ 0		50.0	75.0	87.5	93.8	96.9	98.4	99.2	99.6	99.8	99.9	99.9
0.4	0		40.0	64.0	78.4	87.0	92.9	95.3	97.2	98.3	98.9	99.4	99.6
0.3	0		30.0	51.0	65.7	75.9	83.2	88.3	91.8	94.2	95.9	97.2	98.0
0.2	0		20.0	36.0	48.8	59.0	67.2	73.8	79.0	83.2	86.6	89.3	91.4
0.1	0		10.0	19.0	27.1	34.4	40.9	46.9	52.2	56.9	61.3	65.1	68.6

from the F_1 hybrids (in this particular situation the donor strain must also be inbred). For further matings, animals rejecting the skin grafts most rapidly are used. These animals are presumed to differ from the F_1 hybrid more than those showing prolonged survival of the F_1 grafts and thus to resemble closely the background strain.

If an unknown *H-2* haplotype is being introduced into a background strain and antiserum against this type is not available, the backcross system must be modified. Two such modifications have been described and used (Figs. 2–5 and

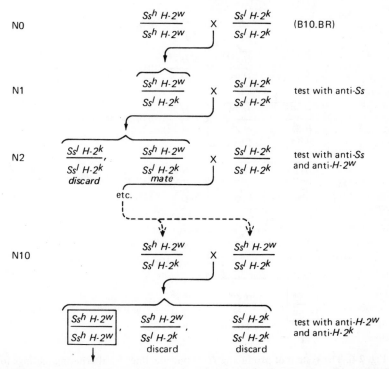

Fig. 2-5. The system of producing *H-2* congenic lines of mice with *Ss* as a marker gene. Explanation in text. $H\text{-}2^w$ = unknown *H-2* haplotype of the donor strain.

2–6). The first modification (J. Klein 1972a) takes advantage of the fact that the middle portion of the *H-2* complex is occupied by a gene coding for a serum protein, *Ss* (see Chapter Nineteen). The *Ss* gene has two alleles, one (Ss^h) for high level and the other (Ss^l) for low level of the protein. The Ss antigen can be used as a marker for the unknown *H-2* haplotype of the donor strain, the only prerequisite being that the background and the donor strains differ in their *Ss* types. For instance, if the donor strain types as Ss^h/Ss^h, it can be backcrossed to an Ss^l/Ss^l background strain and in each backcross generation the Ss^l/Ss^l segregants can be discarded and the Ss^h/Ss^l animals used for further mating (Fig. 2–5). The second modification (Stimpfling and Snell 1968, J. Klein 1973a) requires alternate backcrossing to two already-established CR lines on the same genetic background (Fig. 2–6). The donor animal (e.g., a wild mouse) is crossed to one CR line (e.g., B10.D2, $H-2^d$) and the N1 hybrid to another line (e.g., B10.BR, $H-2^k$); in all following backcrosses, the odd-numbered generations are always mated to the first CR strain (B10.D2) and the even-numbered generations to the second CR strain (B10.BR). In each generation, mice *negative* with one of two antisera (anti-*H-2^d* in even-numbered generations and anti-*H-2^k* in odd-numbered generations) are selected for further mating. This system can be used only if the donor strain does not react with the H-2 antisera used for the selection.

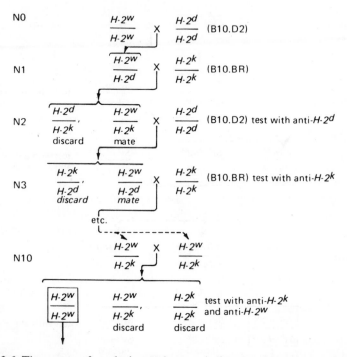

Fig. 2-6. The system of producing *H-2* congenic lines by alternating matings to two already-established congenic lines. Explanation in text. $H-2^w$ = unknown *H-2* haplotype of the donor strain.

3. Nomenclature

A congenic line is designated by a compound symbol consisting of two parts separated by a period or a hyphen. The first part gives either a full or abbreviated symbol of the background strain; the second part gives an abbreviated symbol of the donor strain or a genetic symbol of the differential locus. If necessary, parentheses are added to the compound symbol with additional information about the line, especially in cases where several CR lines derived from the same donor and background strains are available. Substrain symbols are sometimes also added to the congenic line symbol. For example, B10.A(1R)/Sg or C57BL/10Sn-*H-2^{h1}* is a CR line derived in the laboratory of Dr. J. H. Stimpfling (Sg), who transferred the *H-2^a*, a haplotype of the donor strain A/WySn, onto the genetic background of strain C57BL/10Sn (= B10); during the backcrossing, intra-*H-2* crossing-over occurred between the *H-2* haplotypes of the donor and the background strains, and the resulting *H-2^{h1}* haplotype was the first *H-2* recombinant (1R) in Stimpfling's laboratory.

4. Tests of Congenicity

It is important to know whether *H-2* is indeed the sole *H* difference in a given pair of congenic lines or whether some contaminating residual *H* differences might have been carried along with the *H-2* haplotype of the donor. The congenicity of the established CR lines can be tested in two different ways. One way is to produce a F$_2$ generation by crossing the CR line with the background strain (e.g., B10 × B10.A) and challenge the F$_2$ hybrids with two skin grafts, one from each parent (i.e., B10 and B10.A). Theoretically, if the congenic line differs from the background strain in only one *H* gene, three-fourths of the grafts donated by one parent should be permanently accepted. If additional differences segregate in the F$_2$ generation, a significant deviation from the 3:1 ratio ensues. This method, which is both laborious and time consuming, was successfully used by Berrian and McKhann (1960), Linder and E. Klein (1960), J. Klein (1965c), and others.

The second method for testing congenicity of a given pair of CR lines is much simpler. In this case, two CR lines on two different genetic backgrounds are crossed and the resulting F$_1$ hybrids are challenged with skin grafts from the respective background strains. If the CR lines are congenic with their background strains, the grafts are permanently accepted. The test can be illustrated by the following example.

Line C3H.B10 (*H-2^b*) is congenic with C3H (*H-2^k*), and line B10.BR (*H-2^k*) is congenic with B10 (*H-2^b*). In both cases, the CR line should differ from its respective background strain in the *H-2* complex only. If this is true, then the (C3H.B10 × B10.BR)F$_1$ hybrid should permanently accept both B10 and C3H skin grafts. The B10 graft should be accepted because the B10.BR line should carry all the B10 genes except *H-2^b*, provided by the C3H.B10 line. Similarly, the C3H graft should be accepted because the C3H.B10 should carry all C3H genes except *H-2^k*, provided by the B10.BR line.

5. Evaluation

Many currently used CR lines do not meet the criterion of congenicity, namely the requirement of 12 backcrossings to the background strain. Residual differences in addition to the differential locus can therefore be expected and have indeed been reported (Stimpfling and Snell 1968, Herzenberg *et al.* 1963, B. Taylor *et al.* 1973). However, even the lines that meet the criterion do not provide absolute assurance that all differences have been eliminated.

Currently available CR lines differing in the *H-2* complex are listed in Table 2–8; a complete list of all mouse CR lines can be found elsewhere (Klein 1973b).

Table 2-8. Available *H-2* congenic lines

H-2 haplotype	Congenic lines
a	B10.A, C3H.A/Sf, C3H.A/He
a1	A.AL, C3H.AL
an1	A.TFR1
ap1	B10.M(11R)
ap2	A.TFR2
ap3	A.TFR3
ap4	A.TFR4
ap5	A.TFR5
aq1	B10.M(17R)
b	A.BY/Sn, A.BY/Kl, C3H.SW, D1.LP, C3H.B10, D2.B6, AKR.B6/1, AKR.B6/2, BALB.B10, C3H/Bi-*H-2*^{b}
ba	B6.C-*H-2*^{ba}
bb	B6.C-*H-2*^{bb}
bc	B10.129(6M)
bd	B6.M505
by1	B10.BYR
d	B10.D2/n, B10.D2/o, D1.C, C3H.D, B6.C-*H-2*^{d}
da	B10.D2(M504)
f	A.CA/Sn, A.CA/Kl, B10.M
fa	A.CA(M506)
fb	B10.M-*H-2*^{fb}
g	BALB.HTG, B10.HTG, C3H.HTG(77NS)
g1	B10.D2(R101)
g2	D2.GD
g3	B10.D2(R103)
g4	B10.BDR1
g5	B10.BDR2
h1	B10.A(1R)
h2	B10.A(2R)
h3	B10.AM
h4	B10.A(4R)
h15	B10.A(15R)
h18	B10.A(18R)
i3	B10.A(3R)
i5	B10.A(5R)

(Continued)

Table 2-8. (*Continued*)

H-2 haplotype	Congenic lines
i7	B10.D2(R107)
ia1	B10.D2(R106)
j	C3H.JK, BALB.I
ja	B10.WB(69NS)
k	B10.BR, B10.K, B10.CBA, C57BL/6-*H-2ᵏ*, BALB.C3H, B10.AKR, B6.C3H
m	AKR.M, B10.AKM
m1	B10.QAR
o1	C3H.OL
o2	C3H.OH/Sf, C3H.OH/Sn
p	B10.NB, B10.P, B10.CNB, C3H.NB
pa	B10.Y
q	B10.Q, B10.G, B10.D1/Ph, B10.D1/Y, C3H.Q
r	B10.RIII, B10.RIII(71NS), C3H.RIII, LP.RIII
s	A.SW/Sn, A.SW/Kl, B10.ASW, B10.S
sq1	A.QSR1
sq2	B10.QSR2
t1	A.TL
t2	B10.S(7R), A.TH
t3	B10.HTT
t4	B10.S(9R)
u	B10.PL, B10.PL(73NS)
v	B10.SM/Sg, B10.SM/Sn
w1	B10.KPA42
w2	B10.KPB68
w3	B10.SAA48
w4	B10.GAA20
w5	B10.KEA5
w6	B10.TOB1
y1	B10.AQR
y2	B10.T(6R)
?	B10.F(13R), B10.F(14R), B10.P(10R), B10.S(8R)

C. Recombinant Inbred (RI) Strains

"RI strains are those which have been derived from the cross of two unrelated but highly inbred progenitor strains and which have been maintained independently under a regimen of strict inbreeding since the F_2 generation" (Bailey 1971). The principle of developing the RI strains can be explained using Bailey's original experiment as an example (Fig. 2–7). In this experiment, Bailey crossed inbred strains C57BL/6 (abbrev. B) and BALB/c (abbrev. C), which differ in their genes coding for coat color, agouti (*a*), brown (*b*), and albino (*c*), among other differences. The genotype of strain C57BL/6 is *aaBBCC*, that of BALB/c is *AAbbcc*. The intercrossing of the (C57BL/6 × BALB/c)F_1 hybrids leads in the

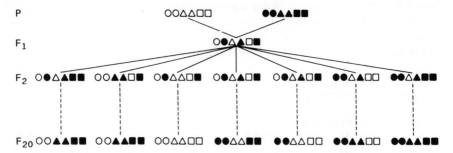

Fig. 2-7. Diagrammatic representation of the genetic principle involved in the production of the recombinant-inbred strains. Circles = agouti (*a*) gene; triangles = brown (*b*) gene; squares = albino (*c*) gene; the two alleles at each locus are indicated by open (BALB/c-derived) and closed (C57BL/6-derived) symbols.

F_2 generation to a segregation of all genes in which the two strains differ, including the coat-color genes. The three genes, since they are not linked, recombine at random into all possible combinations: *aaBBCC*, *AAbbcc*, *AaBbCc*, *AAbbCC*, *aaBBcc*, and so on. (Only 7 of the total 27 possible combinations are shown in Fig. 2–7.) As the F_2 individuals are paired at random and a new line is begun from each pair, fixation of the chance combinations occurs. During the subsequent brother-sister mating, some alleles are lost but no other alleles than those present in the original F_2 pair enter into any of the lines. Because each of the F_2 individuals has a unique combination of genes, the lines derived from them are different from each other. Furthermore, because the nonlinked genes disperse independently of each other among the F_2 mice, they all have unique strain distribution patterns (SDP's). For example, the SDP of gene *a* in Fig. 2–7 is *CCCBBB*, the SDP of *b* is *BBCCCB*, and that of *c* is *BBCBCBB*, where *B* stands for the allele derived from C57BL/6 and *C* for the allele derived from BALB/c.

The seven lines derived by Bailey (1971) from the C57BL/6 × BALB cross were named by him CXBD, CXBE, CXBG, CXBH, CXBI, CXBJ, and CXBK. SDP's of some of the known genes are listed in Table 2–9.

Bailey (1971) suggests at least four different experimental applications of the RI strains:

1. *Identification of histocompatibility (H) loci.* When a new *H* locus is isolated in a congenic line, its relationship to the loci already known can be quickly determined by comparing their respective SDP's.
2. *Search for H gene function.* It is assumed that the *H* genes have functions other than graft rejection. The RI inbred strains may facilitate search for the function by pointing to an association between certain physiological characters and the presence or absence of a particular *H* allele. The RI strains have already proved useful in investigations of the relationship between *H* and *Ir* (immune response) genes (Bailey and Hoste 1971, Merryman *et al.* 1972).

Table 2-9. Strain distribution patterns of genetic loci in the recombinant-inbred strains of Bailey*,**

Locus	Recombinant-inbred strains						
	CXBD	CXBE	CXBG	CXBH	CXBI	CXBJ	CXBK
a	C†	C	C	B	B	B	B
b	B‡	B	C	C	C	C	B
c	B	B	C	B	C	B	B
H-1	B	B	C	B	C	B	B
H-2	C	B	B	C	B	B	B
H-8	C	C	B	B	C	C	C
H-18	C	C	C	C	C	B	C
H-19	B	C	B	C	B	C	B
H-21	B	C	C	C	C	C	B
H-22	B	C	B	C	C	C	B
Ea-4	C	B	B	C	B	B	B
Ea-6	C	B	C	B	B	B	B

* Based on Bailey (1971a), and J. Klein (*unpublished data*).

** Symbols *a*, *b*, and *c* indicate coat-color loci, *H* symbols indicate histocompatibility loci, and *Ea* symbols designate erythrocyte alloantigen loci.

† C = BALB/c origin.

‡ B = C57BL/6 origin.

3. *Analysis of traits dependent on replicative observations.* Genetics of certain traits (for example, virus resistance) is difficult to determine on segregating populations because more than one mouse of the same genotype is required for measurement of such traits. The RI strains, in which a selected number of F_2 segregants can be replicated at will, may circumvent this difficulty.

4. *Detection of linkage.* If a new gene shows the same SDP as a gene already known, the two genes may be linked. However, identical SDP of two unlinked genes can also occur by chance, particularly if the sample of RI strains is relatively small. The suspected linkage must, therefore, be proved by a linkage test.

Part Two

Peripheral Regions of The *H-2* Complex

Section One

Serology

Chapter Three

Introduction to Serological Analysis

I. Basic Terms and Definitions

Exposure of an organism or a cell to certain types of foreign substances (*antigens*) may lead to an *immune response* characterized by two properties, specificity and memory. *Immunological specificity* is the selective reactivity of a given immunological reagent (molecule or cell) with a group of related antigens; *immunological memory* is the ability of an immunological system to recall a previous experience with an antigen and to respond much faster and more powerfully to subsequent exposures to the same antigen. The response to the first exposure is called *primary*, and the exposed animal (or cell) is said to be *primed* or *sensitized*; the response to the second ("booster") exposure is called *secondary* or *anamnestic*. There are two major types of immune response, *humoral*, characterized by secretion of free molecules (*antibodies*) into the body fluids, and *cellular*, characterized by the production of specifically sensitized cells.

Antibodies, responsible for humoral immunity, are structurally related proteins (*immunoglobulins*), synthesized in response to an antigen and capable of specific binding with that antigen. The monomeric antibody (immunoglobulin, abbreviated Ig) molecule consists of two pairs of polypeptide chains joined by disulfide bonds (Fig. 3–1a): longer chains called *heavy* (H), and shorter chains called *light* (L). Each chain has a *constant* (C) *region* displaying little variability from molecule to molecule in amino acid composition and sequence, and a *variable* (V) *region* differing in amino acid sequence among the different molecules. It is through the variable regions that antibodies achieve their specificity and diversity. The different amino acid sequences in the variable regions are responsible for the different shapes of the *combining site*, the portion

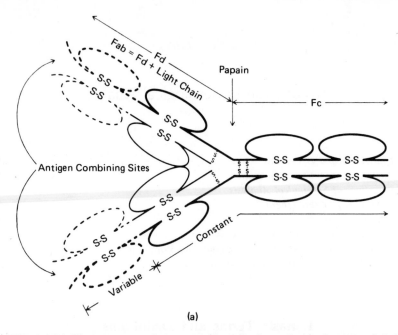

(a)

Fig. 3-1.(*a*) The structure of monomeric antibody molecule (immunoglobulin of class G). Dark line = heavy (H) polypeptide chain; light line = light (L) polypeptide chain; uninterrupted line = constant (C) region; dashed line = variable (V) region; S-S = disulfide bridges. (From F. V. Putnam and H. Kohler: "Plasmocytoma Proteins," *Naturwissenschaften* **56**:439–446, 1969.) (*b*) The structure of pentameric antibody molecule (immunoglobulin of class M). The five monomeric units are joined by disulfide bonds.   [*Fig. 3-1.(b)*→

of the Ig molecule directly involved in the antigen binding. The diversity of shapes of the combining site provides for a range of interactions with a great variety of antigens. At the same time, however, each combining site can interact only with a small number of antigens, namely those whose surfaces are shaped in a complementary fashion. The portion of the antigen molecule to which the antibody is able to become attached is called *antigenic determinant* or *epitope*. The monomeric Ig molecule has two combining sites, one in each of the two duplexes of H and L chains, with one site involving approximately 5–15 amino acids in each chain. Various enzymes can split the Ig molecule into fragments, designated *Fab* ("fragment antigen binding"), *Fc* ("fragment crystalline") and *Fd* (see Fig. 3–1a). The Fc fragment has a site that binds the *complement*, an enzymatic system of serum proteins activated by antigen-antibody reactions, and consisting of several components (C1, C2, C3, etc.).

The constant (C) regions of the different Ig molecules, although very similar in structure, are not completely identical. The differences among the individual C regions can be recognized by antibodies made against them, either in a different species or in the same species but in different individuals. Antibodies made in a different species (e.g., rabbit antimouse) define different *classes* and

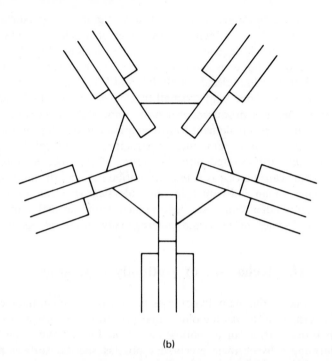

(b)

subclasses of immunoglobulins; antibodies made in different individuals of the same species (e.g., mouse antimouse) define different immunoglobulin *allotypes*. The cross-species antibodies distinguish four types of H chains (μ, γ, α, and δ) and two types of L chains (κ and λ). The four H chains define four Ig classes, IgM, IgG, IgA, and IgD. Each of the four H chains can combine with any of the two L chains, so that, for example, IgM molecules can exist in two forms, IgM (μ, κ) and IgM (μ, λ). The different classes can also be distinguished by their physicochemical properties, such as molecular weight, sedimentation coefficient (S), electrophoretic mobility, content of carbohydrate, and so on. The IgG class is further divided into three subclasses, IgG_1, IgG_{2a}, and IgG_{2b}. Tne two classes of concern here are IgG and IgM. The IgG molecules, constituting approximately 70 percent of normal serum immunoglobulin, occur in the basic monomeric form shown in Fig. 3–1a. The IgM molecules, on the other hand, are pentamers consisting of five subunits, each corresponding to the IgG monomer, and held together by disulfide bonds (Fig. 3–1b). Although an IgM molecule has ten combining sites, only five sites appear to be functional.

The coding for C regions of H and L chains of different classes and subclasses is probably accomplished by different genes. Thus, in the mouse, there are at least eight C region genes, six coding for C regions of H chains μ, γG_1, γG_{2a}, γG_{2b}, α, and δ, and two coding for C regions of L chains κ and λ. Of these, three genes coding for C regions of chains γG_{2a}, γA, and γG_{2b} have been identified using allotype markers and were designated *Ig-1*, *Ig-2*, and *Ig-3* respectively; a fourth gene, *Ig-4*, coding for the γG_1 chain, has been identified on the basis of a difference in electrophoretic mobility. The V regions are presumed to be controlled by a separate set of genes, the number of which is not known. The unique amino acid sequences in the variable regions of the Ig molecules can be recognized as antigens only under special circumstances. In normal animals, the number of Ig molecules with different V regions is so great and the number of molecules of one kind so small that detection of anti-V region antibodies, even if they are produced, is almost impossible. However, if an Ig-secreting cell undergoes a malignant transformation and develops into a plasma cell tumor, *myeloma*, large amounts of structurally identical Ig molecules (*myeloma proteins*) are secreted into the serum of the affected animal. The myeloma proteins can then be isolated and antibodies against antigenic determinants peculiar to an individual Ig molecule (*idiotype*) can be produced. Antiidiotypic antibodies can also be obtained from normal animals after exposure to antibodies of restricted heterogeneity produced against certain antigens.

II. Mechanism of Antibody Formation

It is ironic that of the many hypotheses proposed to explain the mechanism of antibody formation, it was the oldest that proved to be correct in principle. More than three-quarters of a century ago, Paul Ehrlich suggested that the antibody-forming cells or their precursors possess specific surface receptors capable of binding antigens. In normal, nonimmunized animals there are as many cells with different receptors as there are antibodies that the animal can produce. When a foreign antigen enters the bloodstream of an organism, it finds the cell with the proper-fitting receptor, binds to it, and triggers a process leading to the secretion of antibodies. The receptor hypothesis, or rather its modern version, has now been uniformly accepted. The cells bearing the receptors have been identified as *bone marrow-derived lymphocytes* (*B cells*) and the receptors as immunoglobulin molecules. The diversity of the receptors is believed to stem from differences in the variable portion of the Ig molecules—in particular, their combining sites. The mechanism that generates the diversity of the variable regions is not known, but the choice between various hypotheses has been restricted to two: the *germ-line hypothesis* and the *somatic hypothesis*. According to the germ-line hypothesis, an individual has a different gene for each antibody that it is able to produce, and different B cells acquire different receptors by activating different genes. According to the somatic hypothesis, an individual has only a relatively few antibody genes, which are modified (by mutation or translocation, for example) in the course of somatic development into an endless array of allelic forms.

Whatever the mechanism, each B cell (or clone of B cells, where clone means a group of cells derived by binary fission from a single ancestor) appears to be committed to production of one type of antibody. When this commitment occurs is not known. The B cells are derived from *stem cells* (i.e., unspecialized cells capable of extensive proliferation, self-renewal, and differentiation to more mature forms), some of which appear to be pluripotential, in that they can differentiate not only into lymphoid cells but also into hematopoietic cells (erythrocytes, granulocytes, and megakaryocytes). The pluripotentiality seems to argue that the commitment occurs during maturation of stem cells into B cells. On the other hand, the fact that it is easier to induce immunological unresponsiveness (tolerance) in an embryo or a newborn animal than in an adult may be interpreted as an indication that the commitment takes place in early ontogenesis. (It has been postulated that exposure of the embryo to foreign antigens eliminates or inactivates clones of cells precommitted to these antigens.) Obviously, more studies are needed to determine the timing of the commitment process.

In birds, the maturation of B cells occurs in the *bursa of Fabricius*, a saclike protrusion of the cloaca (the posterior end of the gastrointestinal tract). Attempts to find an analogous lymphoid organ in mammals have failed; whether such an organ exists remains unsettled. Mature B cells are found in the thymus-independent areas (areas not affected by the removal of the thymus) of the lymphoid organs: follicles, and medulla of the lymph nodes, peripheral regions of splenic white pulp, and follicles of gastrointestinal lymphoid tissue (see Chapter Six, Fig. 6–1).

The B cells are morpholigically small lymphocytes, characterized by a very narrow rim of cytoplasm and a spherical, indented nucleus with a prominent, tightly packed chromatin. The cells are short-lived, their life span (i.e., the interval between two mitotic divisions or between one division and cell death) being less than ten days. They are sedentary; once they reach their destination in lymph nodes and spleen, they are unable to leave and reenter these organs (recirculate).

Each B cell displays approximately 100,000 receptor molecules, all of one kind. The molecules react with anti-μ antisera and thus must be considered as belonging to the IgM class. However, in contrast to the pentameric (19S) IgM molecules found in the serum, the receptor molecules are in a monomeric (7–8S) form. The IgM monomers are shed from the cell surface and replaced by newly synthesized molecules at a slow but constant rate.

The number of cell types distinguishable by their receptors has been estimated at 10^5. This diversity is apparently sufficient to ensure that almost any antigen entering the blood stream will find a few cells with fitting receptors. To use Edelman's analogy, the receptors "can be likened to ready-made suits. The antigen is a buyer who decides to pick a number of different suits that fit more or less well, rather than instruct the tailor to make one suit to fit him to order. To be well satisfied, the buyer must patronize a store with a very large stock of suits in a great variety of sizes and styles. The immune system is like a store with an almost unlimited stock, one ready to please any possible customer" (Edelman 1970).

It has been estimated that the number of B cells that can find a particular antigen through their receptors is of the order of 10^7. These antigen-binding cells almost certainly represent a mixture consisting of different clones expressing different receptors, some fitting the antigen almost perfectly, others less well, and some only very roughly. The strength of the binding force varies accordingly; cells with perfectly fitting receptors bind the antigens very firmly; those with a less exact fit bind it less firmly or very loosely. When the binding force exceeds a certain threshold, the antigen-receptor interaction triggers a process leading to antibody secretion. The number of B cells capable of immunological response to a given antigen is thus lower than the number of antigen-binding cells, perhaps of the order of 10^5. The triggered B cells respond by increased DNA synthesis (demonstrable by rapid incorporation of tritiated thymidine), morphological transformation, and proliferation. The small lymphocyte transforms into a *blast cell*, that is, a large cell (15 to 20μ in diameter) with abundant basophilic (pyroninophilic) cytoplasm and a voluminous nucleus containing loosely arranged chromatin and prominent multiple nucleoli. The morphological changes (*blast transformation*) are accompanied by rapid synthesis of ribosomes and nuclear as well as cytoplasmic proteins. The blasts then repeatedly divide, expanding the clone and producing progressively smaller cells. The proliferation terminates in the antibody-synthesizing *plasma cell*, characterized by its highly developed endoplasmic reticulum, small, excentrically located nucleus with "cartwheel" distribution of chromatin, and its prominent Golgi area. The proliferation takes place in lymph nodes and spleen, transforming their *primary follicles* into *secondary follicles* with prominent *germinal centers* (see Fig. 6–1).

The plasma cell secretes antibodies which then circulate via the body fluids (*humoral* or *circulating antibodies*). The rate of antibody secretion is about 2000 molecules/second, far greater than the rate of spontaneous receptor shedding. As already indicated, the secreted antibody has the same specificity (the same combining site, the same variable region) as the IgM receptor of the progenitor B cell. Early in the response, the antibody produced by the plasma cells is exclusively of the IgM (19S) type; only later do some cells switch over to IgG (7S) antibody production. There is still a good deal of controversy as to how this IgM $\rightarrow$ IgG switchover is achieved. However, one thing seems certain: the switchover requires help from another type of lymphocyte, the thymus-derived lymphocyte, or T cell. (The T-B cell interaction will be discussed in Chapter Eighteen.) Whether a B cell can develop directly into an IgG-producing plasma cell without an intermediate phase of IgM production is an unsettled question.

During the expansion of the antigen-stimulated clone, some of the proliferating cells, instead of differentiating into plasma cells, revert to the resting state of the small lymphocyte. This new generation of small lymphocytes is, however, qualitatively different from the original B cells; among other things, the new cells have a life span of several months and are capable of recirculation. When they encounter for the second time the same antigen that triggered proliferation of the original clone, they respond by a more rapid proliferation, leading to a much faster and more powerful antibody response. It appears that the cells are able to recall their previous experience with the antigen and thus mount more efficient immunological reaction to it. For this reason they are called *memory cells*. The development of a B cell memory seems to require the collaboration of T cells, and some investigators are even convinced that immunological memory can be mediated *only* by T cells. Immunological memory is demonstrable primarily in terms of IgG antibody response, which, after the second challenge begins more promptly, is heightened in the titer and lasts longer than the IgG response following the primary challenge. IgM memory can be demonstrated only in some systems, and there are even some doubts whether it really exists. The population of antigen-binding cells responsible for the secondary response differs from the one that responds to the primary immunization in that it is larger (contains more cells) and in that it is relatively enriched in cells with high-affinity receptors. Whether this is all there is to the immunological memory is unclear, although some immunologists believe that the memory cells are also different in that they have increased the number or altered the quality of the Ig receptors.

Certain types of antigens (e.g., pneumococcal polysaccharide, *E. coli* lipopolysaccharide, polymerized flagellin, polyvinylpyrrolidone, etc.) stimulate only an IgM response that is not dependent on the presence of the thymus (= *thymus-independent antigens*). The antigens are characterized by polymeric structure, the presence of repeated antigenic determinants, and at least some of them by mitogenic (cell division-stimulating) activity. The great majority of antigens, however, stimulate both IgM and IgG response, with the latter always being *thymus dependent*.

Large proportions (over 50 percent) of B cells can be stimulated nonspecifically (i.e., regardless of the receptors they bear) by *mitogens*, such as *E. coli* endotoxin or by anti-Ig sera. The mitogen-stimulated cells undergo blast transformation and secrete IgM molecules in the form of 19S pentamers (the production of immunoglobulins by the stimulated cells increases 100-fold over that in the resting B cells). The increase of IgM synthesis is selective in that synthesis of other proteins is largely unaffected.

Although morphologically indistinguishable from other small lymphocytes, the B cells can be identified by several surface markers:

1. *High density of immunoglobulins*, demonstrable using anti-Ig sera. Little or no Ig can be detected with these antisera or other small lymphocytes.
2. *Receptors for the Fc fragments of Ig molecules.* The receptors can be detected by incubation of lymphocytes with antibodies combined with an antigen in a radioiodinated form. The antibodies become attached to the Fc receptors on the lymphocytes, and their presence can then be demonstrated by the radioactivity of the antigen. According to some authors, the Fc receptors are present only on mature B cells and absent on stem cells or plasma cells.
3. *Mouse-specific B lymphocyte antigen (MBLA).* The antigen is defined by rabbit antimouse B cell antiserum absorbed with mouse liver, red cells, and thymocytes. The antiserum, however, is not specific for B cells; it also reacts with plasma cells and hematopoietic cells, although it does not react with T cells.

4. *C3 receptor.* The B cells have a receptor for a modified complement component (C3), capable of binding antigen-antibody-complement complexes. The receptor, however, may be present only on a subpopulation of B cells.

5. *Alloantigens.* Two alloantigens (antigens detected with mouse antimouse serum) presumably specific for B cells have been described recently (Ly-4, Ia). These will be discussed later (see Chapter Eight).

III. Limitations of Serological Analysis

Serology is based on the interaction of two entities, antigens and antibodies, or more precisely, antigenic determinants and antibody combining sites. The interaction is mediated by short-range forces such as charge interaction, hydrophobic interaction, van der Waals attraction, hydrogen bond formation, and dipole interaction (for a review, see Pressman and Grossberg 1968). Because of the short range of these forces, the interaction can occur only when the surface of the antibody combining site is complementary to the surface of the antigenic determinant. The complementarity (*stereochemical fit*) must be morphological and/or physicochemical. The morphological complementarity requires a mold-cast type of relationship between the structural contours of the combining site and the antigenic determinant; the physicochemical complementarity requires a correlative arrangement of atomic groupings between the combining site and the antigenic determinant (i.e., negatively charged groups against positively charged groups, proton-donor groups opposite proton-acceptor groups, etc.).

In the past, the interaction between an antigenic determinant and a corresponding antibody combining site has been visualized as a lock-and-key type relationship, with each combining site capable of specifically binding only one antigenic determinant (resembling a key that fits only one lock). This view, however, is almost certainly an oversimplification. Recent data on binding functions of immunoglobulins indicate that the combining sites are polyfunctional in that each site consists of noncontinuous subsites that can bind structurally unrelated determinants (for a review see Richards and Konigsberg 1973). The combining site appears to be a relatively shallow cavity at the end of each of the two arms of the Y-shaped monomeric immunoglobulin unit. The cavity is usually much larger than most of the antigenic determinants, and the binding between the determinant and the site occurs at certain contact points that can be different for different determinants. Thus, rather than being a lock fitting only one key, the combining site is more like a pegboard set with each piece of the set fitting a specific position on the board.

Antibodies for serological analysis are produced by immunization, or exposure of an animal to an antigen it lacks, and are secreted into the serum of such an animal (*antiserum*). Antibodies obtained by immunization of an individuum against antigens from another, genetically different individuum of the same species (*alloantigens*) are called *alloantibodies*, and the sera in which they are contained are called, *alloantisera*.

Serological analysis can best be performed with an antiserum containing one absolutely specific antibody. In reality, of course, this never happens. An antiserum always contains more than one antibody (antibody heterogeneity), and each antibody always reacts with more than one antigen (antibody cross-reactivity). Antibody heterogeneity and cross-reactivity are two sides of the same coin, but for formal reasons they will be discussed separately.

A. Antibody Heterogeneity

Antibody heterogeneity is the result of the presence of more than one determinant on an antigen molecule, and of cross-recognition by B cell receptors.

Most natural antigens carry several determinants that are recognized separately by different clones of B cells. As a result, upon immunization a mixture of antibodies directed against different determinants is produced in situations in which a single antibody against a single antibody determinant is desired. Certain small molecules (*haptens*) are known to carry only one or a few antigenic determinants. These can combine with antibodies, but usually cannot initiate an immune response unless they are attached to a large molecule, a *carrier*.

Heterogeneity due to cross-recognition is achieved in two ways. In one case, a given antigenic determinant interacts not only with a B cell receptor having combining sites precisely complementary to the determinant, but also with receptors showing only partial and incomplete complementarity. Consequently, not one but several different B cell clones are triggered by one determinant, and several different (though similar) antibodies are secreted into circulation. In the second case, only a small area of the antigenic determinant is recognized by a B cell receptor, and different clones of B cells recognize different (probably overlapping) areas of the same determinant. This also results in activation of several B cell clones and production of a family of related, though slightly different antibodies (Fig. 3–2a). It has been shown that even in the case of a simple hapten attached to a synthetic polypeptide carrier containing only one type of amino acid residue, a heterogeneous population of antibodies is produced.

Antibody heterogeneity can be restricted by selecting the recipient for immunization to differ from the donor in a limited number of antigenic determinants. The heterogeneity of an existing mixture of antibodies can be reduced by *absorption* or *elution*. From an antiserum containing antibodies against determinants 1, 2, and 3, the undesired anti-2 anti-3 antibodies can be removed (*absorbed out*) by reacting the mixture with an antigen carrying determinants 2 and 3, but not 1. Alternatively, the antiserum is reacted with an antigen that carries determinant 1, but not determinants 2 and 3, and the bound anti-1 antibody is then released (*eluted*) from the antigen by physicochemical means.

An antiserum from which undesired antibodies have been removed and in

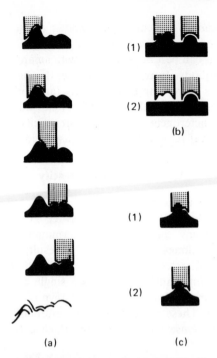

Fig. 3-2. Factors complicating serological analysis. (*a*) Families of antibodies (lower portion of the diagram indicates areas of the complex antigen recognized by individual antibodies). (*b*) Cross-sharing of antigenic determinants: (1) and (2) are two different antigens sharing one determinant. (*c*) Cross-reactivity: (1) and (2) are two slightly different antigens reacting with the same antibody. Solid portions = antigen; dotted portions = antibody.

which only antibodies against one determinant remain is *monospecific* or monovalent. However, the term is misleading, because true monospecificity can never be achieved. A more appropriate term for such an antiserum is *oligospecific* or oligovalent, indicating that the antiserum contains antibodies against a restricted number of antigenic determinants (as opposed to *polyspecific* or polyvalent antiserum, containing antibodies against many antigens).

B. Cross-reactivity

Serological analysis is further complicated by cross-reactivity, defined as reactivity of antibodies with an antigen other than that used for immunization. Cross-reactivity is due either to sharing of determinants by two antigens (Fig. 3–2b) or to stereochemical similarity between two antigens (Fig. 3–2c). Although cross-reactivity can be exhibited by antibodies that appear early in the immune response, it increases progressively with time after immunization, with the most cross-reactive antibodies appearing last. Cross-reactivity is also prominent in secondary response and after multiple immunizations. The gradual loss of specificity in the immune response (*degeneracy*) is directly related to *affinity* and *avidity* of the antibodies (i.e., their ability to form more or less stable complexes with the antigen). The most avid antibodies (antibodies with the highest affinity) also exhibit the highest degree of cross-reactivity. Formation of cross-reactive antibodies seems to depend on the presence of the thymus, indicating that the high-affinity antibodies can be made by B cells only in collaboration with T cells. The increase of antibody affinity with time after immunization (*immunological maturation*) can be explained by competition for the antigen. As the antigen becomes more scarce, B cells with high-affinity receptors have a better chance to bind it, and are therefore preferentially triggered to secrete high-affinity antibodies.

IV. Serological Analysis of a Complex System

Serological analysis of a complex system consists of two steps. In the first step, antibodies are obtained defining individual antigens, and in the second step, the relationship between the antigens and the mode of their inheritance is unraveled. The methods used in such analysis differ according to the genetic status of the population studied, that is, whether the population is genetically heterogeneous or homogeneous.

A. Association Analysis in a Heterogeneous Population

A heterogeneous population consists of genetically different individuals sharing some antigens and differing in others. Immunization between two such individuals leads to production of an antiserum containing a number of different antibodies against antigens of one or more systems (polyspecific antiserum). A polyspecific antiserum, when tested against a random sample (*panel*) of individuals, reacts with some individuals and fails to react with others. When two polyspecific antisera are compared, the following situations can, theoretically, occur:

1. the two antisera may be identical (i.e., they may contain the same antibodies);
2. one antiserum may contain all the antibodies of the second antiserum, as well as some additional ones. Because the second antiserum has no antibodies that the first does not have, it is said to be *included* in the first antiserum;
3. the two antisera share some antibodies but not others;
4. the two antisera have no antibodies in common.

The distinction among these four possibilities is complicated by random factors that may significantly influence the reactivity patterns of the antisera. For example, if two antisera have an identical, or very similar reactivity pattern, it could mean either that they contain similar antibodies or that they contain *different* antibodies that happen to react in such a way as to mimic similarity. To differentiate between the effects of chance alone and a true relationship between the antibodies, one must resort to a statistical analysis of the reactivity patterns. The analysis begins with the construction of a 2×2 contingency table, as shown below:

reactivity with
antiserum 2

		+	−	
reactivity with antiserum 1	+	a	b	$a+b$
	−	c	d	$c+d$
		$a+c$	$b+d$	n

a = number of individuals positive with both antisera;

b = number of individuals positive with first antiserum and negative with second;

c = number of individuals negative with first antiserum and positive with second;

d = number of individuals negative with both antisera;

n = total number of individuals tested $(= a+b+c+d)$.

The following conditional statements can be made about the two antisera:

1. if $b = c = 0$, the two antisera are identical;
2. if $b = 0$, the second antiserum is included in the first;
   if $c = 0$, the first antiserum is included in the second;
3. if $(a+d) > (b+c)$, i.e. there is a significant tendency toward an excess of condordant reactions, the two antisera share some antibodies;
4. if $(a+d) \sim (b+c)$, i.e. the frequency of condordant reactions does not differ significantly from the frequency of discordant reactions, the two antisera are unrelated.

The significance of the association between the two antisera is determined by one of three statistical methods: Fisher's exact test, the χ^2 test, or the correlation coefficient test.

The formula used in Fisher's exact test is

$$p = \frac{(a+b)!(c+d)!(a+c)!(b+d)!}{n!a!b!c!d!} \quad \text{or} \quad \frac{(a+b)!(c+d)!(a+c)!(b+d)!}{n!} \times \frac{1}{a!b!c!d!}$$

where p is the probability of a given distribution of reactivities occurring by chance alone. The test can be used only if one of the figures for the four observations in the 2×2 table (a, b, c, or d) is zero (0). If this is not the case, another 2×2 table must be constructed, in which the smallest figure of the original table has been reduced by one and the three remaining figures adjusted so that the marginal totals $(a+b, c+d$, etc.) remain unchanged. If necessary, this is repeated until 0 is reached. The p values obtained in each reduction step are then added to the p value calculated from the original 2×2 table. The following example illustrates the procedure.

Original 2×2 table:

second antiserum

		+	−	
first antiserum	+	5	2	7
	−	3	6	9
		8	8	16

$$p_1 = \frac{7!9!8!8!}{16!} \times \frac{1}{5!2!3!6!} = 0.1371$$

First reduction step:

second antiserum

		+	−	
first antiserum	+	6	1	7
	−	2	7	9
		8	8	16

$$p_2 = \frac{7!9!8!8!}{16!} \times \frac{1}{6!1!2!7!} = 0.0196$$

Second reduction step:

second antiserum

		+	−	
first antiserum	+	7	0	7
	−	1	8	9
		8	8	16

$$p_3 = \frac{7!9!8!8!}{16!} \times \frac{1}{7!0!1!8!} = 0.0007$$

$[0! = 1$ by definition$]$

Third step:

$$p = p_1 + p_2 + p_3 = 0.1574$$

Conclusion: The probability that the observed reactivity patterns of the two antisera occurred by chance alone is 0.1574.

In cases where a, b, c, and d are relatively large figures, Fisher's exact test becomes inconvenient and must be replaced by another method, most commonly by the χ^2 test.

The χ^2 test cannot be used when the observed figures a, b, c, and d are smaller than 5. With larger numbers, the χ^2 can be calculated using the formula

$$\chi^2 = \frac{(ad-bc)^2 n}{(a+b)(c+d)(a+c)(b+d)},$$

and can reach values of between 0 and n, where n is the number of individuals tested ($= a+b+c+d$). A value of $\chi^2 = 0$ (attainable when $a = b = c = d$) signifies an absence of any association between the two antisera; a value of $\chi^2 = n$ (attainable when $a = d$ and $b = c = 0$, or when $b = c$ and $a = d = 0$) signifies an absolute association between the two antisera, meaning that the antisera are either identical (they contain antibodies reacting with the same antigens) or complementary (they contain antibodies reacting with antithetical antigens).[1] Finally, values of χ^2 higher than zero but lower than n can signify either association or lack of association, the decision between the former and the latter being made by conversion of a given χ^2 value into a probability value (p) using the χ^2 tables. The tables show that for $\chi^2 > 11$, the corresponding p value with one degree of freedom (if the comparison is made between two antisera) is $p < 0.001$. In other words, if the χ^2 value is greater than 11, the reaction pattern observed with the two antigens can occur by chance alone in less than one out of 1000 cases. For this reason, two antisera that give $\chi^2 \geq 11$ when compared by the 2×2 contingency table method are said to be associated (containing antibodies against antigens of the same system). The association can be positive or negative, depending on the sign of the $ad-bc$ value.

The coefficient of correlation (r) represents χ^2 corrected for the number of individuals tested. It can be calculated from the formula

$$r = \frac{ad-bc}{\sqrt{(a+b)(c+d)(a+c)(b+d)}} = \pm \sqrt{\frac{\chi^2}{n}}$$

and can reach values from $+1$ to -1. The value $r = 0$ signifies the absence of an association between two antisera; the value $r = +1$ signifies identity of the two antisera, and $r = -1$ suggests the presence of antithetical antibodies.

If $n \geq 100$, it can be calculated that for

$$r \geq 0.19 \qquad p \leq 0.05$$
$$r \geq 0.23 \qquad p \leq 0.02$$
$$r \geq 0.25 \qquad p \leq 0.01$$
$$r \geq 0.32 \qquad p \leq 0.001$$

The value of positive $r \geq 0.32$ ($p \leq 0.001$) indicates significant positive association; the value of negative $r \geq 0.20$ ($p \leq 0.05$) indicates significant negative association (antithetical relationship between the antibodies of the two antisera).

Thus, the procedure used in the first step of the association analysis can be summarized as follows:

---

[1] Antithetical antigens are those presumably controlled by two alleles at the same locus. In a homozygote at this locus, the presence of one antithetical antigen precludes the presence of the other.

1. Obtain a panel of about 100 different target cell samples from randomly selected individuals.
2. Prepare a battery of 50 or more antisera.
3. Test each antiserum against the whole panel.
4. Compare each antiserum with all other antisera of the battery, one at a time, and arrange the results of this comparison into the 2×2 contingency table.
5. Apply a statistical test (χ^2) to the contingency tables.
6. Arrange the results of the χ^2 test in descending order so that the highest values, indicating the closest association of two antisera, are at the top of the list and the lowest χ^2 values, indicating no association, are at the bottom.
7. Select antisera with the highest mutual χ^2 values for further analysis and discard antisera that show no association. Use $\chi^2 = 11$ as a cutoff point for the associated antisera.

Once the antisera are grouped and the antigens defined by the groups, the analysis can proceed to the second step, namely the definition of the genetic relationship between the antigens. The relationship is determined using the same statistical methods described above (χ^2 test and the coefficient of correlation test), only this time the methods are applied to the antigens rather than to the antisera. A significant positive correlation between antigens indicates that the antigens belong to the same system. A significant negative correlation between two antigens indicates that they are controlled by two alleles at the same locus.

It should be emphasized, however, that association analysis alone does not suffice for full characterization of a complex serological system. The results of such analysis are usually "dirty," in the sense that they possess a high degree of uncertainty. This is due, first of all, to technical limitations, since most serological methods have about 5–10 percent error in reproducibility. Second, association analysis is more prone to error due to serological complexity (multispecificity, cross-reactivity, etc.) than any other type of serological analysis. Finally, the analysis is easily subject to error due to genetic complications such as multiple effect of the same gene, epistatic interaction, departure from random mating, close linkage, and so on. Association analysis may fail to detect relationships that are real and may suggest relationships that do not exist. It should be used only as a first approximation, followed by other methods, such as absorption analysis of selected antisera and family studies.

Although association analysis has been known to immunogeneticists for some time, it became widely used only after its extensive application to the *HL-A* system. It has not been employed in any *H-2* studies, although it may have a potential value for the analysis of wild mouse populations. It is essential for understanding the comparative aspects of the *H-2* and *HL-A* systems, discussed later (cf. Chapter Twenty).

B. Analysis with Inbred Strains of Animals

The principle of serological analysis with inbred strains (or congenic lines) is simple. Animals of strain A are immunized with cells from strain B, and the resulting antiserum is tested against cells from all other available inbred strains. If the antiserum reacts with cells other than those of the donor, absorption is performed with one or more cell types until monospecificity is attained. The absorbed antiserum is then tested with the same panel of inbred strains, and the strain distribution of the antigen defined by antibodies present in the serum is determined. The mode of inheritance of the antigen is established by testing a segregating generation (backcross or F_2). The membership of the antigen in a system of antigens already known is ascertained by a linkage test. Once certain knowledge about the antigenic composition of the strains is gathered, donors and recipients for new immunizations are chosen in a way that minimizes antigenic differences between them and thus ensures the production of antisera containing a small number of antibodies.

The magnitude to which such an analysis can be extended depends on the number of inbred strains available. As pointed out by Gorer and Mikulska (1959), there is a simple mathematical relationship between the number of available strains and the number of antigens detectable in those strains. When only two strains are available (A and B), only two donor-recipient combinations can exist (A anti-B and B anti-A) and two antigens can be detected (1 and 2). With three strains (A, B, and C), the number of donor-recipient combinations is six, and the number of detectable antigens is also six (Table 3-1). The six antigens fall into two categories with three antigens in each category. One category $(n-1)$ contains antigens shared by two strains but absent in the third strain. The second category $(n-2)$ contains antigens specific for a given strain and absent in the remaining two strains. With four strains (A, B, C, and D) the number of possible donor-recipient combinations increases to 12, and the number of possible antigenic differences to 14 (Table 3-2). The antigens fall into three categories: one $(n-1)$ with four antigens, each shared by three strains and absent in the fourth strain; a second $(n-2)$ with six antigens, each present in two strains and absent in two strains, and a third $(n-3)$ with four antigens, each present in only one of the four strains. With five strains there

Table 3-1. Distribution of antigens detectable with three different inbred strains

Strains	Categories of antigens*					
	$n-1$			$n-2$		
A	5	–	7	11	–	–
B	5	6	–	–	12	–
C	–	6	7	–	–	13

* n = number of strains; 5, 6, 7, . . . = presence of antigens; – = absence of antigens.

would be 20 different donor-recipient combinations, 30 different antigens fall-ing into four categories, containing 5, 10, 10, and 5 antigens, and so on. Thus, the general pattern emerges as shown in Table 3-3 (Snell and Stimpfling 1966). The number of antigens in each category is allotted by the coefficients of the binomial expansion, exclusive of the first and last coefficients, which are always equal to one. Because the sum of the coefficients of the binomial expansion is 2^n, and because the first and the last coefficients must be subtracted, the formula for the total number of theoretically possible antigens is $2^n - 2$, where n is the number of different strains available. The number of possible antigens increases very rapidly with the increasing number of available strains. For example, with ten strains, it reaches 1022.

Table 3-2. Distribution of antigens detectable with four different inbred strains

Strains	Categories of antigens*		
	$n-1$	$n-2$	$n-3$
A	$-$ 2 3 4	5 $-$ 7 $-$ $-$ 10	11 $-$ $-$ $-$
B	1 $-$ 3 4	5 6 $-$ $-$ 9 $-$	$-$ 12 $-$ $-$
C	1 2 $-$ 4	$-$ 6 7 8 $-$ $-$	$-$ $-$ 13 $-$
D	1 2 3 $-$	$-$ $-$ $-$ 8 9 10	$-$ $-$ $-$ 14

* n = number of strains; 1, 2, 3, . . . = presence of antigens; $-$ = absence of antigens.

Table 3-3. Relationship between number of available strains and number of detectable antigens in a complex serological system

Number of strains	Number of antigens in categories	Total number of antigens	Number of donor-recipient combinations
2	2	2	2
3	3 3	6	6
4	4 6 4	14	12
5	5 10 10 5	30	20
6	6 15 20 15 6	62	30
.	.	.	.
.	.	.	.
.	.	.	.
n	n n n n $(n-1)$ $(n-2)$ $(n-3)$ ... $(n-n+1)$	$2^n - 2$	$(n-1)n$

The antigens in category $(n-n+1)$ are always restricted to a single strain, and are therefore considered *private*. The antigens in the remaining categories are shared by at least two strains, and are therefore considered *public*.

Antigens belonging to different categories can be arranged into *inclusion groups* or *subtypes*. In each inclusion group, the presence of certain antigens predetermines the presence of other antigens. For instance, the antigens in Table 3-2 can be arranged into four different inclusion groups:

Inclusion group 1	Inclusion group 2	Inclusion group 3	Inclusion group 4
C 1 8 3	A 2 10 11	D 3 9 14	B 4 5 12
D 1 8 –	D 2 10 –	B 3 9 –	A 4 5 –
B 1 – –	C 2 – –	A 3 – –	C 4 – –
A – – –	B – – –	C – – –	C – – –

To detect a maximum number of antigens with a given number of strains, it is not necessary to immunize all donor-recipient combinations. As illustrated in Table 3-4, with three strains, six donor-recipient combinations are possible, and of these, three suffice to detect all six possible antigens. With four strains, 12 donor-recipient combinations exist but four suffice for detection of the 12 possible antigens (Table 3-5), and so on.

As Table 3-5 shows, for $n > 3$ the number of detectable antigens is lower than the number of theoretically possible antigens. With four strains, 14 antigenic differences can exist theoretically, but only 10 can be detected. In this particular case, antigens of the $n - 1$ category (1, 2, 3, 4) escape detection (they remain "hidden") because there is no way to prove the presence of the antibodies directed against them.

The situation just described is purely fictitious. Even if all the theoretically possible antigenic differences among the strains existed, there is no guarantee that they would be detected. Antibodies against different antigens are not

Table 3-4. Absorption analysis with three inbred strains

Antiserum (antibodies)	Absorbed by	Tested against*			
		A	B	C	
A anti-B	A	0	+	+ ⎫	defines antigen 6
(6, 12)	B	0	0	0 ⎬	
	C	0	+	0	defines antigen 12
B anti-C	A	0	0	+	defines antigen 13
(7, 13)	B	+	0	+ ⎫	defines antigen 7
	C	0	0	0 ⎬	
C anti-A	B	+	0	0	defines antigen 11
(5, 11)	C	+	+	0 ⎫	defines antigen 5
	A	0	0	0 ⎬	

* + = positive reaction; 0 = no reaction.

Table 3-5. Absorption analysis with four inbred strains

Antiserum (antibodies)	Absorbed by	Tested against*				
		A	B	C	D	
A anti-B	A	0	+	+	+	
(1, 6, 9, 12)	B	0	0	0	0	
	C	0	+	0	+	defines antigen 9
	D	0	+	+	0	defines antigen 6
	C+D	0	+	0	0	defines antigen 12
B anti-D	A	0	0	+	+	defines antigen 8
(2, 8, 10, 14)	B	+	0	+	+	
	C	+	0	0	+	defines antigen 10
	D	0	0	0	0	
	A+C	0	0	0	+	defines antigen 14
D anti-C	A	0	+	+	0	confirms antigen 6
(4, 6, 7, 13)	B	+	0	+	0	defines antigen 7
	C	0	0	0	0	
	D	+	+	+	0	
	A+B	0	0	+	0	defines antigen 13
C anti-A	A	0	0	0	0	
(3, 5, 10, 11)	B	+	0	0	+	confirms antigen 10
	C	+	+	0	+	
	D	+	+	0	0	defines antigen 5
	B+D	+	0	0	0	defines antigen 11

* + = positive reaction; 0 = no reaction.

produced with equal ease, and some expected antibodies are not produced at all. In contrast, antigens that theoretically cannot be detected (hidden antigens) can be unmasked because of the absence of other antigens.

The analysis of inbred stains and the analysis of heterogeneous populations provide different views of the same system. In the inbred strain, each antiserum can be reproduced *ad libitum* by anyone possessing the strains. Also, the inbred animals can be repeatedly immunized with the same antigen, and even weak antigenic differences can be detected. Furthermore, the specificity of the antisera can be controlled by a careful selection of the donor-recipient combinations. And finally, the inbred strain analysis is usually performed in a cascadelike fashion: information about the antigenic makeup of a given set of strains is used to produce antisera with a higher resolution power; the improved antisera permit recognition of more antigens, the additional antigens permit the production of antisera of even higher resolution power, and so on. Consequently, the inbred strain analysis can go into considerable depth and detail. However, its limiting factor is the fact that inbred strains do not usually represent a cross section of the natural population. In the mouse, for instance, the inbred strains are completely nonrepresentative, because most of them have a common origin. For this reason, the serological findings on inbred strains usually lack generality.

Analysis of heterogeneous populations is complicated by the fact that each antiserum is unique, that most of the antisera are relatively weak, and that antisera that might detect additional differences cannot be used because they are too complex. The analysis is possible only with a high degree of simplification and disregard for details.

The two approaches (association analysis and the analysis of inbred strains) can be compared to the exploration of an unknown city from the ground and from the air. The ground explorer sees only a small section of the city at any one time, but can thoroughly investigate it; the explorer in the air oversees the whole city, quickly grasps its general plan, but misses many interesting details. Obviously, maximum information is obtained by combining the two approaches and exploring the city first from the air and then on foot.

V. Interpretation of Serological Data

Antigens and antibodies, the two entities with which serologists operate, are both unknowns in the serological equation. When an antibody reacts not only with the antigen that induced its formation, but also with some other antigens, there is no way of knowing whether this additional reactivity is due to the heterogeneity of the antibody, the heterogeneity of the antigen, or both. This uncertainty can be illustrated by the following example.

Consider a situation in which an antiserum, Z anti-A, reacts not only with the donor strain A, but also with strains B, C, and D. When an absorption analysis is performed, the results shown in Table 3-6 are obtained. The results can be interpreted as evidence for the presence of three antibodies against three different antigens: anti-1, anti-2, and anti-3 (Fig. 3-3a). The strain distribution of these antigens is as follows:

Strain	Antigens		
A	1	2	3
B	1	—	—
C	—	2	—
D	—	—	3
Z	—	—	—

However, the results can also be interpreted in a different way (Fig. 3-3b). The Z anti-A antiserum could contain four antibodies produced against one antigen of strain A, but cross-reacting with similar, though not identical antigens of strains B, C, and D. The antigenic composition of the four strains can then be written as follows:

Strain	Antigens
A	1 – – –
B	– 2 – –
C	– – 3 –
D	– – – 4
Z	– – – –

Thus, the same serological result can be interpreted in two different ways. In one case, both the antibody and the antigen are considered complex; in the second case, the antigen is considered complex and the antigen simple.[2] The different interpretations are reflected in the symbolism denoting a particular antigenic composition. As long as the symbols remain abstract and have no implications about the molecular structure of the antigen and about the genes coding for the antigen, either interpretation is in order. Unfortunately, serologists usually are not satisfied with the abstraction of the symbolism and tend to go a step further by putting a concrete meaning into the symbols. The imposition of additional meaning can take two forms. On the one hand, implications are made about the biochemistry of the antigen (one molecule with one antigenic determinant versus one molecule with several antigenic determinants), and, on the other hand, about the genetics of the antigen (one gene coding for one antigenic determinant versus one gene coding for several antigenic determinants). Neither form of implication is permissible because each surpasses the limitations of the serological method. The method uses antibodies, themselves totally undefined, to elucidate the nature of the antigen, and the antigen to elucidate the nature of the antibodies. Although several immunogeneticists (Landsteiner 1945, Owen 1959, Hirschfeld 1965) have repeatedly warned that this is a *circulus in definiendo*, the warning is largely being ignored. It should be

Table 3-6. Absorption analysis of antiserum Z anti-A reacting with strains A, B, C and D

Absorbed by strain	Tested against strain			
	A	B	C	D
A	0	0	0	0
B	+	0	+	+
C	+	+	0	+
D	+	+	+	0
Z	+	+	+	+

* + = positive reaction; 0 = no reaction.

[2] For additional interpretations as well as detailed discussion of the different interpretations, see Hirschfeld (1965, 1972).

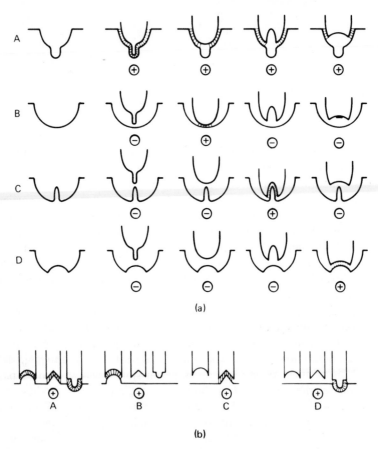

Fig. 3-3.(*a*) One way to interpret serological cross-reactivity. The left portion of the figure shows the configuration of antigenic determinants in strains A, B, C, and D. The right portion shows four types of antibody combining site and how each fits the antigenic determinants in the four strains. (All four antibodies were produced against the antigenic determinant of strain A.) Binding forces between antigen and antibody are indicated by connecting lines. Positive serological reaction is indicated by +, negative by −. (*b*) Another way to interpret serological cross-reactivity. The three antibodies are directed against three different antigenic determinants; strain A carries all three determinants, strains B, C, and D carry only one of the three, a different one in each strain.

clear, however, to anyone working with a complex serological system, that serology alone, without help from biochemistry, cannot determine whether the antibody or the antigen (or both) is complex, and cannot provide information about the organization of the genes coding for a particular array of antigenic determinants.

Chapter Four

Methods of Serological H-2 Typing

I. Production of H-2 Antibodies

H-2 antibodies can be induced by various procedures, the most common of which are tumor transplantation, skin grafting, and inoculation of lymphoid tissue.

A. Tumor Transplantation

Tumor cells derived from strain A are generally rejected when transplanted into strain B, and the rejection is accompanied by the production of anti-H-2 antibodies (Gorer 1937b). The time of appearance and the persistence of the antibodies in the serum depend on the properties of the particular tumor and the strains involved. A description of the results obtained by various investigators with different tumors is beyond the scope of this publication; only one example will be given.

In one of the earliest reports, Mitchison and Dube (1955) inoculated an A strain tumor, Sarcoma 1 (Sal), into C57BR/a recipients and observed that the hosts responded by rejecting the tumor and forming H-2 hemagglutinins. The antibodies first appeared approximately 10 days after the implantation of the tumor and reached a peak 5 days later. A second inoculation of the same tumor led to accelerated rejection of the graft and to earlier peaking of the hemagglutinin titer (7 days after the inoculation). The median survival times of the first- and second-set tumor grafts were 10.8 and 5.5 days, respectively. In both the first- and second-set transplants, the antibodies appeared only during (or shortly after) the breakdown of the tumor tissue.

B. Skin Grafting

The presence of H-2 antibodies (hemagglutinins and leukoagglutinins) in the serum of mice rejecting skin allografts was first demonstrated by Amos *et al.* (1954) in strain combinations C57BL anti-BALB/c and C3H anti-A. Since then, numerous studies, the findings of which parallel those obtained by tumor transplantation, have been reported. Whereas standard serological techniques usually detect H-2 antibodies only at the onset of graft rejection, highly sensitive techniques detect them 2–3 days after grafting, prior to any signs of graft rejection (Hildemann 1967, Sparks *et al.* 1970).

The main disadvantage of skin grafting as a method of antibody production, and the reason it has never been used widely for this purpose, is the relative laboriousness of the procedure.

C. Inoculation of Suspension of Normal Cells

Immunization with cells in suspension is the most commonly used technique for the production of H-2 antibodies. The most frequently used cells are obtained from lymphoid organs such as the spleen, lymph nodes, and thymus, which contain a high concentration of H-2 antigens. Liver cells, although also rich in H-2 antigens, are not recommended as an immunizing stimulus because liver homogenates contain factors that can destroy H-2 antigenicity (Palm and Manson 1965, Hilgert and Krištofová 1966). Although immunization with lyophilized tissue (Snell *et al.* 1948, Snell 1952, Kaliss 1952, Gorer and Kaliss 1959, Jensen and Stetson 1961) or cells incorporated in Freunds adjuvant (Tyan 1965) have been reported, these methods are relatively inefficient for the production of H-2 typing reagents.

A single injection of lymphoid cells usually produces only antibodies against the strongest H-2 antigens; repeated injections are required for production of antibodies against weak antigens. The number of cells per injection, the number of injections, the interval between individual injections, and the time of collection of the serum varies considerably among the different H-2 laboratories. The kinetics of H-2 antibody production vary in accordance with the immunization schedule and the type of antibodies produced. In a typical case, after one injection of lymphoid cells, the H-2 antibodies do not appear until 4–5 days postinjection, the first peak of the antibody titer is reached at about 9 or 10 days after the injection, and additional peaks of lesser magnitude follow on days 17, 27, and 35 (Stimpfling and Richardson 1965). Low levels of the antibodies may persist in the serum for several months. Additional injections usually heighten the titer and shorten the interval between the injection and peaking of the antibody titer.

Adult mice usually serve as both donors and recipients. Females are considered better antibody producers than males, although the difference is negligible.

II. Techniques Used for Detection of H-2 Antibodies

A. Hemagglutination and Leukoagglutination Techniques

H-2 alloantibodies were originally demonstrated through their ability to agglutinate mouse erythrocytes in saline (Gorer 1937b). The saline hemagglutination technique, however, was of limited value in that it was applicable only to certain antisera and often gave unpredictable results. It was clear that even the sera that either were negative in the saline hemagglutination test or became inactive upon storage did contain other types of antibodies, namely those that can combine with an antigen but fail to give a visible reaction. Originally, it was believed that these *incomplete antibodies* had only one combining site (were univalent) and were therefore unable to link red cells into aggregates. However, it was recognized later that incomplete antibodies are able to agglutinate erythrocytes, under the right circumstances. Four major types of techniques developed for the detection of incomplete antibodies are the blocking (and synergic) test, the use of colloidal diluents, the pretreatment of red cells with proteolytic enzymes, and the antiglobulin reaction.

In the *blocking test* (Gorer 1947, Gorer et al. 1959) the cells are suspended in a test serum, incubated, washed, and resuspended in saline. The treated cells are then exposed to antiserum containing complete (saline) antibodies. If the treated cells are no longer agglutinated in the presence of complete antibodies, it is concluded that the test serum contained incomplete antibodies, which blocked the reaction by coating the cells.

The converse of the blocking test is the *synergic test* (Gorer et al. 1959), in which the test serum and the serum containing complete antibodies are mixed and allowed to react with the cells simultaneously. If the test serum contains incomplete antibodies, it will enhance, rather than block the agglutination caused by complete antibodies. Thus, in a typical test, the test serum alone is inactive in saline, the serum containing complete antibodies is active and gives a certain titer, but the test serum plus the complete antibodies give a higher titer than the complete antibodies alone. The major disadvantage of the blocking and synergic tests is that they depend on antisera containing complete (saline) antibodies.

In the second category of techniques, a *colloid* replaces saline as a red cell-suspending agent and antiserum diluent. The main factor behind erythrocytes not being agglutinated by incomplete antibodies in saline is the development in the electrolyte of strong electrostatic forces, which do not allow the cells to come close enough to each other to be bridged by the antibody molecules.

The colloid medium reduces the repulsive forces, bringing the cells closer together and thus permits linkage of the cells by incomplete antibodies. Several media have been used to replace saline as the antibody diluent: normal mouse serum (Gorer 1947), normal guinea pig serum (Gorer 1950), normal human serum absorbed with mouse erythrocytes (Gorer 1950), dextran (Gorer and Mikulska 1954), and *polyvinylpyrrolidone* (PVP) (Stimpfling 1961). Of these, only the dextran and PVP techniques have become established as routine H-2 typing methods. In the *dextran technique*, the red blood cells are suspended in normal human serum, and the antiserum is serially diluted in 2 percent dextran. The human serum must be absorbed with mouse tissue prior to use to remove natural antimouse red cell antibodies. In the *PVP test*, the red cells are suspended in 0.85 percent saline and the antiserum is serially diluted in 1–1.5 percent PVP made in phosphate-buffered saline. The PVP technique is superior to the dextran technique, mainly because it does not require laborious absorption of the human serum and contains one less variable (the human serum).

The third category of hemagglutination methods developed for incomplete antibodies involves treatment of the red cells with *proteolytic enzymes* such as trypsin, papain, bromelin, or ficin (M. Mitchell *et al.* 1969). The mechanism of proteolytic enzyme action is not known, but it appears that the treatment exposes additional antigenic sites and/or makes the sites more readily available for combination with the antibody molecules. To what extent the treatment alters or damages the antigenic sites has not been determined.

The fourth category of techniques, the *antiglobulin tests*, is based on coating the red cells with incomplete alloantibodies (gamma globulin), and then linking together the coated cells with xenogeneic antibodies made against mouse gamma globulin (J. Klein and Iványi 1963). The test is as sensitive as the PVP or dextran technique, but is much more time consuming.

Mouse erythrocytes are generally fragile and usually cannot be stored for more than 24 hr without spontaneous lysis and loss of specific agglutinability. Some erythrocytes are more readily agglutinated than others, the most sensitive strains being C58, YBR, and F/St (Amos 1959). The hemagglutination reaction with F_1 hybrid red cells is usually weaker than the reaction with red cells of the inbred parents (Gorer 1938, Gorer *et al.* 1948), and this difference is interpreted as evidence that the *H-2* heterozygous cells contain only half the concentration of the antigenic sites of the homozygous parents (*dosage effect*).

The original difficulties with the hemagglutination techniques led to attempts at replacing them with white cell tests. Although agglutination of white cells from peripheral blood (granulocytes and lymphocytes) was shown to be a feasible approach to H-2 serology (Amos 1953, Mishell *et al.* 1963, Mishell 1964), the technique never achieved widespread use in H-2 typing laboratories because it offered no advantage over the simpler and less troublesome PVP test.

B. Cytotoxic Test

The cytotoxic test is based upon the killing of cells by antibodies in the presence of complement. The dead cells, unlike the live ones, are

1. unable to exclude vital dyes (such as trypan blue or eosin Y) from their cytoplasm (Gorer and O'Gorman 1956);
2. able to release radioactive chromium (^{51}Cr) bound in their cytoplasm (Sanderson 1964a, b, 1965a, b; Wigzell 1965);
3. able to release ^{14}C-thymidin after trypsin treatment (G. Klein and Perlmann 1963);
4. able to escape detection in an electronic counter because their size falls outside the range for which the counter is set up (Terasaki and Rich 1964).

Of these four assays available for detection of cytotoxic antibodies, only those based on dye exclusion and ^{51}Cr-release are used in routine work. The advantages of the dye-exclusion test are that it is simple, quick, and inexpensive; the ^{51}Cr-release test is advantageous in that it is objective and quantitative. In both the dye-exclusion and ^{51}Cr-release tests, the most troublesome variable is the complement. Because mouse serum has very poor complement activity, normal sera of other species such as rabbit or guinea pig must be used as a source of complement. However, not every rabbit or guinea pig is a suitable donor of complement, and the optimal complement donor and optimal complement dilution must be determined by testing.

The technical aspects of the dye-exclusion test have been discussed in detail by Boyse and co-workers (Boyse *et al.* 1962, 1964a), and those of the ^{51}Cr-release test by Haughton and McGhee (1969). Both tests are available in several modifications listed in Table 4-1.

The cytotoxic test can be used only with cells having a relatively high density of H-2 sites on their cell membranes, such as normal lymphocytes and certain leukemias. [An application of the dye-exclusion and ^{51}Cr-release tests to epithelial cells of the epidermis has recently been described by Scheid *et al.* (1972) and by Cooper and Lance (1971); application of the dye-exclusion test to spermatozoa has been reported by Goldberg *et al.* (1970).] However, this limitation can be circumvented by the *inhibition assay*, in which the antiserum, at a constant dilution known to result in 50–75 percent killing of the target cells, is incubated, in the absence of complement, with doubling dilutions of test cells. After incubation, the antiserum is tested in the presence of complement for residual activity against a constant number of target cells. If the test cells, which can be derived from almost any tissue of the body, share H-2 antigens with the target cells (lymphocytes), they will absorb out some or all of the antibody activity from the antiserum and the antiserum will show lower cytotoxicity against the target cells. The absorbing capacity of the test cells can then be used as an indicator of H-2 antigen concentration on the test cells

Table 4-1. Serological techniques used for detection of *H-2* antigens

Hemagglutination tests

Blocking test	Gorer 1947, Gorer *et al.* 1959
Synergistic test	Gorer *et al.* 1959, Voisin *et al.* 1968, 1969
Hemagglutination in saline	Gorer 1937b
Hemagglutination in normal mouse serum	Gorer 1947
Hemagglutination in normal guinea pig serum	Gorer 1950
Hemagglutination in dextran and human serum	Gorer and Mikulska 1954
Micromodification in plastic trays	Kaliss 1968
Hemagglutination in PVP	Stimpfling 1961
Micromodification in plastic plates	Takasugi and Hildemann 1969
Hemagglutination of enzymatically treated red cells	M. Mitchell *et al.* 1969
Indirect antiglobulin (Coombs) test	J. Klein and Iványi 1963
Migration of red cells in microhematocrit tubes	Severson and Thompson 1968
Hemagglutinin inhibition test	Pizarro *et al.* 1961, 1963
Slide tests	Amos 1953, Mishell *et al.* 1963,
Leukoagglutination test	Mishell 1964
Migration of leukocytes in microhematocrit tubes	Severson and Thompson 1968

Hemolytic tests

With visual reading	Hildemann 1957
With spectrophotometric reading	Winn 1962, 1964
With ^{51}Cr-labeled red cells	G. Möller 1965

Localized hemolysis (plaque-formation) in gel

With mouse erythrocytes as target cells	Hildemann and Pinkerton 1966
With lymphoblasts as target cells	Fuji *et al.* 1971a, b
With ascites lymphoma as target cells	G. Taylor and Bennett 1973

Cytotoxic tests

Dye exclusion tests	
Tube test	Gorer and O'Gorman 1956
Slide test	Boyse *et al.* 1962, 1964a
Microtitration with wire loops on siliconized slides	Spooner *et al.* 1965
With epidermal cells	Scheid *et al.* 1972
With spermatozoa	Goldberg *et al.* 1970
Microtitration in plastic plates	Takasugi and Hildemann 1969
Blocking test	Boyse *et al.* 1968a
Inhibition test	Basch and Stetson 1962
Test based on electronic counting of live cells	Terasaki and Rich 1964
Test based on trypsin digestion of ^{14}C-thymidine-labeled cells	G. Klein and Perlmann 1963
^{51}Cr-release assay	Wigzell 1965
Direct assay with lymph node cells	Sanderson 1964a, b, 1965a, b
Direct assay with spleen cells	Boyle 1968
Direct assay with epidermal cells	Cooper and Lance 1971
Microassay in plastic trays	Kaliss 1969
Inhibition assay	Sanderson 1965a, b

Table 4-1. (*Continued*)

Inhibition assay with blood cells	David and Shreffler 1972b
Two-stage test	Haughton and McGhee 1969
Cytotoxic antiglobulin technique	Harder and McKhann 1968, Fass and Herberman 1969

Fluorochromasia assays

With cells embedded in agarose	Celada and Rotman 1967
With cells in suspension	Edidin and Church 1968

Fluorescent antibody tests

Direct	Neauport-Sautes *et al.* 1973
Indirect	
With suspension of living cells	G. Möller 1961a, 1964, Barth and Russell 1964, Cerottini and Brunner 1967
Quantitative—from papain-digested samples	Strom and E. Klein 1969
With frozen sections	Cerottini and Brunner 1967, G. Möller 1961a, Barth and Russell 1964, Gervais 1968, 1970, 1972a
With paraffin-embedded sections	Vojtíšková and Pokorná 1971, 1972a, b

Complement fixation tests

Qualitative test (alloantiserum is serially diluted; hemolysis is measured visually)	Batchelor 1960
Quantitative test (concentration of alloantiserum is held constant; hemolysis is measured photometrically)	Winn 1962, 1964, 1965b

Radioimmunoassays

Antibodies labeled with titrated D,L-alanine	U. Hämmerling *et al.* 1969b, U. Hämmerling and Eggers 1970
Antiglobulin serum labeled with ^{125}I	Harder and McKhann 1968, Sparks *et al.* 1969
Antigen labeled with ^{125}I	Foschi and Manson 1970

Colony inhibition test

With tumor cells	I. Hellström and Sjögren 1965

Adherence tests

Immune adherence test with monolayer cells	Tachibana and E. Klein 1970
Mixed hemadsorption test with monolayer cells	Tachibana *et al.* 1970, Barth *et al.* 1967
Rosette (allocluster) formation with sensitized lymphocytes	Micklem and Staines 1969

relative to the target cells. The inhibition test has been applied to both the dye-exclusion (Basch and Stetson 1962) and the ^{51}Cr-release tests (Sanderson 1965a, b).

In a standard *one-stage cytotoxic test*, the antiserum, complement, and target cells are incubated together in one mixture. In a *two-stage test* the antiserum is incubated with the target cells, the sensitized cells are separated by centrifugation, washed, and exposed to the complement. The two-stage test must be used in cases where the antiserum shows anticomplementary activity; it is applicable to both the dye-exclusion and ^{51}Cr-release assays (Haughton and McGhee 1969).

A combination of a cytotoxic test and an antiglobulin test has been described by Fass and Herberman (1969). In this technique the target cells are incubated with an alloantiserum, washed, incubated with an antiglobulin serum (rabbit antimouse immunoglobulin), washed again, and finally incubated with complement. The cytotoxicity is estimated by trypan blue exclusion.

C. Hemolytic Tests

Incubation of red cells with antibodies in the presence of complement results in lysis and a release of the red cell content (hemolysis). The hemolysis can be observed visually (Hildemann 1957) or measured photometrically (Winn 1962, 1964); alternatively, the erythrocytes can be labeled with radioactive chromium (^{51}Cr) and the amount of lysis estimated from the release of the radioactive label into the medium (G. Möller 1965). The two main drawbacks of the hemolytic test are that variation exists among cell suspensions obtained from mice of the same inbred strain and that many alloantisera known to contain hemagglutinating antibodies fail to show hemolytic activity (Winn 1964).

D. Complement Fixation Test

The complement fixation test is based on the observation that an antibody, on reacting with an antigen, binds (fixes) complement. The test is carried out in two stages. In the first stage, the antigen (test cells), the alloantiserum, and the complement (normal guinea pig serum) are incubated together; in the second stage, indicator cells (sheep erythrocytes coated with horse or rabbit antisheep hemolysins) are added to the mixture. Hemolysis, which can be measured either visually (Batchelor 1960) or photometrically (Winn 1962, 1964, 1965b), indicates that free complement, unbound by the alloantiserum, remained in the mixture after the first stage. Absence of hemolysis indicates that the complement has been fixed by the alloantibodies reacting with the H-2 antigens on the test cells.

E. Fluorochromasia Assays

Fluorochromasia assays (Celada and Rotman 1967, Edidin and Church 1968) resemble the cytotoxic test in that they are also based on the distinction of live cells from cells killed or damaged by an antibody in the presence of complement. The distinction is facilitated by fluorescein diacetate, a nonpolar substance that rapidly penetrates the cell membrane and is converted in the cytoplasm of living cells into polar fluorescein, emitting bright fluorescence when exposed to ultraviolet light. Because of their polarity, molecules of fluorescein can leave live cells only by an active transport across the membrane, which proceeds at a much slower rate than the passive flow of nonpolar molecules into the cells. As a consequence, live cells accumulate fluorescein, thereby becoming brightly fluorescent, whereas cells with damaged membranes do not exhibit fluorochromasia, due to a rapid loss of fluorescein by passive diffusion.

F. Fluorescent Antibody Techniques

Fluorescent antibody techniques (direct or indirect) are advantageous in that they can be applied to practically all types of tissues. In the *indirect (sandwich) techniques*, the cells are first incubated with H-2 alloantibodies and then with xenoantibodies produced in rabbits, goats, or horses against mouse gamma globulin. The xenoantibodies are conjugated with either fluorescein isothiocyanate (FITC) or rhodamine B. Cells sensitized with the H-2 alloantibodies bind the labeled xenoantibodies and display an intense green-yellow (FITC) or reddish (rhodamin B) fluorescence in ultraviolet light. The technique can be applied either to cells in suspension (G. Möller 1961a, 1964) or to sections of frozen (G. Möller 1961a, Gervais 1968, 1970, 1972a) and paraffin-embedded (Vojtišková and Pokorná 1971, 1972b) tissue. In the *direct test* (Neauport-Sautes *et al.* 1973), the alloantibodies are conjugated with FITC or rhodamine B and applied directly to the cells without exposure to xenoantibodies.

G. Radioimmunoassays

Radioimmunoassays involve attachment of a radioactive isotope to an antibody (or an antigen) and determination of the radioactivity by scintillation counting. A common method of radiolabeling is radioiodination, in which the antibody molecules are labeled with ^{125}I or ^{131}I. Although this method has been successfully applied to many antigen-antibody systems, it has met with limited success in H-2 serology because radioiodination of mouse alloantibodies drastically increases the specific binding activity of the antibodies. An alternative to radioiodination, which involves attachment of ^{3}H-D,L-alanine to mouse IgG antibodies by peptide linkage, has been proposed by U. Hämmerling and coworkers (Hämmerling *et al.* 1969b, Hämmerling and Eggers 1970). The labeled antiserum is incubated with viable target cells, the cells are digested, and the radioactivity of the digested samples is determined.

Another alternative is the use of an antiglobulin technique with the label attached to the xenoantibody rather than the alloantibody (Harder and McKhann 1968, Sparks *et al.* 1969). In this test, the target cells are incubated first with the H-2 alloantibodies, then with goat antimouse IgG serum labeled with ^{125}I. After washing, the radioactivity of the cell pellets is determined.

In the radioimmune assay of Foschi and Manson (1970), the ^{125}I label is attached to solubilized and partially purified H-2 antigens rather than H-2 antibodies. The H-2 alloantibody is absorbed irreversibly onto polysterene test tubes, the isotope-labeled antigen is bound to it, and the radioactivity of the rinsed tubes is determined.

H. Immune Adherence Assay

The immune adherence assay is based on the adhesion of normal human erythrocytes in the presence of complement to cells coated with H-2 alloantibodies and estimation of the reaction from the degree of clustering (rosette formation, cf. Tachibana and E. Klein 1970). The mechanism of the reaction is not known.

I. Mixed Hemadsorption Test

The mixed hemadsorption test as applied to the *H-2* system (Tachibana *et al.* 1970) involves the coating of target cells with H-2 alloantibodies and of indicator cells (sheep erythrocytes) with mouse antibodies against sheep red blood cells, and linking the two types of cells together with goat antimouse gamma globulin serum. The intensity of the reaction is determined microscopically from the degree of rosette formation.

J. Hemolytic Plaque-Formation Assay

In the hemolytic plaque-formation assay (Fuji *et al.* 1971a, b), donor mice are immunized by grafting with allogeneic skin, the immune spleen cells are mixed in melted agar with cells from a mouse lymphoblast line, the agar is spread on a microscopic slide and incubated with a rabbit complement. The immune spleen cells continue to produce antibodies which, in the presence of complement, lyse the target lymphoblast cells in their vicinity and thus form clear areas (plaques) in the agar. A similar technique described for mouse erythrocytes as target cells (Hildemann and Pinkerton 1966) proved to be difficult to reproduce.

K. Colony Inhibition Assay

In the colony inhibition assay (I. Hellström and Sjögren 1965), cultured tumor cells are incubated with H-2 alloantiserum in the presence of complement and plated, and the colonies formed are enumerated. The alloantiserum reduces the number of colonies by 60–100 percent as compared to the control group exposed to normal mouse serum. Treatment with complement alone decreases the number of colonies by approximately 25 percent.

Even though, as indicated above, there is a large variety of techniques available to H-2 serologists, the majority of them are highly specialized and seldom used outside the laboratory of their origin. Only four techniques are in general use: the PVP hemagglutination test of Stimpfling (1961), the cytotoxic test of Gorer and O'Gorman (1956), the cytotoxic test of Sanderson (1964a, b,

1965a, b) and Wigzell (1965), and the indirect fluorescent antibody test of G. Möller (1961). Because all four techniques have both advantages and disadvantages, the serologist must select his technique on the basis of the problem to be solved.

A negative result in any of the described techniques does not necessarily prove the absence of an antigen, and a positive result does not always indicate the presence of an antigen. In the former case, concentration of the antigen on the cell surface could be so low that not enough antibodies are bound to cause a detectable reaction; in the latter case, antibodies can be bound to an antigen nonspecifically. Because of the possibility of obtaining false negative or false positive results, *absorption analysis* should always be used in addition to a direct serological test.

Absorption analysis can be used not only for the confirmation of the results obtained by direct testing, but also for removal of undesired antibodies from a polyspecific serum, and for detection of H-2 antigens on cells that cannot be tested by a direct test. The absorption can be performed either *in vitro* or *in vivo*. *In vitro* absorption involves incubation of cells with alloantiserum and testing of the absorbed serum for remaining activity against target cells. In the *in vivo* absorption technique, the alloantiserum is injected into a live mouse, recovered after a period of time by bleeding of the animal, and tested. *In vivo* absorption is more efficient than the *in vitro* technique, but is disadvantageous in that it substantially dilutes the serum.

III. Nature of H-2 Antibodies

Alloantigens of the H-2 system can stimulate the production of antibodies of at least three different classes: IgM, IgA, and IgG (G. Möller 1966, Andersson *et al.* 1967, Voisin *et al.* 1966, 1969; J. Klein *et al.* 1974c). The IgM (19S) antibodies appear 3–5 days after primary immunization with living lymphoid cells, peak at about 6–7 days, and then disappear rapidly, usually before the end of the second week (Fig. 4-1a). The IgG antibodies appear 5–7 days after immunization, peak about 12–16 days, and persist for over 1 month. The kinetics of the primary response seem to be similar in different strains of mice, in that all those tested first produce IgM antibodies and then switch over to IgG. The kinetics of the anamnestic (secondary) response (Fig. 4-1b), on the other hand, show marked strain differences (Andersson *et al.* 1967), with A.CA and A.SW mice responding primarily with IgG antibodies, and C57BL mice responding with both IgG and IgM antibodies. Similar strain differences are also found after hyperimmunization with sheep red blood cells (Winn 1965a). The mouse antisheep cell sera fall into three categories. In one category are antisera from strains that, even after hyperimmunization, produce high levels of short-lived IgM antibodies and only small or undetectable amounts of IgG antibodies. Mice of other strains respond initially with the production of IgM antibodies but, upon secondary stimulation, their response consists solely or predominantly

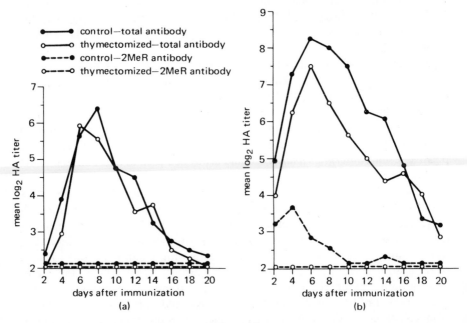

Fig. 4-1.(a) Primary antibody response to H-2 antigens as measured by PVP hemagglutination (HA) test. The immunizing tissue was from B10.A mice. The recipients were C57BL/10Sn (B10) normal and thymus-deprived mice. The antisera were treated with 2-mercaptoethanol to distinguish IgG (2Me-resistant) from IgM (2Me-sensitive) antibodies. (b) Secondary antibody response to H-2 antigens as measured by PVP hemagglutination (HA). (Reproduced with permission from J. Klein, S. Livnat, V. Hauptfeld, L. Jeřábek, and I. Weissman: "Production of anti-H-2 antibodies in thymectomized mice." *Europ. J. Immunol.* 4:41–44. Copyright © 1974 by Verlag Chemie GmbH. All rights reserved.)

of long-lived IgG antibodies. In the third category are antisera from strains that, upon repeated stimulation, produce mixtures of IgM and IgG antibodies. F_1 hybrids between high and low IgM producers are high IgM producers (Andersson *et al.* 1967), suggesting that the kinetics of the anamnestic response are regulated by a dominant genetic factor(s).

Neonatal thymectomy or adult thymectomy combined with lethal irradiation and transfusion of bone marrow cells treated with anti-Thy-1 serum abolishes the IgG type of anti-H-2 response, but does not influence the IgM response (Fig. 4-1; cf. J. Klein *et al.* 1974c). Apparently, the IgM type of anti-H-2 response is thymus independent, whereas the IgG type is thymus dependent.

The efficiency of the various immunoglobulin classes of H-2 antibodies in the different serological tests is summarized in Table 4-2. The IgM antibodies function well in direct hemagglutination, cytotoxic and hemolytic tests, and poorly or not at all in the fluorescent antibody test (Andersson *et al.* 1967). IgG antibodies function in all four tests (G. Möller 1966, Andersson *et al.* 1967,

Table 4-2. Efficiency of immunoglobulin classes in serological assays

	Class		
Assay	IgM	IgG	IgA
hemagglutination { direct	+	+	−
synergic	−	−	+
cytotoxic	+ +	+	−
hemolytic	+ +	+	−
fluorescent antibody	− ?	+	− ?

Irvin *et al.* 1967, Chard 1968, Voisin *et al.* 1966, 1969; J. Klein *et al.* 1974c). IgA antibodies are active in the synergic hemagglutination test (Voisin *et al.* 1969), but not in the cytotoxic test (Schlesinger *et al.* 1969). The cytolytic and agglutinating titers of the IgM and IgG antibodies seem to be strain dependent (G. Möller 1966). Antisera prepared in strains A, A.BY, A.SW, C57BL, and B10.129(5M) against strain A cells contain IgM and IgG antibodies; the IgM antibodies have slightly higher titers in hemolytic than in agglutination tests,

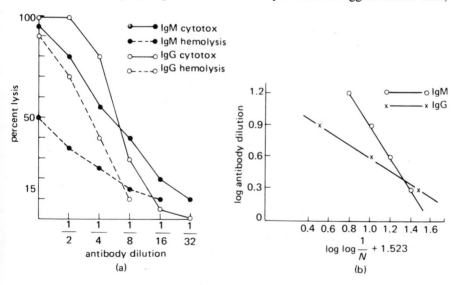

Fig. 4-2.(*a*) Cytolytic efficiency of IgM and IgG H-2 antibodies in antiserum A.SW anti-A obtained 7 days after primary immunization. The IgG and IgM antibodies were separated by Sephadex G-200 gel filtration. (*b*) The order of reaction in a cytotoxic system of IgM and IgG C57BL/10 anti-A antibodies based on the formula of Weinrach. The reciprocal of the slope of the line obtained by plotting log antibody dilution against log log $1/N$ (N = fraction of live cells) is the order of reaction of that antibody. (Reproduced with permission from B. Andersson, H. Wigzell, and G. Klein: "Some characteristics of 19S and 7S mouse isoantibodies *in vivo* and *in vitro.*" *Transplantation* **5**:11–20. Copyright © 1967 by Williams & Wilkins Co. All rights reserved.)

whereas IgG antibodies are potent agglutinins but poor hemolysins. In contrast, in A.CA anti-A sera the agglutinating and hemolytic titers run parallel for both IgM and IgG fractions. The cytolytic efficiency (percent lysis) of IgM antibodies, when plotted against antibody dilution, decreases less sharply than that of IgG antibodies (Fig. 4-2a, Andersson *et al.* 1967). Using an end point of 50 percent, IgG antibodies show a higher titer than IgM antibodies, whereas the opposite occurs with an end point of 15 percent. When the order of antibody reaction is calculated according to the formula of Weinrach *et al.* (1958), IgG antibodies show a value close to 2 and IgM antibodies a value close to 1 (Fig. 4-2b), suggesting that in the cytolytic reactions IgM antibodies are more efficient per molecule than IgG antibodies. This suggestion agrees with electronmicroscopic studies of hemolytic antibodies against sheep red blood cells, indicating that 2–4 IgM molecules suffice to lyse a cell, whereas 200–4000 IgG molecules are required to produce the same result (Humphrey and Dourmashkin 1965).

Chapter Five

Current Status of H-2 Serology

H-2 serology is based almost entirely on analysis of inbred strains and congenic resistant lines of the laboratory mouse; analysis of H-2 antigens in populations of wild mice has begun only recently, and has not significantly altered the view of the system. Since relatively few different *H-2* haplotypes exist in the laboratory mouse, H-2 analysis can be intensive rather than extensive, leading to a thoroughness not otherwise possible.

I. Principles of Serological H-2 Typing

The ultimate goal of serological analysis is the characterization of a given *H-2* haplotype. This *H-2 typing* is performed differently today than it was in the early period of H-2 serology.

A. Early Studies

Most of the early work on H-2 serology was done by P. A. Gorer's group in England and G. Hoecker's group in Chile. The approach used by Gorer and his associates was similar to the one described in Chapter Four. The authors selected four inbred strains (A, C57BL, BALB/c, and C3H), cross-immunized them in all possible donor-recipient combinations, and scrutinized the antisera by absorption analysis (Amos *et al.* 1955). To simplify the description of these studies, we shall ignore for a moment one of the four strains (A) and proceed as if the analysis were done with only three strains. The three strains can be arranged into six donor-recipient combinations, of which three suffice to identify the maximum number of different antigens (see Chapter Three). The three critical combinations are BALB/c anti-C3H, C57BL anti-BALB/c, and C3H anti-C57BL (Table 5-1). The first combination, BALB/c anti-C3H, produced an antiserum that reacted with red cells of the donor strain (C3H) and cross-reacted with red cells of the third strain (C57BL). Absorption with C57BL tissue removed the activity against C57BL cells but not the activity against C3H cells. These results were interpreted by Amos and his co-workers as evidence for the presence in the unabsorbed antiserum of two antibodies reacting with two different antigens, one antibody reacting with an antigen shared by C3H and C57BL (antigen E or 5), and another antibody reacting with an antigen restricted to C3H (antigen K or 11). In a similar manner, the authors demonstrated that antiserum C57BL anti-BALB/c reacted with antigens 3 and 4, and antiserum C3H anti-C57BL with antigens 6 and 2 (Table 5-1). Altogether, the three antisera defined six antigens, of which three were limited to a single strain and three were shared by two strains (Table 5-2).

Table 5-1. Serological analysis of three inbred strains of mice*

| | | Tested against** | | | |
Antiserum	Absorbed by	C57BL	BALB/c	C3H	Antigen identified
BALB/c anti-C3H	—	+	0	+	5
	C57BL	0	0	+	11
C57BL anti-BALB/c	—	0	+	+	3
	C3H	0	+	0	4
C3H anti-C57BL	—	+	+	0	6
	BALB/c	+	0	0	2

* Based on Amos *et al.* 1955.
** + or 0 = positive or negative result in a hemagglutination test.

Because the three antisera were produced in strain combinations that differ in many genes, the six antigens could not automatically be assumed to be members of the same system. Their genetic relationship, therefore, had to be examined by a linkage test. The association of antigens 2 and 5 was determined from a backcross (BALB/c × C57BL)F_1 × BALB/c which was tested with antiserum BALB/c anti-C57BL containing anti-2 and anti-5 antibodies. In a direct hemagglutination test, the antiserum reacted with 71 of 140 tested backcross animals, suggesting that the genetic determinants for antigens 2 and 5 were closely linked. (A 3:1 ratio of positive to negative animals instead of the observed 1:1 ratio would be expected if the two antigens segregated independently.) The linkage was then confirmed by an absorption test, in which 32 of the 140 backcross animals were injected with the BALB/c anti-C57BL antiserum. The mice were bled 24 hr later, and the absorbed antisera were tested against C57BL (test for antigen 2) and C3H (test for antigen 5) red blood cells. Thirteen animals removed neither anti-2 nor anti-5, 18 removed both, and one female removed anti-2 but not anti-5. Hence, in the large majority of the progeny, the two antigens segregated together as if they were indeed members of the same genetic system. In similar tests, antigen 2 was shown to segregate with antigen 4 and antigen 4 to segregate with antigens 3, 6, and 11. Clearly, all six antigens behaved as members of the same system, which became known as the *H-2 system*.

Table 5-2. H-2 antigens detected by analysis of three inbred mice

Strain	*H-2* haplotype	H-2 antigens					
		2	4	11	3	5	6
C57BL	*b*	2	–	–	–	5	6
BALB/c	*d*	–	4	–	3	–	6
C3H	*k*	–	–	11	3	5	–

The three-strain analysis is summarized in Table 5-2, which can be regarded as an embryonic *H-2 chart*, that is, a summary of a momentary status of H-2 serology. The actual H-2 chart constructed by Gorer's group in 1955 was more complicated, because the analysis included a fourth strain, A, which was unique in the sense that it did not carry any H-2 antigens not carried either by BALB/c or C3H. The explanation offered by Gorer and Mikulska (1959) postulated that the *H-2* haplotype of strain A arose by recombination between *H-2* haplotypes *d* and *k*. The inclusion of one recombinant type in the original quartet of inbred strains allowed Gorer and his co-workers to "split" some antigens that would otherwise have behaved as units.

An approach similar to the one just described was employed by Hoecker and his associates (Hoecker *et al.* 1954), who used a large number of inbred strains (17) but did not analyze all the theoretically possible donor-recipient combinations. Instead, they concentrated on a few combinations selected at random. This selectivity, dictated by purely practical reasons, later became a common practice among *H-2* serologists.

It must be emphasized that the H-2 chart shown in Table 5-2 reflects only one particular interpretation of the serological results and that alternative interpretations are also possible, as was discussed earlier and will be discussed again later in this chapter. The interpretation adopted by Gorer's and Hoecker's groups was based on the assumption of a one-to-one relationship between H-2 antibodies and H-2 antigens (i.e., one antibody reacting with one antigen.); a precedent that has led to a highly one-sided view of the *H-2* system was set by that interpretation.

In the period following the original studies by Gorer and Hoecker and their respective co-workers, the H-2 chart was gradually expanded both by the addition of new *H-2* haplotypes and antigens and by splitting of the existing *H-2* haplotypes and antigens. New H-2 antigens were discovered by typing additional strains, as demonstrated by the following example.

In 1958 Snell described a new line, AKR.M, which was congenic with strain AKR (Snell 1958b). An antiserum prepared by immunization of AKR (H-2^k) mice with AKR.M tissue was analyzed by Stimpfling and Pizarro (1961) and shown to contain at least five new H-2 antibodies (Table 5-3). The unabsorbed serum reacted with a number of different strains, including A.CA, A.SW, C57BL, DBA/2, DBA/1, and AKR.M. Absorption with strain A.CA removed the activity against the absorbing strain but not against other strains. It was therefore concluded that A.CA cells shared at least one antigen with AKR.M [antigen A^1 (27)]. Strains able to absorb hemagglutinating activity for A.CA cells were presumed to possess A^1, and since the strain distribution of A^1 was different from all known H-2 antigens, it was assumed that A^1 was a new antigen.

Table 5-3. Reactions of AKR anti-AKR.M serum after absorption with different inbred strains*

| Absorbed by | Tested against** | | | | | | | Antigens detected |
	AKR	A.CA	A.SW	C57BL	DBA/2	DBA/1	AKR.M	
AKR	0	+	+	+	+	+	+	
A.CA	0	0	+	+	+	+	+	27
A.SW	0	+	0	+	+	+	+	28
A.CA + A.SW	0	0	0	+	+	+	+	27, 28
C57BL	0	0	0	0	+	+	+	27, 28, 29
DBA/2	0	0	0	0	0	+	+	27, 28, 29, 13
DBA/1	0	0	0	0	0	0	0	27, 28, 29, 13, 30
AKR.M	0	0	0	0	0	0	0	27, 28, 29, 13, 30

* Based on Stimpfling and Pizarro 1961.
** + or 0 = positive or negative reaction in a hemagglutination test.

Absorption with strain A.SW removed the hemagglutinating activity for the absorbing strain but not for other strains. The reaction with A.SW was therefore attributed to a new antigen shared by A.SW and AKR.M [antigen B^1 (28)].

Absorption with the combined tissues of strains A.SW and A.CA removed activity against these two absorbing strains but not against C57BL red cells. This suggested that strain C57BL had another antigen in common with AKR.M, in addition to A^1 and B^1 (C57BL tissue was able to absorb out anti-A^1 and anti-B^1 activity), and this third antigen was designated C^1 (29).

Because absorption with strain DBA/2 removed hemagglutinins reacting with C57BL cells (but absorption with C57BL tissue did not remove hemagglutinins reacting with DBA/2 cells), it was postulated that the DBA/2 strain shared with AKR.M another antigen in addition to A^1, B^1, and C^1. Because the strain distribution of this antigen was identical with the strain distribution of an antigen previously designated M (13), no new symbol was assigned to it.

Finally, absorption of the AKR anti-AKR.M serum with strain DBA/1 removed hemagglutinins for both DBA/1 and AKR.M cells, indicating that the two strains shared an antigen absent in other strains [antigen D^1 (30)].

The unique combination of H-2 antigens of strain AKR.M was designated *H-2^m*. Thus, one new strain and one new antiserum led to the identification of four new H-2 antigens (27, 28, 29, 30) and one new *H-2* haplotype (*H-2^m*).

The discovery of new *H-2* recombinants is usually accompanied by the splitting of the existing *H-2* haplotypes and antigens, as illustrated by the following example. To demonstrate a linkage between genetic determinants for antigens 4 and 11, Amos and his co-workers (1955) tested a progeny from a backcross $(C57BL \times A)F_1 \times C57BL$ with anti-4 and anti-11 sera. (Strain A is $+4, +11$; strain C57BL is $-4, -11$.) Among 194 mice tested, 97 were $+4$, $+11$; 95 were $-4, -11$, and one each was $+4, -11$ and $-4, +11$ (Gorer and Mikulska 1959). The two aberrant animals were further backcrossed to C57BL and the progeny tested with the same two antisera. The mice derived from the $+4, -11$ animal were either $+4, -11$ or $-4, -11$; those derived from the $-4, +11$ animals were $-4, +11$, or $-4, -11$, indicating that the new combinations of H-2 antigens (haplotypes) were inheritable. Gorer and Mikulska (1959) explained the origin of the new *H-2* haplotypes by a genetic exchange (recombination, crossing-over) between the two parental *H-2* chromosomes in the F_1 hybrid, and designated them $H-2^h$ ($-4, +11$) and $H-2^i$ ($+4, -11$). The heterozygotes were then mated *inter se* and homozygous lines HTH ($H-2^h$) and HTI ($H-2^i$) were obtained.

These new lines revealed that some of the antigens previously considered simple could be split into two or more. For example, antiserum A anti-C57BL was originally specific for an antigen called B (Gorer 1959). The unabsorbed antiserum reacted with C57BL cells and cells from both recombinant lines, HTH and HTI. Absorption with HTH tissue removed activity against the absorbing strain but not against strains C57BL and HTI. Absorption with HTI tissue removed activity for HTI but not for C57BL and HTH (Table 5-4).

Table 5-4. Reactions of A anti-C57BL serum following absorption with *H-2* recombinant strains*

Absorbed by	Tested against**		
	C57BL	HTH	HTI
—	+	+	+
HTH	+	0	+
HTI	+	+	0
C57BL	0	0	0

* Based on Gorer 1959.
** + or 0 = positive or negative reaction in a hemagglutination assay.

Table 5-5. Recommended combinations for production of oligospecific antisera against H-2 antigens

Target antigens	Recipient	Donor	H-2 haplotype combination	Tested against Strain	H-2 haplotype	Target antigens	Reference
1 (11, 23, 25)	(DBA/2 × B10)*	B10.A	(d × b)a	B10.P	b	1	Amos 1959**
2	(5R × LP.RIII)	B10	(i5 × r)b	B10		2	M. Cherry and G. D. Snell, personal communication
3 (1, 12, 19, 36, 45)	(A.BY × B10.M)	B10.S	(b × m)s	B10.D2	s	3(36)	Stimpfling and Richardson 1965
4 (41, 42, 43)	(B10.AKM × 129)	B10.A	(m × bc)a	B10.A	a	4(41, 42, 43)	M. Cherry and G. D. Snell, personal communication
5 (33, 39, 45)	(DBA/2 × B10.HTG)	B10	(d × g)b	B10.A	a	5(45)	J. Klein et al. 1970
6 (2, 33, 34, 35, 39, 46)	(C3H.OH × B10.BR)	B10	(o2 × k)b	71NS	r	6	J. Klein, unpublished
7 (9, 37)	(A × B10)	B10.M	(a × b)f	B10.S	s	7	J. Klein, unpublished
8 (9, 37)	(A.BY × B10.S)	B10.M	(b × s)f	71NS	r	8	G. D. Snell, personal communication
9 (37)	(DBA/2 × B10.S)	B10.M	(d × s)f	B10.M	f	9(37)	G. D. Snell, personal communication
11 (17, 30)	(DBA/2 × B10.S)	B10.Q	(d × s)q	B10.BR	k	11	M. Cherry and G. D. Snell, personal communication
12 (36, 42)	(B10 × DBA/1)	DA	(b × q)qp1	DA	qp1	12(36, 42)	M. Cherry and G. D. Snell, personal communication
13 (43, 30)	(A.BY × B10.BR)	B10.AKM	(b × k)m	B10.D2	d	13(43)	Stimpfling and Richardson 1965
15 (38)	(2R × A.CA)	B10.WB	(h2 × f)ja	B10.WB	ja	15(38)	M. Cherry and G. D. Snell, personal communication
16 (38)	(B10.A × A.CA)	B10.P	(a × f)p	B10.P	p	16(38)	G. D. Snell, personal communication
17	(DBA/2 × B10.AKM)	B10.Q	(d × mq)	B10.Q	q	17	G. D. Snell, personal communication
18	(B10 × C3H)	71NS	(b × k)r	71NS	r	18	J. Klein, unpublished
19 (7)	(B10.A × DA)	B10.S	(a × qp1)s	B10.S	s	19(17)	J. Klein, unpublished
20	(DBA/2 × B10.BR)	B10.PL	(d × k)u	B10.PL	u	20	Snell et al. 1971a
21	(B10.A × C3H)	B10.SM	(a × k)v	B10.SM	v	21	M. Cherry and G. D. Snell, personal communication
23	(B10 × LP.RIII)	2R	(b × r)h2	2R	h2	23	M. Cherry and G. D. Snell, personal communication

No.	Cross*					Ref.**	Reference
25 (18)	(DBA/2 × B10.Q)	71NS	(d×q)r	B10.BR	k	25	Snell et al. 1971a
27 (9)	(C3H × B10.S)	B10.M	(k×s)f	B10	b	27	G. D. Snell, personal communication
28 (19, 36)	(C3H × B10.M)	B10.S	(k×f)s	B10	b	28	Snell et al. 1974
29 (31)	(C3H × B10.P)	C3H.OH	(k×p)o2	B10	b	29	Snell et al. 1974
30	(B10.A × LP.RIII)	B10.AKM	(a×r)m	B10.AKM	m	30	M. Cherry and G. D. Snell, personal communication
31 (34)	(A × B10)	B10.D2	(a×b)d	B10.D2	d	31(34)	G. D. Snell, personal communication
32	(A × B10)	B10.BR	(a×b)k	B10.BR	k	32	G. D. Snell, personal communication
33 (39)	(A × B10.D2)	5R	(a×d)i5	5R	i5	33(39)	G. D. Snell, personal communication
34 (31)	(A × B10)	B10.D2	(a×b)d	B10.P	p	34	D. Davies 1971
35 (16, 34, 38, 41)	(2R × A.CA)	B10.P	(h2×f)p	B10	b	35	M. Cherry and G. D. Snell, personal communication
36 (19, 42)	(2R × A.CA)	B10.S	(h2×f)s	B10	b	36	M. Cherry and G. D. Snell, personal communication
37 (9)	(DBA/2 × B10.S)	B10.M	(d×s)f	B10.P	p	37	Démant et al. 1971a
38 (16, 34)	(A × B10.M)	B10.P	(a×f)p	B10.WB	ja	38	Démant et al. 1971a
39 (33)	(A × B10.D2)	5R	(a×d)i5	B10.M	f	39	Démant et al. 1971a
40 (49)	B10.D2(M504)	B10.D2	(da)d	B10.D2	d	40(49)	Dishkant et al. 1973
41 (16, 34, 35, 38)	(2R × A.CA)	B10.P	(h2×f)p	B10.D2	d	41(42)	Démant et al. 1971b
42 (7, 12, 19, 36)	(B10.BR × A.BY)	B10.S	(k×b)s	B10.D2	d	42(36)	Démant et al. 1971b
43 (21, 27, 28, 29)	(C3H × B10.P)	B10.SM	(k×p)v	B10.D2	d	43(27, 28, 29)	Démant et al. 1971b
44 (7, 15, 38)	(B10 × C3H)	B10.WB	(b×k)ja	B10.D2	d	44	Čapková and Démant 1972
45 (15, 38, 44, 47)	(A.CA × B10)	B10.WB	(f×b)ja	DBA/1	q	45	Čapková and Démant 1972
46 (2, 33, 39)	A	B10	(a)b	B10.D2	d	46	D. Davies 1971
47 (3, 4, 8, 13, 31, 34, 41, 42, 43, 44)	B10	B10.WB	(b)d	B10.WB	ja	47(44)	D. Davies 1971
49 (40)	B10.D2(M504)	B10.D2	(da)d	B10.D2	d	49(40)	Dishkant et al. 1973
50	B10.D2	B10.D2(M504)	(d)da	B10.D2(M504)	da	50	Dishkant et al. 1973

* F$_1$ hybrids. For abbreviations of strain symbols, see Table 5-7.
** The reference is to the haplotype combination; the strain combination can be different.

Apparently, the antiserum contained at least two antibodies against two different antigens, one shared by C57BL and HTH but absent in HTI (antigen 2), and the other shared by C57BL and HTI but absent in HTH (antigen 33).[1] Hence, an antigen (B) that previously appeared to be simple was shown to consist of at least two components, 2 and 33. Although both anti-2 and anti-33 antibodies were apparently present in the A anti-C57BL serum, they were inseparable in the absence of $+2$, -33 or -2, $+33$ haplotypes.

B. Modern Approach

The current methods of serological H-2 typing differ from those used in the early period of H-2 studies. A strain with an unknown *H-2* haplotype is typed in the following way. First, the presence or absence of known H-2 antigens is determined; second, the strain is tested for the presence of new, previously unidentified H-2 antigens; third, the identity of the analyzed *H-2* haplotype is confirmed by transplantation methods.

The presence or absence of known H-2 antigens is determined by using a battery of oligospecific alloantisera, listed in Table 5-5. The strain combinations for the production of these antisera have been selected according to five criteria.

1. The donor differs from the recipient in a small number (preferably only one) of H-2 antigens. A substantial restriction of antisera specificity is achieved by using F_1 hybrids (rather than standard inbred strains) as recipients for immunization. To give an example, immunization of C57BL/10(*H-2^b*) mice with C3H(*H-2^k*) tissue theoretically can produce at least 11 different H-2 antibodies (anti-1, 3, 8, 11, 23, 24, 25, 32, 45, 47, and 49); in contrast, (C57BL/10 × A)F_1 hybrids theoretically produce only one H-2 antibody (anti-32) when immunized with C3H tissue.

2. The donor-recipient combinations are as close as possible to the original ones used to define the H-2 antigens. If every laboratory used a different strain combination to define a particular H-2 antigen, communication problems would soon develop, because it is unlikely that the same antiantibody can be produced in more than one haplotype combination. In the absence of any official definition of individual H-2 antigens, the tacit agreement among H-2 serologists is to use the original combinations through which the antigens were described (Table 5-6). In cases where this is not possible because the original antisera contained too many antibodies, closely related combinations are chosen.

3. The *H-2* haplotypes of the donor is on the same genetic background as that of one of the recipient's parents, thus precluding non-H-2 antibody formation by the recipient.

4. The genetic background of the second parent of the F_1 recipient is different from that of the donor. The introduction of an unrelated genetic

---

[1] The second antibody in the A anti-C57BL antiserum was originally identified as anti-22. However, since antigen 22 probably does not exist, it is assumed that the antibody was anti-33.

Table 5-6. Antisera used originally to define individual H-2 antigens

Antigen	Recipient	Donor	H-2 combination	Absorbed with Strain	Absorbed with H-2 haplotype	Tested against Strain	Tested against H-2 haplotype	Reference
1	(DBA/2 × C57BL)F_1	A	(d×b)a	—	—	F/St	n	Amos 1959
2	A	C57BL	(a)b	HTI	i	C57BL	b	Amos et al. 1955, Gorer 1959
3	C57BL/10-H-2^d	C57BL/10	(d)b	C3H	k	C57BL/10	b	Hoecker et al. 1954
	C57BL/10	C57BL/10-H-2^d	(b)d	C3H	k	C3H	k	Hoecker et al. 1954
4	C57BL	A	(b)a	—	—	DBA/2	d	Gorer et al. 1948
	C3H	A	(k)a	C57BL	b	BALB/c	d	Amos et al. 1955
	C3H	BALB/c	(k)d	C57BL	b	BALB/c	d	Amos et al. 1955
	A.SW	A	(s)a	C3H	k	C57BL/10-H-2^d	d	Hoecker et al. 1954
5	BALB/c	C57BL	(d)b	—	—	A	a	Amos et al. 1955
	C57BL/10-H-2^d	C57BL/10	(d)b	—	—	A	a	Hoecker et al. 1954
6	C3H	C57BL	(k)b	—	—	A	a	Amos et al. 1955
7	A	A.CA	(a)f	—	—	A.SW	s	Hoecker et al. 1959
8	A.SW	A	(s)a	—	—	A.CA	f	Hoecker et al. 1959
9	A.SW	A.CA	(s)f	A	a	A.CA	f	Hoecker et al. 1959
[10	DBA/1	DBA/2	(q)d	?	?	I?	j	Amos 1959]
11	BALB/c	A	(d)a	C57BL	b	A	a	Amos et al. 1955
	B^{A}LB/c	C3H	(d)k	C57BL	b	A	a	Amos et al. 1955
	(BALB/c × C57BL)F_1	A	(d×b)a	—	—	A	a	Amos et al. 1955
12	A.SW	A	(s)a	DBA/2	d	AKR	k	Hoecker et al. 1954
	(DBA/1 × SWR)F_1	DA	(q×q)qp1	—	—	—	—	Snell and Cherry 1974
13	AKR	AKR.M	(k)m	—	—	DBA/2?	d	Amos 1959
	AKR	AKR.M	(k)m	C57BL	b	DBA/2	d	Stimpfling and Pizarro 1961
[14	C3H	DBA/2	(k)d	?	?	?	?	Amos 1959]

Table 5-6. (*Continued*)

Antigen	Recipient	Donor	H-2 combination	Absorbed with Strain	Absorbed with H-2 haplotype	Tested against Strain	Tested against H-2 haplotype	Reference
15	(C57BL/10 × C3H)F₁	C3H.JK	(b×k)j	—	—	—	—	Snell et al. 1971a
	(B10.Y × C3H.B10)F₁	I	(pa×b)j	—	—	—	—	J. Klein 1971a
16	C3H	P	(k)p	C3H	k	P	p	Hoecker et al. 1954
17	DBA/1B-H-2^d	DBA/1	(d)q	A	a	DBA/1	q	Hoecker et al. 1954
18	C3H	C3H.RIII	(k)r	—	—	—	—	Shreffler and Snell 1969
19	A	A.SW	(a)s	A	a	A.SW	s	Hoecker et al. 1954
20	(AKR × DBA/2)F₁	PL	(k×d)u	—	—	—	—	Démant et al. 1971b
21	(C3H × BDP)F₁	SM	(k×p)v	—	—	—	—	Snell et al. 1971a
[22	BALB/c	C57BL	(d)b	HTH	h	C57BL	b	Gorer and Mikulska 1959
23	C3H	C57BL	(k)b	—	—	JK	j	Amos 1959]
23	RIII	C3H	(r)k	A.CA	f	C3H	k	Hoecker et al. 1959
24	(PL × A.CA)F₁	C3H.NB	(u×f)p	?	r	?	a or h	Snell et al. 1971a
25	[A.SW	A	(s)a	—	—	STOLI	e(= q)	Hoecker et al. 1959]
	(B10.D2 × DBA/1)F₁	B10.RIII(71NS)	(d×q)r	—	—	B10.BR	k	Snell et al. 1971a
27	AKR	AKR.M	(k)m	A.CA	f	A.CA	f	Stimpfling and Pizarro 1961
28	AKR	AKR.M	(k)m	A.SW	s	A.SW	s	Stimpfling and Pizarro 1961
29	AKR	AKR.M	(k)m	A.CA + A.SW	f+s	C57BL	b	Stimpfling and Pizarro 1961
30	AKR	AKR.M	(k)m	DBA/1	q	AKR.M	m	Stimpfling and Pizarro 1961

No.								Reference
31	A	BALB/c	(a)d	—	—	—	—	Amos et al. 1955
32	AKR.K	AKR	(a)k	—	—	—	—	Hoecker et al. 1954
	A	C3H	(a)k	—	—	—	—	Gorer and Mikulska 1959
33	HTH	C57BL	(h)b	—	—	—	—	Gorer and Mikulska 1959
34	(C57BL/6×A)F$_1$	B10.D2	(b×a)d	—	—	P	*p*	D. Davies 1971
35	(C3H×A.CA)F$_1$	C3H.NB	(k×f)p	—	—	C57BL/10	*b*	Démant et al. 1971b
36	(FL×LP.RIII)F$_1$	A.SW	(k×r)s	—	—	C57BL/10	*b*	Démant et al. 1971b
37	(B10.D2×A.SW)F$_1$	B10.M	(d×s)f	—	—	C3H.NB	*p*	Démant et al. 1971a
38	(C3H×A.CA)F$_1$	C3H.NB	(k×f)p	—	—	WB/Re	*ja*	Démant et al. 1971a
	(B10.A×A.CA)F$_1$	B10.Y	(a×f)pa	B10.BR	—	WB/Re	*ja*	Démant et al. 1971a
39	(A×B10.D2)F$_1$	B10.A(5R)	(a×d)i	—	*k*	B10.M	*f*	Démant et al. 1971a
40	B10.D2(M504)	B10.D2	(da)d	—	—	B10.D2	*d*	Dishkant et al. 1973
41	[B10.A(2R)×A.CA]F$_1$	B10.Y	(h2×f)pa	—	—	B10.D2	*d*	Démant et al. 1971b
42	(FL×C57BL/10)F$_1$	A.SW	(k×b)s	—	—	B10.D2	*d*	Démant et al. 1971b
43	(B10.BR×C3H.NB)F$_1$	B10.SM	(k×p)v	—	—	B10.D2	*d*	Démant et al. 1971b
44	(C57BL/10×C3H)F$_1$	I	(b×k)j	—	—	B10.D2	*d*	Čapková and Démant 1972
45	(A.CA×C57BL/10)F$_1$	WB/Re	(f×b)ja	—	—	DBA/1	*q*	Čapková and Démant 1972
46	A	C57BL/10	(a)b	—	—	B10.D2	*d*	D. Davies 1971
47	C57BL/10	DBA/2	(b)d	—	—	WB/Re	*ja*	D. Davies 1971
49	B10.D2(M504)	B10.D2	(da)d	—	—	B10.BR	*k*	Dishkant et al. 1973
50	B10.D2	B10.D2(M504)	(d)da	—	—	—	—	Dishkant et al. 1973
101	B10.A	B10.KPA42	(a)w1	—	—	—	—	J. Klein 1972a
102	(C3H×B10.D2)F$_1$	B10.KPB68	(k×d) w2	—	—	—	—	J. Klein 1972a
103	C3H	B10.SAA48	(k)w3	—	—	—	—	J. Klein 1972a
104	C3H	B10.GAA20	(k)w4	—	—	—	—	J. Klein 1972a
105	B10.A	B10.KEA5	(a)w5	—	—	—	—	J. Klein 1972a
106	BALB/c	T7WF	(d)w6	—	—	—	—	J. Klein 1971b

Table 5-7. Recommended strain panel for testing H-2 antisera

H-2 haplotype	Strain	Abbreviation	Alternate strains
a	B10.A	—	A
an	A.TFR1	—	—
ap	B10.M(11R)	11R	A.TFR2
aq	B10.M(17R)	17R	—
b	C57BL/10	B10	A.BY, 129
by	B10.BYR	—	—
d	B10.D2	—	DBA/2
da	B10.D2(M504)	M504	—
df	LG/Ckc	—	—
f	B10.M	—	A.CA
g	B10.HTG	—	—
h	B10.A(2R)	2R	—
i	B10.A(5R)	5R	—
ja	B10.WB	—	—
k	B10.BR	—	C3H/He
m	B10.AKM	—	AKR.M
o2	B10.OH	—	C3H.OH
p	B10.P	—	B10.Y
q	B10.Q	—	DBA/1
qp	B10.DA	—	DA
r	B10.RIII(71NS)	71NS	LP.RIII
s	B10.S	—	A.SW
sq	A.QSR1	QSR1	—
t2	B10.S(7R)	7R	—
u	B10.PL	—	PL
v	B10.SM	—	SM
y	B10.AQR	—	B10.T(6R)
z	NZW	—	—

background into the donor-recipient combination may strengthen the immune response through hybrid vigor (Stimpfling and Pandis 1969).[2]

5. The total number of strains involved in the antisera production is minimized by using the same strain in as many different donor-recipient combinations as possible, thus reducing animal colony expenses.

Each antiserum of the battery must be tested against a panel of strains representing major *H-2* haplotypes (Table 5-7) and only antisera displaying the expected pattern of reactivity can be used for H-2 typing.

Once the presence or absence of known H-2 antigens in the typed strain is determined, a search is launched for previously undetected antigens using the typed strain as a donor of tissue for immunization. The choice of the recipient

---

[2] Hybrid vigor (heterosis) is the superiority of heterozygous over homozygous individuals with respect to one or more characters.

is purely empirical; however, avoidance of recipients lacking many antigens carried by the donor is recommended. Otherwise, the produced antisera may contain a large number of antibodies and thus be too complex for analysis. An antiserum defines a new H-2 antigen if it contains only a small number (preferably one) of unknown antibodies, if the antigen defined by the new antiserum belongs to the *H-2* system, and if the strain distribution pattern of the antigen differs from the distribution patterns of all known H-2 antigens.

Membership of the new antigen in the *H-2* system is considered automatic if the new antiserum is produced in a combination differing only in the *H-2* complex. In all other instances, a linkage test must be performed.

In cases where the antigenic configuration of the tested strain resembles that of some known strain, an F_1 test (see Chapter Seven) is used to support further the similarity between the two *H-2* haplotypes. If the *H-2* haplotype of the tested strain cannot be distinguished serologically and by tissue grafting from one of the known *H-2* haplotypes, it is designated by the same *H-2* symbol as the known haplotype; if the *H-2* haplotype of the tested strain is different from all known *H-2* haplotypes, it is given a new symbol.

II. H-2 Antigens

A. Nomenclature

The H-2 antigens were originally designated by capital letters (A, B, C, etc.), but the number of antigens increased so rapidly that it soon exceeded the number of letters in the alphabet, and so it became necessary to use compound symbols such as A^1, B^1, C^1, and so on. Because such symbols were awkward and confusing, a committee of H-2 serologists (Snell *et al.* 1964) abandoned the letter symbols in favor of the numerical system of nomenclature originally proposed by Rosenfield and co-workers (1962) for the Rh blood group complex of man. In this system, each antigen is designated by an Arabic numeral, and the absence of an antigen by a minus sign $(-)$ before the appropriate number. In charts where there is no risk of confusion, the absence of an antigen is simply indicated by the minus sign (without the number). Antigens belonging to different systems are distinguished by combining the antigen symbol with the system symbol. For example, H-2.1, H-2.2, and H-2.3 are antigens of the *H-2* system, while Ea-2.1 and Ea-2.2 are antigens of the *Ea-2* system. The advantages of the numerical system are that it is simple, open-ended, and free of any biochemical and genetic implications.

A letter-to-number conversion table is given below.

A = 1	C = 3	D^b = 2	F = 6	J = 10	N = 14	V = 22
A^1 = 27	C^1 = 29	D^k = 32	G = 7	K = 11	P = 16	W = 23
B = 2	D = 4	E = 5	H = 8	K^b = 33	Q = 17	Y = 25
B^1 = 28	D^1 = 30	E^d = 31	I = 9	M = 13	S = 19	

Letters R and Z (Hoecker *et al.* 1959) designated antigens that have since been shown not to belong to the *H-2* system; letters L, O, T, and U (Amos 1959) designated antigens so poorly defined that they were not included in the H-2 chart.

The assignment of letter symbols to individual antigens was at first arbitrary. Some antigens were assigned letters according to the *H-2* haplotype in which they were discovered (e.g., antigens D, K, P, Q, and S were found in *H-2* haplotypes *d*, *k*, *p*, *q*, and *s*, respectively), others were designated simply by picking up unassigned letters (e.g., A, C, E, etc.). The current tendency is to assign numbers to newly discovered antigens in consecutive order, the only exception being that the antigens of wild mice are designated by symbols higher than 100 (J. Klein 1972a), in spite of the fact that the last number used for antigens in the inbred stains is 56.

B. Public and Private Antigens

As more strains were H-2 typed and new antigens added to the growing list, it was noticed that some antigens were present in only one *H-2* haplotype while others were shared by several unrelated haplotypes. The haplotype-specific antigens were called *private* (Hoecker *et al.* 1954) and the shared ones *public* (J. Klein 1971a). It was tacitly assumed that the division of H-2 antigens into private and public was an artifact that would disappear once a more representative sample of the natural mouse population was obtained. However, this proved not to be the case. Studies on wild mice indicated that antigens rare among inbred strains were also rare among wild mice, and antigens frequent among inbred strains were also frequent among wild mice (J. Klein 1970a, 1971a).

To qualify for the *private* category, an antigen must be limited to a single major unrelated *H-2* haplotype; the same antigen, however, can be present in several additional haplotypes derived from the original haplotype either by recombination or recent mutation. The total number of currently known private antigens is 20 (Table 5-8). All known *H-2* haplotypes (except *H-2ᶻ*) carry at least one private antigen, and most carry two. The antigens are usually strong in that they generate relatively high-titered antisera, particularly when measured by the cytotoxic test. The antiprivate antibodies are very specific and show no evidence of cross-reactivity.

The *public* H-2 antigens are present in more than one unrelated *H-2* haplotype. The most recent H-2 chart contains 27 such antigens, 11 present in two *H-2* haplotypes, three in three, and the remaining 13 shared by four or more *H-2* haplotypes (Table 5-9). Snell and his co-workers (Snell *et al.* 1973a) suggest division of the public antigens into two groups: short and long. The category of short antigens contains 14 antigens, most of which are present in only two *H-2* haplotypes. Some of the short antigens (e.g., 11, 25, 41, 42, 43) are relatively strong generators of antibodies; others (e.g., 24 and 13) are relatively weak (Snell *et al.* 1973a). Most of the short antigens are controlled by a single gene

Table 5-8. A simplified version of the H-2 chart

H-2 haplotype symbol	Private antigens determined by regions*	
	K	*D*
H-2 haplotypes of independent origin		
b (*ba, bb, bc, bd, be*)	33	2
d (*da*)	31	4
f (*fa*)	?	9
k	23	32
p (*pa, n*)	16	?
q	17	30
r	18	
s	19	12
w1	101	
w2	102	
w3	103	
w4	104	
w5	105	
w6	106	
z	?	?
H-2 haplotypes derived by recombination		
a (*a1*)	23	4
an1	19	9
ap1 (*ap2, ap3, ap4, ap5*)	?	4
aq1	23	9
by1	17	2
df	31	?
g (*g1, g2, g3, g4, g5*)	31	2
h (*h1, h2, h3, h4, h15, h18*)	23	2
i (*i3, i5, i7, ia1*)	33	4
j (*ja*)	15	2
m (*m1*)	23	30
o1 (*o2*)	31	32
qp1	17	12
sq1 (*sq2*)	19	30
t1 (*t2, t3, t4, t5*)	19	4
u	20	4
v	21	?
y1 (*y2*)	17	4

* Antigens not yet assigned to either the *K* or *D* regions are placed in between.

or gene cluster. Long public antigens are characterized by wide distribution, complexity, and cross-reactivity. They can be classified as weak (e.g., H-2.7) to moderately strong (e.g., H-2.1), and most appear to be controlled by two genes in different regions of the *H-2* complex.

Table 5-9. Public H-2 antigens grouped according to the number of unrelated *H-2* haplotypes in which they occur*

		Number of *H-2* haplotypes					
2	3	4	5	6	7	8	9
H-2 antigens							
13	11	7	47	8	1	3	5
25	34	42		27	27	29	6
37	35			29	49		28
38	36			45			
39				46			
41							
42							
43							
44							
Total 9	4	2	1	5	3	2	3

* Modified from Snell *et al.* 1973a.

The structural significance of the division into private, short and long public antigens is not clear, but several possibilities can be contemplated. First, the distinction has no structural meaning at the level of the antigen and the entire phenomenon is a serological artifact caused by cross-reacting antibodies. Second, the phenomenon is merely a reflection of the manner in which serological analysis is performed (see Chapter Four). Third, the division into private and public antigens has a real meaning, which is as follows:

1. the private and public H-2 antigens are controlled by different genes and the different serological behavior of the antigens is due to their biochemical peculiarities;
2. the antigens are controlled by the same genes (i.e., one gene codes for both private and public antigens) and the division is the result of the evolution of these genes. The long public antigens are the result of ancient mutations, whereas the private antigens reflect the most recent genetic changes.

Whatever the explanation, an overemphasis on the division of the H-2 antigens into different categories would be unwise, because the boundaries between the categories are already obscure. For example, antigen H-2.11 is shared by at least two unrelated *H-2* haplotypes and is therefore classified as public, although in other respects it behaves as a typical private antigen. Further analysis will probably show that the H-2 antigens form a continuum, with the sharpest, least cross-reactive and most restricted ones at one end and the most cross-reactive and widely shared antigens at the other end.

The terms *private* and *public antigens* have been used in human blood grouping to convey a different meaning (see Race and Sanger 1968). To a human serologist, a public antigen is one that occurs with a high frequency, meaning that individuals lacking it are extremely rare. Private antigens in human blood grouping are antigens that are so rare that they are considered "curiosities of no particular value" (Zmijewski 1968). Also, human private and public antigens are usually orphans that have not been assigned to any particular blood group system. Once an antigen is shown to belong to an established system, it is removed from the private and public categories. This is all diametrically opposite to the usage of the terms in H-2 serology.

C. Antigenic Series

The complexity of H-2 serology stimulated efforts to bring some order into the system and to find a relationship among H-2 antigens. The simplest relationship between any two antigens is an antithetical one. Two antigens are considered antithetical if the presence of one precludes the presence of the other in genetically homozygous individuals. Two antithetical antigens are presumed to be controlled by two alleles at the same locus. In the early period of H-2 serology, several antithetical relationships were described. For example, antigens 2, 4, and 32 were considered members of one series, and antigens 11 and 33 members of another series. The antithetical relationships of these antigens were reflected in the original nomenclature: antigens 2, 4, and 32 were designated by the capital letter D and distinguished by small superscript letters (D^b, D, and D^k, respectively); antigens 11 and 33 were designated K and K^b respectively. Later, as H-2 serology grew in complexity, such simple relationships were lost in the intricacies of the H-2 chart. An isolated attempt by Egorov (1967b) to compare the H-2 antigens of unrelated strains through dispersion analysis led to some interesting conclusions, but was generally regarded as a statistical extravaganza by those aware of the H-2 chart's unreliability. Paradoxically, it was only after H-2 serology was greatly expanded by the addition of new *H-2* haplotypes that some order in the system began to emerge. The realizations that not all H-2 antigens were equally important and that some characterized the individual *H-2* haplotypes better than others were crucial factors in the recognition of such order. It became apparent that each major *H-2* haplotype was fully characterized by its two private antigens, and that the private antigens of the different haplotypes could be arranged into two series—D and K (Snell *et al.* 1971b).

Antigens in the two series are mutually exclusive, meaning that each *H-2* homozygote carries one private antigen from each series (D and K), but never two from the same series. Assignment of the individual antigens to the K or D series is based on the *H-2* recombinants. The starting point for the D-K serialization is a combination of *H-2* haplotypes *d*, *k*, and *a*. The *H-2^d* haplotype carries private antigens 31 and 4, and the *H-2^k* haplotype carries antigens 23 and 32. The *H-2^a* haplotype was derived from *H-2^d* and *H-2^k* by genetic recombination in such a way that it received antigen H-2.4 from *H-2^d* and antigen

H-2.23 from $H\text{-}2^k$. Antigen 4 (formerly D) is therefore assigned as the first member of the first, or D series, and antigen 23 as the first member of the second, or K series. (In earlier studies, it was antigen 11 or K rather than 23 that was considered the private antigen of $H\text{-}2^k$.) Assignment of antigen 4 to the D series puts antigen 31, the second private antigen of $H\text{-}2^d$, in the K series, and antigen 32, the second private antigen of $H\text{-}2^k$, in the D series. The serialization is then continued by taking one $H\text{-}2$ recombinant after another and weighing its private antigens against those already assigned. For example, the $H\text{-}2^g$ recombinant received antigen 31 from $H\text{-}2^d$ and antigen 2 from $H\text{-}2^b$; because 31 is in the K series, antigen 2 must be in the D series (and antigen 33, the second private antigen of $H\text{-}2^b$, in the K series). An $H\text{-}2$ recombinant that does not involve any of the already serialized private antigens cannot be serialized, and $H\text{-}2$ haplotypes that have not been involved in any known $H\text{-}2$ recombination behave as if they possess only one private antigen. The serialized private H-2 antigens are listed in Table 5-8, in which the unserialized ones are placed in the middle between the D and the K series.

Serialization of public H-2 antigens is carried out in conjunction with the serialization of private antigens. Whenever a public antigen is inherited together with a private one, it is assumed that the two antigens belong to the same series. For example, antigen 8 is considered a member of the K series because it has been inherited together with the K series private antigen 31 in the $H\text{-}2^g$ recombinant. However, the serialization is complicated by the fact that some public antigens seem to belong to both series at the same time (Section 5.II.D).

Whether the public antigens within each series (D or K) also show some degree of negative correlation is not clear; the sample of unrelated $H\text{-}2$ haplotypes may be too small to show any such relationship if it were to exist. Mutual exclusiveness between antigens 1 and 28, and 3 and 7 has been postulated by Snell *et al.* (1973a).

D. D-K Cross-reactivity

In 1966 Shreffler and his co-workers (Shreffler *et al.* 1966) described the $H\text{-}2^o$ recombinant derived from haplotypes $H\text{-}2^d$ and $H\text{-}2^k$. Because both $H\text{-}2^d$ and $H\text{-}2^k$ types possess antigen H-2.3, it was expected that $H\text{-}2^o$ would also be 3-positive. However, typing for H-2.3 gave ambiguous results: the recombinant reacted weakly with anti-3 antisera, yet immunization in a combination of $H\text{-}2^o$ anti-$H\text{-}2^k$ produced an antibody that behaved in all respects like an anti-3. The authors therefore concluded that $H\text{-}2^o$ possessed an anomalous "3" different from the antigen 3 in both $H\text{-}2^d$ and $H\text{-}2^k$. They proposed several explanations for how such an anomalous 3 could have arisen, one being that different $H\text{-}2$ haplotypes carry determinants for antigen 3 in different regions of the $H\text{-}2$ complex. Shreffler later reiterated this point and postulated a similar situation for antigens 1 and 5 (Shreffler 1970, Shreffler *et al.* 1971). Similar postulates were made by Snell and his colleagues (Snell *et al.* 1971a, Snell and Cherry 1974, Démant *et al.* 1971b). The indirect evidence in support of the concept of duplicate 1, 3, and 5 antigens provided by the two groups of investigators and reinterpreted according to the present concept of the *H-2* system is summarized below. But before the evidence is considered, three points need clarification.

The first point concerns the genetic definition of the D and K series. There is ample evidence (to be discussed in Chapter Ten) that the two antigenic series are controlled by two separate segments of the chromosome known as the *D* and *K* regions. The genetic fine structure of the *D* and *K* regions is irrelevant for most considerations discussed here. Although we assume that each region consists of only one gene or gene cluster coding for the known serologically detectable H-2 antigens, disproving this assumption would not affect the validity of the conclusions about the duplicate sites.

The second point concerns the method of antigen assignment to the D and K series. As explained above, the assignments can be made *directly* if appropriate *H-2* recombinants are available. If appropriate *H-2* recombinants are not available, the D-K assignments can be made *indirectly* on the basis of the serological behavior of the relevant antisera. Two approaches can be used. One is to obtain an oligospecific antiserum known to be directed against either a D or K series antigen. If the antiserum reacts with the tested *H-2* haplotype, it can be hypothesized that this haplotype carries the same antigen in the same series as the immunizing donor. The second approach is to obtain an oligospecific antiserum against an antigen of the tested *H-2* haplotype, examine the antiserum against a panel of strains, and determine by comparison with known antisera whether it behaves more like an anti-D or an anti-K series reagent. It should be emphasized, however, that the indirect D-K assignments are of dubious value. They are based on the assumption that cross-reactivity is more likely to occur between antigens of the same series than between antigens of different series, an assumption for which there is no experimental evidence.

Finally, the third point concerns the nomenclature of the cross-reactive antigens. Following the suggestion of Snell and his co-workers (Snell *et al.* 1973a, 1974, Snell and Cherry 1974), membership of an antigen in one of the two series is indicated by prefix D or K, and its origin by a small-letter suffix. For example, symbol K1k stands for antigen 1 in the K series of the *H-2^k* haplotype. The suffix designation stresses that antigens of the same family are slightly different in unrelated *H-2* haplotypes (e.g., H-2.1 in *H-2^k* is different from H-2.1 in *H-2^s*; H-2.3 in *H-2^d* is different from H-2.3 in *H-2^q*, etc.).

The individual cross-reacting antigens can now be described.

H-2.1. Recombinant *H-2^h*, whose K series is derived from *H-2^a* and D series from *H-2^b* (Gorer and Mikulska 1959), carries antigen 1 (Amos 1959), which behaves exactly like the strong 1 of the parental *H-2^a* haplotype (Snell *et al.* 1971a). Because *H-2^b* is 1-negative, antigen 1 of *H-2^h* must be regarded as a member of the K series, and furthermore, because the K series of *H-2^a* is derived from *H-2^k*, it seems reasonable to assume that H-2.1 or *H-2^h* is actually a K1k-antigen.

Recombinant *H-2^o*, which has its K series derived from *H-2^d* and its D series from *H-2^k* (Shreffler *et al.* 1966), carries a weak (Shreffler *et al.* 1966) or intermediate 1 (Snell *et al.* 1971a). Because H-2^d is 1-negative and H-2^k is 1-positive, the weak 1 of H-2° must be derived from the D series of H-2^k (D1k).

Thus, H-2^k carries two H-2.1 antigens, one in the K series (K1k) and another in the D series (D1k). If the two antigens are sufficiently different, it should be possible, using the *H-2* recombinants, to block K1 and produce antibodies against D1 and vice versa. For example, *o* anti-*k* should produce anti-K1k, and *h* (or *a*) anti-*k* should produce anti-D1k. Such antibodies, however, have not been reported, suggesting that K1k and D1k *are not* sufficiently different and the blockage of one antigen in the recipient cross-blocks the other antigen.

Additional support for the existence of 1-like antigens in both the K and D series was obtained by Snell and his co-workers (1971a). Their anti-1 antiserum AS-373, which was ($u \times f$) anti-*p*, reacted with *H-2* haplotypes *p, h, o,* and *r*. Absorption with *r* tissue removed activity against *r, q,* and *o*, but did not remove activity against *a, h, k,* and *m*. The authors interpreted this as an indication that the original antiserum contained two anti-1 antibodies: one reacting with *r, q,* and *o* and therefore presumably directed against D1 antigens in these *H-2* haplotypes, the other reacting with *a, h, k,* and *m* and therefore presumably directed against the K1k antigen. The K1 detected by AS-373 was designated by Snell and his colleagues as H-2.24, but a more accurate designation is K1.

The presence of K1 in H-2^q and H-2^s is supported by the fact that *H-2* recombinants *y* and *t*, which carry the K series of *q* and *s*, respectively, are typed as 1-positive. The presence of K1 in *r* and *v* is postulated simply because the K site seems to be more common for this antigen.

H-2.3. Evidence for two distinct 3-sites, K and D, is provided by *H-2* recombinants B10.A(4R) (H-2^{h4}) and HTI (H-2^i). The former recombinant carries the K series of H-2^a (which in turn is derived from H-2^k) and the D series of H-2^b; the latter recombinant carries the K series of H-2^b and the D series of H-2^a (H-2^d). Because the H-2^b haplotype is 3-negative and H-2^a, H-2^d, H-2^k, H-2^h, and H-2^i haplotypes are all 3-positive, the 3 of H-2^{h4} must be derived from the K series of H-2^k (K3k), the 3 of H-2^i from the D series of H-2^d (D3d) and the 3 of H-2^a from both the K series of H-2^k and the D series of H-2^d.

Antibodies against the two different sites, K3k and D3d, were produced by Shreffler and his co-workers (1966). The anti-K3k antibody was obtained in combination *o* anti-*k*, in which the D3k site was blocked from inducing antibodies by the presence of the D^k series in both the donor and the recipient. The anti-D3d antibody was produced in combination *o* anti-*d*, in which the K3d site was blocked by the presence of the K^d series in the donor and the recipient.

The *H-2* recombinants allow the following assignments: *K3d* to *d, g,* and *o*; *K3k* to *k, a, h,* and *m*; *D3d* to *d, a, i, t, ap2, u,* and *y*; *D3k* to *k* and *o*. On the basis of a serological analysis of a number of different anti-3 antisera, Snell and his co-workers (Démant *et al.* 1971b, Snell *et al.* 1973a, Snell and Cherry 1974) make the following additional assignments:

D3s. Because antiserum ($b \times ja$) anti-*s* is not absorbed by *h* cells, which carry the K3k antigen, anti-3 in this antiserum probably detects the D series antigens. The presence of D series 3 in *s* is also supported by the finding that antiserum ($m \times ja$) anti-s contains an anti-3 antibody. This should be anti-D3, because a K series 3 (K3k) is present in the recipient.

D3p. Because antiserum ($b \times f$) anti-p is not absorbed by h (K3k) cells, the antibody in this antiserum is probably directed against a D series 3. This assumption is supported by the observation that p does not absorb anti-K3k sera and that p is present in producers of antisera containing anti-K3k antibodies.

K3r. Antiserum ($b \times p$) anti-r behaves like anti-K3k, suggesting that it may contain a 3-like antibody against the K series antigen of r.

D3q. Antiserum ($b \times o$) anti-m seems to contain two 3-like antibodies, anti-K3k and anti-D3q.

D3v. The 3v antigen is assigned to the D series simply because D seems to be a more common position for 3.

H-2.5. Recombinant H-2^g, which has its K series derived from 5-negative H-2^d and its D series from 5-positive H-2^b, is 5-negative, suggesting the existence of a K5 site in H-2^b. Recombinant H-2^o, which has its D series derived from 5-positive H-2^k and its K series from 5-negative H-2^d, is 5-positive (Shreffler et al. 1966), suggesting the existence of a D5 site in H-2^k.

Because the H-2^a recombinant inherited H-2.5 from H-2^k, together with other K series antigens, the H-2^k must carry two 5-like sites, one associated with the K series (K5k) and the other associated with the D series (D5k).

The presence of 5 in y indicates that q carries a K series 5 (K5q) which should also be present in *ap1*.

An indication of the existence of D series 5 in r comes from an antiserum ($d \times f$) anti-i (Snell et al. 1971a), which reacts with o. Cells from H-2° absorb the antiserum well for target haplotype r and poorly or not at all for a, h, m, and u. Snell and his co-workers (1971a) interpret this finding as evidence for the presence of two antibodies reacting with two 5-sites. However, the serum should contain only one anti-5 antibody, namely anti-K5b, because o carries D5k but not K5b. The positive result with the H-2° haplotype is probably due to cross-reaction of the anti-K5b antibody with the D5k site. The fact that absorption with o cells removes the anti-r activity may mean that r carries a D series 5.

In the *H-2* haplotypes p, u, v, and z, a K series 5 is postulated simply because that seems to be its more common position.

H-2.27, 28, 29. Because in the original k anti-m serum used to define the 28-family antigens (Stimpfling and Pizarro 1961) the recipient and the donor shared their K ends, all the antibodies in this serum were directed against the D end of H-2^q. This places the 28-family of q in the D series. The presence of 28-sites in the D series of a, h, u, and y is required on the basis of the genetic origin of these haplotypes.

The H-2° recombinant seems to carry at least some antigens of the 28-family (Shreffler et al. 1966). Because H-2° shares the D end with the H-2^k, the reactivity of k anti-m antibodies with o cells must be ascribed to a 28-site in the K end of o. Similar K28 sites have been postulated in the H-2^d haplotype.

Presence of the K28 site in H-2^b is required on the basis of biochemical data of Shimada and Nathenson (1967), who reported that in the purified H-2^b

preparation, the 28-family antigens were found in the same peak as H-2.33, which is a K-series antigen.

H-2.35 and H-2.36. Recombinants $H\text{-}2^a$ and $H\text{-}2^o$ place 35 and 36 of $H\text{-}2^d$ in the D series; recombinants $H\text{-}2^g$, $H\text{-}2^h$, and $H\text{-}2^i$ place 35 and 36 of $H\text{-}2^b$ in the K series. Recombinant $H\text{-}2^{qp1}$ places 36 of $H\text{-}2^s$ in the D series. Antigen 35 of $H\text{-}2^b$ is tentatively assigned to the D series, where most of the 35-sites seem to be located.

A deliberate search for D-K cross-reactive antibodies described by David and his co-workers (1973b) was successful in at least two instances. One antiserum, C57BL/10 $(K^b D^b)$ anti-B10.A(5R) $(K^b D^d)$, was expected to contain anti-D^d antibodies, and it behaved as if it did. However, the antiserum also reacted with the B10.A(4R) $(K^k D^b)$ strain, which shares the D^b antigens with the recipient, indicating that at least some of the anti-D^d antibodies cross-reacted with the K^k antigens. Serological analysis of the antiserum suggested that the cross-reacting antibody was probably anti-3. The second antiserum, B10.A(2R) $(K^k D^b)$ anti-B10.A $(K^k D^d)$, reacted not only with strains carrying D^d antigens but also with strain C57BL/10 $(K^b D^b)$, which shares the D^b end with the recipient. The positive result with the C57BL/10 cells was attributed to cross-reaction of the anti-D^d antibodies with K^b antigens. Though the cross-reacting antibodies were not identified, the most likely candidates were anti-35 and 36.

E. Families of Antigens

One might expect that a battery of different antisera produced in different donor-recipient combinations against the same antigen would have the same range of reactivity, but this is not always the case. Several examples of antisera that should have been uniform but were actually quite diverse were provided by Snell and his co-workers (Snell *et al.* 1971a, Démant *et al.* 1971b). In one case (Fig. 5-1), the authors selected eight strain combinations that, according to the H-2 chart, should have produced antibodies against antigen 1 (Table 5-10). They tested all antisera produced in these combinations by hemagglutination

Table 5-10. Antisera produced by Snell *et al.* (1971a) against antigen H-2.1

Antiserum no.	Recipient	Donor	Recipient-donor H-2 haplotypes	Antibodies present
AS-343	(5R × A.CA)F₁	BDP	$(i \times f)p$	1, 16, 38, non-H-2
AS-344	(5R × A.CA)F₁	B10.Y	$(i \times f)pa$	1, 16, 38
AS-370	(C3H.SW × B10.M)F₁	C3H.NB	$(b \times f)p$	1, 16
AS-373	(PL × A.CA)F₁	C3H.NB	$(u \times f)p$	1, 24, 16, Ly-1.1
AS-361	(BALB/c × 41N)F₁	SM	$(d \times b)v$	1, 21
AS-346	(C3H.SW × B10.M)F₁	SM	$(b \times f)v$	1, 21, 43
AS-402	(C3H.SW × A.CA)F₁	C3H-$H\text{-}2^o$	$(b \times f)o$	1, 3, 31, 32
AS-290	(B10.D2 × D1.LP)F₁	DBA/1	$(d \times b)q$	1, 11, 17, 30?

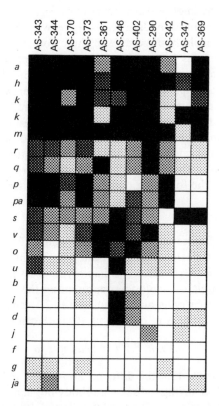

Fig. 5-1. Strength of reactions of antisera directed against the 1-family of H-2 antigens. The strength is indicated by the degree of shading. Symbols on the top are code numbers of antisera, small letters on the left are *H-2* haplotypes. Explanation in the text. (Reproduced with permission from G. D. Snell, P. Démant, and M. Cherry: "Hemagglutination and cytotoxic studies of H-2. I. H-2.1 and related specificities in the EK crossover regions." *Transplantation* 11:210–237. Copyright © 1971 by Williams & Wilkins Co. All rights reserved.)

and cytotoxic tests against a panel of strains representing major *H-2* haplotypes and some also by *in vivo* or *in vitro* absorption. A summary of these tests is shown in Fig. 5-1, in which the strength of the reaction is indicated by different degrees of shading. All eight antisera are similar in the range of their reactions, but they also exhibit differences, especially in the strength of the reaction. According to their reactivity with the anti-1 antisera, the *H-2* haplotypes were divided into three groups: 1-complete, 1-intermediate, and 1-negative (Snell *et al.* 1971a). The *1-complete group* (+1, +23) is so designated because the *H-2* haplotypes in this group all possess antigen H-2.23 in addition to H-2.1, a fact that Snell and his co-workers consider important. The 1-complete *H-2* haplotypes react strongly with all the anti-1 antisera. The *1-intermediate H-2* haplotypes (+1, −23) give moderate to strong reactions with some antisera and inconsistent (sometimes positive, sometimes negative) reactions with other antisera. The difference in strength of reactivity between 1-complete and 1-intermediate types is particularly noticeable in the cytotoxic absorption tests. The *1-negative* H-2 haplotypes (-1, -23) are either completely negative or only weakly and inconsistently positive. The 1-complete group is comprised of *H-2* haplotypes *a*, *h*, *k*, and *m*, which all have one of the two series of antigens in common (K^k). The group could actually be considered to be represented by one *H-2* haplotype ($H-2^k$), explaining why it behaves so uniformly. In the 1-intermediate group, on the other hand, only two *H-2* haplotypes are clearly related (*p* and *pa*), and correspondingly, the H-2.1 antigens in this group are heterogeneous. Based on the quantitative cytotoxic absorption data, the antigens can be arranged into the following order of decreasing strength:

$$1r, 1p, 1q, 1o$$

It seems that each of these antigens is unique and differs both quantitatively and qualitatively from all the other H-2.1 antigens. In this sense, the distinction into 1-complete and 1-intermediate *H-2* haplotypes loses its meaning. The $H-2^k$, which is the only unrelated haplotype representing the 1-complete group, can be regarded simply as carrying another unique H-2.1. The order of *H-2* haplotypes carrying H-2.1 antigens of decreasing strength can then be written as

$$k \ (a, h, m), r, p \ (pa), q, s, o$$

An important point is that the different anti-1 sera are "neither sufficiently alike to be regarded as having the same antibody nor sufficiently different to be regarded as defining distinct specificities" (Snell *et al.* 1971a). Antigen H-2.1 can therefore be considered a family of closely related, though distinct, determinants (*1-family*).

Snell and his colleagues (1971a) also demonstrated that immunization of a 1-positive strain with another 1-positive strain led to an induction of antibodies that resembled anti-1 in many respects. They called such antibodies "blocked," to distinguish them from "unblocked" antibodies produced in 1-negative strains. Three such antisera are shown in Fig. 5-1:

Antiserum no.	Recipient	Donor	Recipient-donor H-2 haplotypes	Antibodies present
AS–342	(A.SW × B10.M)F$_1$	BDP	$(s \times f)p$	1, 16, non-H-2
AS–347	(5R × BDP)F$_1$	A.SW	$(i \times p)s$	1 ?, 19
AS–369	(B10.D2 × C3H.NB)F$_1$	A.SW	$(d \times p)s$	1, 19, non-H-2 ?

The authors explain the highly unorthodox behavior of the blocked antibodies in the following way:

The 1 region of the H-2 antigen can have not only 1-positive and 1-negative sites but also sites which are reactive but which have varying degrees of difference from each other. Alleles s and v may be supposed to give rise to two of the more nearly identical sites; alleles s and p, to two of the most unlike sites. Yet s and p are enough alike so that anti-p sera react with s. In these circumstances, the antisera produced against different alleles would not be identical but would have a recognizable family relationship (Snell *et al.* 1971a).

An alternative explanation is that the whole phenomenon is a serological artifact.

Antigen H-2.3 is the principal figure in another family of antigens, the 3-family (Démant *et al.* 1971b). In contrast to the 1-family, the antigens of the 3-family are sufficiently distinct to justify the assignment of different symbols to each of them. The members of the 3-family are antigens 13, 41, 42, and 43, demonstrable by hemagglutination, and antigens H-2.35 and 36, demonstrable by cytotoxicity (Table 5-11). All five antigens are present in the H-2^d haplotype and its derivatives carrying the D^d antigens (H-2^a, H-2^i, H-2^u). Antigens 13, 41, 42, 43, and 44 are each present in one additional 3-positive haplotype. Antigen H-2.35 is present in H-2^p, which is positive for 41, and H-2^b, which is 3-negative, and a similar relationship exists between antigens H-2.42 and H-2.36. Démant and his co-workers (1971b) also believe that there seem "to be cytotoxic specificities corresponding to hemagglutinating specificities 13 and 43, the difference being again the reaction of the cytotoxic antibody with b." In combinations where b is not present in the recipient, immunization with q, p, s, or v tissue produces anti-13, anti-41, anti-42, and anti-43, respectively, and also the cytotoxic counterparts of these antibodies. In combinations where b is present in the recipient, only the respective hemagglutinating antibodies are produced. The cytotoxic and the hemagglutinating antibodies seem to be reacting with different antigens. This conclusion is supported by the observation that the hemagglutinating antigens are members of the D series, whereas the cytotoxic

Table 5-11. Distribution of 3-family antigens among relevant *H-2* haplotypes

H-2 haplotype	3-family antigens							
d (a, i, u)	3	13	41	42	43	44	35	36
q (m)	3	13	–	–	–	–	–	–
p	3	–	41	–	–	–	35	–
s	3	–	–	42	–	–	–	36
v	3	–	–	–	43	–	–	–
j	3	–	–	–	–	44	–	–
r	3	–	–	–	–	–	–	–
k (h)	3	–	–	–	–	–	–	–
o	3	–	–	–	–	–	–	–
b	–	–	–	–	–	–	35	36

antigens are members of the K series. (Interestingly, other antigens of the K^b series—namely H-2.5 and H-2.33—are also difficult to detect by hemagglutination, suggesting that the K^b gene(s) is poorly expressed in the erythroid cell sequences.)

Antibodies against the 3-family antigens react strongly with and are fully absorbed by the immunizing *H-2* haplotype (*p* in the case of anti-41, *s* in the case of anti-42, etc.) and by the *H-2* haplotypes possessing D^d antigens (*d*, *a*, *i*, and *u*). The antibodies also react weakly, both directly and by absorption, with a number of other 3-positive *H-2* haplotypes which, however, cannot completely absorb for the indicator *H-2* haplotype. The weak reactivity with other 3-positive haplotypes is seen by Démant and his co-workers (1971b) as evidence that all these antibodies are directed against a family of antigens (*3-family*). They interpret the family as a group of similar and cross-reacting antigens. An anti-serum made against one of the 3-positive haplotypes, "e.g., an anti-13 made against *q*, possesses a family of antibodies formed against the 13 site. All of these react quite strongly with this site and are fully absorbed by it. The corresponding site in allele *pa* is similar but not identical. It reacts to some degree but may not produce a demonstrable absorption" (Démant *et al.* 1971b).

F. Inclusion Groups and Subtype Systems

According to Snell and his colleagues (Snell *et al.* 1971a, Démant *et al.* 1971b), members of an antigenic family such as 1 and 3 are related not only among themselves but also to certain other antigens. The relationship outside the family can take the form of an inclusion or subtype grouping. An *inclusion group* is a cluster of antigens distributed among the different haplotypes so that the less frequent ones are present only when the more frequent ones are also present (i.e., the less frequent antigens are *included* in the more frequent ones).

The 1-family antigens form a *23-inclusion group*, so designated because the least frequent antigen of this group is H-2.23:

H-2 haplotype	H-2 antigens
k (*a, h, m*)	23 25 11 1 5
r	25 11 1 5
q (*y, qpl*)	11 1 5
p	1 5
b(*i*)	5

(The *H-2* haplotypes in parentheses are those derived by recombination from the haplotype preceding the parentheses.)

The 23-inclusion group can be interpreted in several ways, the simplest interpretation being that the grouping is coincidental and has no real meaning. This can easily happen as the sample of known unrelated *H-2* haplotypes is still very small. However, even if the 23-inclusion group holds after analysis of a sufficiently large population sample, it will still be possible to argue that the grouping does not necessarily reflect an internal relationship between the antigens involved. As was previously explained (see Chapter Three), inclusion groups are a natural consequence of the performance of serological analysis in a complex system. They can occur even among completely unrelated antigens. On the other hand, the grouping could have some structural basis and reflect a genuine relationship at the level either of antibodies or of antigens. The structure of the antigens in an inclusion group can be such that it could lead to unidirectional cross-reaction. For example, the 23-inclusion system can be explained by assuming that anti-25 cross-reacts with 23 but anti-23 does not cross-react with 25; anti-11 cross-reacts with 25 and 23, but anti-25 and anti-23 do not cross-react with 11, and so on. Unilateral cross-reaction between antigens 1 and 23, and between 5 and 25, has been postulated by Snell and his co-workers (1971a) as an explanation of the strong reaction of anti-1 with 23-positive haplotypes, and of anti-5 with 25-positive haplotypes.

The 3-antigen family shows only a hint toward an inclusion system (Démant *et al.* 1971b): antigen 4 is included in 13 and 3, antigen 13 is included in 3, but antigens 41, 42, 43, 44, 35, and 36 do not include 13 or each other (although they include 4 and are included in 3). This complicated interrelationship has been termed the *4-subtype system* by Snell's group. Speculations about the nature of the 23-inclusion group apply also to the 4-subtype system.

G. Description of Individual H-2 Antigens

What follows is a brief description of the known H-2 antigens, the manner in which they were defined, their serological properties, and their membership in the antigenic series. The antigens follow in numerical order. The antisera defining them are listed in Table 5-6.

H-2.1. Amos (1959) observed that antiserum (DBA/2 × C57BL)F$_1$ anti-A reacted with red cells of strain F/St, and he attributed the reaction to the presence of antigen A (1). The antigen was later shown to be complex, consisting of similar but not identical sites (see Section 5.II.E), and controlled by at least two genes or gene complexes (see Section 5.II.D). Anti-1 antibodies are usually formed only after hyperimmunization, but the antibodies are moderately strong in both hemagglutination and cytotoxic tests.

H-2.2. Amos (1953) and Amos *et al.* (1955) obtained three antisera by the immunization of BALB/c, C3H, and A recipients with C57BL leukosis E.L.4. The A anti-E.L.4 serum was specific for C57BL red cells, whereas the C3H anti-E.L.4 and BALB/c anti-E.L.4 sera became specific after absorption with BALB/c and C3H tissue, respectively. The target antigen of these antisera was designated B. The authors' original suspicion that the B antigen was complex was confirmed after the *H-2^h* and *H-2^i* recombinants became available (Gorer and Mikulska 1959). Absorption of BALB/c anti-E.L.4 antiserum with HTH (*H-2^h*) tissue removed the anti-HTH but not the anti-C57BL activity. The antibody removed by the HTH absorption was designated anti-D^b to emphasize that the corresponding antigen (H-2.2) was a member of the D series. The H-2.2 antigen is specific for the $H-2^b$ haplotype and its genetic derivatives, but a similar antigen is also present in $H-2^j$. The anti-2 antibodies are easily produced and react in both hemagglutination and cytotoxic tests.

H-2.3. An antiserum C57BL/10 anti-C57BL/10-$H-2^d$ produced by Hoecker et al. (1954) was expected to contain anti-H-2.4 antibodies and react only with $H-2^a$ and $H-2^d$ cells. However, the antiserum also reacted with $H-2$ haplotypes k, p, q, and s. The additional reactivity could be removed by absorption with $H-2^k$ tissue. Hoecker and his co-workers therefore concluded that the antiserum contained, in addition to anti-H-2.4, another antibody, anti-C (3), reacting with k, p, q, and s. Subsequent studies revealed that antigen 3, like antigen 1, was complex, consisting of a family of similar sites, and controlled by at least two genes. Anti-3 antibodies are moderately strong hemagglutinins and poor cytotoxins.

H-2.4. Anti-4 antibodies were probably present in the rabbit antiserum produced by Gorer (1938) against mouse A strain erythrocytes, and antigen H-2.4 is probably identical with Gorer's antigen II, which gave the $H-2$ complex its name. Anti-4 antibodies were also present in C57BL anti-A serum shown by Gorer and his co-workers (1948) to agglutinate A strain red blood cells in saline. The antibody was identified by Amos and his co-workers (1955) in antisera C3H anti-A and C3H anti-BALB/c. The hyperimmune antisera contained additional antibodies, but absorption with C57BL tissue rendered them specific for A and BALB/c cells. Antigen 4 is serologically one of the strongest H-2 antigens, inducing both hemagglutinating and cytotoxic antibodies. It is specific for the $H-2^d$ haplotype and its genetic derivatives.

H-2.5. Antiserum BALB/c anti-E.L.4, produced by Amos and his co-workers (1955), reacted not only with the donor strain (C57BL) but also with strains A and C3H. Absorption with A or C3H tissue removed the cross-reacting antibody but not the C57BL-specific antibody. The cross-reacting and the specific antibodies were designated anti-E (5), and anti-B (2), respectively. A similar antibody was obtained independently by Hoecker and his co-workers (1954) in strain combination C57BL/10-$H-2^d$ anti-C57BL/10, and was designated anti-X (X for unknown). H-2.5 is a strong antigen, which easily induces both hemagglutinating and cytotoxic antibodies. Quite often, however, the anti-5 sera fail to agglutinate the donor (C57BL) red cells, although they react strongly with C57BL lymphocytes. The H-2.5 is one of the most widely shared H-2 antigens, common among wild mice (J. Klein 1971a) and present in all inbred $H-2$ haplotypes except d and f. The 5-sites of the different $H-2$ haplotypes are probably different (Snell et al. 1973a) and are controlled by at least two genes. Complexity of the 5-antigen site was also suggested by studies of wild mice (J. Klein 1971a).

H-2.6. The reactivity of the C3H anti-E.L.4 antiserum (see H-2.2) with A and BALB/c (but not C57BL) cells can be absorbed out with A or BALB/c tissue (Amos 1953, Amos et al. 1955), indicating that the antiserum contains, in addition to the C57BL-specific antibody, another antibody against an antigen shared by A, BALB/c, and C57BL (antigen F or 6). Of the independent *H-2* haplotypes, antigen 6 is absent in only *k*, *u*, and *v*. The weak, low-titer anti-6 antibody is difficult to induce even after heavy hyperimmunization. It is formed more easily after immunization with *H-2ᵇ* than with *H-2ᵈ* or *H-2ᵃ* haplotypes (Amos *et al.* 1955).

H-2.7. Antiserum A anti-A.CA reacts with A.CA and cross-reacts with A.SW red blood cells (Hoecker *et al.* 1959). Absorption with A.SW tissue removes the A.SW but not the A.CA activity, indicating that the antiserum apparently contains two antibodies, one directed against an antigen shared by A.CA and A.SW (antigen G or 7) and another reacting with an antigen specific for A.CA (antigen I or 9). Antigen 7 is restricted to *H-2* haplotypes *f*, *s*, *j*, and *p* (and their derivatives) (Shreffler and Snell 1969). It induces only weak, predominantly hemagglutinating antibodies. Recent studies (Stimpfling 1973, C. S. David, *personal communication*, J. Klein, *unpublished data*) suggest that anti-7 hemagglutinating antibodies detect an antigen controlled by a region distinct from *K* and *D*, and located between *S* and *D* (region *X*).

H-2.8. Antiserum A.SW anti-A (Hoecker *et al.* 1959) contains antibodies against antigens H-2.4 and 11, as indicated by its reaction with *H-2ᵈ* and *H-2ᵃ*, and at least one additional antibody (anti-H or 8), which reacts with −4, −11 strain A.CA (*H-2ᶠ*). The relatively weak antigen 8, shared by *H-2* haplotypes *d*, *f*, *k*, *p*, and *r*, induces both hemagglutinating and cytotoxic antibodies.

H-2.9. The reactivity of antiserum A.SW anti-A.CA (Hoecker *et al.* 1959) with strains carrying antigen 8 (A, C57BL/10-*H-2ᵈ* and C3H) is absorbed with A strain tissue. However, the absorbed antiserum still reacts with A.CA (*H-2ᶠ*) tissue, indicating that it contains an *H-2ᶠ*-specific antibody, anti-I (9). H-2.9 is a strong private antigen of the *H-2ᶠ* haplotype. It induces both hemagglutinating and cytotoxic antibodies. At present it is not clear whether the antigen belongs to the K series, the D series, or both. Stimpfling *et al.* (1971) described two apparently reciprocal *a/f* recombinants which placed antigen 7 in the K series and antigen 9 in the D series. Shreffler and his co-workers (*personal communication*), on the other hand, obtained three *H-2* recombinants from *t2/f* and two from *t1/f* heterozygotes. These recombinants placed antigen 7 into the D series and antigen 9 into the K series. These conflicting results can be explained by assuming that antigens 7 and 9 are controlled by both the K and D regions of the *H-2* complex, although, were this the case, all −*/f* recombinants would be expected to be +7 and +9, which they are not.

H-2.10. Antigens J (10) and N (14) were described by Amos (1959) as follows:

During the course of an experiment performed by Dr. T. S. Hauschka, a number of mice of a backcross between the hybrid (C3H/He × DBA/2) and C3H/He were injected with the DBA/2 lymphoma (Dalton). The surviving homozygous H-2ᵏ animals were hyperimmunized with a second injection of tumor and their serum used for antibody testing. The backcross appeared to give a higher titre serum than was normally found in the serum C3H/He anti-DBA/2 and a number of additional antigens were first detected with this antibody. In the strongest samples, the serum reacted against six H-2 antigens. Four were identified as D, F, M and N. The other two resembled each other rather closely. One is probably the same as antigen J detected in the serum DBA/1 anti-DBA/2, the other has been provisionally called L, and has not been included in the Tables as it has not yet been confirmed in another serum of lesser complexity.

Anti-N has proved disappointing. It should serve to differentiate H-2^q from H-2^b in a genetic mating in the absence of data on Q or B, but in practice anti-N, like anti-A, is very variable and many samples of serum do not contain the detectable antibody. This whole collection of antigens, D, F, M, N, J and L is also found in the A strain cell.

In his H-2 chart, Amos (1959) assigned to antigens J and N the following haplotype distribution:

J-positive: *H-2^a*, *H-2^d*, *H-2^l*, and *H-2^n*

J-negative: *H-2^b*, *H-2^e*, *H-2^h*, *H-2^j*, *H-2^k*, and *H-2^q*

N-positive: *H-2^a*, *H-2^b*, *H-2^d*, *H-2^g*, and *H-2^n*

N-negative: *H-2^j*, *H-2^k*, *H-2^l*, and *H-2^q*

Because no other information exists on antigens J and N and because antisera against these antigens are no longer available, the antigens probably should be dropped from the H-2 chart and numbers 10 and 14 reassigned to new antigens.

H-2.11. Antigen 11 (originally designated K) was defined by Amos and his co-workers (1955) with antisera BALB/c anti-C3H and BALB/c anti-A rendered specific for *H-2* haplotypes *k* and *a* by absorption with C57BL tissue. Antigen 11 has a relatively narrow distribution, being present in only three independent *H-2* haplotypes, *k*, *q*, and *r* (see H-2.25). It is a strong antigen, easily producing hemagglutinating and cytotoxic antibodies of relatively high titers. The antigen is placed in the K series by several *H-2* recombinants (*a*, *m*, *y*, and others).

H-2.12. Antigen 12 is a relatively recent addition to the H-2 chart (Snell and Cherry 1974). It is defined by antiserum (DBA/1 × SWR)F$_1$ anti-DA, which contains at least three antibodies: one weak hemagglutinating antibody reacting with B10.A, BALB/c, and A.SW (probably anti-42); one weak cytotoxic antibody reacting with B10, B10.A, and BALB/c (probably anti-36), and one moderately strong cytotoxic antibody reacting only with A.SW and DA (anti-12). The anti-12 antibody is also present in Snell's antisera (DBA/1 × C3H)F$_1$ anti-DA, (DBA/1 × LP)F$_1$ anti-DA and (B10 × C3H.OH)F$_1$ anti-DA. Because strains DBA/1 and DA share the K series, H-2.12 must be a D-series antigen. The antigen is restricted to *H-2^s* and its derivative, *H-2^{qp1}*. Anti-12 is a predominantly cytotoxic antibody.

H-2.13. Antiserum AKR anti-AKR.M, originally obtained by Snell and analyzed by Amos (1959), reacted with *H-2^m* of the donor strain and cross-reacted with *H-2* haplotypes *a*, *d*, *i*, and *q*. The cross-reactivity was attributed to an antibody defining a new antigen, antigen M or 13. Anti-13 antibodies are predominantly of the hemagglutinating type. Antigen 13 has a rather restricted distribution among the unrelated *H-2* haplotypes, being present in only *d* and *q*. Several *H-2* recombinants (e.g., *a*, *i*, *m*, *y*) place the antigen in the D series.

H-2.14. See H-2.10.

H-2.15. The *H-2^j* haplotype of strains JK and I carries, in addition to H-2.2^j, another private antigen that was identified simultaneously by Snell *et al.* (1971b) and J. Klein (1971a). The former investigators used antiserum (B10 × C3H)F_1 anti-C3H.JK and called the antigen 15; Klein (1971a) used antiserum (B10.Y × C3H.B10)F_1 and called the antigen 24. Since the 24 symbol was used simultaneously for a different antigen by Snell *et al.* (1971a), Klein adopted the H-2.15 symbol for the new *H-2^j* antigen. Because H-2.2 is a D-series antigen, it must be assumed that antigen 15 belongs to the K series. Antigen 15 induces relatively strong hemagglutinating and cytotoxic antibodies.

H-2.16. Antiserum C3H anti-P produced by Hoecker *et al.* (1954) reacted with red cells of strains P and A. The anti-A activity was nonspecific, because it was absorbed with C3H tissue. The remaining activity with P cells was attributable to a P-specific antigen (antigen P or 16). Anti-16 antibody was later produced by Shreffler and Snell (1969) in the combination (C3H × AKR.M)F_1 anti-C3H.NB. In addition to anti-16, the antiserum contained at least two hemagglutinins: anti-7 reacting with A.CA and one unidentified antibody reacting with A, D1.C, and DBA/2. Antigen 16 is very weak, and the anti-16 antibody is difficult to produce. In the present H-2 charts, H-2.16 is tentatively assigned to the K series, although it might actually be a complex of two antigens, one in the K series and the other in the D series.

H-2.17. Anti-17 (or Q) was identified by Hoecker *et al.* (1954) in antiserum DBA/1-*H-2^d* anti-DBA/1, which reacted with all *H-2* haplotypes carrying antigen 5, in addition to *H-2^q* of DBA/1. The anti-5 activity was removed by absorption with A strain tissue and this rendered the antiserum specific for DBA/1. Antigen 17, one of the two private antigens of *H-2^q*, is placed in the K series by *H-2* recombinants *m*, *y*, and *qp1*. The anti-17 is a moderately strong hemagglutinating and cytotoxic antibody.

H-2.18. Letter R, corresponding to number 18, was originally used by Hoecker *et al.* (1959) to designate an antigen detected by antiserum C3H anti-RIII. The antigen was first believed to be a member of the *H-2* complex (Hoecker *et al.* 1959), but was later shown to belong to a different system, *Ea-2* (see Chapter Eight). An antibody against an *H-2^r*-specific antigen (antigen 18) was obtained by Shreffler and Snell (1969) in antiserum C3H anti-C3H.RIII. Antigen 18, tentatively assigned to the D series, is the only known private antigen of *H-2^r*, and is likely, therefore, to be split when the appropriate recombinants become available. Anti-18 is a weak hemagglutinating and cytotoxic antibody.

H-2.19. Anti-19 (S) antibody was identified by Hoecker *et al.* (1954) in antiserum A anti-A.SW, which reacted nonspecifically with several strains. Absorption with A tissue removed the nonspecific reactivity and rendered the antiserum specific for A.SW. The antigen is placed in the K series by *H-2* recombinants *sq1*, *an1*, *t1*, and *t2*. Anti-19 is a strong hemagglutinating antibody.

H-2.20. Antigen 20 is a new private antigen of $H-2^u$ identified by antiserum (B10.AKM × WB)F_1 anti-PL (Démant *et al.* 1971b). The antiserum contains at least three antibodies: anti-4, anti-20, and an unidentified non-H-2 antibody. Antigen 20, capable of inducing both hemagglutinins and cytotoxins, must belong to the K series, because the D series of $H-2^u$ seems to be identical to that of $H-2^d$.

H-2.21. Antigen 21 is another new private antigen detected by antiserum [BALB/c × B10.C(41N)]F_1 anti-SM (Snell *et al.* 1971a). The antiserum contains at least two antibodies, anti-1 and anti-21. The anti-1 can be removed by absorption with any 1-positive strain (e.g., $H-2^h$ or $H-2^m$), leaving the antiserum specific for $H-2^v$ of SM. Anti-21, which is also present in antiserum (C3H.SW × B10.N)F_1 anti-SM, is a moderately strong hemagglutinating antibody. The presence of a known private D-series antigen (H-2.30) in $H-2^v$ places antigen 21 in the K series.

H-2.22. Antigen V was originally defined with two antisera, BALB/c anti-C57BL (Gorer and Mikulska 1959) and C3H anti-C57BL (Amos 1959), both known to contain anti-H-2.2 antibody. The only strain supposedly distinguishing between anti-H-2.2 and anti-H-2.22 was JK($H-2^j$), typed as −2, +22. Recent retyping of this strain, however, shows it to be H-2.2 positive. Consequently, at present there is no antiserum or strain that would differentiate between V and H-2.2, and thus, for all practical purposes, antigen V ceases to exist. Number 22 should therefore be reassigned to a new antigen.

H-2.23. Hoecker *et al.* (1959) produced antiserum RIII anti-C3H, which reacted with C3H, A, A.CA, A.SW, B10.D2, B10, and STOLI. Absorption in A.CA or STOLI removed anti-A, -A.CA, -STOLI, -A.SW, -B10.D2, and -B10 activity, but not the activity against C3H and A. The antibody absorbed by A.CA or STOLI was called anti-Z and the remaining antibody anti-W. Antigen Z later proved to belong to the *Ea-2* system (see Chapter Eight); antigen W seemed identical with antigen A described by Amos (1959), and for this reason was not included in the 1964 H-2 chart (Snell *et al.* 1964). However, it later became apparent that the anti-W antibody indentified an antigen distinct from 1 (A), and the antigen, its symbol changed to 23, was reinserted into the H-2 chart. Antigen 23 is placed in the K series by several *H-2* recombinants (e.g., *a, m, h,* and others). It is a relatively strong antigen and can be detected by both hemagglutination and cytotoxicity assays. The antigen is limited to $H-2^k$ and its genetic derivatives.

H-2.24. The symbol 24 was used by J. Klein (1971a) for a private antigen of $H-2^j$, later called 15. The same symbol was also used by Snell *et al.* (1971a) for an antigen defined by antiserum (PL × A.CA)F_1 anti-C3H.NB and considered to be a member of the 1-family (see Section 5.II.D). The antigen is present in $H-2^k$ (and its derivatives) and in $H-2^p$. Anti-24 is primarily a cytotoxic antibody.

H-2.25. Antigen 25 was originally defined by antiserum A.SW anti-A, which reacted with all strains carrying antigen 11 and also with strain STOLI typed as 11-negative (Hoecker *et al.* 1959). Because Shreffler and Snell (1969) later showed that the *H-2* haplotype of STOLI was identical to the *H-2^q* haplotype of DBA/1, the *H-2^q* haplotype should have been listed as -11, $+25$. However, in the meantime, Amos (1962) published an H-2 chart in which the DBA/1 strain was listed as 11-positive. This set a precedent that was then followed by a number of investigators, including Hoecker. Consequently, the antigen that was originally K (11) is now 25 (Y), and the original Y (25) is now 11 (K). The differentiating haplotypes are *r* ($+11$, $+25$) and *q* ($+11$, -25). Antigen 25, which is a moderately strong antigen inducing both hemagglutinating and cytotoxicity antibodies, is shared by *k* and *r*. It is placed in the K series by *H-2* recombinants *a*, *h*, and *m*.

H-2.26. This number is unassigned, because the original Z of Hoecker *et al.* (1959) proved to be a non-H-2 antigen (Snell *et al.* 1967).

H-2.27, 28, 29. These three antigens were identified by Stimpfling and Pizarro (1961) in a manner already discussed (see Section 5.I.A). All three antigens, probably controlled by both the D and K subdivisions, behave similarly and apparently belong to the same family (Snell *et al.* 1974). The antibodies against these antigens (both hemagglutinating and cytotoxic) are usually very weak and difficult to induce.

H-2.30. An anti-30 (D^1) was present in the AKR anti-AKR.M antiserum analyzed by Stimpfling and Pizarro (1961). Antigen 30 is a private antigen of *H-2^q*, placed by *H-2* recombinants *m* and *sq1* in the D series. It is moderately strong, especially in the hemagglutination test.

H-2.31. Antigen 31 (E^d) was defined by Amos *et al.* (1955) with antiserum A anti-BALB/c. The antigen induces strong cytotoxic but poor hemagglutinating antibodies, is limited to the *H-2^d* type and its genetic derivatives, and belongs to the K series, because *H-2* recombinants *g* and *o* are 31-positive. Recently, Lilly (1974) reported that some anti-31 sera have a high prozone[3] in the hemagglutination test, whereas others do not. Genetic analysis revealed that the prozone effect was caused by a single dominant gene, identical to or closely linked with the *Ea-4^b* allele (see Chapter Eight) of the C57BL strains.

H-2.32. Anti-32 (D^k) antibody was probably present in the AKR.K (*H-2^a*) anti-AKR(*H-2^k*) antiserum produced by Hoecker *et al.* (1954). However, the antibody was very weak in the hemagglutination test and could not be analyzed to establish its identity. Gorer and Mikulska (1959) tested the same antiserum in the cytotoxic assay and obtained a strong reaction with C3H lymphocytes. A similar antibody was produced by these investigators in combination A anti-C3H. Antigen 31 induces strong cytotoxins and only traces of hemagglutinins, is limited to *H-2^k* and its derivatives, and belongs to the D series because the *H-2°* recombinant carrying the D antigens of *k* is 32-positive.

H-2.33. Antigen 33 (K^b) was identified with antiserum HTH anti-E.L.4 (C57BL) (Gorer and Mikulska 1959), which occasionally gave a weak reaction in the hemagglutination test and a consistently strong reaction in the cytotoxic

[3] Prozone is defined as the absence or weakness of serological reactivity (e.g., hemagglutination) at high concentration of antibodies in tests in which reactivity is observed when the antibodies are more diluted.

test with C57BL(H-2^b) target cells. The antigen is placed by the H-2^i recombinant in the K series.

H-2.34. Antigen 34 was identified with antiserum (A × C57BL)F$_1$ anti-BALB/c (D. Davies 1969), which contained at least two cytotoxic antibodies, one specific for H-2^d (anti-31) and the other (anti-34) cross-reacting with F/St (H-2^n) and DBA/1(H-2^q). Absorption with F/St or DBA/1 tissue removed the anti-34 but not the anti-31.

H-2.35. Antigen 35 was defined by antiserum (C3H × A.CA)F$_1$ anti-C3H.NB (Démant *et al.* 1971b), reacting with H-2 haplotypes *a, d, i, u, b,* and *p,* among others. Absorption with *b* cells removed not only the anti-*b* activity, but also the activity against *a, d, i,* and *u.* Absorption with *a, i,* or *u* removed the anti-*a,* -*i,* and -*u* activity, but not the anti-*b* activity. Apparently, the antiserum contained one antibody (anti-35) reacting with *a, d, i, u,* and *p,* but not *b.* Antigens 35 and 41 have the same distribution except for H-2^b, which carries 35 but lacks 41. The two antigens also differ in that one (35) induces primarily cytotoxins and the other (41) primarily hemagglutinins. Antigen 35 is probably present in both the D and K series (see Section 5.II.D); antigen 41 is a member of the D series, as evidenced by its presence in H-2 recombinants *a, i,* and *u.*

H-2.36. Antigen 36 was defined by antiserum (FL × LP.RIII)F$_1$ anti-A.SW (Démant *et al.* 1971b), reacting with H-2 haplotypes *a, d, i, u, b,* and *s.* Absorption with *b* cells removed both anti-*b* and anti-*a,* -*d,* -*i,* and -*u* activity. Presence of H-2.36 was therefore postulated in H-2 haplotypes *s, b, a, d, i,* and *u.* Another antigen, H-2.42, has the same distribution except for its absence in H-2^b. Also, anti-36 is a cytotoxic antibody, whereas anti-42 is a hemagglutinating antibody. Like 35, antigen 36 is probably present in both the D and K series.

H-2.37. Anti-37 was detected in antiserum (B10.D2 × A.SW)F$_1$ anti-B10.M (Démant *et al.* 1971a), which, in the hemagglutination test, reacted only with the donor type (H-2^f) while in the cytotoxic test, it reacted also with strains C3H.NB (H-2^p) and B10.Y(H-2^{pa}). The hemagglutination reaction was due to the presence of anti-9, the cytotoxic reaction to the presence of anti-37. The anti-37 (but not anti-9) was absorbed by C3H.NB or B10.Y tissue. Anti-37 was also present in antisera (B10 × A.SW)F$_1$ anti-B10.M and (B10.A × C3H.SW)F$_1$ anti-C3H.NB. Antigen 37 induces only cytotoxic antibodies, is shared by H-2 haplotypes *f* and *d,* and belongs to the K series, as indicated by its presence in H-2 recombinant *ap2,* and absence in H-2^a.

H-2.38. Antigen 38 was defined by two complex antisera, (C3H × A.CA)F$_1$ anti-C3H.NB and (B10.A × A.CA)F$_1$ anti-B10.Y (Démant *et al.* 1971a), which reacted with a number of strains, among them WB(H-2^{ja}). Absorption with WB tissue removed the anti-WB (anti-38) activity. Antigen 38 is shared by H-2^j(H-2^{ja}) and H-2^p. Like 37, antigen 38 has been detected only by the cytotoxic test and has tentatively been assigned to the K series, although there is no evidence to support such an assignment.

H-2.39. Anti-39 antibody is present in antiserum (A × B10.D2)F$_1$ anti-B10.A(5R) (Démant *et al.* 1971a), reacting with H-2 haplotypes *i* (donor type), *b,* and *f.* Absorption by *f* tissue removes only the anti-*f* activity, but not the anti-*i* or anti-*b* activities. The antiserum apparently contains two antibodies, one specific for *b* and its derivative *i* (anti-33), and another cross-reacting with *f* (anti-39). Because *i* (in the donor) and *a* (in the recipient) share the D*ᵈ* series of antigens, antigen 39 must belong to the K series. Anti-39 is a strong cytotoxic and weak hemagglutinating antibody.

H-2.40. Antigen 40 was detected by Dishkant *et al.* (1973) in antiserum B10.D2(M504) anti-B10.D2, which reacted strongly with *H-2* haplotypes *a*, *d*, *i*, and *u* and weakly with *h*, *k*, *m*, *o*, *p*, *q*, *r*, and *s*. Absorption with *h* or *k* tissue removed the weak but not the strong activity, indicating that the antiserum contained two antibodies, one (anti-49) reacting with *a*, *d*, *u*, *h*, *k*, *m*, *o*, *p*, *q*, *r*, and *s*, and the other (anti-40) specific for *d* and its derivatives (*a*, *i*, and *u*). The anti-40 and anti-49 resembled anti-4 and anti-3, respectively, except that they were produced in a 4- and 3-positive recipient. Both anti-40 and anti-49 are primarily hemagglutinating antibodies. Antigen 40 seems to belong to the D series on the basis of its presence in *H-2* recombinants *a*, *i*, and *u*, antigen 49 belongs to both the *K* and the *D* on the basis of its presence in *H-2* recombinants *h*, *m*, and *o*.

H-2.41. See H-2.35.

H-2.42. Antigen 42 is defined by antiserum (FL × B10)F₁ anti-A.SW (Démant *et al.* 1971b), containing at least two antibodies, one (anti-19) specific for A.SW and the other (anti-42) cross-reacting with *H-2* haplotypes *a*, *d*, *i*, and *u*. Absorption in *a*, *d*, *i*, or *u* removes the anti-*a*, -*i*, and -*u*, but not the anti-*s* activity. Antigen 42 induces primarily hemagglutinating antibodies, has the same distribution as antigen 36 except for *H-2ᵇ*, which is 36-positive and 42-negative, and belongs to the D series, as indicated by its presence in *H-2* recombinants *a*, *i*, and *u*.

H-2.43. Antigen 43 is defined by antiserum (B10.BR × C3H.NB)F₁ anti-B10.SM (Démant *et al.* 1971b), reacting with *H-2* haplotypes *a*, *d*, *i*, *u*, and *v*. Absorption with *a* cells removes the *a*, *d*, *i*, and *u* activity, but not the *v* activity, indicating that the antiserum apparently contains at least two antibodies, one (anti-43) reacting with all the positive *H-2* haplotypes, and another (anti-21) specific for the *H-2* haplotype of the donor. Anti-43 is predominantly a hemagglutinating antibody. The membership of 43 in the D series is documented by its presence in *H-2* recombinants *a*, *i*, and *u*.

H-2.44. Hyperimmune antiserum (B10 × C3H)F₁ anti-I (Čapková and Démant 1972) reacts with the donor *H-2* haplotype (*j*) and cross-reacts with *a*, *d*, *i*, and *t*. Absorption with *a*, *d*, or *i* cells removes the cross-reactive antibody (anti-44) but not the *j*-specific antibody (anti-15). Anti-44 is predominantly a hemagglutinating antibody. Presence of 44 in *d*, *a*, *i*, *t*, *u*, and *y* places the antigen in the 3-family of the D series.

H-2.45. Antigen 45 is defined by antiserum B10 anti-WB (Čapková and Démant 1972), reacting with the donor *H-2ʲᵃ* haplotype and cross-reacting with a number of other *H-2* haplotypes (*a*, *h*, *k*, *m*, *n*, *o*, *p*, *q*, *r*, *s*, and *t*). Absorption with *a*, *h*, or *k* cells removes the cross-reacting antibody (anti-45), but not the *ja*-specific antibody (anti-15). Presence of 45 in *a*, *h*, *m*, and *k* places the antigen in the 1-family of the K series. Anti-45 is predominantly a cytotoxic antibody.

H-2.46. Antigen 46 is defined in terms of the cross-reactivity of antiserum A anti-B10 with *H-2* haplotypes *b*, *d*, *f*, *p*, and *ja* (D. Davies 1971). The anti-46 is predominantly a cytotoxic antibody. The presence of 46 in *H-2* recombinants *g*, *i*, and *o* places the antigen in the K series.

H-2.47. Antigen 47 is defined in terms of cross-reactivity of antiserum B10 anti-DBA/2 with *H-2* haplotypes *d*, *k*, *a*, *r*, and *j* after absorption with DBA/1 tissue (D. Davies 1971). Like anti-46, anti-47 is also predominantly a cytotoxic antibody. The presence of 47 in *H-2* recombinants *g*, *h*, and *m* places the antigen in the K series.

H-2.48. Unassigned.

H-2.49. Antigen 49 is defined by antiserum B10.D2(M504) anti-B10.D2 (Dishkant *et al.* 1973). See H-2.40.

H-2.50. Antigen 50, identified with antiserum B10.D2 anti-B10.D2(M504) (Dishkant *et al.* 1973), is restricted to the mutant donor haplotype ($H-2^{da}$). Since the mutation apparently occurred in the *H-2D* region, antigen 50 is most likely a member of the D series. Anti-50 is a strong hemagglutinating and weak cytotoxic antibody.

Six new H-2 antigens have been tentatively identified by P. Démant, G. D. Snell, and M. Cherry (*personal communication*) and designated 51 through 56. Their strain distribution is shown in Table 5-13.

H-2.101 through H-2.106. Antisera against these antigens were obtained by the immunization of inbred strains with strains carrying different wild-derived *H-2* haplotypes (J. Klein 1972a, b). The antigens are restricted to the donor strains and the antibodies are predominantly hemagglutinins.

III. H-2 Haplotypes

A. Nomenclature

A particular combination of H-2 antigens controlled by a single chromosome is called the *H-2 haplotype* and designated by small letters and numbers in superscript position. For example, $H-2^a$ is a combination of antigens 1, 3, 4, 5, 6, 8, 11, 13, 23, 24, 25, 27, 28, 29, 35, 36, 40, 41, 42, 43, 44, 45, 47, 49, and 52; $H-2^b$ is a combination of antigens 2, 5, 6, 27, 28, 29, 33, 35, 36, 39, 46, 53, 54, and 56, and so on. Because the number of known *H-2* haplotypes has already outrun the alphabet, it has been necessary to utilize double superscript letters (e.g., $H-2^{ba}$, $H-2^{bc}$ etc.). For the second letter of the superscript, the first 15 letters of the alphabet (*a* through *o*) are reserved for minor variants (e.g., $H-2^{ba}$ is a minor variant of $H-2^b$), whereas the remaining 11 letters (*p* through *z*) can be used for new major variants (e.g., $H-2^{ap}$ is entirely different from $H-2^a$).

An *H-2* recombinant that is different from any previously known haplotype is considered a new major variant. According to the original nomenclatorial rules (Snell *et al.* 1964), a series of similar *H-2* recombinants obtained from the same *H-2* heterozygote was designated by compound superscript symbols, consisting of a letter, serial number of the recombinant, and abbreviation of the discoverer's name. For example, $H\text{-}2^{h\text{-}2Sg}$ was the second *H-2* recombinant of the $H\text{-}2^h$ series discovered by Stimpfling. To avoid confusion of the numeral 1 with the letter *l*, any first recombinant in a series was left unnumbered. Because such a notation was cumbersome and awkward, it was replaced by a simplified symbolism (J. Klein *et al.* 1974a) in which the *H-2* recombinants with identical *H-2K* and *H-2D* regions were designated by a single or double letter, followed by an Arabic numeral distinguishing members of the same recombinant family (e.g., $H\text{-}2^{h1}$, $H\text{-}2^{h2}$, $H\text{-}2^{ap1}$, $H\text{-}2^{ap2}$, etc.).

The assignment of the double-letter symbols for both major and minor *H-2* haplotypes should follow alphabetical order, and so symbols *bp* or *bq*, for example, should not be used before symbols *ap* through *az* have been exhausted. However, this rule has not been strictly followed, and the symbols in current use are scattered throughout the alphabet.

The *H-2* haplotypes derived from wild mice were originally designated *wa*, *wb*, *wc*, and so on (J. Klein 1972a), but this was later changed to *w1*, *w2*, *w3*, and so on (J. Klein *et al.* 1974a).

Symbols $H\text{-}2^c$, $H\text{-}2^e$, $H\text{-}2^l$, $H\text{-}2^n$, and $H\text{-}2^w$ were dropped from the H-2 charts for the following reasons:

$H\text{-}2^c$. Congenic line D1.C was developed by Snell (1958b) from strains DBA/1 and BALB/c by the cross-intercross mating system, in which the selection was carried out with a DBA/1 tumor. When Snell (1958b) observed that a B10.D2 ($H\text{-}2^d$) tumor was rejected by 40 percent of (C57BL/10 × D1.C)F$_1$ hybrids, whereas an A($H\text{-}2^a$) tumor was accepted by all (AKR × D1.C)F$_1$ hybrids, he concluded that the D1.C line carried a new haplotype, $H\text{-}2^c$, derived by recombination from $H\text{-}2^d$. However, J. Klein (*unpublished data*) later reexamined the D1.C line and found that B10.D2 and D1.C skin grafts survived indefinitely on (C57BL/10 × D1.C)F$_1$ and (BALB/c × DBA/1)F$_1$ hybrids, respectively, suggesting that $H\text{-}2^c$ and $H\text{-}2^d$ were identical. This identity was then confirmed by serological typing.

$H\text{-}2^e$. The $H\text{-}2^e$ haplotype was assigned by Hoecker *et al.* (1959) to strain STOLI, which carried a combination of H-2 antigens different from all combinations then known. However, subsequent serological analysis of STOLI by other investigators revealed a conspicuous similarity of the $H\text{-}2^e$ haplotype with the $H\text{-}2^q$ haplotype of strain DBA/1, which was not included in the original study by Hoecker *et al.* (1959). The only difference between $H\text{-}2^e$ and $H\text{-}2^q$ was in antigens H-2.25 and 11, with the $H\text{-}2^e$ typed as 11-negative, 25-positive, and the $H\text{-}2^q$ typed as 11-positive, 25-negative (Amos 1959). Reexamination of the two strains by Shreffler and Snell (1969) showed that both strains carried antigen 25 and lacked antigen 11, that they were serologically indistinguishable by more than 60 antisera, that they failed to produce H-2 antibodies after cross-immunization, and that (D1.C × STOLI)F$_1$ hybrids accepted DBA/1 tumor grafts. These findings suggested that $H\text{-}2^e$ and $H\text{-}2^q$ were identical.

$H\text{-}2^l$. The $H\text{-}2^l$ haplotype was identified by Amos (1959) as a new combination of H-2 antigens carried by strains I/St and probably also N/St. Serologically, the H-2^l haplotype closely resembled the H-2^j haplotype of strain JK/St, the only difference being the presence of antigen J (10) in l and its absence in j. Since anti-J is no longer available, it is not possible to reexamine the difference between the two strains. However, extensive tests in several laboratories indicate that H-2^l and H-2^j are serologically indistinguishable, except for antigens H-2.28 and possibly also 29 (Shreffler and Snell 1969). The H-2 haplotype of I/St therefore appears to be just a minor variant of H-2^j.

H-2^n. The H-2^n haplotype was defined by Amos (1959) in strain F/St and typed as H-2.3 negative, which differentiated it from strain P (H-2^p). Subsequent tests, however, showed that both F/St and P shared not only H-2.3 but also 16 (private antigen of H-2^p), 1, 7, and 8 (Shreffler and Snell 1969), thus making the H-2 haplotypes of these two strains serologically indistinguishable. The H-2^n and H-2^p haplotypes were transferred onto the same genetic background of strain C57BL/10 by Stimpfling and Reichert (1970), and the resulting congenic lines, B10.F and B10.P, were compared by skin grafting. Grafts from B10.P to B10.F survived indefinitely, whereas grafts from B10.F to B10.P were rejected, suggesting that the H-2^p haplotype does not determine any antigens not determined by H-2^n, but that H-2^n determines some antigens not determined by H-2^p (provided that the rejections were not due to residual background differences). The H-2 haplotype of the F/St strain seems, therefore, to be a minor variant of the H-2^p haplotype.

H-2^w. See H-2^{ja} in Section 5.III.C.

B. Classification of H-2 Haplotypes

The 68 reported H-2 haplotypes (Table 5-12) can be classified into four groups:

1. Unrelated: b, d, f, k, p, q, r, s, z, $w1$, $w2$, $w3$, $w4$, $w5$, and $w6$.
2. Partially related: j, u, and v.
3. Fully related: a, $a1$, $an1$, $ap1$, $ap2$, $ap3$, $ap4$, $ap5$, $aq1$, $by1$, df, g, $g1$, $g2$, $g3$, $g4$, $g5$, h, $h1$, $h2$, $h3$, $h4$, $h15$, $h18$, i, $i3$, $i5$, $i7$, $ia1$, m, $m1$, $o1$, $o2$, $qp1$, $sq1$, $sq2$, $t1$, $t2$, $t3$, $t4$, $t5$, $y1$, and $y2$.
4. Minor variants: ba, bb, bc, bd, be, da, fa, fb, ja, and pa.

The *unrelated group* contains 15 H-2 haplotypes, nine from laboratory mice and six from wild mice. The number of unrelated wild-derived H-2 haplotypes is likely to increase. In this writer's laboratory, 25 additional unrelated haplotypes are being analyzed (J. Klein 1973a), and some 25 more haplotypes are being extracted from wild populations. A number of wild-derived H-2 haplotypes are also being analyzed by Iványi and his co-workers (Micková and Iványi 1971).

The *partially related group* contains three H-2 haplotypes, all of which carry unrelated H-$2K$ and related H-$2D$ regions. The H-$2D$ region of H-2^j resembles H-$2D^b$, H-$2D^v$ resembles H-$2D^q$, and H-$2D^u$ seems identical to H-$2D^d$. The resemblance between H-$2D^j$ and H-$2D^b$ and between H-$2D^v$ and H-$2D^q$ is in the sharing of similar private antigens and some (but not all) public antigens. The origin of H-2^u can be explained by recombination between H-2^d and an unknown H-2 haplotype. Similarly, it can be postulated that H-2^j and H-2^u were derived respectively from H-2^b and H-2^q by recombination and mutational differentiation.

The *fully related group* consists of 43 H-2 haplotypes, each of which can be explained by recombination that took place between H-$2K$ and H-$2D$ regions of two unrelated haplotypes. For example, H-2^a is a postulated recombinant presumably derived from unrelated H-2 haplotypes d and k. It carries the H-$2K$ region of H-2^k and the H-$2D$ region of H-2^d and has no antigens not carried by either d or k. H-2^a grafts are accepted by the H-$2^d/H$-2^k heterozygotes (Snell 1953, J. Klein 1966a).

The *group of minor variants* consists of 10 H-2 haplotypes, each of which can be derived from one unrelated H-2 haplotype. This derivation probably occurred by mutation, which in some variants (e.g., *ba*, *bb*, *bc*, etc.) is well documented, while in others (e.g., *be*, *ja*, etc.) it is merely postulated. In most variants, the difference between the variant haplotype and the corresponding unrelated haplotype is detected by skin grafting, but not serologically. In some variants (e.g., *pa*, *ja*, and others) the difference may actually be in the loci closely linked to H-2 rather than in the H-2 complex itself.

C. Minor Variants

H-2^{ba}. The H-2^{ba} variant, originally designated H(z1), is the result of a spontaneous mutation that occurred in the H-2^b haplotype of the H-$2^b/H$-2^d heterozygote (Bailey *et al.* 1971). The *ba* and *b* haplotypes can be distinguished only by transplantation methods. Attempts to find a qualitative serological difference between the two haplotypes have failed.

H-2^{bb}. H-2^{bb}, formerly H(z49), is another mutation obtained by Bailey (1969) in the same experiment that produced H-2^{ba}. This mutation is also detectable only by skin grafting.

H-2^{bc}. Snell and his co-workers (1971d) typed [B10.A(H-2^a) × B10.129(6M)]F$_1$ × B10.129(6M) backcross segregants with an anti-H-2^a antiserum, and then challenged them with B10.129(12M) skin grafts. The grafts were permanently accepted by the H-2^a-positive animals and rejected by the H-2^a-negative animals, suggesting a difference in the H-2 complex between lines B10.129(6M) and B10.129(12M). Because line B10.129(12M) is known to carry the H-2^b haplotype and because the H-2 haplotype of B10.129(6M) is serologically indistinguishable from H-2^b, the authors concluded that the B10.129(6M) line possesses a minor variant of H-2^b, which they called H-2^{bc}. They also postulated the presence of the H-2^{bc} haplotype in strain 129 from which the B10.129(6M) line received its H-2 complex. They explained the survival of the skin grafts in H-$2^a/H$-2^{bc} heterozygotes of the backcross population by a complementary action of H-2^a and H-2^{bc} haplotypes.

Table 5-12. *H-2* haplotypes (major and minor) and strains carrying them

Standard	Synonym	Prototype strain	Other strains	Reference for prototype strain
a	dk	A	A/He, A/Sn, A/Wy, AKR.K, AL/N, A2G, B10.A, C3H.A/Sf, C3H.A/Ha	Gorer et al. 1948, Snell and Higgins 1951, Hoecker et al. 1954, Amos et al. 1955
a1	al	A.AL	C3H.AL, B10.AL	Shreffler and David 1972, David and Shreffler 1972a
an1	te	A.TFR1		D. C. Shreffler, personal communication
ap1	ap	B10.M(11R)		Stimpfling et al. 1971
ap2	ta	A.TFR2		D. C. Shreffler, personal communication
ap3	tb	A.TFR3		D. C. Shreffler, personal communication
ap4	tc	A.TFR4		D. C. Shreffler, personal communication
ap5	td	A.TFR5		D. C. Shreffler, personal communication
aq1	aq	B10.M(17R)		Stimpfling et al. 1971
b		C57BL/10	ABP/Le, A.BY, AKR.B6, BALB.B10, BAN/Re, BLPBR, C3H.SW, C3H/Bi-H-2^b, C3H.B10, C57BL/6, C57L, CC57BR, CC57W, DW/J, D1.LP, D2.B6, HG/Hu, SB/Le, ST/a, V/Le	Gorer et al. 1948, Snell and Higgins 1951, Hoecker et al. 1954, Amos et al. 1955
ba		B6.C-H-2^{ba}		Bailey et al. 1971
bb		B6.C-H-2^{bb}		Bailey 1969
bc		B10.129(6M)		Snell et al. 1971d
bd		B6.M505	129, LP/J	Egorov and Blandova 1971
be		C57BL/LiA		Dux et al. 1971
by1		B10.BYR		J. Klein, unpublished data
[c		D1.C		Snell 1958b]
d	d	DBA/2J	BALB/c, C6.C-H-24, B10.D2, C3H.D, C57BL/Ks, Dancer/Le, D1.C, LG/J, NBL/N, NZB, SEA/GnJ, SEC/1Gn, ST.T6, WH, YBL/Rr, YBR/Wi	Gorer et al. 1948, Snell and Higgins 1951, Hoecker et al. 1954, Amos et al. 1955
[d'	d	YBL/Rr		Snell et al. 1953]
da		B10.D2(M504)		Egorov 1967a
df		LG/Ckc		M. Cherry, G. D. Snell and C. S. David, personal communication
[e	q	STOLI		Hoecker et al. 1959]
f		A.CA	B10.M, RFM/Un	Allen 1955b, Hoecker et al. 1959
fa		A.CA(M506)		Egorov and Blandova 1971
fb		B10.M-H-2^{fb}		Mobraaten and Bailey 1973
g	g-Go, ga	HTG	B10.HTG	Gorer and Mikulska 1959
g1	g-Eg, gb	B10.D2(R101)		Vedernikov and Egorov 1973
g2	gd	D2.GD		Lilly and J. Klein 1973
g3	g-2Eg, gc	B10.D2(R103)		Vedernikov and Egorov 1973
g4	ge	B10.BDR1		H. C. Passmore, personal communication
g5	gf	B10.BDR2		H. C. Passmore, personal communication
h	h-Go, ha	HTH		Gorer and Mikulska 1959
h1	h-Sg, hb	B10.A(1R)		Stimpfling and Richardson 1965
h2	h-2Sg, hc	B10.A(2R)		Stimpfling and Richardson 1965
h3	hg	B10.AM		B. D. Amos, personal communication
h4	h-3Sg, hd	B10.A(4R)		Stimpfling and Richardson 1965
h15	h-4Sg, he	B10.A(15R)		Stimpfling et al. 1971
h18	h-5Sg, hf	B10.A(18R)		J. H. Stimpfling, personal communication

			Determinants	Reference
i3	*i-Sg, ib*	B10.A(3R)		Stimpfling and Richardson 1965
i5	*i-2Sg, ic*	B10.A(5R)		Stimpfling and Richardson 1965
i7	*i-Eg, ie*	B10.D2(R107)		Vedernikov and Egorov 1973
ia1	*id*	B10.D2(R106)		Vedernikov and Egorov 1973
j		JK		Amos 1959
ja	*w*	WB/Re		Snell and Stimpfling 1966
k		CBA	BALB.I, C3H.JK, I/St, N/St(?) B10.WB(69NS), WC/Re, WK/Re AKR, BALB.AKR, BALB.C3H, B6.C3H, B10.BR, B10.K, B10.CBA, CE, CHI, C3H/HE, C3H/B, C3H/St, C3H/Sn, C3H/Di, C3H/An, C3HA, C57BL/6-H-2^κ, C57BR/a, C57BR/ed, C58, DE/J(?), D1.ST, FL/2Re, FL/6Re, FSF/Gn, HRS/J, L/St, MA/J, PH/Re, RF/J, ST/bJ, 101	Snell 1951, Hoecker et al. 1954, Amos et al. 1955
[k'	*k*	AKR		Snell et al. 1953]
[kf	*k*	FL/2Re		Snell et al. 1971a]
[l'	*j*	I/St		Amos 1959]
m		AKR.M	B10.AKM	Snell 1958b, Stimpfling and Pizarro 1961
ml		B10.QAR1		J. Klein, *unpublished data*
n	*p?*	F/St		Amos 1959
ol	*ol*	C3H.OL	B10.F/Sg, B10.F/Eg, B10.F/Y, B10.F/Ao	Shreffler et al. 1966
o2	*oh*	C3H.OH		Shreffler and David 1972, David and Shreffler 1972a
p		P/Sn	BDP/J, B10.NB, B10.CNB, B10.P, C3H.NB	Snell and Higgins 1951, Hoecker et al. 1954
pa		B10.Y		Snell et al. 1971a
q		DBA/1	AU/SsJ, BUB/Bn, B10.D1/Ph, B10.D1/Y, B10.G, B10.Q, C/St, C3H.Q, C3H/HeNRe, STOLI, SWR/J, TF/Gn, T138, T190	Snell et al. 1953, Hoecker et al. 1954
qp1	*qs*	DA/HuSn	B10.DA(80NS)	G. D. Snell, *personal communication*
r		RIII/Wy	B10.RIII(71NS), B10.RIII, C3H.RIII, LP.RIII, RIII/J	Snell et al. 1953, Hoecker et al. 1954
s		A.SW	B10.ASW, B10.S, SJL, TN	Hoecker et al. 1954, Snell 1958b
sq1	*ar*	A.QSR1		McDevitt et al. 1972
sq2	*as*	B10.QSR2		McDevitt et al. 1972
tl	*tl*	A.TL	A.TH	Shreffler and David 1972, David and Shreffler 1972a
t2	*th*	B10.S(7R)	B10.PL, B10.PL(73NS)	Stimpfling and Reichert 1970
t3	*tt*	B10.HTT	B10.SM/Sg, B10.SM/Sn	Meo et al. 1973b, J. Klein et al. 1974b
t4		B10.S(9R)		Stimpfling and Reichert 1970
t5		BSVS		Shreffler and David 1974
u		PL/J		Snell et al. 1971a
v		SM/J		Snell et al. 1971a
[w	*ja*	WB/Re		Snell and Stimpfling 1966]
w1	*wa*	B10.KPA42		J. Klein 1972a
w2	*wb*	B10.KPB68		J. Klein 1972a
w3	*wc*	B10.SAA48		J. Klein 1972a
w4	*wd*	B10.GAA20		J. Klein 1972a
w5	*we*	B10.KEA5		J. Klein 1972a
w6	*wf*	B10.T7WF		J. Klein 1971b
y1	*y-Kli, ya*	B10.AQR	AQR	J. Klein et al. 1970
y2	*y-Sg, yb*	B10.T(6R)		Stimpfling and Reichert 1970
z		NZW		D. Davies 1971a

Because lines C57BL/10 and B10.129(12M) on the one hand, and 129 and B10.129(6M) on the other are known to carry different alleles at the *Tla* locus, the skin grafting results can also be explained by assuming that the rejections were not due to a difference at the *H-2* complex, but to a difference at a locus outside *H-2*, close to or identical with the *Tla* locus.

A minor variant of *H-2^b*, possibly identical with *H-2^{bc}*, was postulated by Snell and Bunker (1965) in strain LP.

H-2^{bd}. Egorov and Blandova (1971) described an *H-2^{bd}* mutation that occurred in a male of strain C57BL/6 (*H-2^b*). The mutant (B6.505) and the parental (C57BL/6) lines reject each other's skin graft, but do not show any qualitative serological difference. The *H-2^{bd}* variant is different from the *H-2^{ba}* mutation (Blandova *et al.* 1972).

H-2^{be}. The presence of the *H-2^{be}* variant has been postulated by Dux and her co-workers (Dux *et al.* 1971, Dux and Corduwener 1972) in the C57BL/LiA strain maintained at the Netherlands Cancer Institute in Amsterdam. The strain has been separated from C57BL/10Sn for about 200 generations. The two strains are histoincompatible but serologically indistinguishable.

H-2da. The *H-2da* mutant was obtained by Egorov (1967a) after treatment of B10.D2(*H-2^d*) mice with diethylsulphate. The mutant line, B10.D2(M504), differs from B10.D2 serologically as well as histogenetically.

H-2$^{d'}$. Snell and his co-workers (1953a) observed that segregants from cross (BALB/c × A-T)F$_1$ × YBL/Rr inoculated with a BALB/c tumor displayed 36 percent recombination between the gene for tumor susceptibility (*H-2*) and the gene for tail length (*T*). Segregants of a similar cross, (DBA/2 × A-T)F$_1$ × YBL/Rr, inoculated with a DBA/2 tumor displayed 38.9 percent recombination. The authors viewed these results as an indication that strain YBL/Rr carries an *H-2$^{d'}$* haplotype, similar to but not identical with *H-2^d* of BALB/c and DBA/2. (The principle of the linkage test involved in these experiments is described in Chapter Seven). Indirect evidence supporting this view was obtained by Amos (quoted by Gorer 1956), who observed that antigen H-2.4 of YBR (a strain closely related to YBL) was serologically different from H-2.4 of strains BALB/c and DBA/2. In spite of these results, strains YBL and YBR were later included in the *H-2^d* group, and the *H-2$^{d'}$* symbol was dropped (Snell and Stimpfling 1966). However, the two strains should be retyped by both serological and transplantation methods.

H-2^{fa}. The *H-2^{fa}* symbol was used by Egorov and Blandova (1972) for a spontaneous *H-2* mutation that occurred in a A.CA(*H-2^f*) female. The mutant (A.506) and the parental (A.CA) lines reject each other's skin grafts, and can be distinguished serologically (Egorov 1974).

H-2^{fb}. The *H-2^{fb}* variant arose by spontaneous mutation from *H-2^f* in a [B10.M × B10.RIII(71NS)]F$_1$ male (Mobraaten and Bailey 1973). The variant is now present in strain B10.M-*H-2^{fb}*, which rejects B10.M(*H-2^f*) skin grafts.

H-2^{ja}. Serological analysis of strains WB/Re and WC/Re by Stimpfling and Snell (quoted by Snell and Stimpfling 1966) revealed that the two strains carried an *H-2* haplotype that seemed different from all previously defined *H-2* haplotypes. A new symbol, $H-2^w$, was therefore assigned to the combination of antigens present in these strains. Subsequent analysis (Snell *et al.* 1971a, Démant *et al.* 1971a, b), however, revealed a conspicuous similarity between $H-2^w$ and $H-2^j$, both of which possess the same private antigens (2^j and 15) and a similar array of public antigens. According to Snell (*personal communication*), antiserum (B10.AKM × WB)F_1 anti-A.SW reacts in a hemagglutination test with C3H.JK ($H-2^j$) cells, and this reaction does not seem to be due to non-H-2 antibodies because the antiserum does not react with C3H.NB($H-2^p$) cells. Because strain WB is present in the recipient, the $H-2$ haplotypes of WB and C3H.JK must be different. Reactions with some additional antisera seem to suggest that the difference between the $H-2$ haplotypes of WB and C3H.JK involves the 28-family site. However, in spite of the apparent serological differences, the $H-2^j$ and $H-2^{ja}$ haplotypes are only weakly histoincompatible, because in combinations B10.WB →(B10 × C3H.JK)F_1, C3H.JK→(C3H.NB × WB)F_1, B10.WB→(B10.BR × I)F_1, and C3H.JK→(C3H × WB)F_1, only some grafts showed signs of rejection, usually not earlier than 60 days after transplantation. Neither the serological nor the transplantation results necessarily mean that the presumed difference is in the $H-2$ complex. The delayed rejections, in particular, could be due to minor differences in the background. The data warrant replacement of the $H-2^w$ with the $H-2^{ja}$ symbol, because the difference between the $H-2$ haplotypes of JK and WB is only minor.

$H-2^{k'}$. The $H-2^{k'}$ symbol was assigned by Snell *et al.* (1953a) to the AKR strain on the basis of a linkage test (see Chapter Seven) involving three different segregating populations: (C57BR/a × A-T)F_1 × AKR, (AKR × T^h)F_1 × CBA and (C3H × A-T)F_1 × AKR. The test indicated linkage between the T and $H-2$ genes in the first population, and an absence of linkage in the other two populations. Snell and his co-workers concluded from this result that the AKR carries a minor variant of $H-2^k$. However, because no other differences between $H-2^k$ and $H-2^{k'}$ were found, the latter symbol was later dropped.

$H-2^{pa}$. Snell (1958b) produced a congenic line, B6.Y, that carried an $H-2$ haplotype derived from Y, a noninbred stock, on the C57BL/6 background. Because (D1.ST × B6.Y)F_1 hybrids were 100 percent susceptible to a DBA/1 ($H-2^q$) tumor, he concluded that the B6.Y line carried the $H-2^q$ haplotype. When the line was later backcrossed to strain C57BL/10, and a new line, B10.Y, produced, serological analysis of this new line (Stimpfling and Reichert 1970, Snell *et al.* 1971a) revealed its $H-2$ haplotype to be different from $H-2^q$ but indistinguishable from $H-2^p$. Transplantation analysis of B10.Y (Snell *et al.* 1971a) indicated a minor $H-2$-associated histoincompatibility between strains C3H.NB ($H-2^p$) and B10.Y. Because of this minor difference, Snell and his co-workers (1971a) designated the $H-2$ haplotype of B10.Y as *pa*. Stimpfling and Reichert (1970) exchanged skin grafts between strains B10.Y and B10.P ($H-2^p$) and observed indefinite survival even after preimmunization, suggesting that B10.Y and B10.P were $H-2$ identical. The discrepancy between the results of the two laboratories can be explained by assuming either that the rejections observed by Snell and his co-workers were not due to $H-2$ differences, or that C3H.NB strain rather than B10.Y carries a minor variant of $H\text{-}2^p$. To explain why B6.Y was originally typed as $H\text{-}2^q$, Snell and his co-workers (1971a) speculated that the line was segregating for both p and q, and that the newer B10.Y line became fixed for p.

IV. The H-2 Chart

The H-2 chart is the summary of a momentary status of H-2 serology that lists the individual *H-2* haplotypes, their antigenic composition, and the strains carrying the haplotypes. Although it is now clear that the *H-2* complex consists of at least two series of antigens (D and K), it is still customary to pool the information on both series into one chart. Due to a steady increase in the number of H-2 antigens (Table 5-13), the chart has become rather complex and has lost its usefulness as a quick source of information. The chart can be simplified by listing only the unrelated and the partially related *H-2* haplotypes (Table 5-14). Such a simplification is based on the assumption that the K and D

Table 5-13. The *H-2* chart of inbred strains*

H-2 haplotype	Prototype strain	1	2	3	4	5	6	7	8	9	11	12	13	15	16	17	18	19	20	21	23	24	2
a	A/J	1	—	3	4	5	6	—	8	—	11	—	13	—	—	—	—	—	—	—	23	24	
an	A.TFR1	1	—	?	—	·	6	7	—	—	—	—	·	—	·	—	—	·	19	·	—	·	
ap	B10.M(11R)	—	—	3	4	—	·	7	8	—?	—	·	13	·	·	·	·	·	·	·	·	—	·
aq	B10.M(17R)	1	—	—	—	5	·	—	8	9	11	·	—	·	·	·	·	·	·	·	23	·	
b	C57BL/10	—	2	—	—	5	6	—	—	—	—	—	—	—	—	—	—	—	—	—	—	—	—
by	B10.BYR	1	2	3	—	5	6	—	—	—	11	—	—	—	—	17	—	—	—	—	—	—	·
d	DBA/2	—	—	3	4	—	6	—	8	—	—	—	13	—	—	—	—	—	—	—	—	—	—
da	B10.D2(M504)	—	—	3	4	—	·	·	8	—	—	·	13	—	—	—	—	—	—	—	—	—	·
f	A.CA	—	—	—	—	6	7	8	9	—	—	—	—	—	—	—	—	—	—	—	—	—	—
g	HTG	—	2	—?	—	—	6	—	8	—	—	—	—	—	—	—	—	—	—	—	—	—	—
h	HTH	1	2	3	—	5	6	—	8	—	11	—	—	—	—	—	—	—	—	—	—	23	24
i	HTI	—	—	3	4	5	6	—	—	—	—	—	13	—	—	—	—	—	—	—	—	—	—
j	JK/St	1?	2	—	—	—	6	7	—	—	—	—	—	15	—	—	—	—	—	—	—	—	—
k	C3H/He	1	—	3	—	5	—	—	8	—	11	—	—	—	—	—	—	—	—	—	—	23	24
m	AKR.M	1	—	3	—	5	6	—	8	—	11	—	13	—	—	—	—	—	—	—	—	23	24
o	C3H.OH	1	—	3	—	5	—	—	8	—	—	—	—	—	—	—	—	—	—	—	—	—	—
p	P/J	1	—	3	—	5	6	7	8	—	—	—	—	—	16	—	—	—	—	—	—	—	24
q	DBA/1	1	—	3	—	5	6	—	—	—	11	—	13	—	—	17	—	—	—	—	—	—	—
qp	DA	·	—	·	—	·	·	·	·	—	11	12	·	—	—	17	—	—	—	—	—	—	—
r	RIII	1	—	3	—	5	6	—	8	—	11	—	—	—	—	—	18	—	—	—	—	—	—
s	A.SW	1	—	3	—	5	6	7	—	—	—	12	—	—	—	—	—	19	—	—	—	—	—
sq	B10.QSR1	1	—	3	—	5	6	—	—	—	—	·	—	·	—	—	·	19	·	·	—	—	
t2	B10.S(7R)	1	—	3	4	5	6	7	—	—	—	—	13	—	—	·	—	19	—	—	—	—	
t4	B10.S(9R)	·	·	·	4	—	—	·	·	·	·	·	·	·	·	·	19	·	·	—	—		
u	PL/J	c	—	3	4	5	·	—	8?	—	—	—	13?	·	—	—	—?	—	20	—?	—	—	
v	SM/J	1	—	3	—	5?	·	·	—	—	—	—	—	—	—	—	—?	—	—	21	—	·	
y	B10.AQR	1	—	3	4	5	6	—	—	—	11	·	·	—	—	17	—	—	—	—	—	—	
z	NZW	—	—	—	—	5	6	—	—	—	—	·	—	·	—	—	·	—	—	·	—	·	·

* $(-)$ = absence of an antigen; $(\cdot)$ = unknown; $(?)$ = presence or absence of antigen is uncertain; (c) = some

series of antigens behave as blocks that are inherited in their entirety, and that the recombinant *H-2* haplotypes represent nothing more than rearrangements of these blocks. Any recombinant *H-2* haplotype can be reconstructed from the simplified chart by combining the appropriate K and D series blocks. For example, the antigenic configuration of *H-2^g*, a $K^d D^b$ recombinant, can be reconstructed from the H-2 chart in Table 5-14 by combining the K series of *d* with the D series of *b*. The H-2 chart can be further simplified by omitting the public and listing only the private antigens (Table 5-8).

The choice among the three graphic representations of the H-2 antigens depends on the specific needs of an investigator and on his personal preferences. In some ways, the three charts complement each other in the information they provide. But regardless of the form used, a graphic representation is always inadequate, simplistic, and somewhat misleading, because it is impossible to condense all the available serological information into a two-dimensional diagram. The diagram not only instantly freezes a system that is normally in a permanent state of change, but it also "cross sections" it. The fact that antisera

s

29	30	31	32	33	34	35	36	37	38	39	40	41	42	43	44	45	46	47	49	50	51	52	53	54	55	56
29	—	—	—	—	—	35	36	—	—	—	40	41	42	43	44	45	—	47	49	—	—	52	—	—	—	—
·	·	·	·	·	·	·	·	·	·	·	·	·	·	·	·	·	—	·	·	·	·	·	·	·	·	·
·	·	·	·	·	·	·	·	37	·	·	·	·	·	·	·	·	·	·	·	·	·	·	·	·	·	·
·	·	·	·	·	·	·	·	·	·	·	·	·	·	·	·	·	·	·	·	·	·	·	·	·	·	·
29	—	—	—	33	—	35	36	—	—	39	—	—	—	—	—	—	46	—	—	—	—	—	53	54	—	56
29	—	—	—	—	—	—	—	—	—	—	—	—	—	—	—	45	—	—	—	—	·	·	·	·	·	·
29	—	31	—	—	34	35	36	—	—	—	40	41	42	43	44	—	46	47	49	—	—	—	—	—	—	—
·	—	31	—	—	·	35	·	—	·	·	—	·	·	·	44	—	·	—	50	·	·	·	·	·	·	·
—	—	—	—	—	—	—	—	37	—	39	—	—	—	—	—	—	46	—	—	—	—	—	53	—	—	—
29	—	31	—	—	34	—	—	—	—	—	—	—	—	—	—	—	46	47	—	—	—	—	—	—	—	56
29	—	—	—	—	·	—	—	—	—	—	—	—	—	—	—	45	—	47	49	—	—	52	—	—	—	56
29	—	—	—	33	·	35	36	—	—	39	40	41	42	43	44	—	46	—	49	—	—	—	53	54	—	—
29	—	—	—	—	—	—	—	—	38	—	—	—	—	—	44	45	46?	47?	—	51	—	—	—	—	56	
—	—	—	32	—	—	—	—	—	—	—	—	—	—	—	—	45	—	47	49	—	—	52	—	—	—	—
29	30	—	—	—	·	—	—	—	—	—	—	—	—	—	—	45	—	47	49	—	—	52	—	—	55	56
29	—	31	32	—	34	—	—	—	—	—	—	—	—	—	—	—	46	47	49	—	—	—	—	—	—	—
—	—	—	—	—	34?	35	—	37	38	—	—	41	—	—	—	—	46?	·	49	—	—	—	—	—	—	—
29	30	—	—	—	34	—	—	—	—	—	—	—	—	—	—	45	·	—	49	—	—	52	—	54	55	56
·	—	—	—	—	·	·	36	·	·	·	·	42	·	·	·	·	·	·	—	52	—	54	—	—		
—	—	—	—	·	—	36	—	—	—	—	—	42	—	—	45	·	47	49	—	—	52	—	54	—	—	
—	—	—	—	·	—	36	—	—	—	—	—	42	—	—	45	·	—	49	—	51	—	—	—	—		
29	30	—	—	—	·	·	·	·	·	·	·	·	·	·	45	·	·	·	·	·	·	·	·			
29	—	—	—	—	·	35	36	·	·	·	40	41	42	43	44	—	·	49	·	·	·	·	·	·		
·	·	·	·	·	·	·	·	·	·	·	·	·	·	·	·	·	·	·	·	·	·	·	·	·		
29	—	—	—	—	·	35	36	—	—	—	40	41	42	43	·	·	·	·	49	·	—	52	53	—	—	—
?	30	—	—	—	·	—	—	·	·	·	—	—	—	43	·	45?	·	·	·	·	—	—	—	—	55	—
29	—	—	·	·	·	·	·	·	—	40	·	·	·	·	·	·	49	·	·	·	·	·	·			
29	—	—	—	—	·	·	·	·	·	·	·	·	·	46	47	·	·	·	·	:	·	·				

eact with the indicated *H-2* haplotype.

Table 5-14. H-2 chart of the K and D series (*H-2* haplotypes of independent origin only)*

Antigens of the K series — Public and Private; Antigens of the D series — Public and Private.

H-2 haplotype	K 1	3	5	7	8	11	25	27	28	29	34	35	36	37	38	39	42	45	46	47	K Private	D 1	3	5	6	13	27	28	29	35	36	41	42	43	44	49	D Private
b	—	—	5	—	—	—	—	27	28	29	—	35	36	—	—	39	—	—	46	—	33	—	—	—	6	—	27	28	29	—	—	—	—	—	—	—	2
d	—	3	—	—	8	—	—	27	28	29	34	—	—	—	—	—	—	—	46	47	31	—	3	—	6	13	27	28	29	35	36	41	42	43	44	49	4
j	1?	—	c	7	8	—	—	27?	28?	29?	—	—	—	37	38	39	—	45	46	47?	15	—	—	—	6	—	27	–?	–?	—	—	—	—	—	—	—	9
k	1	3	5	7	8	11	25	—	—	—	34?	—	—	—	38	—	—	45	46?	47	23	1	3	5	6	—	—	28	29	—	—	—	—	—	44	—	32
p	1	—	5	—	8	—	—	—	—	—	—	—	—	37	38	—	—	45	46?	·	16	1	3	—	6	—	—	—	—	35	—	41	42	43	—	—	?
q	1	3	5	—	—	11	—	—	—	—	—	—	—	—	—	—	—	45	46?	—	17	—	—	5	6	—	—	28	29	c	c	41	42	43	—	49	30
r	1	3	5	—	8	11	25	—	—	—	34	—	—	—	—	—	—	45	—	47	·	1	—	5	6	13	27	—	—	35	c	—	—	—	—	49	18?
s	1	—	5	7	—	—	—	—	—	—	—	35	36	—	—	—	42	45	·	—	19	1	—	5	6	—	c	—	—	c	36	42	—	—	—	49	12
u	c	—	5	—	8?	—	—	—	—	—	—	—	36	—	—	—	—	45	·	·	20	1	3	—	6	13?	27?	28	29	—	—	41	42	43	—	49	4
v	1	3	5	—	—	—	—	—	—	—	—	—	—	—	—	—	—	45?	—	·	21	1	3	—	·	·	–?	28?	29	—	—	—	—	43	—	49	30
z	—	·	5	—	—	—	—	27	—	29	—	—	—	—	—	—	—	—	46	47	·	—	—	6	—	—	—	·	28?	—	—	—	—	—	—	·	·

*(—) = absence of an antigen; (·) = unknown; (?) = presence or absence of antigen is uncertain; (c) = some antisera cross-react with the indicated *H-2* haplotype.

against the same antigen often "see" this antigen differently cannot be reflected in the H-2 chart. Instead, the individual entries into the chart are made on the basis of either single antisera or an abstract "average" obtained from a number of antisera. In both cases the antigens are misrepresented.

These qualifications should serve as a warning against a literal interpretation of the H-2 chart. Although the chart is regarded with ultimate respect by many, it is an unreliable source of information. If it predicts the presence of certain antibodies in specific combinations, it does not necessarily guarantee that such antibodies will indeed be formed. Any departure from traditional donor-recipient combinations, even with the H-2 chart in hand, always means an excursion into an unexplored territory.

V. Interpretation of H-2 Serology

H-2 serology has traditionally been based on the assumption of a one-to-one relationship between antibodies and antigens (*simple-complex* interpretation, cf. Hirschfeld 1965). An attempt to explain the *H-2* system from the point of view of *complex-simple* interpretation (complex antibodies cross-reacting with a simple antigen) was recently made by Thorsby (1971). Although his general approach was correct, the author grossly distorted the specifics of the *H-2* system (J. Klein and Shreffler 1971, 1972b). A more realistic H-2 chart, based on the assumption of a complex-simple relationship between the antibodies and antigens, is shown in Table 5-8, which is simply a list of the private H-2 antigens (i.e., the most restricted antigens, defined by the sharpest and least cross-reactive antisera). According to the complex-simple interpretation, the private are the "true" antigens, whereas the remaining (public) antigens are merely serological illusions.

It is erroneous to believe that a serologist can actually prove one or the other interpretation. To a serologist, an antigenic molecule is a Kantian *Ding an sich*, impenetrable by serological methods. A discussion as to whether public H-2 antigens actually exist is, therefore, purely academic, because serology alone can contribute very little to it. However, it is probably reasonable to predict that neither the traditional simple-complex nor the newer complex-simple interpretation of the *H-2* system is correct (J. Klein and Shreffler 1971, 1972b), but that the truth lies somewhere between. Some of the public antigens will probably prove to be nothing more than illusions created by cross-reactive antibodies, while others will be shown to represent specific sites, distinguishable from the private sites, on the antigenic molecule.

Section Two

Histocompatibility

Chapter Six

Introduction to Histocompatibility

I. "Transplantese"

Transplantation or *grafting* is the transfer of living cells, tissues, or organs from one part of the body to another or from one individual to another. The cell, tissue, or organ being transferred is the *graft* or *transplant*. Grafts placed in the same anatomical position normally occupied by the transplanted tissue are called *orthotopic*, and those placed in an unnatural position are called *heterotopic*. For example, a piece of skin taken from the tail of the donor mouse and placed on the tail of another mouse is an orthotopic graft, whereas the same tissue placed on the dorsum of the recipient is a heterotopic graft. Grafts taken from and placed on the same individual are called *autogeneic (autografts)*; grafts transplanted between genetically identical individuals (for instance, between mice of the same inbred strain) are called *syngeic (syngrafts or isografts)*; grafts transplanted between genetically different individuals of the same species (for example, between two different inbred strains of the mouse) are called *allogeneic (allografts or homografts)*; and finally, grafts transplanted between individuals of two different species are referred to as *xenogeneic (xenografts or heterografts)*.

The fate of a graft is determined by the genetic relationship between the donor and the host. Each species has a set of genes coding for antigens that determine compatibility or incompatibility of tissue transplants [*histocompatibility (H) genes* or *antigens*]. In general, grafts exchanged between animals that do not differ in the histocompatibility genes are *accepted* (i.e., they heal in and survive indefinitely), whereas those transplanted between individuals differing in the *H* genes are *rejected* (destroyed). The rejection is caused by a specific immune response against the histocompatibility (transplantation) antigens (*allograft reaction*). The complex of immunological phenomena associated with the rejection of grafts in unsensitized recipients is the *first-set reaction*; immunological response to a graft by a sensitized recipient is the *second-set reaction*. Under certain conditions, the recipient may be rendered immunologically unresponsive to foreign H antigens of the graft. The state of immunological unresponsiveness is known as *immunological tolerance*. Nonreactivity associated with the presence in the recipient of high-titered circulating antibodies against the H antigens of the graft is referred to as *immunological enhancement*. Whether the mechanisms of tolerance and enhancement are principally different is not known.

With most grafts, the allograft reaction is a one-way process: the host reacts against the graft, but the graft cannot react against the host (*host-versus-graft reaction*). However, grafts containing significant numbers of immunocompetent lymphoid cells are capable of mounting a *graft-versus-host reaction*.

II. Mediators of the Allograft Reaction

A. The T Cell Saga

A central figure in the graft rejection process is the *thymus-derived lymphocyte* or *T cell*, which originates from stem cells of the hematopoietic organs and migrates into the thymus (Fig. 6-1). The first hematopoietic organ to appear in the mouse is the yolk sac, an extraembryonic membrane, composed of mesoderm and endoderm (see Chapter Eleven). The first hematopoietic islets develop

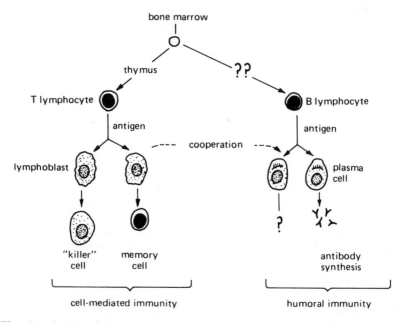

Fig. 6-1. Origin of T and B cells and their relationship to different forms of immunity.

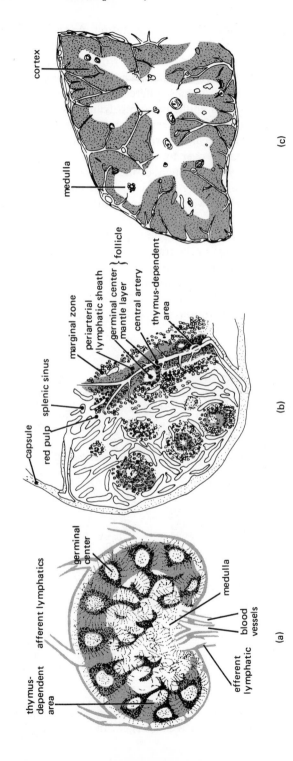

Fig. 6-2. Anatomy of the lymph node (a), spleen (b), and thymus (c). (a, reproduced with permission from P. B. Medawar: Antilymphocytic serum: its properties and potential. *Hospital Practice* **4**:26–33. Copyright © 1969 by Hospital Practice Co. All rights reserved.) (b, reproduced with permission from L. Weiss: *The Cells and Tissues of the Immune System*. Copyright © 1971 by Prentice-Hall. All rights reserved.)

in the wall of the yolk sac about $7\frac{1}{2}$ days into gestation. At about 11 days, the hematopoietic function of the yolk sac begins to decline and is taken over by the fetal liver. At about the same time, stem cells from either the yolk sac or the fetal liver first appear in the thymus anlage, which is composed of epithelial cells. In the fetal thymus, the stem cells differentiate, presumably under the inductive influence of the thymus epithelium, into lymphocytes (thymocytes), which later (beginning on about the sixteenth day of gestation) become the predominant component of this organ. Shortly before birth, the hematopoietic function of the fetal liver is taken over by the bone marrow, which continues sending stem cells into the thymus throughout the rest of the mouse's life. In adults, however, the process of seeding the thymus with bone marrow-derived stem cells proceeds at a much slower rate than in the fetus or the newborn animal.

The differentiation of T cells in the thymus proceeds in two steps. In the first step, the large basophilic stem cells transform by a series of cell divisions into progressively smaller cells, finally coming to rest as typical small lymphocytes. This morphological change is accompanied by the acquisition of at least six new alloantigens: Thy-1, Tla, Gv-1, Ly-1, Ly-2, 3, and Ly-5. The thymocyte, having just completed its first maturation step, shows a relatively low content

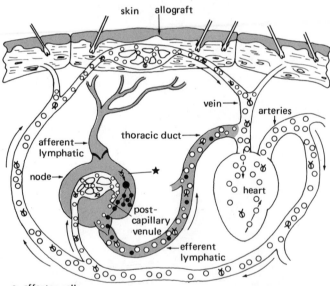

- • effector cells
- ○ small lymphocytes
- ✻ immunologically competent cell with antigen—receptor sites

★ immunologically competent cell that has been "triggered" by antigen and will transform into a large pyroninophilic cell

Fig. 6-3. Recirculation of T lymphocytes and their sensitization to a skin allograft. (Reproduced with permission from R. Billingham and W. Silvers: *The Immunobiology of Transplantation.* Copyright © 1971 by Prentice-Hall. All rights reserved.)

of H-2 antigens and a sensitivity to normal guinea pig serum, corticosteroid hormones, and X-rays. The transformation of the stem cells into a thymocyte begins in the peripheral regions of the cortex, and continues as the differentiating cells descend deeper into the cortex and finally pass into the medulla, the central portion of the thymus (Fig. 6-2c). The second maturation step, the transformation of the thymocyte into a typical T cell, takes place in the medulla. During this process, the thymocytes lose their Tla antigens, reduce their content of Thy-1 antigens, increase their content of H-2 antigens, and become less sensitive to guinea pig serum, corticosteroids, and X-rays. The mature T cells then leave the thymus and migrate to the peripheral lymphoid organs, primarily the lymph nodes and spleen. The point of entry of the cells into the thymus and the point of departure of the mature T cells from the thymus are not known. It appears, however, that the thymus is highly selective as to which cells it allows entry. This selectivity is attributed to the morphological blood-thymus barrier, impenetrable for most blood cells. The forces behind the differentiation of a stem cell into a thymocyte and of a thymocyte into a T cell are largely unknown, although many believe that an important role in these processes is played by a thymic hormone or hormones.

After leaving the thymus, the T cells begin to recirculate. They are carried by blood to the spleen and lymph nodes, enter these organs, percolate through them, and return to the blood, directly from the spleen and indirectly—via lymphatics—from the lymph nodes. The T cells continue to recirculate in this fashion throughout their life span, which is at least several months in the mouse (Fig. 6-3).

In the lymph nodes, the T cells tend to accumulate in the deep portions of the cortex (*paracortical area*), often conglomerated into distinct follicles (Fig. 6-2a); in the spleen, T cells are found primarily in the *white pulp*, a sheath of lymphocytes surrounding splenic arteries (Fig. 6-2b). Follicles similar to those occurring in lymph nodes may also be found in the outer layers of the white pulp. Because these areas are severely depleted of lymphocytes following surgical removal of the thymus, they are called *thymus dependent*.

The highest concentration of mature T cells is found in the thoracic duct lymph, followed by peripheral blood, lymph nodes, and spleen. Bone marrow is relatively free of T cells (Table 6-1).

B. Properties of T Cells

Morphologically, T cells resemble the second major class of lymphocytes, the B cells. The two classes differ in the following properties:

1. *Life span*. The T cells are long-lived, with a life span of several months; the majority of B cells are short-lived, with a life span of a few days or weeks.

2. *Recirculation*. The majority of T cells recirculate continuously between blood and lymph, passing through the peripheral lymphoid organs, lymph nodes, and spleen. Most B cells do not recirculate, and those that do,

Table 6-1. Frequency of T and B cells in various tissues of the mouse*

Tissue	Percent T cells	Percent B cells
thymus	100	0–1
lymph node	68	21
spleen	35	42
blood	70	19
thoracic duct lymph	85	17
Peyer's patches	25	61
bone marrow	0	15

* Reproduced with permission from A. Basten and J. G. Howard: "Thymus dependency." *Contemporary Topics in Immunobiology* 2:266. Copyright © 1973 by Plenum Press. All rights reserved.

pass with a slower transit time through different areas of lymphoid tissue.

3. *Distribution.* T cells are concentrated in the thymus-dependent areas of the peripheral lymphoid organs; B cells concentrate in the thymus-independent areas.

4. *Physical properties.* The average T cell is slightly larger, denser, less adherent to glass, plastic, or nylon, and more negatively charged than the average B cell. T cells are also less sensitive to cytotoxic drugs (e.g., cyclophosphamide), corticosteroids, and irradiation.

5. *Response to mitogens.* T cells can be stimulated to undergo blast transformation and proliferation by exposure to phytohemagglutinin (PHA) or concanavalin A (Con A), mitogens that do not stimulate B cells. The latter, on the other hand, can be stimulated by *E. coli* endotoxin or lipopolysaccharide (LPS), which are ineffective on T cells.

6. *Antigenic properties.* T cells do not react with anti-Ig and anti-MBLA sera and have a lower content of Fc and C3 receptors. They do carry at least one antigen, the Thy-1 antigen, absent in B cells (see Chapter Eight). It is difficult to prove that all T cells and no B cells possess the Thy-1 antigen, but this is true in the great majority of the cells in the two classes.

7. *Function.* T cells are known to be involved in at least three functions: they mediate allograft reaction (and cellular immunity in general[1]), they act as helper cells in humoral immunity (see Chapter Eighteen), and they are involved in immunological memory of both cellular and humoral immunity. B cells serve primarily as precursors of antibody-forming cells in humoral immunity and probably also as memory cells for humoral immunity.

[1] Other forms of cellular immunity are delayed hypersensitivity, and tuberculine test reaction.

C. Separation of T and B Cells

Many experiments require "pure" T or B cell populations, and a number of ways are now available for achieving the physical separation of the two.

1. Methods of T Cell Deprivation

a. Use of Congenitally Athymic Mice. In 1966 Flanagan described a recessive mutation that, in the homozygous state, caused a complete loss of hair over the body of the mouse (Flanagan 1966). The mutation was called *nude*, and the *nu* locus was later mapped in chromosome 11 (LG VIII). The *nu/nu* homozygotes are retarded in their growth and often die at an early age; the heterozygotes are normal. In 1968 Pantelouris reported that *nu/nu* mice were lacking a thymus (Pantelouris 1968), a discovery that launched the nude mice to stardom among laboratory animals. An abnormal thymus anlage can be observed in the *nu/nu* embryo on the fourteenth day of gestation, but the rudiment is never seeded by lymphocytes. The absence of the thymus means that the stem cells lack a site at which to differentiate into T cells, and that T cells are therefore absent in *nu/nu* mice. The maturation of B cells is apparently unaffected by the *nu* mutations. Arguments continue as to whether the nude mice are completely deprived of T cells (it is possible, for instance, that some T cells may differentiate outside the thymus under certain physiological stresses, and there is some evidence to support this possibility), but there is no doubt that these mice are closer to yielding a pure B cell population than any others.

b. Thymectomy. Surgical extirpation of the thymus (thymectomy) removes the source of new T cells but not those already in circulation. Since the majority of T cells are long-lived, the effects of thymectomy, if performed in an adult animal, are delayed; hence thymectomy must be performed at birth or very shortly after, before the animal develops a sizable T cell pool. If thymectomy is performed on an adult animal, the T cells already present in the circulation and in the lymphoid organs must be destroyed. This is achieved by lethal irradiation of the thymectomized mice. Such mice must then be protected against radiation death by a transfusion of syngeneic cells, usually bone marrow cells treated *in vitro* with anti-Thy-1 serum in the presence of complement (to ensure that no mature T cells are transferred with the inoculum). In the absence of the thymus, the stem cells of the bone marrow transplant are unable to differentiate into new T cells, and the thymectomized animal should therefore contain only B cells. In practice, however, this result is almost never achieved, because the thymectomy is not always complete, some T cells may survive the irradiation, and some may escape the anti-Thy-1 treatment. Thymectomy, therefore, achieves at best only a severe depletion of T cells, rather than their complete removal.

c. Treatment with ALS. Treatment with ALS is the least specific method of T cell deprivation. It consists of repeated injections of ALS (*antilymphocyte serum*), obtained by immunizing a different species (e.g., horse) with mouse lymphocytes, into a normal mouse. The antiserum preferentially destroys the circulatory pool of lymphocytes, particularly T cells.

d. *In vitro* Treatment of Lymphocytes. T lymphocytes can be selectively destroyed *in vitro* by incubating a cell suspension with anti-Thy-1 serum in the presence of complement and removing the dead cells, by centrifugation in a density gradient.

2. Methods of B Cell Deprivation

In birds, deprivation of B cells can be achieved by *bursectomy*, that is, surgical extirpation of the bursa of Fabricius. Because no bursa equivalent has been identified in mammals, in the mouse, B cell deprivation is much more difficult to achieve than T cell deprivation. Several investigators have reported that B cells can be selectively depleted by the action of certain drugs (e.g., cyclophosphamide), but the depletion in these cases is only partial.

Depletion of B cells *in vitro* can be achieved by the treatment of lymphocytes with anti-Ig sera in the presence of complement, by retention of B cells on a column, by a cell sorter, and by electrophoretic fractionation.

III. Mechanism of Graft Rejection

Graft rejection is an extremely complex and versatile process which may express itself in many different forms, depending on the specific circumstances of each case. In a very simplified way, the process can be divided into three phases: recognition, proliferation, and killing (Fig. 6-3). Both the recognition and killing phases seem to occur directly in the graft, whereas the proliferation phase takes place in the regional lymph nodes draining the graft area. The recognition of H antigens of the graft is apparently the function of the T lymphocytes. These cells constantly browse through the tissues of the body, scanning the cell surfaces for any unfamiliar changes or aberrations. The sudden emergence in the host of transplanted cells displaying foreign H antigens is quickly spotted by the patrolling T cells. Exactly how the T cells recognize the foreign H antigens is not known, but many believe that the recognition involves a direct cell-to-cell contact mediated by receptors on the T cells. The problem of the T cell receptor will be discussed in detail in the later sections of this monograph (see Chapter Eighteen); here it suffices to say that, despite an enormous effort toward its identification, the receptor remains purely hypothetical. Although most immunologists accept the existence of the receptor, they cannot agree on whether it belongs to one of the known classes of immunoglobulins, to a new class of immunoglobulins (IgX), or to a completely new type of recognition molecule. Whatever its nature, the T cell receptor, like the B cell receptor, has a high degree of specificity. In each lymphocyte population, only a small fraction of cells can recognize a particular antigen; once this fraction is removed, the remaining cells are unable to respond to the same antigen, although they are able to respond to other, unrelated antigens. It seems likely, therefore, that

T cells, like B cells, exist in clones, each clone reacting with only a limited range of related antigens. The recognition of foreign antigens by T cells may be aided by macrophages, which may modify the form of the antigen so that it will stimulate T cells.

The T cells that make contact with the alloantigens of the graft apparently return to the regional lymph nodes, there entering proliferation, the second phase of the rejection process. This phase closely resembles the blast transformation process observed after the stimulation of B cells. The small T lymphocytes begin synthesizing DNA, RNA, and proteins, enlarge into pyroninophilic blasts, and begin to divide. The dividing cells produce lymphocytes of progressively decreasing size, ending with small lymphocytes. Whether the new generation of small lymphocytes is qualitatively different from the original T cell clone is still debatable, although one thing seems certain: the former can carry out functions that the latter apparently cannot. The majority of new lymphocytes leave the lymph nodes, enter the blood, invade the graft, and begin to destroy it; they become *killer cells*. A minority of the lymphocytes remain in circulation as *memory cells*, capable of initiating much more potent second-set reaction when the sensitized recipient is reexposed to the same alloantigen.

The killing mechanism is almost totally obscure. An interpretation favored by many is that the killing is based on a direct contact between the killer and the target cells. In addition, however, several other phenomena are apparently involved. The lymphocytes, at least in *in vitro* situations, are known to release a number of factors aiding the rejection process: lymphotoxin (a factor capable of killing cells), chemotactic factor, a factor stimulating mitosis in other lymphocytes, a factor increasing the permeability of blood vessels, and others. An additional aid is probably provided by macrophages, which contribute to the cytopathic reactions and scavenge and digest cellular debris in the graft. In at least some cases (particularly with certain types of grafts), the rejection process may also involve the B cells. These cells, too, can be stimulated by the H alloantigens and triggered to secrete antibodies that can help to destroy the graft.

All three phases of the rejection process have counterparts in certain *in vitro* phenomena. The recognition and proliferation phases have their counterpart in the *mixed lymphocyte reaction* (MLR), observed where lymphocytes from genetically different individuals are cultivated together in tissue culture (see Chapter Eighteen). The killing phase has its counterpart in the *cell-mediated cytotoxicity* (CML) phenomenon, in which target cells can be lysed *in vitro* by specifically sensitized lymphocytes (see Chapter Eighteen).

IV. Laws of Transplantation

The primary rule of transplantation is that a graft is rejected whenever it possesses H antigens absent in the recipient. This rule can be expanded into five *laws of transplantation* (Snell and Stimpfling 1966):

1. Grafts within an inbred strain (syngeneic grafts) succeed.

2. Grafts between different inbred strains (allografts) fail.
3. Grafts from either inbred parent strain to the F_1 hybrid succeed, but grafts in the reverse direction fail.
4. Grafts from F_2 or subsequent F generations to F_1 hybrids succeed.
5. Grafts from either inbred parent strain succeed in some members of an F_2 generation but fail in others. Also, grafts from one inbred parent strain succeed in some members and fail in others of a backcross produced by crossing the F_1 hybrid to the opposite parent strain.

The laws are based on the assumption that the *H* genes are codominant, and that an F_1 hybrid therefore expresses both alleles at each *H* locus. This assumption is supported by a large body of experimental data. (For a discussion of recessive histocompatibility genes, see Chapter Nineteen.)

There are many exceptions to the laws, the most important being that they do not apply to transplantation between individuals of different sexes. Since both the Y chromosome (Eichwald and Silmser 1955) and the X chromosome (Bailey 1963) determine H antigens, the presence or absence of sex-linked histocompatibility genes must be taken into account in any grafting experiment. The outcome of transplantation across the sex-linked histocompatibility barrier is shown diagrammatically below:

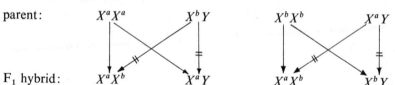

parent: $X^a X^a$ $X^b Y$ $X^b X^b$ $X^a Y$

F_1 hybrid: $X^a X^b$ $X^a Y$ $X^a X^b$ $X^b Y$

(XX = female; XY = male; a, b = alleles at the X-linked histocompatibility locus; $\rightarrow$ = graft accepted in the indicated direction; $\nrightarrow$ = graft rejected in the indicated direction.)

To provide for the sex difference, the laws of transplantation must be modified as follows:

1. Within an inbred strain, grafts from females to males are accepted, whereas grafts from males to females may be rejected. [Whether they are actually rejected depends on the presence of a particular allele at an *H-2*-linked immune response (*Ir*) gene, among other factors; see Chapter Seventeen.]
2. Grafts from female parent to male or female F_1 recipient are accepted, whereas grafts from male parent to male or female F_1 recipient may be rejected.

Chapter Seven

Methods of Histocompatibility Testing

Tissue and organ transplantation has two main aspects: surgical, concerned with the performance of technically successful transplants, and genetic, concerned with the inherited factors determining the fate of the transplants. Accordingly, this chapter is divided into two parts, each dealing with one of the two aspects.

I. Surgical Techniques

Theoretically, a graft can be derived from almost any part of the body and can consist of either normal or neoplastic tissue. Because tumor grafting played an important role in the formulation of the genetic theory of transplantation (see Chapter One), it will be considered first.

A. Tumor Transplantation

The advantage of the tumor method is that it is rapid and technically simple; the disadvantage is that it is not always specific. In the mouse, the most commonly used tumor transplants are *sarcomas* (tumors arising in connective tissue), *carcinomas* (tumors developing from epithelial cells), *lymphomas* (tumors of lymphoid tissue), and *myelomas* (bone marrow-derived tumors). The tumors can be of *spontaneous* origin (occurring without any intentional intervention by the investigator) or *induced* by *carcinogens* (e.g., chemical reagents, X-rays, viruses, etc.). Only some newly arisen tumors are transplantable; others may never take in new hosts, or may die off during the first few transplant generations. Tumors may not be transplantable because of the presence of a tumor-specific transplantation antigen, the requirement of specific physiological conditions for tumor growth, infection of the neoplastic tissue with bacteria, and other factors. Some tumors may undergo a period of adjustment in the first transplant generations and grow only sporadically, but later they become consistently lethal to their synegenic hosts. Once established, transplantable tumors can be maintained indefinitely by serial transfers (*passages*) on individuals of the same strain. Some mouse tumors have been maintained by serial transplantation for over half a century.

However, with successive passages from host to host, the tumors may change progressively: they may undergo morphological alterations, shifts in chromosome number, and display variations in growth rate and invasiveness; they may also change their antigenic characteristics. Many tumors become less specific in later transplant generations and may override histocompatibility barriers that would cause rejection of normal tissues.

Tumor transplants can grow either as *solid* tissues or as *ascites* (i.e., a suspension of single cells growing in the fluid-filled peritoneal cavity). Many solid tumors can be *converted* into ascitic forms either directly or by repeated selection. Ascitic tumors can be transplanted by suction of the ascitic fluid from the peritoneum of tumor-bearing mice and intraperitoneal inoculation of the cells into the new host. Solid tumors can be transplanted either as small pieces with a special needle (trocar) or as a cell suspension, obtained by mincing of the solid tissues. The latter technique is advantageous in that an accurately measured number of cells can be administered. The cell suspension can be inoculated in almost any part of the body, the more commonly used methods being subcutaneously on the flank, intramuscularly into the thigh, or intraperitoneally. The ultimate indication of graft acceptance is the tumor's causing the death of the host; the ultimate indication of rejection is the host's survival.

For further information and references on tumor transplantation, see reviews by Hauschka (1952), Kaliss (1961, 1966), Snell (1958a, c), and G. Klein (1959).

B. Transplantation of Normal Tissues

1. Skin Grafting

Skin grafting is by far the most popular technique for normal tissue transplantation in the mouse. Its advantages include great sensitivity, easy assessment of the graft survival, and relative resistance to transplantation trauma. A major disadvantage of this technique is its relative laboriousness; even in its simplest version, the technique is still considerably more time consuming than, for example, tumor transplantation.

The standard skin-grafting technique, developed by Billingham and Medawar (1951), consists of two steps: preparation of the graft and preparation of the grafting site (*graft bed*). The graft can be taken from the trunk, from the tail, or from the ear. Grafts from the trunk can be obtained by killing and skinning the donor and cutting the skin into pieces of desirable size and shape (*full-thickness grafts*). Thin sheets of skin can be sliced off with a scalpel from a living donor (*split-thickness grafts*), or the skin can be lifted up into a conical elevation with forceps and cut free at the base with a scalpel (*pinch grafts*). Grafts from the tail can be obtained by slicing off thin sheets of skin with a scalpel, or by amputating the tail, skinning it, and trimming the skin to the required size. Grafts from the ear are easily produced by cutting off the pinna at its base and peeling away the thin skin from the underlying cartilage. Full-thickness grafts consist of epidermis and complete—or almost complete—dermis; split-thickness grafts consist of epidermis and only superficial dermal layers, and pinch grafts are comprised, at least in the center, of not only the epidermis and dermis, but also the underlying layers of fat (*panniculus adiposus*) and muscle (*panniculus carnosus*).

The usual grafting site in the mouse is the dorsal or lateral skin of the trunk, which has the advantages of being relatively inaccessible to the animal's teeth and having the firm support of the thoracic ribs. The graft bed can be prepared by cutting off the skin in small pieces with scissors until the desired shape and size of the area is cleaned off, or by pinching off the skin with a scalpel. During the cutting, care must be taken not to damage the *panniculus carnosus* and the blood vessels overlying it. The bed can be of the same size as the graft (*fitted grafts*), or it can be larger (*open-fit grafts*). The grafts are protected from misplacement and from physical damage by a gauze dressing and bandage, both of which are removed 7–10 days later.

In the first few days after transplantation, incompatible skin grafts are grossly and microscopically indistinguishable from compatible grafts. In the first 2 days after the operation, the graft depends on diffusion of nutrients from the host through intercellular spaces. Blood supply is reestablished 2–3 days after grafting, primarily by the linking (anastomoses) of the host and graft capillaries, but also by an ingrowth of new capillaries into the graft. At about 5–6 days after transplantation, the compatible graft contains considerably more blood vessels than normal skin, and this hypervascularity causes the graft's characteristic pink color. The increase in vascularity is accompanied by intense mitotic activity in the epidermis, reaching its peak 6–8 days after grafting and then slowly declining over a period of several weeks. At 6 days the graft epidermis is at least three times thicker than normal skin, and this epidermal hyperplasia causes the graft to appear swollen and soft to the touch. Later, the upper layer of the original epidermis hardens and eventually peels off as a "ghost graft." The hair follicles, damaged as a result of transplantation trauma, regenerate and begin to grow a new hair crop after the reestablishment of a blood supply. The space between the surfaces of the graft and the graft bed is filled with healing tissue, so that the 6-day graft is already firmly attached to the host. When the compatible graft has merged imperceptibly with the host's skin and remains in that condition throughout the life of the recipient, it is said to be permanently *accepted*.

Incompatible grafts differ from compatible ones in that they develop an allograft reaction that damages or destroys the transplanted tissue. The destruction (*rejection*) can be either acute (its duration being relatively short, usually not more than a week) or chronic (prolonged over a period of several weeks or months), depending on the strength of the histocompatibility barrier. The onset of the allograft reaction is determined by the strength of H antigens, with strong antigens causing the reaction to begin as early as 5–6 days postoperatively (in first-set grafts).

The earliest sign of *acute rejection* is dilation of blood vessels and their engorgement with erythrocytes, followed by hemorrhages, and by invasion through the vessel walls of a mixed population of lymphoid cells, primarily small lymphocytes (*lymphocytic* or *round cell infiltration*). This inflammatory reaction spreads upward through the dermis, around the blood vessels, toward the epidermis. In addition to cells, large quantities of fluid also pass through the damaged vessels, causing the graft to swell and change color from pink to red and then to yellow or brown. The cells of vessel walls become pycnotic and lose their cytoplasm, and their nuclei fragment into small pieces. Necrosis and breakdown of the remaining tissue quickly follow, and the graft transforms into a scablike mass that ultimately sloughs.

A second-set reaction across strong *H* differences usually follows the same pattern as the first-set reaction, only in a hastened and more pronounced manner. Occasionally, however, when the reaction is very strong and begins very early, the graft fails to establish the initial blood anastomoses and degenerates without the transient period of healing in. Such *white grafts* do not show any lymphocytic infiltration in histological sections. Some believe that the white-graft phenomenon is associated with the presence of humoral antibodies directed against the donor-tissue antigens.

Chronic rejection is extremely variable in appearance and duration, its signs being gradual hair loss, scaliness or balding of the graft surface, scar formation, thinning of the epidermis, and weakening of the attachment to the dermis. Histologically, chronic rejection is usually accompanied by mild inflammatory reactions in the graft dermis. The rejection may be complete, followed by replacement of the graft with the host tissue, or partial, followed by recovery of the graft. Grafts of the latter type are said to have undergone a "cosmetic crisis."

Skin grafts can be appraised visually (by naked-eye observation) or histologically. For first-set grafts, particularly those with relatively long survival times, the former usually suffices; for second-set grafts transplanted across a strong *H* barrier, the latter is often imperative, as naked-eye observation may not distinguish between the late effects of surgical trauma and the early effects of allograft reaction. The visual scoring is based on observation of macroscopic changes in the graft, such as variations in color, thinning or loss of the hair crop, balding, swelling, "wetness," ulceration, and scar formation. The grafts should be scored once a day in the early posttransplantation period (first 4 weeks) and once a week thereafter. The histological scoring is based on sections of grafts removed at varying intervals after transplantation (Fig. 7-1). Although the histological scoring must take into account the whole status of the graft, two main criteria are used in appraising the sections: the survival of epidermis

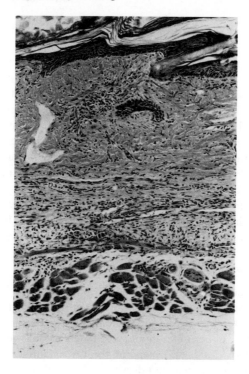

(a)

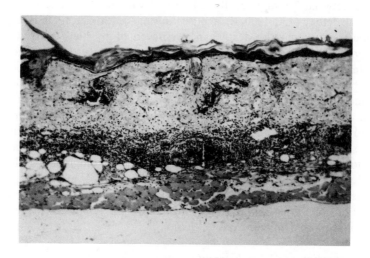

(b)

Fig. 7-1. Histological sections through syngeneic (a) and *H-2* allogeneic (b) skin grafts 8 days after transplantation. In the syngeneic graft, epidermis is well preserved and lymphocytic infiltration is minimal; in the allogeneic graft, epidermis is almost completely destroyed and dermis is heavily infiltrated with lymphocytes.

(expressed as percentage) and the degree of lymphocytic infiltration (expressed in arbitrary units, usually on a scale from one to four).

Even when transplanted under exactly the same conditions, across the same *H* difference and to genetically homogeneous recipients, all grafts are not rejected at the same time. The rejection process is influenced by many environmental factors, which cause some grafts to be rejected sooner than others. The range of individual survival times can vary from a few days in the case of strong H antigens to several months in the case of weak H antigens. It has become customary to express the length of the graft duration in terms of the *median survival time* (MST), which is the time that passes between transplantation and rejection of 50 percent of the grafts.

For further information on skin grafting, see articles by Medawar (1944), Billingham and Medawar (1951), Billingham *et al.* (1954), Bailey and Usama (1960), Billingham and Silvers (1961), and Eichwald *et al.* (1966).

2. Transplantation of Lymphoid Tissues

Lymphoid tissues can be transplanted in the form of single-cell suspensions prepared by homogenization of the donor organ (bone marrow, lymph nodes, spleen, thymus, or fetal liver) and inoculated intraperitoneally or intravenously. The recipient can be either untreated or irradiated with X-rays or gamma rays. The irradiation provides *Lebensraum* for the transplanted cells by destroying the recipient's lymphoid tissue, and decreases the host's capability for immunological response to the graft. Depending on the dose, the irradiation can be sublethal (between 250 and 750 R, a dose that will allow most of the animals to recover), lethal (750–1000 R, a dose causing death due to failure of the hematopoietic system—the death can be prevented by bone marrow transplantation), or supralethal (> 1000 R, a dose causing irreparable damage to the gastrointestinal and nervous systems—at this dose the animals cannot be saved even by bone marrow transplantation). The survival of the transplanted cells can be monitored radiologically (in cases where the donor and the host cells differ in their capability to incorporate radioactive isotopes), cytologically (provided that the donor and the host differ in the morphology of their chromosomes), serologically (when the donor and the host differ antigenically), immunologically (when the donor cells secrete immunoglobulins that are immunologically distinguishable from those of the host), or electrophoretically (when the donor and the host differ in an isozyme, serum protein, or hemoglobin). For references and further information on lymphoid tissue transplantation, see Micklem and Loutit (1966).

3. Transplantation of Other Normal Tissues

Any other normal tissue can be transplanted heterotopically, most commonly either subcutaneously or under the kidney capsule. Orthotopic transplantation of most mouse organs is technically difficult, and is therefore rarely performed.

II. Histogenetic Methods

The purpose of histocompatibility testing is to determine the *H* gene makeup of an individual. For the purpose of H-2 typing, four histogenetic methods[1] have been developed: allotransplantation, the F_1 test, the component test, and analysis by linkage.

A. Allotransplantation Test

Theoretically, the simplest way to identify the *H-2* haplotype of a new strain is to exchange grafts between that strain and another strain carrying a known *H-2* haplotype. If the grafts are accepted, the two strains are *H-2* identical; if they are rejected, the strains are *H-2* different. In practice, however, such a procedure can seldom be used. In the case of skin allografts, the allotransplantation test is limited only to situations involving congenic lines; in the case of tumor allografts, the method is applicable to tumors that transgress minor *H* barriers but do not transgress the *H-2* barrier. The suitability of this approach to H-2 analysis was explored by Snell *et al.* (1953b). Although the authors were able to show a strong correlation between *H-2* and the behavior of tumor allografts, they found so many exceptions that they did not consider the use of the method for actual H-2 typing feasible.

B. F_1 Test

The F_1 test always involves three strains: one used as a transplant (usually skin or tumor) donor, the others as parents of an F_1 hybrid (Snell 1958b). The donor strain must be congenic with at least one of the hybrid's parents. The test is based on the assumption that one of the two parental strains provides the hybrid with all *H* genes present in the graft donor, that is, all except *H-2* (Table 7-1). If the donor carries an *H-2* haplotype identical to the *H-2* haplotype

Table 7-1. Principle of the F_1 test: If grafts are accepted in both donor-recipient combinations, then $H\text{-}2^x = H\text{-}2^a$

	Test I	Test II
Donor	B.$H\text{-}2^x$ B.$H\text{-}2^x$	A $H\text{-}2^a$ A $H\text{-}2^a$
F_1 recipient	A $H\text{-}2^a$ B $H\text{-}2^b$	X $H\text{-}2^x$ A.$H\text{-}2^b$

* A, B or X = different genetic backgrounds; B.$H\text{-}2^x$ = congenic line carrying $H\text{-}2^x$ on B background.

[1] The term *histogenetic methods* was coined by Snell (1958b) to designate genetic methods applied to studies of tissue compatibility. In its broadest sense it is synonymous with the term *transplantation methods*.

of this parent, the grafts are accepted; if the donor possesses a different *H-2* haplotype, the grafts are rejected. The use of the F_1 test can be illustrated by the following example.

A congenic resistant line called D1.C was originally typed as carrying a new haplotype, $H\text{-}2^c$ (Snell 1958b). However, subsequent serological analysis showed a great similarity between $H\text{-}2^c$ and $H\text{-}2^d$, suggesting that the two haplotypes were actually identical. To test the possible identity of $H\text{-}2^c$ with $H\text{-}2^d$, J. Klein (*unpublished data*) crossed strains D1.C ($H\text{-}2^c$) and C57BL/10Sn or B10 ($H\text{-}2^b$), and challenged the resulting F_1 hybrids with B10.D2 ($H\text{-}2^d$) skin grafts. The F_1 hybrids received all the genes carried by strain B10.D2, except *H-2*, from B10. Since the grafts were permanently accepted, the author concluded that the F_1 hybrid received all the H-2 antigens carried by strain B10.D2 from D1.C. This suggested but did not prove identity between the D1.C and B10.D2 *H-2* haplo-types. It was still possible that strain D1.C carried some H-2 antigens that were not present in the B10.D2 strain, in addition to the shared ones. To rule out this possibility, Klein produced another F_1 hybrid by crossing strains DBA/1 ($H\text{-}2^q$) and B10.D2 ($H\text{-}2^d$), and challenged the hybrid with D1.C skin grafts. In this case, the DBA/1 strain had the same genetic background as the D1.C donor but the two strains differed in their *H-2* haplotypes. The D1.C grafts could therefore be accepted by the F_1 hybrids only if the B10.D2 strain carried all the H-2 antigens carried by the D1.C strain. In the actual experiment, the grafts were indeed accepted. Combined together, acceptance of the grafts in both types of F_1 hybrids indicated that D1.C and B10.D2 carried the same sets of H-2 antigens and hence that the $H\text{-}2^c$ and $H\text{-}2^d$ haplotypes were identical.

Luckily, in this particular case, the right strains were available for carrying out the F_1 test in both directions, once with the D1.C strain as a donor, and a second time with this strain as one parent of the F_1 hybrid. In cases where the test can be carried out only in one direction, graft acceptance by the F_1 hybrid does not prove identity but merely shows substantial similarity between the compared *H-2* haplotypes. The grafts can be accepted by the F_1 hybrid even if the donor does not possess an *H-2* haplotype identical with that of one of the hybrid's parents. This can happen under two circumstances. First, as already indicated, one of the hybrid's parents may possess all the H-2 antigens of the donor plus some that the donor does not have. Second, neither of the hybrid's parents alone possesses all the H-2 antigens of the donor but together the two parents make up the full antigenic complement of the donor. This principle of complementarity is utilized in the component test.

C. Component Test

In 1951, Snell observed that mice of the heterozygous genotype $H\text{-}2^d/H\text{-}2^k$ succumbed to an $H\text{-}2^a$ tumor, and he concluded that the $H\text{-}2^a$ haplotype is comprised of two components, *d* and *k*, complementing each other genetically. This so-called *dk effect* is now explained on the basis of $H\text{-}2^a$'s being a recom-binant derived from $H\text{-}2^d$ and $H\text{-}2^k$. As such, $H\text{-}2^a$ should not carry any antigens that haplotypes H-2^d and H-2^k do not carry, and H-2^a grafts, therefore, should be accepted by the H-$2^d/H$-2^k heterozygote. The phenomenon can be used in H-2 typing in the following way.

A strain carrying an unknown H-2 haplotype is crossed to an H-2^d (or H-2^k) strain and the resulting F_1 hybrids are transplanted with H-2^a grafts. If the grafts are accepted, it can be concluded that the H-2 haplotype of the tested strain is probably similar to H-2^k (or H-2^d). For the actual grafting, either tumor (Snell 1951) or skin transplants (J. Klein 1965c) can be used. This method, known as the *component test*, was used by Snell (Snell 1951, Snell *et al.* 1953a) as a source of supportive evidence for results obtained with other methods of H-2 typing. It did not become a widely used method mainly because of its limitation to a single combination of H-2 haplotypes. However, the test should now be applicable to many other combinations involving other H-2 recombinants. For instance, it can be expected that heterozygotes H-$2^b/H$-2^d, H-$2^a/H$-2^b, H-$2^a/H$-2^q, and so on, will accept grafts from donors H-2^g, H-2^h (and H-2^i), H-2^y, respectively, and the test could therefore be potentially useful for testing H-2 haplotypes a, b, d, k, q, and many others.

D. Analysis by Linkage

The linkage test, introduced by Snell and his co-workers (Snell and Higgins 1951, Snell *et al.* 1953a), takes advantage of the fact that the H-2 complex is linked to dominant genes for tail abnormalities, *Brachyury* (*T*), *Kinky* (*Ki*), and *Fused* (*Fu*). The test is based on a double cross,

$$(M \times T) \times N$$

where M and N are any two inbred strains and T is a strain carrying T (or Ki or Fu). The offspring of this cross is classified for tail length and inoculated with a tumor native to the strain in the M position. The test can answer the question of whether the two inbred strains, M and N, carry the same or different H-2 haplotypes. If the H-2 haplotypes of all three strains entering the cross are not known, then any one of the following five possibilities could theoretically occur:

1. $M = H$-2^m; $T = H$-2^m; $N = H$-2^m (all three strains have the same H-2 haplotype).
2. $M = H$-2^m; $T = H$-2^t; $N = H$-2^m (strains M and N have the same H-2 haplotype, but strain T has a different haplotype).
3. $M = H$-2^m; $T = H$-2^m; $N = H$-2^n (strains M and T have the same H-2 haplotype, but strain N has a different haplotype).

    If any of these three possiblities occur, all the progeny of the $(M \times T) \times N$ cross will carry the H-2^m haplotype, and therefore will be susceptible to the M-strain tumor.
4. $M = H$-2^m; $T = H$-2^n; $N = H$-2^n (strains N and T have the same H-2 haplotype, but strain M has a different haplotype).

5. $M = H-2^m$; $T = H-2^t$; $N = H-2^n$ (each strain carries a distinct $H-2$ haplotype).

If one of the last two possibilities occurs, the cross $(M \times T) \times N$ will produce two types of progeny: short-tail, resistant to the M tumor and normal-tail, susceptible to the M tumor.

If the result of the test is such that most of the normal-tail offspring succumb to the M-strain tumor whereas most of the short-tail progeny reject the tumor, a conclusion can be made that strains M and N carry different $H-2$ haplotypes. (Theoretically, normal-tail animals that reject the tumor and short-tail animals that succumb to the tumor should represent recombinants between T and $H-2$). Strain T, in this case, can have either an $H-2$ haplotype identical with strain N or one distinct from both M and N; the test does not distinguish between these two possibilities. If, on the other hand, the progeny are all susceptible to the M-strain tumor, the only conclusion that can safely be made is that two of the three strains have identical $H-2$ haplotypes. The test does not identify these two strains, but this shortcoming can be circumvented by setting up another cross,

$$(N \times T) \times M$$

and inoculating the progeny with an N-strain tumor. A comparison of the results from the two types of cross can provide information about the $H-2$ haplotypes of all three strains involved.

The results of the linkage test can be distorted by several factors (Snell *et al.* 1953a):

1. The genes for tail abnormalities do not show a complete penetrance; among the segregating progeny a small fraction of animals can carry the mutant gene (T, Fu, and Ki) and still have normal tails (*normal overlaps*).
2. Certain transplantable tumors occasionally grow in animals that are genetically resistant (*false positives*) or fail to grow in hosts that are genetically susceptible (*false negatives*).
3. H genes other than $H-2$ segregate in the progeny of the double cross and influence the ratio of susceptible and resistant animals.

The linkage test was very useful in the early stages of H-2 typing, but has recently been replaced by more accurate assays.

Chapter Eight

Histocompatibility System of the Mouse

Histocompatibility (*H*) genes are members of a large family of loci controlling *cell-membrane alloantigens*. Some 60 loci belonging to this family have been identified in the mouse (46 loci definitely, 14 tentatively), and it is more than likely that the total number is much higher, perhaps several hundred. The loci can be divided into three groups on the basis of the methods used for their identification (Snell and Cherry 1972):

1. erythrocyte alloantigen (*Ea*) loci, detected by classical blood-typing methods with erythrocytes as target cells;
2. lymphoid-tissue alloantigen loci, detectable by the cytotoxic test on nucleated cells of various lymphoid organs, lymphocytes (*Ly* loci),

thymocytes (*Thy* loci), thymocytes and leukemias (*Tla* loci), and plasma cells (*Pca* loci);

3. histocompatibility (*H*) loci, detectable by tissue, primarily skin and tumor transplantation.

A somewhat special group are loci controlling alloantigens that are associated in one way or another with murine viruses (*Gv* and *X* loci). This classification is unnatural in that some loci can be detected by all three methods, and superficial in that it may not reflect true differences and similarities between the different loci, but it is convenient and practical. The strain distribution of antigens controlled by the cell membrane loci is shown in Tables 8-1 and 8-2, and the localization of these loci in the mouse genome (if known) is shown in Fig. 8-1.

I. Erythrocyte Alloantigen (*Ea*) Loci

Seven loci have been described in this group and designated *Ea*-1 through *Ea*-7.

Ea-1. Three alleles are known at the *Ea-1* locus: *Ea-1ᵃ*, controlling antigen Ea-1.1 (A); *Ea-1ᵇ*, controlling antigen Ea-1.2 (B), and *Ea-1ᵒ*, controlling the absence of antigens 1 and 2 (Singer *et al.* 1964). Alleles *a* and *b* have been found so far only in wild mice; all inbred strains carry the *o* allele. The antibody

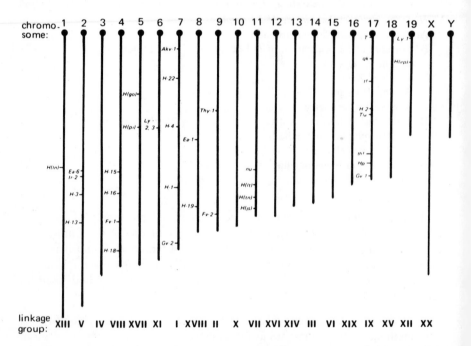

Fig. 8-1. Location of membrane alloantigen loci (as well as other loci discussed) in the mouse genome.

response to the *Ea-1* antigens is controlled by the *immune response-2* (*Ir-2*) locus in chromosome 2 (LG V; see Gasser 1969); the *Ea-1* gene is in chromosome 8 (LG XVIII; see Foster *et al.* 1968). The responder strains are YBR/He, SEC/Re, and C57BR/cd; the nonresponders are C3H/J, CBA/J, DBA/2J, C57BL/10, and others.

Ea-2 (R, Z, rho, H-14). The *Ea-2* is the most controversial among the *Ea* loci, because of the uncertainty surrounding the questions of the linkage of *Ea-2* with *H-2* and the role of *Ea-2* in skin-graft rejection.

In 1959 Hoecker and his co-workers (Hoecker *et al.* 1959) described two antisera, C3H anti-RIII and RIII anti-C3H, which they believed identified two new antigens of the *H-2* system, R and Z. Subsequent studies (Hoecker and Pizarro 1962), however, demonstrated that the R and Z antigens were controlled by a separate locus, thought to be linked to *H-2*. The R antigen was also detected by Popp (1967, 1969) with antisera C3H anti-RFM and A.CA anti-RFM. Popp designated the antigen "rho" and the corresponding locus *H-14*. In 1967 Snell and his co-workers demonstrated that R and Z were controlled by alleles at the same locus, which was later designated *Ea-2* (Snell 1971). Although Snell and his co-workers (1967b) observed linkage between *Ea-2* and *H-2* in some of the backcross generations designed to produce an *Ea-2* congenic line, in the final analysis the two loci seemed to have segregated independently. The authors therefore concluded that *H-2* and *Ea-2* were not linked, and the same conclusion was also reached by Popp (1967) concerning the *H-14* locus. Recently, however, Pizarro and Vergara (1973) published the results of a careful linkage study that indicated a clear linkage between *Ea-2* and *H-2* with recombination frequency of 14.8 percent between these two loci, 20.4 percent between *tf* and *Ea-2*, and 26 percent between *T* and *Ea-2*, and with the order of loci *T—tf—H-2* *—Ea-2*. The discrepancy among the results of the various authors remains unexplained. An obvious possibility—that the different laboratories are not detecting the same antigen—seems to be ruled out by the fact that Pizarro and Vergara (1973) used Snell's anti-Ea-2 sera as well as their own, and did not report any discordance in the results of their testings. Another possibility is that the Brachyury stock used by Pizarro and Vergara (1973) carried a *t* factor with a crossing-over suppressing effect; however, this too is unlikely, as the recombination frequency observed by these authors for the *T-tf* and *tf-H-2* intervals was not significantly different from that observed in normal mice (see Chapter Eleven).

The role of the *Ea-2* locus in graft rejection is even more puzzling. The Ea-2 antigens are present in relatively high concentration on various tissues of the body (liver, spleen, brain, testis, kidney, thymus, and lungs, cf. Popp 1967, 1969), and yet skin grafts exchanged between *Ea-2* congenic lines are rejected only under certain circumstances. Popp (1969) observed no rejections of grafts transplanted among congenic lines C57/Ha, C57.F-*H-14*^{a} and C57.F-*H*-14^b, even after preimmunization. Stimpfling (1973), on the other hand, observed rapid rejections (in less than 3 weeks after grafting) of B10.RIII(R) skin grafts by B10.RIII(R) × LP)F$_1$ hybrids, but no rejections of grafts in combination

Table 8-1. Strain distribution of antigens controlled by cell-membrane alloantigen loci, exclusive of H loci*

Strain	H-2	Ea-1	Ea-2	Ea-3	Ea-4	Ea-5	Ea-6	Ea-7	Ly-1	Ly-2	Ly-3	Ly-4	Ly-5	Pca-1	Thy 1 (θ)	Tla	Gv-1	X.1
A	a	·	2	–	1	1	1	2	2	2	2	–	1	+	2	1, 2, 3	+ +	–
C57BL	b	–	2	–	2	–	1	2	2	2	2	2	1	–	2	–	+	–
C57L	b	·	2	1	1	·	·	2	2	2	·	2	1	·	2	–	·	·
LP	b	·	2	·	1	·	·	·	·	·	·	·	·	·	·	·	·	·
129	bc	2	2	·	1	1	·	1	2	2	2	·	1	·	2	2	+ + +	1
BALB/c	d	·	2	–	1	·	2	2	2	2	2	–	1	–	2	2	+ + +	–
DBA/2	d	–	2	·	1	–	2	2	1	1	2	–	1	+	2	2	–	–
C57BL/Ks	d	·	2	·	2	·	·	2	2	2	·	–	·	–	·	2	+	·
SEC/1Re	d	–	2	·	1	–	·	·	2	2	·	·	·	·	2	2	·	·
NZB	d	·	·	·	·	1	1	2	2	·	2	·	·	+	·	1, 2, 3	·	1
YBR	d	–	2	·	1	1	·	·	2	2	·	·	·	·	·	·	–	·
RFM	f	·	1	·	·	·	·	·	·	·	·	·	·	·	1	·	–	·
HTG	g	·	2	·	1	·	2	2	2	2	2	–	1	–	2	·	–	·
HTI	i	·	·	·	·	·	·	·	2	2	·	·	·	·	·	1, 2, 3	·	·
JK	j	·	2	1	1	–	2?	·	1	1	2	·	1	·	·	·	·	·
I	j	·	2	·	1	1	1	2	2	1	·	·	·	–	2	–	·	–
WB/Re	ja	·	2	·	1	·	·	2	2	1	2	2	1	–	2	–	·	·
C3H/He	k	–	2	·	1	1	1	1	1	2	·	–	·	·	2	–	+ +	–
C3H/St	k	·	·	·	·	1	2?	1	1	2	·	·	·	+	2	–	·	·
CBA/J	k	–	2	·	1	1	1	1	1	1	·	·	·	·	2	–	·	·

Strain	Haplotype																
AKR	*k*	—	+ +			1	+ +	—			1	1	2	2	1?	·	1	·	2	·
RF/J	*k*	·	+			1	+	—	2	1	1	2	2?			1	·	1
ST/bJ	*k*	·			1, 2, 3	2	·	—	2	2	2	2	·	·	1	·	2
C57BR/cd	*k*	·			1, 2, 3	·	·	—	2	2	2	2	·	·	1	·	2
FL/2Re	*k*	·	+ + +		2	·	·	·	2	1	1	2	·	·	1	·	2
HRS	*k*	·			·	·	·	·	·	·	·	2	·	·	1	·	2
CE/J	*k*	·	+ +	1, 2, 3	2	+	·	2	2	2	2	·	·	1	·	2
C58	*k*	—	+ + +	1, 2, 3	2			—	2	1	2	1	—	1	·	1	·	2
MA/J	*n*	·			1?	+	·	·	1	—	1	2	·	—	1	·	1
F/St		·			1?	1, 2, 3	+	·	·	1	·	·	·	—	1	·	2
BDP	*p*	·			1	·	·	·	2	2	2	2	2?	·	1	·	2
DBA/1	*q*					1, 2, 3	2	·	—		2	2	2	2		1	·	2
SWR	*q*	·			1, 2, 3	1?	·	—		2	2	2	·		1	·	2
BUB/Bn	*q*	·				1?	·	·		2	2	1	·	·	1	·	2
DA/HuSn	*qp1*	·				2	·	·		2	2	2	·	·	1	·	2
RIII	*r*	·			·	·	·	·	·	2	2	2	·	·	1	·	·
SJL	*s*			+	1, 2, 3	2	+ +	2	·	2	2	2	2	·	1	·	2
PL	*u*	·			1, 2, 3	1	+	·	·	2	1	2	2	·	1	·	2
SM/J	*v*	·			—	2	·	·	·	2	1	2	2	·	1	·	2

* Based on Snell and Cherry (1972).

B10.RIII(R)→B10,   B10.RIII(R)→(LP × B10)F$_1$,   B10.RIII(R)→(B10.RIII ×
B10)F$_1$ and B10→(LP × B10.RIII)F$_1$. [B10.RIII(R) is H-2^bEa-2^a, B10.RIII
is H-2^rEa-2^b, and B10 and LP are H-2^bEa-2^b]. A possible explanation of this
unusual rejection pattern is that the rejections are mediated almost exclusively by humoral antibodies that are produced only in the presence of certain
immune response (*Ir*) genes. Such an interpretation is supported by recent
findings (Stimpfling 1973; Snell 1971) that the Ea-2 antibody response is
controlled by *H-2*-associated *Ir* genes, and by the observation of Popp
and Davis (1971) that immunization across the *Ea-2* barrier leads to a
strong lymphocyte transformation reaction in the thymus-independent areas of
spleen and lymph nodes; no such reaction can be observed in thymus-dependent
areas.

In another *Ea-2* congenic line, B6-*Ea-2*^{a}, derived from Popp's C57.F-*H-14*^{a}
strain, Flaherty and Bennett (1973) observed rejections of skin grafts from the
inbred partner, C57BL/6, but only after preimmunization. The rejections were
not accompanied by production of anti-Ea-2 antibodies, and Ea-2 antigens
could not be detected on epidermal cells either by a direct cytotoxic test or by
absorption. These authors postulated the existence of another locus, *H(Ea-2)*,
linked to, but distinct from *Ea-2*, to explain the observed histoincompatibility.

The *Ea-2* locus has two alleles: *Ea-2*^{a}, present in strains RIII, F/St, RF/J,
and RFM, and *Ea-2*^{b}, present in all other typed strains. The antigens controlled
by the *a* and *b* alleles are Ea-2.1 (R) and Ea-2.2 (Z), respectively.

Ea-3 (lambda). The *Ea-3* locus was identified by Egorov (1965) with antiserum C57BL/10 anti-C57L. The only antigen known to be controlled by this
locus is Ea-3.1, present in strain C57L (allele *Ea-3*^{a}); the antithetical antigen
presumably controlled by the *Ea-3*^{b} allele of strains C57BL/10, A, BALB/c,
and C3H/He has not been identified.[1] The reactivity of the Ea-3.1 antibodies
seems to be controlled by a locus segregating independently of *Ea-3*.

Ea-4 (BL, D). The *Ea-4* locus, discovered by Shreffler (1966), was identified
with a (C3H/HeJ × DBA/2)F$_1$ anti-C57BL/10 serum, from which the H-2 antibodies were removed by absorption with C3H.B10 (*H-2*^{b}) tissue. Another
antiserum identifying the *Ea-4* locus was obtained by J. Klein and Martínková
(1968) in a combination NZB anti-B10.D2. The two known alleles at this locus,
Ea-4^a and *Ea-4*^{b}, code for antigens Ea-4.1 and Ea-4.2, respectively. The *b* allele
is present in the C57BL strains, the *a* allele in the rest of the typed inbred
strains. The Ea-4.2 antigen is present in a large quantity on red blood cells,
moderate quantity on lymph node cells, small quantity on lung and kidney cells
and in a very small quantity on thymus and gut cells; it is absent from liver,
spleen, brain, muscle, heart, testis and uterus (Shreffler 1966). Congenic lines
differing only at the *Ea-4* locus accept reciprocally exchanged skin grafts
indefinitely (D. C. Shreffler and J. Klein *unpublished*). The *Ea*-locus is not
closely linked with *Hbb*, *a*, *b*, *c*, *d* or *H-2* (Shreffler 1966, J. Klein and Martínková

---

[1] However, antiserum C57L anti-C57BL/10-lymphoma was reported by G. Möller
and E. Möller (1962a) to contain non-*H-2* antibodies detectable by the fluorescent antibody
technique. The relationship of these antibodies to the Ea-3 system has never been examined.

1968). Recent observation by Lilly (1974) suggests that the antigens controlled by the *H-2* and *Ea-4* loci may intereact (see p. 113).

Ea-5 (alpha). The antiserum identifying the *Ea-5* locus was obtained by Amos and his co-workers (1963b) after inoculation of C3H/St lymphoma 6C3HED into C57BL mice and absorption of the immune serum with C3H/He liver cells. All attempts to produce a similar antiserum by immunization with normal tissues failed. Of the two *Ea-5* alleles known, only the *a* allele codes for an antigen (Ea-5.1). The antigen is present in high concentration on erythrocytes and kidney cells, moderate concentration on testis, lung, and 6C3HED lymphoma, low concentration on spleen, brain, and muscle, and is absent on liver cells. Since the anti-Ea-5.1 antibodies are difficult to produce, knowledge of this locus is limited.

Ea-6 (delta). The anti-Ea-6.1 antibody was originally produced after immunization of (C3H/St × DBA/2)F_1 hybrids with C57BL leukemia EL4 (Amos 1958). Subsequently, a similar antibody was found in the serum of C3H/St mice hyperimmunized against C3H/He ascites sarcoma MC1M (Amos *et al.* 1963b). An antithetical antigen, controlled by the *Ea-6^b* allele, has recently been identified by Lilly (1974), using an antiserum produced by immunization of A mice with BALB/c sarcoma MethA. The Ea-6.1 antigen is present in high concentration on red cells and MC1M tumor cells, moderate concentration on testis, brain, feces, and perhaps spleen, low concentration on lung and liver, and in very low concentration on kidney and muscle. Skin grafts exchanged between congenic lines differing at the *Ea-6* locus are permanently accepted (F. Lilly *personal communication*). The *Ea-6* locus is in chromosome 2 (LG V), seven map units from *pallid* (Lilly 1967b).

Ea-7 (T). Amos (1959) reported that antiserum 129 anti-C57 contained at least two antibodies, which he termed anti-T and anti-U. The same antiserum was later obtained by Stimpfling and Snell (1968), who showed that the stronger hemagglutinating antibody present therein identified an antigen segregating independently of *H-2*. The locus coding for this new antigen was later designated *Ea-7*. The two alleles at this locus, *Ea-7^a* (present in 129, LP, C3H/He, CBA/J, and C58) and *Ea-7^b* (present in the remaining tested strains), determine antigens Ea-7.1 and Ea-7.2, respectively. The locus does not seem to play any role in skin or tumor transplantation. There is some similarity between the *Ea-7* and *Ea-5* loci, and the identity of these loci has not been ruled out. The humoral antibody response evoked by antigen Ea-7.2 is enhanced by the simultaneous presence of an H-2 incompatibility between the donor and the recipient (Stimpfling and Reichert McBroom 1971). The *Ea-7* locus is not closely linked to loci *p*, *c*, or *A*. Anti-Ea-7.1 is also present in antiserum C57BR/cd anti-C3H/He.

II. Lymphoid Tissue Alloantigen Loci

This group consists of seven loci (Table 8-1), but the number is rapidly growing. Some of these loci are expressed only in certain types of lymphoid cells, and their products thus represent true differentiation antigens.

Ly-1 (Ly-A, mu). Two antigens controlled by the *Ly-1* locus have been identified: Ly-1.1, controlled by the *Ly-1ᵃ* allele, and Ly-1.2, controlled by the *Ly-1ᵇ* allele (Boyse *et al.* 1968d). The former was detected with C57BL/6 anti-DBA/2-leukemia SL2 serum, absorbed first *in vivo* in DBA/2 mice to remove anti-*H-2ᵈ* antibodies and then *in vitro* with AKR thymus or leukemia to remove anti-Ly-2.1 antibodies, and tested against C3H or DBA/2 thymocytes. Antibodies against the Ly-1.2 antigen were produced by immunization of DBA/2 mice with C57BL leukemia EL4 and testing the antiserum against BALB/c thymocytes. The Ly-1.1 antigen was independently detected by Cherry and Snell (1969), using antiserum (RF/J × RIII)F₁ anti-C3H/He. The Ly-1.1 antigen is restricted to lymphocytes of the thymus, lymph nodes, spleen, and peripheral blood; it is absent from erythrocytes, brain, lung, liver, and kidney cells.

Thymocytes have a considerably higher concentration of Ly-1 antigens than other lymphocytes. Bone marrow absorbs anti-Ly-1 sera slightly, probably because of the presence of mature lymphocytes. The *Ly-1* locus is in chromosome 19 (LG XII) at a distance of 27 map units from *ruby eye* (Itakura *et al.* 1971). According to M. Cherry (quoted by Snell 1971), the *Ly-1* locus is without histocompatibility effect. However, the Ly-1 congenic lines produced by Boyse and his co-workers reject mutually exchanged skin grafts (Flaherty and Bennett 1973), indicating that there must be a histocompatibility locus on the same chromosome as is occupied by *Ly-1*. The distinctiveness of the putative *H (Ly-1)* locus from *Ly-1* is supported by observations that *Ly-1* congenic lines do not produce anti-Ly-1 antibodies after the rejection of skin grafts, and that Ly-1 antigens cannot be detected on epidermal cells (Scheid *et al.* 1972).

Ly-2 (Ly-B). This locus has two alleles: *Ly-2ᵃ*, coding for antigen Ly-2.1, and *Ly-2ᵇ*, coding for antigen Ly-2.2 (Boyse *et al.* 1968d). The Ly-2.1 antigen was detected with an antiserum produced by inoculation of AKR leukemia K36 into C57BL/6 mice, *in vivo* absorption of the anti-*H-2ᵏ* antibodies in (C57BL/6 × AKR)F₁ hybrids, and testing the absorbed antiserum against I thymocytes. Anti-Ly-2.2 was produced by inoculation of C57BL/6 leukemia EL4 into (C3H/An × I)F₁ mice and testing the antiserum against C57BR thymocytes. The tissue distribution, as well as other properties of the Ly-2 antigens, are similar to those of the Ly-1 antigens. The *Ly-2* locus is in chromosome 6 (LG XI) at a distance of seven map units from *mi, microphthalmia* (Itakura *et al.* 1972). Skin grafts exchanged between congenic lines differing at the *Ly-2* locus are rejected, and this very weak histocompatibility is attributed to three separate but linked *H* loci, tentatively designated *H(Ly-2-N8)*, *H(Ly-2-N16)*, and *H(Ly-2, 3)* (Flaherty and Bennett 1973).

Ly-3 (Ly-C). Boyse and his co-workers (Boyse *et al.* 1971) identified two antithetical antigens, Ly-C.1 and Ly-C.2 (later changed to Ly-3.1 and Ly-3.2), with antisera (CBA/T6 × SJL)F₁ anti-C58 and C58 anti-CE/J, respectively. The *Ly-3* locus was shown to be closely linked or identical to *Ly-2* (no recombinants between *Ly-2* and *Ly-3* were found among 370 segregants). The properties of Ly-3 antigens are very similar to those of Ly-2 and Ly-1 antigens.

Ly-4. The *Ly-4* locus was identified by Snell and his co-workers (1973b) with

(BALB/c × SWR)F$_1$ anti-B10.D2, as well as several other antisera. The *Ly-4^b* allele, present in the C57BL strain, controls antigen Ly-4.2; the antithetical antigen, Ly-4.1, has not been described. The strain distribution of *Ly-4* alleles is similar to *H-3* alleles and the two loci might possibly be identical. The Ly-4.2 antigen can be detected only on lymph node lymphocytes, and is presumably expressed predominantly in B cells (Aoki *et al.* 1974), although anti-Ly-4.2 sera can be produced by immunization with the thymus.

Ly-5. The *Ly-5* locus was identified by Komuro *et al.* (1974) using antisera SJL/J anti-A.SW spleen and lymph node cells (reacting with antigen Ly-5.1 controlled by allele *Ly-5^a*) and (B6-*H-2^k* × A.SW)F$_1$ anti-SJL/J spleen and lymph node cells (reacting with antigen Ly-5.2 controlled by allele *Ly-5^b*). From the former antiserum, thymocyte autoantibodies were removed by absorption with SJL/J thymocytes; from the latter antiserum, T1a antibodies were removed by absorption with A strain leukemia RADA1. The Ly-5 antigens appear to be specific for T cells. The *Ly-5* locus is not closely linked to *Ly-1*, *Ly-2/Ly-3*, *c*, *p*, *Thy-1*, *H-2* and *Ldr-1*.

Pca-1. Only one antigen controlled by the *Pca-1* locus has been identified so far (Takahashi *et al.* 1970). The identifying antiserum DBA/2 anti-BALB/c myeloma MOPC-70A, is cytotoxic to myeloma cells in the presence of complement, and this cytotoxicity can be removed by absorption with liver, kidney, spleen, brain, and lymph nodes but not with peripheral blood lymphocytes, bone marrow cells, leukemias, and sarcomas. The presence of the Pca-1.1 antigen on plasma cells is inferred from the observation that anti-Pca-1.1 serum abrogates the production of antibodies by these cells.

Thy-1 (*θ*, theta). The Thy-1 antigens 1 and 2, originally called *θ*-AKR and *θ*-C3H, respectively, were first detected by Reif and Allen (1963, 1964) with antisera prepared by reciprocal immunization of C3H and AKR strains. The antigens can be detected by the cytotoxic test on thymocytes, thymus-derived lymphocytes, some leukemias, and epidermal cells (Scheid *et al.* 1972), and by absorption on nervous tissues. Congenic lines differing at the *Thy-1* locus are weakly skin incompatible, with many grafts never rejected; however, the grafting leads, in most cases, to Thy-1 antibody production (John *et al.* 1972). The *Thy-1* locus is in chromosome 9 (LG II) at a distance of 15 map units from *dilute* (Itakura *et al.* 1972, Blankenhorn and Douglas 1972).

Tla. See Chapter Eleven.

III. Virus-Associated Alloantigen Loci

Two loci have been identified in the group of virus-associated alloantigen loci.

Gv-1. See Chapter Eleven.

X.1. Sato and his co-workers (1973) discovered that BALB/c radiation-induced leukemias are rejected by hybrids of BALB/c with certain other mouse strains and that the sera of such hybrids contain antibodies cytotoxic to the tumors. They designated the antigen(s) detected by these antibodies X.1, in recognition of the fact that it resembled antigen X, previously described by Gorer (1961). The X.1 antigen is present on the surface of both leukemia cells and the virions harbored by these cells. The presence of this antigen on the surface of normal cells (lymphocytes) is indicated by the capacity of certain strains to absorb anti-X.1 activity. However, the concentration of X.1 on normal lymphocytes is so low that the antigen cannot be demonstrated by any direct technique.

IV. Histocompatibility (H) Loci

A. Number of H Loci

The methods used to estimate the number of H loci can be divided into four categories, based on the principle involved: segregation, association, mutation, and isolation (Bailey 1970).

1. Methods Based on Segregation

In an F_2 generation, a certain proportion of individuals should have H genotypes identical with those of one parent, and should therefore permanently accept its skin grafts. The proportion of individuals with permanently surviving grafts depends on the number of segregating H loci; in general, the greater the number of segregating H loci, the smaller the proportion of permanently accepted grafts. The proportion of accepted $P{\rightarrow}F_2$ grafts can thus be used to estimate the number of H loci. The same applies to combinations $P{\rightarrow}B$, $F_1{\rightarrow}F_2$, $F_2{\rightarrow}F_2$, $F_2{\rightarrow}P$, $B{\rightarrow}B$, and $B{\rightarrow}P$ [P = parental (inbred) strain, $F_1 = F_1$ hybrid, $F_2 = F_2$ hybrid, and B = first backcross generation]. A simple formula can be derived for each combination, and this formula can then be used to calculate the number of segregating H loci. The formula for the $P{\rightarrow}F_2$ combination can be derived as follows.

Consider two inbred strains differing in one H locus, for example, *H-1*. If one strain is *aa* and the other *bb* (where *a* and *b* are alleles at the *H-1* locus), then in the F_2 generation the following segregation occurs:

F_1 parent one

		a	*b*
F_1 parent two	*a*	*aa*	*ab*
	b	*ab*	*bb*

If the F_2 mice are now grafted with skin from the *aa* strain, the *aa* and the *ab* segregants will accept the grafts, and the *bb* segregants will reject them. Thus, three-quarters or $(\frac{3}{4})^1$ of the F_2 mice accept the grafts from one of the two inbred grandparents.

If the two inbred strains differ at two H loci (*H-1* with alleles *a* and *b* and

H-2 with alleles x and y) and if the strains' genotypes are $aaxx$ and $bbyy$, then the F_2 animals segregate as follows:

F$_1$ parent one

		ax	ay	bx	by
	ax	**$aaxx$**	**$aaxy$**	**$abxx$**	**$axby$**
F_1 parental two	ay	**$aaxy$**	$aayy$	**$abxy$**	$abyy$
	bx	**$abxx$**	**$abxy$**	$bbxx$	$bbxy$
	by	**$abxy$**	$abyy$	$bbxy$	$bbyy$

After grafting with skin from the $aaxx$ strain, only those F_2 segregants carrying both the a and x alleles (boldface in the table above) accept the grafts; all the others reject them. Thus, nine-sixteenths or $(\frac{3}{4})^2$ of the F_2 mice accept the parental graft.

In this manner it can be shown that for three H genes the proportion of accepted grafts is $(\frac{3}{4})^3$, for four genes $(\frac{3}{4})^4$, and for L genes $(\frac{3}{4})^L$. The relationship between the number of successful grafts (S) and the number of H loci (L) in the P$\rightarrow$F$_2$ grafting combination can therefore be expressed as

$$S = (\tfrac{3}{4})^L$$

and from this, L can be calculated:

$$L = \frac{\ln(S)}{\ln(\frac{3}{4})}$$

where ln is the natural logarithm.

In an early attempt to estimate the number of H loci in the mouse, Prehn and Main (1958) grafted (BALB/c $\times$ DBA/2)F$_2$ hybrids with BALB/c skin and found that out of 120 transplanted mice, three retained the graft for more than 200 days. From this, the authors calculated that the number of H loci in which the two inbred strains differ is

$$L = \frac{\ln(\frac{3}{120})}{\ln(\frac{3}{4})} = 13$$

Using the same approach, formulas for other donor-recipient combinations can be derived:

P $\rightarrow$F$_2$:	$S = (\frac{3}{4})^L$		F$_2\rightarrow$F$_2$:	$S = (\frac{5}{8})^L$
P $\rightarrow$B :	$S = (\frac{1}{2})^L$		B $\rightarrow$B :	$S = (\frac{3}{4})^L$
F$_1\rightarrow$F$_2$:	$S = (\frac{1}{2})^L$		B $\rightarrow$P :	$S = (\frac{1}{2})^L$

Somewhat more complicated formulas must be used when the segregating populations are more complex. Examples are given below.

1. *nth backcross to parent generation.* Instead of using the first backcross generation, one can also use the second, the third, or the nth generation

and transplant grafts from these mice to the recurrent parent (the parent used for backcrossing). The formula for this type of grafting is

$$S = [1 - (\tfrac{1}{2})^n]^L$$

where n is the number of generations backcrossed ($n = 0 = F_1$; cf. Bailey and Mobraaten 1969, Elandt-Johnson 1969).

2. *Partially inbred strains.* Similarly, instead of exchanging grafts between F_2 mice, one can also use F_n mice, where n is the generation of brother-sister inbreeding (Chai and Chiang 1963).

3. *Second-set grafts in a backcross generation.* Owen (1962) devised a method for estimating the number of H genes from the frequency of second-set reaction to grafts exchanged between mice of a backcross generation. He showed that the probability (p) of a backcross individual's rejecting a graft from one donor in a second-set fashion after it has rejected a graft from another donor is

$$p = (\tfrac{7}{8})^L$$

where L is the number of H loci.

4. *Wild mice.* The number of H loci segregating in wild mice can be determined by crossing each mouse to an inbred strain and exchanging skin grafts among the sibs derived from these crosses (Iványi *et al.* 1969). If the wild mouse differs from the inbred strain at both alleles of any given H locus, the cross is

$$aa \times bc$$

and the probability of graft survival among the sibs is

$$S = (\tfrac{1}{2})^L$$

If the wild mouse shares one allele at a particular H locus with the inbred strain, the cross is

$$aa \times ab$$

and the probability of graft survival is

$$S = (\tfrac{3}{4})^L$$

In the former case, $L = \log S / \log 0.5$; in the latter case, $L = \log S / \log 0.75$ (Micková and Iványi 1972).

Equations for calculating the effective number of alleles per locus and the effective number of segregating H loci were derived by J. Klein and Bailey (1971).

2. Methods Based on Association

The number of H loci can also be estimated from the proportion of histo-incompatible lines among the congenic lines that differ at mutant non-H loci. The histoincompatibilities can be presumed to be due to H loci introduced concomitantly with the mutant loci. The incidental introduction of such "contaminating" genes has a certain probability, which can be used to calculate L. For the derivation of the formula for such calculation, the reader is referred to the article by Bailey (1970).

3. Methods Based on Mutation

The mutation rate of *all* H loci is estimated by Bailey and Kohn (1965) at 5.4×10^{-3}/gamete (see Chapter Ten), whereas the mutation rate of a *single* non-H locus in the mouse is 7.5×10^{-6}/gamete. Assuming that the mutation rates of all loci are the same, the ratio of total H gene mutation rate to the mutation rate of a single gene, $[(5.4 \times 10^{-3})/(7.5 \times 10^{-6})]$, should give the number of H loci (Bailey 1968, 1970).

4. Methods Based on Isolation

The most reliable method for estimating the number of H loci involves their isolation and identification in congenic lines. The number of H genes derived by the different methods are given in Table 8-3. The minimum number is 35, because that many H loci have already been identified. The upper estimate, obtained by the mutation rate method, is 720, possibly more. This latter method is based on a number of assumptions (for example, that the mutation rate of H loci is not higher than that of other loci), most of which cannot, at present, be tested and can easily lead to an inaccurate estimate. However, from the rate at which new H loci have recently been identified, a safe bet is that the total number of these loci is probably several hundreds.

B. Nomenclature

Histocompatibility loci identified as distinct from other known loci are designated by the prefix H, followed by a serial number in the order of their discovery (i.e., *H-1*, *H-2*, *H-3*, etc.). Histocompatibility loci identified only tentatively and not yet definitely proved to be distinct from other loci are designated by the prefix H followed by an arbitrary symbol. For example, the H locus known to be linked to the *leaden* (*ln*) gene in chromosome 1 (LG XIII) is designated $H(ln)$; H mutants were designated by Bailey and Kohn (1965) $H(z1)$, $H(z2)$, $H(z3)$, and so on. The provisional symbols are changed to standard symbols once the identity of the H loci is definitely established. Symbols *H-5* and *H-6*, originally used for loci now designated *Ea-5* and *Ea-6*, respectively, have not been reassigned to new loci. The H loci carried by the sex chromosomes X and Y are designated *H-X* and *H-Y*, respectively. The known H loci and their congenic lines are listed in Table 8-2.

C. Major and Minor H Loci

In 1956 Counce and her co-workers described marked differences in the intensity of the allograft reaction directed against the antigens controlled by the

Table 8-2. Non-*H-2* loci and their identifying strains

Locus	Identifying strains	Reference
H-1	C3H.K, B10.BY, B10.129(5M)	Snell 1958b
H-3	B10.LP-a	Snell 1958b
H-4	B10.129(21M)new	Snell and Stevens 1961
H-7	B10.C(47N)	Snell and Bunker 1965
H-8	B10.D2(57N)	Snell and Bunker 1965
H-9	B10.C(45N), B10.C(44N)	Snell and Bunker 1965
H-10	B10.129(9M)	Snell and Bunker 1965
H-11	B10.129(10M), B10.D2(55N)	Snell and Bunker 1965
H-12	B10.129(12M), B10.129(6M)	Graff *et al.* 1966a, Snell *et al.* 1971d, Snell *et al.* 1967a
H-13	B10.129(14M)	Snell *et al.* 1967a
H-15	B6.C-*H-15*	
H-16	B6.C-*H-16*	
H-17	B6.C-*H-17*	
H-18	B6.C-*H-18*	
H-19	B6.C-*H-19*	
H-20	B6.C-*H-20*	
H-21	B6.C-*H-21*	
H-22	B6.C-*H-22*	D. W. Bailey *Mouse News Letter 45*: 15–16, 1972
H-23	B6.C-*H-23*	
H-24	B6.C-*H-24*	
H-25	B6.C-*H-25*	
H-26	B6.C-*H-26*	
H-27	B6.C-*H-27*	
H-28	B6.C-*H-28*	
H-29	B6.C-*H-29*	
H-30	B6.C-*H-30*	
H-Y		Eichwald and Silmser 1955
H-X		Bailey 1963

Tentatively identified loci

Locus	Identifying strains	Reference
H(ep)	B6-*ep*	D. W. Bailey and H. P. Bunker *Mouse News Letter 47*:18, 1972
H(Eh)	B6-*Eh*	
H(go)	B6-*go*	
H(js)	B6-*js*	
H(ln)	B6-*ln*	D. W. Bailey and H. P. Bunker *Mouse News Letter 47*:18, 1972
H(lt)	B6-*lt*	
H(pi)	B6-*pi*	
H(tn)	B6-*tn*	
H(Tla)	A-*Tla^b*, B6-*Tla^a*	
H(Ly-1)	B6-*Ly-1^a*	
H(Ly-2-N8)	B6-*Ly-2^a*(N8)	Flaherty and Bennett 1973
H(Ly-2-N16)	B6-*Ly-2^a*(N16)	
H(Ly-2, Ly-3)	B6-*Ly-2^{a}Ly-3^a*	
H(Ea-2)	B6-*Ea-2^a*	

Table 8-3. Estimates of the number of histocompatibility loci in different strains of mice*

Donor	Recipient	S/T** (at day)	No. of H loci	Reference
A CBA	$(A \times CBA)F_2$ $(A \times CBA)F_2$	2/120(100) 1/154(100)	15	Barnes and Krohn 1957
BALB/c BALB/c	$[BALB/c \times DBA/2)F_1 \times DBA/2]BC$ $(BALB/c \times DBA/2)F_2$	0/99(60) 3/120	>6 13	Prehn and Main 1958
CBA A	$(A \times CBA)F_2$ $(A \times CBA)F_2$	10/105(100) 14/151(100)	8–9	Hicken and Krohn 1960
$[(C57BL \times CBA)F_1 \times C57]BC$	$[(C57BL \times CBA)F_1 \times C57BL]BC$	23/137†	13	Owen 1962
LG(N13–N19)	LG(N13–N19)	198/312(90)	20	Chai and Chiang 1963
C57BL/6 BALB/c $(BALB/c \times C57BL/6)F_{11}$ $[(BALB/c \times C57BL/6) \times C57BL/6]BC_5$	$(BALB/c \times C57BL/6)F_2$ $(BALB/c \times C57BL/6)F_2$ $(BALB/c \times C57BL/6)F_{11}$ C57BL/6	0/207(60) 0/200(60) 193/879(60) ?	≥17	Bailey and Mobraaten 1969
DBA/2	$(DBA/2 \times C57BL/6)F_3$	♂♂10/63(240) ♀♀7/120(24)	28 44	Brambilla et al. 1970
$(Wild \times C57BL/10)F_1$	$(Wild \times C57BL/10)F_1$	31/202(100)	<6	Iványi and Démant 1970
$(Wild \times C3H/He)F_1$	$(Wild \times C3H/He)F_1$	7/350(150)	4–7	J. Klein and Bailey 1971
$(Wild \times C57BL/10)F_1$ $(Wild \times C3H/He)F_1$ $(Wild \times A)F_1$	$(Wild \times C57BL/10)F_1$ $(Wild \times C3H/He)F_1$ $(Wild \times A)F_1$	34/299(200) 9/195(200) 5/253(200)	2–4 4 4–6	Micková and Iványi 1972

* All estimates except one are calculated from the number of rejected skin grafts transplanted in the indicated combinations; the one exception (Hicken and Krohn 1960) is calculated from the number of rejected ovarian grafts.

** Number of mice with surviving grafts at indicated day/total number of grafted mice.

† Number of mice not showing second-set reaction/total number of mice transplanted with two grafts.

first three identified H loci—$H-1$, $H-2$, and $H-3$. For example, a tumor of C57BL/10($H-2^b$) origin, transplanted in a dose of 1000 cells/mouse to the B10.D2($H-2^d$) congenic line, was rejected by all recipients; however, the same tumor in the same dose killed 90 percent of the B10.LP mice, which differ from the C57BL/10 strain at the $H-3$ locus. In the former case, the $H-2$ apparently was such a strong histocompatibility barrier that the tumor was unable to overcome it; in the latter case, the $H-3$ barrier was much weaker and so was overcome by the tumor in a large number of the inoculated mice. The distinction between a "strong" $H-2$ locus and a "weak" $H-3$ locus was confirmed by the results of a skin-grafting experiment. Skin grafts exchanged between mice differing in the $H-2$ system survived an average of 8.5 days, whereas grafts exchanged between mice differing at the $H-3$ (or $H-1$) locus survived an average of 24 days or more.

On the basis of these results, Counce and her co-workers defined a *strong H locus* as "a locus such that a difference between donor and host at this locus will prevent the progressive growth of nearly all tumor homotransplants and cause the rapid rejection of skin homografts," and a *weak H locus* as "a locus such that a difference between donor and host at this locus will permit the progressive growth of various tumor homotransplants and fail to cause the rapid rejection of skin homografts" (Counce et al. 1956). Because all subsequently discovered H loci were weak by this definition, and because the $H-2$ complex remained the sole representative of the strong category, the weak loci are also called *non-H-2* loci.

It is difficult to prove that $H-2$ is the only strong locus in the mouse, although this is very likely true, at least for the inbred strains. If another strong H locus were to exist, it would almost certainly have been detected in the numerous crosses designed to produce various congenic lines. In many of these lines, the selection for the differential H locus was random, and the chances were much better for picking up a strong locus than a weak one, especially in cases where the selecting agent was a tumor.

The absence of a second strong H locus is also supported by results obtained by Micková and Iványi (1969), who grafted B10 mice with skin from $H-2^b/H-2^b$ homozygotes produced by an $(A \times B10)F_1 \times B10$ backcross. Animals whose grafts were rejected within 20 days after grafting were used for further backcrossing to the B10 strain, and this process was repeated for six generations. Had a strong locus existed, it would have been picked up through such selection. In the actual experiment, the number of animals whose skin grafts were rapidly rejected by the parental B10 strain progressively decreased during the backcrossing until, in the N5 generation, all graft rejections occurred after 20 days. The authors concluded that among the non-$H-2$ loci in which strains A and B10 differ, none is so strong as the $H-2$ complex, and that the observed rapid rejections in the first five generations of backcrossing were due to the cumulative effect (cf. below) of multiple weak loci.

Later it became apparent that strength was not the only property distinguishing the $H-2$ system from the non-$H-2$ loci. A number of other fundamental differences confirming the unique position of the *H-2* complex in the histocompatibility system of the mouse have been discovered. To emphasize this uniqueness, the *H-2* complex has been designated as major (*major histocompatibility complex*, MHC) and the weak *H* loci as minor [*minor histocompatibility* (MIH) *loci*]. The properties that distinguish MHC and MIH loci are briefly enumerated below.

1. Skin and other tissue grafts, when transplanted across MHC differences, are rejected by an acute process in less than 3 weeks; skin grafts transplanted across MIH differences are usually rejected later than in 3 weeks, often by a chronic process lasting many days, and some grafts are not rejected at all. Grafts of other tissues (e.g., tumors, ovaries, teeth) may completely overcome the MIH barrier. With an MHC difference, second-set grafts are often rejected as white grafts, whereas this type of rejection is very rare with an MIH difference (Eichwald *et al.* 1966).

2. The MHC is extremely complex genetically, consisting of perhaps several hundred loci (cf. Chapter Ten); no such complexity has yet been reported for any of the MIH loci.

3. The MHC is extremely polymorphic genetically, and can probably exist in several hundred different forms (cf. Chapter Twelve); the most polymorphic MIH locus has only three alleles.

4. The MHC is intimately associated with genes controlling the immune response to a variety of antigens (cf. Chapter Seventeen); no *close* association of MIH and *Ir* loci has been reported so far.

5. The MHC is strongly involved in the mixed lymphocyte and graft-versus-host reactions (cf. Chapter Eighteen); the MIH loci have only minor, if any effect on these reactions, with a few exceptions.

6. The number of lymphocytes capable of reacting to MHC antigens in mixed lymphocyte culture or in the graft-versus-host reaction is substantially higher than the number of lymphocytes capable of reacting with antigens controlled by the MIH loci (Wilson *et al.* 1968, Simonsen 1967).

7. Preimmunization of the donor against the antigens of the host increases graft-versus-host reactivity if the donor and host differ in MIH loci, but does not substantially alter the reaction if the donor and host differ in the MHC (Lind and Szenberg 1961, Simonsen 1962a, b).

8. Immunization across the MHC barrier induces both cellular and humoral immunity; humoral immunity across MIH loci is much more difficult to prove.

9. The MHC is involved in physiological cooperation between T and B cells (cf. Chapter Eighteen); incompatibility at MIH loci seems to have no effect on this cooperation.

10. It is much more difficult to induce tolerance to antigens controlled by the MHC than to those controlled by MIH loci (Uphoff 1961).

11. The immune response to MHC antigens is more difficult to control by immunosuppression than the response to MIH loci (Silvers *et al.* 1967).

D. Properties of Minor *H* Loci

1. Strength

The strength of minor *H* loci, as defined by the median skin-graft survival times, is extremely variable. The grafts can be rejected as early as 3 weeks after transplantation or as late as 300 days. Some may never be rejected. In general, the weaker the *H* barrier, the greater the interval between the onset and completion of graft rejection, and the broader the range of rejection times of the individual grafts. The variability in rejection times of individual grafts is due to environmental rather than genetic factors. Progeny of mice rejecting grafts relatively early show the same spectrum of rejection times as progeny of mice rejecting grafts relatively late (J. Klein 1967). The MST is influenced by antigen dose, sex of the recipient, and allelic combination.

a. Antigen Dose. Small skin grafts are often rejected faster than large ones (Lapp and Bliss 1966, McKenzie 1973, Hildemann *et al.* 1970). It is conceivable that large grafts induce transient tolerance in the host, particularly in very weak combinations. Antigen dose is probably also responsible for the slower rejection of grafts from heterozygous, as opposed to homozygous donors (Lapp and Bliss 1966).

b. Sex of the Recipient. Grafts exchanged between females are often rejected faster than grafts exchanged between males (Graff *et al.* 1966a).

c. Allelic Combination. It has been shown repeatedly that antigenic strength is not so much a function of a particular *H* locus as of its particular allele. Alleles at the same locus are known to differ considerably in their effect on skin-graft survival, and may often be arranged in hierarchical order of decreasing immunological potency. For example, alleles at the *H-1* locus can be arranged in the following order (Hildemann 1970):

$$H\text{-}1^c \rightarrow H\text{-}1^b \ (15) > H\text{-}1^b \rightarrow H\text{-}1^a \ (25) > H\text{-}1^a \rightarrow H\text{-}1^b \ (100) > H\text{-}1^b \rightarrow H\text{-}1^c > (250)$$

The numbers in parentheses indicate MST's.

According to Hildemann (1970), the relative importance of these three factors is

allelic combination > graft dosage > recipient sex

Preimmunization of the host with tissue of the prospective donor usually shortens the MST of the subsequent skin transplants, and this second-set reaction is particularly pronounced in strain combinations having a very weak *H* difference. In general, the weaker the *H* barrier, the greater the effect of preimmunization on graft survival.

The basis for the varying strengths of H antigens is not known. Theoretically, late rejection can be due to a longer antigen recognition phase, to the induction of quantitatively less intense immune response, or to the development of a qualitatively different immune response. Although it is interesting to speculate on the various mechanisms that might be responsible for the differences in antigenic strength, such speculations are purely academic, as there is little data on which to base any conclusion. The subject has been thoroughly discussed by Lengerová (1969), G. Möller (1970), and Batchelor and Brent (1972).

2. Cumulative Effect

In 1964, McKhann reported that skin grafts transplanted across $H-1 + H-3$ barriers were rejected more rapidly than those transplanted across $H-1$ or $H-3$ alone. It appeared as if the effects of the two loci accumulated when the antigens they controlled occurred together. This phenomenon, confirmed later by J. Klein (1965c) and by Graff *et al.* (1966b), became known as the *cumulative* or *additive effect*. It was tacitly assumed that the cumulative effect was caused by some sort of synergistic interaction of the immune responses to the two antigens that occur concomitantly on the target cells. An alternative explanation of the cumulative effect has recently been proposed by Bailey (1971b), who explains that it is not necessary to postulate synergy between the responses to the two antigens, that, on the contrary, the shortening can be explained as an independence of the two responses. His argument goes as follows.

Consider two H loci, one weak, the other strong, but with considerable overlapping in their graft survival time distribution. In the overlapping interval, the rejection of a graft with a double difference can be due either to the strong or to the weak antigen; sometimes the weak and sometimes the strong antigen is first to provoke a rejection of grafts in this interval. Each time the weak antigen provokes the rejection before the strong does, the survival curve is shifted to the left, to a time earlier than that corresponding to the strong difference. Mathematically, if the probability of graft survival on a certain day after transplantation is S_1 for $H-1$ and S_2 for $H-3$, then the probability for $H-1 + H-3$ is $S_1 S_2$, a product that is lower than either S_1 or S_2. (For example, if $S_1 = 0.20$ and $S_2 = 0.15$, then $S_1 S_2 = 0.03$.) Bailey's hypothesis of independent effect predicts that the shift to the left will be greater the closer the MST's of the two single antigenic differences are to coinciding, and that the greatest shift will be obtained with two very weak H loci of approximately coinciding MST's and of broad-range rejection times. The results obtained by Graff and his co-workers (1966b) are in agreement with this prediction.

3. Humoral Versus Cellular Immunity

In contrast to the H-2 antigens that can be detected through cellular as well as humoral immunity, the antigens controlled by MIH loci have so far been detected primarily through cellular immunity. Although reports have been published describing serological detection of H-1, H-3, and some other non-H-2 antigens, attempts to reproduce these results have either failed completely, or have, at best, met with only partial success. Consequently, a serology of the weak H antigens is practically nonexistent. The reasons for the difficulty in obtaining workable antisera against MIH antigens are obscure. It may be that the antibodies are actually produced, but the antigens are present in a form not easily detectable by existing serological methods (the antigens may be buried deep in the membrane or even inside the cells, their concentration on the cell surface may be low, they may be present on tissues other than those used as a source of target cells for serological tests, etc.); alternatively, the properties of the MIH loci may be such that the antigens activate only the cellular and not the humoral branch of the immune response. Some evidence supporting the first possibility has recently been obtained by Mariani *et al.* (1973) and by Baldwin and Cohen (1974). The former authors observed that skin grafting across multiple non-*H-2* barriers (strain combination DBA/2→BALB/c) produced a significantly greater number of germinal centers in the lymph nodes and spleen than did grafting across a strong *H-2* barrier (C57BL→A). The centers were found as early as 1 day after grafting. Because germinal center formation is usually attributed to a proliferation of B cells, it seems logical to assume that the non-*H-2* loci provide a stimulus for humoral as well as cellular immunity. The more intensive germinal center response in the non-*H-2* differences is explained by Mariani and his co-workers as the consequence of earlier graft vascularization:

> In order for the antigenic stimulus from the skin graft to be effective in the production of germinal centers, it must be transmitted from the site of grafting to the lymph nodes and other lymphoid sites. . . . Because good vascularization existed in the weak non-*H-2* barrier group, this resulted in better transmission of the antigenic stimulus and hence a greater production of germinal centers (Mariani *et al.* 1973).

Baldwin and Cohen (1974) went one step further and demonstrated that sera from mice sensitized against *H-3* + *H-13* antigens were able either to prolong or shorten graft survival when passively transferred into recipients grafted across the same antigen barrier.

Hence, it appears that humoral immunity across non-*H-2* differences is induced almost as easily as, or even more easily than across *H-2* differences, but that the antibodies produced are not easily detected by present serological methods.

V. Histocompatibility Loci in the H-2 Complex

A. *H-2* and Organ Transplantation

As a rule, incompatibility in the *H-2* complex causes the rapid rejection of organ or tissue transplants such as skin (Billingham *et al.* 1954), bone marrow (Morgado *et al.* 1965), heart (Corry *et al.* 1973), ovaries (Krohn 1959; Linder 1961; Goldman 1974), teeth (J. Klein and Secosky 1971), and others. One exception to this rule seems to be orthotopic kidney transplants, which have been reported to survive in *H-2* allogeneic hosts for over 100 days (Skoskiewicz *et al.* 1973). The reason for the exceptional behavior of kidney transplants is not known, but one of the factors involved might be immunological enhancement. In most of the other organ transplants, *H-2*-incompatible grafts are rejected within 3 weeks after the operation.

With skin, first-set rejections occur between 10 and 14 days after grafting in lines that differ in the whole *H-2* complex but are compatible at all MIH loci. A difference in *H-2* and multiple non-*H-2* loci may lead to even earlier rejection, between 8 and 10 days (Billingham *et al.* 1954, Graff and Bailey 1973). Second-set rejections across the *H-2* complex occur between 6 and 8 days after the second grafting. The variability of MST's among the different congenic strain combinations suggests either that some *H-2* haplotypes (antigens) are stronger than others, or that genes in the *H-2* complex control the strength of the immune response to H-2 antigens.

B. Number and Localization of *H* Loci in the *H-2* Complex

It was originally believed that *H* loci were distributed evenly throughout the entire *H-2* complex, but this belief was shaken when it was demonstrated by Démant and his co-workers (1971c, 1972) and by J. Klein and Shreffler (1972a) that there are portions of the *H-2* complex that are either not at all involved in skin-graft rejection or play only a minor role. Testing of the involvement of different regions and subregions of the *H-2* complex in graft rejection is possible because of the availability of *H-2* recombinant strains. Using recombinants in which the genetic exchange took place at different positions within the *H-2* complex in combination with each other and with the parental strains, situations can be created in which the host can react against only a portion of the complex. Rejection or nonrejection of the grafts then indicates whether that particular portion contains histocompatibility loci. This type of analysis revealed that rejections occurred whenever the donor differed from the recipient in the peripheral regions of the *H-2* complex, and did not occur when the donor and the recipient differed in the central *H-2* regions. Hence, it appears that *H* loci responsible for skin-graft rejection are concentrated in or near the *K* and *D* regions; the central segment of the complex, particularly the *S* region and the segment between *Ss* and *H-2D*, do not seem to contain any *strong H* loci. However, the existence of weaker *H* loci, particularly those requiring pre-immunization to be detected, has not been excluded.

At present, three regions with strong histocompatibility effects are known to exist in the *H-2* complex: *K*, *I*, and *D*.

1. The K Region

"Pure" *K* differences, presumably uncontaminated by other *H* loci, are known so far in only two strain combinations, B10.AQR ↔ B10.A and A.TL ↔ A.AL. These combinations provide information about *K* regions derived from three *H-2* haplotypes, *k*, *q*, and *s*. Skin grafts transplanted across the *H-2K* barrier are rejected during the third week after transplantation (J. Klein, *unpublished data*).

2. The I Region

The *I* region loci are located close to the *K* region on the genetic map of the *H-2* complex, and they have only recently been recognized as separate from the *K* region *H* loci (J. Klein *et al.* 1974b). "Pure" *I* region differences exist in strain combinations B10.AQR ↔ B10.T(6R), A.TL ↔ A.TH, B10.HTT→ (A.TL × B10)F$_1$ and A.TL→(A.CA × B10.HTT)F$_1$. In the first four combinations, the donor and the recipient differ in the entire central portion of the *H-2* complex (from *H-2K* to *H-2D*), in the last two combinations the difference is restricted to the *I* region. It is postulated, but not proved, that all six strain combinations involve the same *H* locus difference and that this difference resides in the *IA* subregion. If so, the six strain combinations provide information about *H-2I* alleles derived from *H-2* haplotypes *k*, *q*, and *s*. Skin grafts exchanged between strains differing at the *H-2I* locus are rejected with about the same speed as those transplanted across the *K* region, that is, during the third postoperative week (J. Klein *et al.* 1974b).

3. The D Region

Because the majority of *H-2* recombinants were derived by crossing-over in the chromosomal segment between the *S* and *D* regions, a number of combinations are available for testing the involvement of the *H-2D* locus (loci) in graft rejection. In addition, mutation *H-2da*, presumably affecting the *H-2D* locus, probably provides the "purest" known *D*-region difference. The majority of skin grafts transplanted across the *H-2da* barrier are rejected between 16 and 17 days postoperatively, but occasionally a few grafts survive much longer, often for several months (cf. Chapter Ten). Grafts transplanted across the *D* region differences provided by the *H-2* recombinant strains are usually rejected during the third postoperative week (J. Klein 1972b, McKenzie and Snell 1973).

C. The K-D Asymmetry

Although the three histocompatibility loci of the *H-2* complex seem to have approximately equal effects on graft survival, the two ends of the *H-2* complex, *K* and *D*, display a certain asymmetry. The asymmetry was first pointed out by Rychlíková and her co-workers (1970), who noted that in the mixed lymphocyte culture, *K*-end differences caused strong activation of lymphocytes, whereas *D*-end differences seemed to be totally inert. Stimulated by this report, several investigators found *K-D* asymmetry in a number of other phenomena (Table 8–4), among them the tempo of graft rejection. J. Klein (1972b) and McKenzie and Snell (1973) reported that skin grafts transplanted across *K*-end differences were rejected more rapidly than those transplanted across *D*-end differences. (Although this is *generally* true, a large number of exceptions exist, and the variability among different strain combinations and different *H-2* haplotypes is considerable.)

In all instances in which *K-D* asymmetry was reported, the *K*-end difference always included a difference in the *I* region, and there is now little doubt that in several phenomena it is the *I* region that is responsible for the asymmetry. For instance, in the mixed lymphocyte reaction, the *I* region causes far greater stimulation than any other region of the *H-2* complex (Bach *et al.* 1972a, b; Meo *et al.* 1973a), thus explaining why the *K* end appears stronger than the *D* end. This explanation of *K-D* asymmetry, however, does not seem to apply to skin grafting, because the *I* region causes no stronger graft rejection than the *K* or *D* regions. (All three regions cause graft rejection in the third postoperative week.) In this case the asymmetry is perhaps better explained by postulating a cumulative effect between *H-2K* and *H-2I*. Because *H-2K* and *H-2I* loci are so close together, they act as a unit in most *H-2* recombinants, and the two *K*-end loci compared to a single locus at the *D* end, provide for the different strength of the two ends.

Table 8-4. Reports on asymmetrical behaviour of the *K* and *D* ends in different functions attributable to the *H-2* complex

Function	Responses of the		Reference
	K end	*D* end	
Activation in mixed lymphocyte culture	strong	weak	Rychlíková *et al.* 1970
Graft-versus-host reaction measured by splenomegaly	strong	weak	Démant 1970
Graft-versus-host reaction measured by chronic allogeneic disease	strong	weak	Gleichmann and Gleichmann 1972
Blast transformation *in vivo*	early	late	Popp 1973
Skin-graft rejection	rapid	slow	J. Klein 1972b, McKenzie and Snell 1973
Cytotoxic antibodies after grafting	present	absent	McKenzie and Snell 1973
Cytotoxic antibodies after hyperimmunization	strong	weak	McKenzie and Snell 1973
Passive enhancibility of skin grafts	difficult	easy	McKenzie and Snell 1973
Lymphoma graft rejection	rapid	slow	Bonmassar *et al.* 1971
Bone marrow-graft rejection in irradiated hosts	absent	present	Bonmassar *et al.* 1971
Degree of immunosuppression after ALS treatment	low	high	Démant and Nouza 1971, Němec *et al.* 1973

D. Relationship Between Antigens
Detectable by Serological and Transplantation Methods

The relationship between serologically detectable and histogenetically detectable antigens must be explored at two levels, genetic (Are the histogenetically and the serologically detectable antigens controlled by the same set of loci?) and molecular (Are the determinants of the serologically detectable antigens identical with those of the histogenetically detectable antigens?).

1. Genetic Relationship

Although the loci for the histogenetically and serologically detectable antigens map in the same regions of the *H-2* complex, it does not stand to reason that they are identical. It may be argued that genetic analysis of the mouse is still too crude to separate loci that occur next to each other or are very closely linked. In fact, the results of the early work with purified H-2 antigens were interpreted as evidence for genetic duality in the *H-2* complex (Medawar 1959). Some 15 years ago, many investigators believed that the complex was comprised of at least two types of gene, one type coding for H antigens detectable by serological methods (at that time primarily by hemagglutination, hence the name), and another type coding for T antigens capable of inducing transplantation immunity. (Some investigators insisted on a third type of gene coding for E antigens involved in immunological enhancement.) The H antigens were believed to be expressed primarily on erythrocytes, to be stable to lyophilization, to appear relatively late in ontogenetic development and, when purified, to be capable of inducing humoral but not cellular immunity. The T antigens, on the other hand, were believed to be absent from erythrocytes, to be stable to lyophilization, to appear early in development, and to be capable of inducing cellular but not humoral immunity. It is now clear that there is no basis for such a distinction. Several investigators have repeatedly demonstrated that the same antigenic preparations can induce both cellular and humoral immunity, while the other presumed differences between H and T antigens have proved to be artifactual.

However, one can argue that the purified preparation of H-2 antigens contains a mixture of H and T molecules and, therefore, that the biochemistry has not proved that H and T genes are the same. This argument is difficult to refute, especially because H-2 biochemistry is still in a Paleolithic stage. At present, the strongest argument for the identity of H and T loci is provided by the $H\text{-}2^{da}$ mutant. Assuming that the $H\text{-}2^{da}$ haplotype is indeed the result of a single mutation in the $H\text{-}2D$ gene, the two functions must be controlled by the same locus, because the genetic change in the mutant strain is not only serologically detectable but also leads to skin-graft rejection (see Chapter Ten).

2. Molecular Relationship

A commonly held view is that serologically and histogenetically detectable antigens are not only coded for by the same genes, but that they also represent the same determinants of the antigenic molecule. Many believe that if the H-2 chart indicates a difference between the donor and the recipient, for example, in antigen 3, then the observed graft rejection is caused by antigen 3. However, this belief is totally without foundation. Not only is there no experimental evidence for it, but it is not something one would expect *a priori*. It is now well established that the two basic elements of humoral and cellular immunity, the B and T lymphocytes, recognize different portions of the same antigenic molecule, and there is no reason to presume that this process is any different with H-2 antigens. One might, therefore, expect that the antigens recognized by the serological and transplantation methods *are not* the same.

With this background information, one can then ask two specific questions. First, are all the histocompatibility antigens detectable serologically (and vice versa)? And second, do the histocompatibility antigens display the same degree of cross-reactivity as the serologically detectable antigens?

a. **The Problem of Serologically Undetectable H Antigens.** The answer to the first question is not clear-cut. In the inbred strains, all the major *H-2* haplotypes, as well as all the single serologically detectable antigens that have been tested, cause skin-graft rejection. The opposite, however, is not true. There are differences in the *H-2* system that cause graft rejection but have not been detected serologically. This applies to most of the minor variants, particularly those known to be derived from recent mutations. In some of these, the absence of serological detectability might be simply a matter of insufficient effort on the part of the investigators; others have been scrutinized thoroughly, and still no qualitative differences have been found.

The *I* region differs from the *K* and *D* regions in that it has not been associated with the production of typical H-2 antibodies. Although the region does code for serologically detectable antigens (Ia), these differ from the *K* and *D* series antigens in tissue distribution, biochemical properties, involvement in mixed lymphocyte reaction, and other characteristics (see Chapter Nineteen). The only evidence *suggesting* identity of the *H-2I* locus with the loci coding for these antigens is the observation that skin rejection across the *H-2I* barrier is accompanied by the production of anti-Ia antibodies (J. Klein *et al.* 1974b). Because most of the minor variants have not been tested for their ability to induce the Ia (rather than H-2) type of antibodies, it is possible that at least some of them may represent mutations in the *I* region.

Should the antigenic differences in the minor variants prove to be controlled by the *K* and *D* regions, two alternatives will have to be considered. First, minor structural changes such as those caused by recent point mutations may be sufficient to induce cellular immunity, whereas more extensive alterations may be required for the induction of humoral immunity. Second, the available major *H-2* haplotypes may represent a biased sample, because practically all of them were identified by serological methods. Serological typing may select only a certain class of *H-2* haplotypes, and the serologically indistinguishable-histogenetically distinguishable haplotypes may escape detection.

The above considerations emphasize the importance of complementing serological identification of new haplotypes with histogenetic analysis, using the F_1 test in both directions or, preferably, an exchange of skin grafts between congenic lines. In the past, this was seldom done. There has been no systematic attempt to analyze, for example, all strains carrying the H-2^k haplotype by both serological and histogenetical methods. Most of these strains were identified as H-2^k either on the basis of serology or on the basis of the F_1 test, but very few were tested by both methods. It is possible that a systematic comparative study of the "identical" haplotypes carried by various inbred strains would reveal minor differences in either serologically or histogenetically detectable antigens.

b. **Cross-reactivity of Histocompatibility Antigens.** As shown in the preceding section, H-2 haplotypes cross-react extensively when tested by serological methods. For example, antibodies obtained by immunization of an H-2^b strain with H-2^d tissue may react not only with H-2^d but also with H-2^k, H-2^s, H-2^p, H-2^q, and other target cells. Does a similar cross-reactivity exist among the antigens detectable by transplantation methods? This question can be answered by sensitizing a recipient to a certain H-2 haplotype and testing the same recipient with a graft from yet another H-2 haplotype. Specific accelerated rejection of the second graft would indicate cross-reactivity between the H-2 haplotypes of the two donor strains.

One of the first experiments of this type was performed by Mitchison (quoted by Hoecker et al. 1954), who immunized B10.D2 mice against B10 tissue, challenged the presensitized recipients with a C3H tumor, and demonstrated that the pretreated mice rejected the tumor more rapidly than the unsensitized controls. A more extensive study was described by Berrian and Jacobs (1959), who tested in a similar way all the possible permutations of recipients, first donors, and second donors, which were derived from four inbred strains: A, B10, B10.D2, and C3H. The recipients were presensitized either with viable spleen cells or with antigenic extracts prepared from spleen cells. In several combinations the authors observed accelerated rejections of the second grafts and interpreted this observation as evidence of shared H-2 antigens among the different H-2 haplotypes. Their experiments were, however, complicated by two factors. First, in at least some combinations the accelerated rejections might have been due to sharing of non-H-2 antigens, and second, the A strain carries a recombinant H-2 haplotype (H-2^a), which shares genetic regions with B10.D2 (H-2^d) and C3H (H-2^k).

Both of these complications were eliminated in the experiments of J. Klein and Murphy (1973), in which permutations of strains B10 (H-2^b), B10.D2 (H-2^d), and B10.BR (H-2^k), all on the same genetic background, were tested. In all tested combinations the authors observed significantly poorer graft survival in the experimental combinations than in the first-set controls (as determined by semiquantitative evaluation of histological sections prepared from the grafts). The degree of destruction of the experimental grafts was intermediate between the first- and second-set control grafts, suggesting cross-reactivity at the level of cellular immunity between unrelated H-2 haplotypes. One objection left unanswered by these experiments is that the observed accelerated rejections of the third-party grafts could be due to cross-reacting antibodies rather than cross-reacting cells. The antibodies produced during the rejection of the first grafts could contribute to and accelerate the rejection of the second grafts. In mice, this objection is difficult to answer, as it is not possible to eliminate completely the humoral branch of the immune response.

It is interesting to note that when similar experiments are performed *in vitro*, cross-sensitization is usually not observed (see Chapter Eighteen).

Section Three

Genetics

Chapter Nine

Principles of Genetic Analysis

I. Basic Terms and Definitions

The basic unit of hereditary material is the *gene*. "The word 'gene' does not imply any hypothesis; it expresses only the established fact that many properties of the organism have their origins in some particular, distinctive and thereby independent elements ... present in the gametes" (Johannsen 1909, p. 130). This definition, provided in 1909 by W. Johannsen, who introduced the term gene into modern biology, is, admittedly, a vague one. But in the 65 years since this proposal, geneticists have failed to agree on any more exact description; consequently, it may be best to preserve the original denotation of the gene as an abstract unit of genetic information. The term sometimes used as a substitute for gene is *cistron*, defined as a segment of nucleic acid coding for one polypeptide chain.

A particular combination of genes is called a *genotype*; a particular combination of traits or observable characteristics determined by the genotype is called a *phenotype*. In the genetic material of an organism, genes are arranged in a linear order, each gene occupying a fixed position, the *locus*. A gene may exist in several alternate forms, or *alleles*, designated by letters *A*, *a*, *B*, *b*, and so on. Alleles most frequently found in natural populations are called *wild type*; those derived from wild-type alleles by *mutation* are called *mutant*.

In a somatic cell of a higher organism, such as the mouse, each gene is represented twice, and the cell is therefore said to be *diploid*. In a germinal cell of such an organism, only one gene from each pair is present, and the cell is therefore said to be *haploid*. A diploid organism (or cell) is *homozygous* if the two genes (*alleles*) of a given pair are identical or very similar (e.g., *AA, aa, BB, bb*), and *heterozygous* if they are different (e.g., *Aa, Bb*). Often only one of the two alleles of a heterozygote is phenotypically *expressed* (manifested). An allele that produces the same phenotype when it is heterozygous as when it is homozygous is *dominant* and is designated by capital letter symbols (e.g., *A, B, C*); an allele that is phenotypically expressed only when it is homozygous is *recessive* and is designated by small letter symbols (e.g., *a*, *b*, *c*); two alleles that are both phenotypically expressed in a heterozygote are *codominant*. Dominance and recessivity are historical terms that will eventually become unnecessary, because it appears that, in the majority of cases, both alleles at a given locus are expressed, even though only one might be causing a visible effect. If a trait controlled by dominant gene *A* is not always expressed in the *Aa* heterozygote, the *penetrance* (manifestation, expression) of the gene is considered *incomplete* (partial), as opposed to *complete penetrance* of genes always exhibiting the dominant character.

The physical bearers of genes are *chromosomes*, threadlike bodies the number of which is constant in each cell and is characteristic for a given species. Each chromosome is represented twice in a diploid cell and once in a haploid cell. The reduction from the diploid to haploid status occurs at *meiosis*, the division of the nucleus preceding the formation of gametes; the restoration of diploid status occurs during fertilization, when two haploid gametes fuse together. Each chromosome in a dividing somatic cell consists of two *chromatids* held together by the *centromere*. Chromosomes with centromeres located in the middle are called *metacentric*, those with the centromere at the end are called *telocentric* (or *acrocentric*); the free ends of the chromosome are *telomeres*. In meiosis, the corresponding (*homologous*) chromosomes come together and pair along their lengths, forming the *bivalents*. At a certain meiotic stage, two of the four chromatids in each bivalent (the nonsister chromatids) break at corresponding positions and rejoin reciprocally (Fig. 9–1). The process of breakage and reunion of the chromatids during meiosis is called *crossing-over*, and the observed physical crossing of the two chromatids is known as the *chiasma*. In general, each bivalent undergoes at least one crossing-over per meiosis and may undergo more than one (i.e., double or triple crossing-over, resulting in two or three chiasmata). The number of chiasmata in early meiosis is equal to the

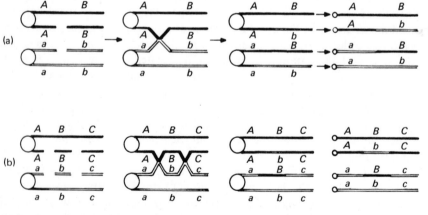

Fig. 9-1. Interpretation of single (a) and double (b) crossing-over. (*A, B, C* are linked loci; centromeres are depicted by circles.)

number of crossing-overs in each bivalent. As shown in Fig. 9–1, crossing-over leads to an exchange of genes (*recombination*) between the two homologous chromosomes.

Genes located in different (nonhomologous) chromosomes are distributed randomly among the progeny (they *segregate independently*), whereas genes located in the same chromosome may remain associated for many generations (they are *linked*). *Linkage* is defined as the tendency of two genes in the same chromosome to remain together through the inheritance process. However, the linkage of two genes is not absolute; they can eventually be separated by crossing-over. The probability of a separation of two linked genes depends on the probability of crossing-over between them. Because, in a simplified situation, the position of the break leading to crossing-over is determined by chance, genes located close together in the chromosome have a lower probability of being separated by recombination than genes located farther apart. In other words, the nearer two loci are, the closer (stronger) their linkage. The probability of recombination between two loci, the *recombination frequency* (f), is determined by the number of recombinants (i.e., individuals bearing recombinant chromosomes) divided by the total number of offspring scored.

Since the recombination frequency reflects the closeness or remoteness of two loci in the chromosome, it can be used as a measure of the distance between the two loci. A linear representation in which distances between genes are proportional to the recombination frequency is called the *genetic* (*recombination* or *chromosome*) *map*. The genetic map is usually drawn as a straight line, with genes represented as "points" separated by intervals corresponding in length to the observed recombination frequency. The length of each interval in the genetic map is expressed as a percentage of recombination, 1 percent being called one *centimorgan* (cM) or one *map unit* (*crossover unit*). The distance of 50 cM (0.5 morgan) corresponds to a recombination probability of 1.0, which means that two genes at this distance apart always recombine. Such genes are indistinguishable from independently segregating genes, and the only way to show that they are located in the same chromosome is to prove that they are both linked to a third gene located between them. All genes carried by a pair of homologous chromosomes are said to belong to the same *linkage group*, and the number of linkage groups in each species is equal to the number of chromosomes in the haploid cells.

Genetic analysis of an immunogenetic system consists of two steps. In the first step, the mode of inheritance of a particular trait is elucidated, and in the second step, the position of the newly discovered gene in the genome is determined.

II. Segregation Analysis

The manner of inheritance of the studied trait is determined by segregation analysis, in which conclusions are drawn from the segregation of the trait among the progeny of an appropriate cross. Specifically, one usually wants to know: Is the trait genetically controlled, and if so, how many genes are involved? Are the genes codominant, dominant, or recessive? Are the genes fully penetrant? Answers to these questions can usually be obtained from a single cross, provided that the cross is set up in an appropriate manner. The most commonly used cross is a *single backcross*, in which two parental strains (or individuals), P_1 and P_2, are *intercrossed*, and the resulting F_1 *hybrid* is backcrossed to either P_1 or P_2. Using a locus with two alleles, A and a, the cross can be diagrammed as follows:

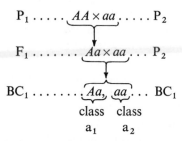

If both A and a are expressed in the F_1 hybrid, the alleles at the $A(a)$ locus are codominant; if only A is expressed, A is dominant and a recessive. Because the F_1 hybrid produces two types of gamete (A and a) in an equal proportion, and because the P_2 parent produces only one type of gamete (a), the backcross generation is expected to consist of two classes of individuals, Aa (class a_1) and aa (class a_2), in a proportion of $\frac{1}{2}:\frac{1}{2}$, or 1:1.

Consequently, to estimate the number of genes involved in the control of the trait under consideration, a backcross is set up and the number of classes, the number of individuals in each class, and the *segregation ratio* are determined. If only two classes are obtained and the observed ratio does not differ significantly from the expected 1:1 ratio, one concludes that the trait is controlled by a single locus with two alleles and complete penetrance (*simple Mendelian inheritance*). The significance of the difference between the observed and expected values is determined by a statistical test, most commonly the χ^2 test. For two classes of individuals, the χ^2 is calculated from a formula:

$$\chi^2 = \frac{(\text{observed } a_1 - \text{expected } a_1)^2}{\text{expected } a_1} + \frac{(\text{observed } a_2 - \text{expected } a_2)^2}{\text{expected } a_2}$$

The general formula for any number of classes is

$$\chi^2 = \sum \frac{(\text{observed} - \text{expected})^2}{\text{expected}}$$

where $\sum$ indicates the summation of $(\text{observed} - \text{expected})^2 / \text{expected}$ values calculated separately for each class.

The calculated χ^2 value must be converted into a P value by consulting a χ^2 table or χ^2 graph. In the χ^2 table, the P value is determined by finding the χ^2 value closest to the calculated value under a given number of degrees of freedom. The number of degrees of freedom is equal to the total number of classes minus one. Because there are only two classes in the cross described above (a_1, a_2), the number of degrees of freedom is one. By convention, if

$P > 0.05 (\chi^2 < 3.841)$ ⎫ the difference ⎫ not significant

$P \leq 0.05 (\chi^2 \geq 3.841)$ ⎪ between the ⎪ significant

$P \leq 0.01 > 0.001 (\chi^2 \geq 6.635 < 10.828)$ ⎬ observed and expected values ⎬ highly significant

$P \leq 0.01 (\chi^2 \geq 10.828)$ ⎭ is ⎭ very highly significant

(A probability of 0.05 means that a chance deviation as large as or larger than that observed would be obtained only once in 20 repeats.)

If the calculated value of χ^2 in the single backcross experiment is lower than 3.841, the conclusion that the trait under consideration is controlled by a single Mendelian gene with two alleles is justified. If the χ^2 value is equal to or greater than 3.841, the single Mendelian locus hypothesis must be rejected and alternative hypotheses tested (e.g., segregation of more than one gene, non-Mendelian nature of the gene segregation).

In cases with two classes (a_1 and a_2), such as the single backcross, a simpler formula for the calculation of χ^2 can be used:

$$\chi^2 = \frac{(a_1 - ma_2)^2}{mn}$$

where n = the total number of individuals ($a_1 + a_2$) and m is the expected proportion of the two classes, $a_1 : a_2$. In the single backcross where m = 1, the formula can be further simplified to

$$\chi^2 = \frac{(a_1 - a_2)^2}{n}$$

The use of the two formulas can be illustrated by an experiment in which the segregation of the *thin fur* (*thf*) gene was followed (J. Klein, *unpublished data*).

A single backcross *thf/+ × thf/thf* gave the following results:

	thf/+	*thf/thf*	total
observed number	148	137	285
expected proportion	$\frac{1}{2}$	$\frac{1}{2}$	—
expected number	142.5	142.5	285

From these results, the χ^2 value can be calculated as follows:

first variant: $\quad \chi^2 = \dfrac{(148 - 142.5)^2}{142.5} + \dfrac{(137 - 142.5)^2}{142.5} = 0.424 (P \sim 0.5)$

second variant: $\quad \chi^2 = \dfrac{(148 - 137)^2}{285} = 0.424 (P \sim 0.5)$

For one degree of freedom, the deviation from the expected results is not significant, so the *thin fur* trait is concluded to be controlled by a single recessive gene.

III. Linkage Analysis

The second step in the genetic analysis of an immunogenetic system is the determination of the location in the genome of the genes controlling the studied trait. This is achieved by determining the linkage relations of the studied genes with other genes in the genome. The aims of linkage analysis are to detect linkage, to estimate the linkage strength, and to determine the linear order of the linked genes.

A. Detection of Linkage

The condition for determining presence or absence of linkage between two genes is their simultaneous segregation in an appropriate cross. The most frequently used cross is the *double backcross* (test cross), so termed because a double heterozygote is mated with a doubly recessive animal. The two genes entering the cross can be in one of two phases, coupling or repulsion. Two genes are said to be in the *coupling phase* if they have been contributed by the same parent, and they are in the *repulsion phase* if contributed by two different parents. Another, but less accurate way of defining the two phases is to say that in coupling, the two dominant or wild-type alleles, *A* and *B*, are located in one chromosome and the two recessive or mutant alleles, *a* and *b*, in another, whereas in repulsion, both the dominant and recessive genes are in different chromosomes. Coupling and repulsion are sometimes also called *cis-* and *trans*-configurations, respectively:[1]

$$\text{coupling (}cis\text{-configuration):} \quad \frac{AB}{ab} \quad \text{or} \quad AB/ab$$

$$\text{repulsion (}trans\text{-configuration):} \quad \frac{Ab}{aB} \quad \text{or} \quad Ab/aB$$

Each cross designed for testing linkage should be set up in both coupling and repulsion phases. This is particularly important in cases where inviability or interaction between the genes entering the cross is suspected.

In the mouse, the recombination frequency is often higher in females than in males, although with some genes the opposite is true (Dunn and D. Bennett 1967). It is therefore important to set up the linkage test with equal numbers of male and female heterozygotes.

Considering the two genes A/a and B/b in coupling, the double backcross can be depicted as follows:

$$P_1 \cdots AB/AB \times ab/ab \cdots P_2$$
$$\downarrow$$
$$F_1 \cdots\cdots\cdots AB/ab \times ab/ab \cdots P_2$$

---

[1] The convention in writing genetic symbols is to underline linked loci with one continuous line $\left(\frac{AB}{ab}\right)$ and each independently segregating locus with a separate line $\left(\frac{A}{a} \frac{B}{b}\right)$. A noncommittal way of writing the symbols is AB/ab.

Because the F_1 parent produces four types of gamete (AB, Ab, aB, and ab), while the P_2 parent produces only one type (ab), there will be four classes of offspring:

class	a_1	a_2	a_3	a_4
genotype	AB/ab	Ab/ab	aB/ab	ab/ab

where ($a_1 + a_2 + a_3 + a_4 = n$). Of these, two ($a_1$ and a_4) represent the parental types, and the other two (a_2 and a_3) the recombinant types. (If the cross were set up in repulsion, the parental types would have been a_2 and a_3 and the recombinant types a_1 and a_4.)

If the two genes $A(a)$ and $B(b)$ segregate independently, the frequency of the recombinant types should be the same as that of the parental types:

$$\tfrac{1}{4}AB:\tfrac{1}{4}Ab:\tfrac{1}{4}aB:\tfrac{1}{4}ab$$

In other words, there should be 50 percent of the parental types and 50 percent of the recombinant types. On the other hand, if the two loci are linked, the frequency of the recombinant types should be significantly lower than that of the parental types (that is, less than 50 percent). The linkage of loci $A(a)$ and $B(b)$ can therefore be established by showing that the observed ratios of the parental and recombinant types differ significantly from the ratios expected under the assumption of independent segregation. The significance of the deviation is determined by the χ^2 test. The χ^2 formula for detection of linkage in a double backcross experiment is

$$\chi^2 = \frac{[(a_1 + a_4) - (a_2 + a_3)]^2}{n}$$

where a_1, a_2, a_3, and a_4 are the numbers of individuals in classes a_1, a_2, a_3, and a_4, and n is the total number of individuals. Although there are four classes of individuals in the experiment, the comparison is made only between *two* groups, the parental ($a_1 + a_4$), and the recombinant ($a_2 + a_3$), and so there is only one degree of freedom. The calculated χ^2 value is located in the χ^2 tables under one degree of freedom and the P value is determined. A P value of 0.05 or less (χ^2 value of 3.841 or more for one degree of freedom) indicates that the observed deviation from the expected frequencies is significant and that the two loci are linked. However, before the conclusion is finalized, one must ascertain that the deviation is not caused by factors other than linkage. This certainty is achieved by proving that each of the two loci, taken separately, shows undisturbed segregation ratios. The χ^2 formulas for testing the segregation of loci $A(a)$ and $B(b)$ in a double backcross are

$$\chi^2_{Aa} = \frac{[(a_1 + a_2) - (a_3 + a_4)]^2}{n}$$

$$\chi^2_{Bb} = \frac{[(a_1 + a_3) - (a_2 + a_4)]^2}{n}$$

Because in each of these two calculations two groups are formed from four classes, and because the final comparison is made only between the two groups, there is, again, only one degree of freedom in each case. If the P values corresponding to the calculated χ^2_{Aa} and χ^2_{Bb} values indicate a significant difference between the observed and expected segregation ratio under the single gene hypothesis, the linkage hypothesis is accepted.

The practical use of the three χ^2 formulas in linkage analysis can be illustrated by the data obtained in the double backcross

$$H\text{-}2^b + / H\text{-}2^d thf \times H\text{-}2^d thf / H\text{-}2^d thf$$

The results of this cross were the following (J. Klein, *unpublished data*):

	$H\text{-}2^b+$	$H\text{-}2^b thf$	$H\text{-}2^d+$	$H\text{-}2^d thf$	total
observed number	132	13	16	124	285
expected proportion	$\frac{1}{4}$	$\frac{1}{4}$	$\frac{1}{4}$	$\frac{1}{4}$	—

$$\chi^2_{H\text{-}2} = \frac{[(132+13)-(16+124)]^2}{285} = \frac{25}{285} = 0.088 \qquad (P > 0.8)$$

$$\chi^2_{thf} = \frac{[(132+16)-(13+124)]^2}{285} = \frac{121}{285} = 0.424 \qquad (P > 0.5)$$

$$\chi^2_{H\text{-}2-thf} = \frac{[(132+124)-(13+16)]^2}{285} = \frac{51529}{285} = 180.803 \qquad (P < 0.001)$$

This statistical analysis permits the following conclusions to be drawn. First, the observed segregations of $H\text{-}2$ and thf loci taken separately are not significantly different from segregations expected under the single-gene hypothesis. Second, the difference between the observed segregation and that expected under the hypothesis of independent assortment of $H\text{-}2$ and thf loci is very highly significant. Third, loci $H\text{-}2$ and thf are linked.

The χ^2 formulas shown above can be used only for double-backcross experiments; they must be modified for other types of cross. The general χ^2 formula for any type of cross is

$$\chi^2 = \sum \left[\frac{(a-mn)^2}{mn} \right] - n$$

where a is the observed number of individuals in class a, m is the expected proportion, n the total number of individuals, and mn the expected number of individuals in class a. The same formula can also be written as

$$\chi^2 = \sum \left(\frac{a^2}{mn} \right) - n$$

which is somewhat easier to compute.

B. Estimation of Linkage Strength

Having established linkage between two genes, the next step is to determine the *strength* of the linkage. As indicated earlier, the linkage strength is expressed as the *recombination frequency* (f).

$$\text{in coupling:} \quad f = \frac{a_2+a_3}{a_1+a_2+a_3+a_4} = \frac{a_2+a_3}{n}$$

$$\text{in repulsion:} \quad f = \frac{a_1+a_4}{a_1+a_2+a_3+a_4} = \frac{a_1+a_4}{n}$$

From this, the standard error (S.E.) of f is calculated, using the formula

$$\text{S.E.} = \pm \sqrt{\frac{f(1-f)}{n}}$$

As an example, the calculation of f and S.E. in the experiment cited above is shown below:

Female heterozygotes:

$$f_{H\text{-}2-thf} = \frac{8+11}{82+8+11+75} = \frac{19}{176} = 0.108 \quad \text{or} \quad 10.8 \text{ percent}$$

$$\text{S.E.} = \pm \sqrt{\frac{0.108(1-0.108)}{176}} = \pm\sqrt{0.000547} = \pm 0.0234 \quad \text{or} \quad 2.3 \text{ percent}$$

Male heterozygotes:

$$f_{H\text{-}2-thf} = \frac{5+5}{50+5+5+49} = \frac{10}{109} = 0.0917 \quad \text{or} \quad 9.17 \text{ percent}$$

$$\text{S.E.} = \pm \sqrt{\frac{0.0917(1-0.0917)}{109}} = \pm\sqrt{0.000764} \text{ or } \pm 0.0276 \text{ or } 2.8 \text{ percent}$$

For $F_1 \times F_1$ crosses, other methods, such as the maximum likelihood methods, must be used. These are described by M. C. Green (1963) and by Robinson (1971).

C. Determination of Gene Order

The final step in linkage analysis is the determination of the linear order of the linked loci. The order of three loci, $A(a)$, $B(b)$, and $C(c)$, in the same linkage group can be determined in two ways: by comparing their recombination frequencies, and by a three-point cross. In the first method, if the recombination frequency between A and B is f_1, between B and C is f_2, and between A and C is f_3, and if $f_1 < f_3 > f_2$, then the order of loci is A—B—C. In other words, the largest f indicates that the corresponding loci are farthest apart. With closely linked loci, however, the error in estimates of the recombination frequencies may be so large that the method becomes unreliable. In this case, the order of loci must be determined by a three-point cross. The cross is actually a linkage test with three loci ("points"). A cross

$$\frac{A\ B\ C}{a\ b\ c} \times \frac{a\ b\ c}{a\ b\ c}$$

can, theoretically, produce eight classes of offspring, two parental and six recombinant (four derived by single and two by double crossing-over; see Table 9–1). Since the frequency of double crossing-over in any given interval is always lower than that of single crossing-over, the two least frequent classes obtained in a three-point cross are assumed to be double recombinants. As Table 9–1 shows, the genotypes of the double recombinants depend on the

Table 9-1. Recombinant classes obtained with three different orders of loci A, B, and C

Crossing-over in interval	Recombinant classes obtained with indicated order of loci							
	I*	II*		I	II		I	II
	A	B	C	A	C	B	B	A	C
	a	b	c	a	c	b	b	a	c
I	A	b	c	A	b	c	a	B	c
	a	B	C	a	B	C	A	b	C
II	A	B	c	A	b	C	A	B	c
	a	b	C	a	B	c	a	b	C
I+II	A	b	C	A	B	c	a	B	C
	a	B	c	a	b	C	A	b	c

* I and II indicate intervals between genes.

order of genes in the chromosome, so the gene order can be inferred from the genotypes of the two least frequent classes.

The same example used earlier will illustrate the two methods. To determine the order of loci T, H-2, and thf, a three-point cross was set up:

$$\frac{T\ H\text{-}2^b\ +}{+\ H\text{-}2^d\ thf} \times \frac{+\ H\text{-}2^d\ thf}{+\ H\text{-}2^d\ thf}$$

The following results were obtained (J. Klein, *unpublished data*):

class:	$T\,H\text{-}2^b\,+$	$+\,H\text{-}2^d\,thf$	$T\,H\text{-}2^d\,thf$	$+\,H\text{-}2^b\,+$
observed number:	111	103	21	21
class:	$T\,H\text{-}2^b\,thf$	$+\,H\text{-}2^d\,+$	$T\,H\text{-}2^d\,+$	$+\,H\text{-}2^b\,thf$
observed number:	13	16	0	0

The recombination frequencies were

$$f_{T\text{-}H\text{-}2} = \frac{42}{285} = 0.147 \quad \text{or} \quad 14.3 \text{ percent}$$

$$f_{H\text{-}2\text{-}thf} = \frac{29}{285} = 0.102 \quad \text{or} \quad 10.2 \text{ percent}$$

$$f_{T\text{-}thf} = \frac{71}{285} = 0.249 \quad \text{or} \quad 24.9 \text{ percent}$$

Because the largest recombination frequency is between T and thf, these two loci must be farthest apart, and $H\text{-}2$ must be located between them. Furthermore, because the two least frequent classes are $\underline{T\,H\text{-}2^d\,+}$ and $\underline{+\,H\text{-}2^b thf}$, they must represent double crossovers, making the order $T \cdots H\text{-}2 \cdots thf$.

Chapter Ten

Recombination and Mutation in the *H-2* Complex

I. Recombination

A. Principle

Consider two inbred strains, A and B, and their respective haplotypes, *H-2ᵃ* coding for antigens H-2.23 and 4, and *H-2ᵇ* coding for antigens H-2.33 and 2. A single backcross

$$\frac{H\text{-}2^a}{H\text{-}2^b} \times \frac{H\text{-}2^b}{H\text{-}2^b}$$

should produce two classes of offspring, $H\text{-}2^a/H\text{-}2^b$ and $H\text{-}2^b/H\text{-}2^b$, distinguishable by typing with anti-H-2.23 and anti-H-2.4 antisera. Animals in the former class should react positively with the two antisera, those in the latter class should react negatively. An overwhelming majority of the backcross animals will, indeed, follow these expectations, but approximately one out of each 300 tested mice will be exceptional; it will type positively with one antiserum but negatively with the other, and thus will behave as if it had lost one of the two antigens. If it can be shown by breeding the exceptional mouse that the loss of the antigen persists in the next generation, it may be concluded that a genetic change has occurred. A progeny test with the exceptional animal will usually show that the loss of an antigen has been accompanied by a gain of an antigen(s) from the second *H-2* haplotype of the heterozygote. For example, if the exceptional mouse types is $+23$, -4, a progeny test will show that the haplotype that lost the H-2.4 determinant gained the H-2.2 determinant from the *H-2^b* haplotype, making the phenotype $+23$, $+2$. The process that produced the exceptional haplotype apparently resulted in a *recombination* of the genetic material of the *H-2* complex by crossing-over within the complex (intra-*H-2* recombination or crossing-over). The intra-*H-2* recombination may be diagrammed as follows:

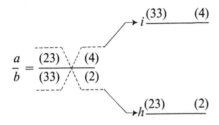

In this diagram, the horizontal lines indicate the *H-2* chromosomes and the interrupted lines the direction and position of the genetic crossing-over; the numbers indicate the genetic determinants of the corresponding antigens.

The new combination of *H-2* determinants is referred to as the *H-2 recombinant haplotype* and is assigned a new symbol, as will be discussed below.

B. Methods of Detection

H-2 recombinanus can be detected by serological testing, skin grafting, or tumor transplantation of a segregating population.

1. Serological Testing

The principle of serological detection of *H-2* recombinants was described in the previous section. In the above example, segregation of the *H-2* haplotypes was achieved by *backcrossing* the F_1 hybrid to one of the two parental strains. Segregation may also be achieved by *intercrossing* two F_1 hybrids or by *outcrossing* an F_1 hybrid to a third strain. The intercrossing produces an F_2 generation consisting of the following genotypes:

$$(F_1) \quad \frac{(23)(4)}{(33)(2)} \quad \times \quad \frac{(23)(4)}{(33)(2)} \quad (F_1)$$

$$F_2: \quad \frac{(23)(4)}{(23)(4)}, \quad \frac{(23)(4)}{(33)(2)}, \quad \frac{(33)(2)}{(33)(2)}, \quad \frac{(23)(2)}{(33)(2)}, \quad \frac{(23)(2)}{(23)(4)}, \quad \frac{(33)(4)}{(23)(4)}, \quad \frac{(33)(4)}{(33)(2)}$$

parental types   recombinant types

In this case the segregants must be tested with antisera against all four antigens (2, 4, 23, and 33) to detect the *H-2* recombinants; typing with only two antisera would not distinguish the recombinant from the parental types.

In an outcross, the F_1 hybrid is mated to a third strain, C, carrying an unrelated *H-2* haplotype:

$$(F_1) \quad \frac{(23) \quad (4)}{(33) \quad (2)} \times \frac{(17) \quad (30)}{(17) \quad (30)} \quad (C)$$

$$\frac{(23) \quad (4)}{(17) \quad (30)}, \quad \frac{(33) \quad (2)}{(17) \quad (30)}, \quad \frac{(23) \quad (2)}{(17) \quad (30)}, \quad \frac{(33) \quad (4)}{(17) \quad (30)}$$

parental types   recombinant types

In this case, typing with two antisera suffices, but typing for all four antigens is preferred.

Of the three mating types, outcross is clearly the most suitable for detecting *H-2* recombinants, because it lowers the chances of mistyping. In the backcross system, an animal typed as $+23$, -4 could be a recombinant, but it could also be a parental type in which antigen 4 escaped detection. In an outcross, such an animal, if it is indeed a recombinant, should type as 2-positive. (In the backcross progeny, all animals are $+2$, $+33$.)

Mistypings do occur frequently in the search for *H-2* recombinants and, for this reason, an *H-2* recombinant cannot be considered as having been proved until it has been confirmed by a progeny test. In this test, the presumed recombinant animal is mated to an appropriate strain and the progeny is typed for the antigens involved in the suspected recombination. If the exceptional phenotype persists in the next generation, the genetic nature of the change has been established. Once progeny from the exceptional animal is obtained, the heterozygotes are intercrossed and a homozygous line carrying the recombinant *H-2* haplotype is produced.

2. Skin Grafting

The skin-grafting method can be applied only to a segregating population obtained from a cross between congenic lines differing in the *H-2* complex. The method has been used in two modifications. In the first modification (J. Klein, *unpublished data*), animals of an (A × A.B) × A.C outcross (A, A.B, and A.C are three congenic lines with *H-2* haplotypes *a*, *b*, and *c*, respectively) each receive two grafts, one from the A and the other from the A.B parental strain. The parental-type segregants reject one of the two grafts, the recombinants reject both.

H-2 haplotype of skin-graft donor: *aa*

H-2 haplotype of segregants: *ac*   *bc*   *rc*

H-2 haplotype of skin-graft donor: *bb*

(*r* = recombinant *H-2* haplotype; → = direction of grafting, graft accepted; ⇸ = direction of grafting, graft rejected).

In the second modification (Vedernikov and Egorov 1973), the animals of an (A × A.B)F$_1$ × A.B backcross are grafted with either A or (A × A.B)F$_1$ hybrid grafts. The *ab* segregants accept the *aa* or *ab* grafts, the *bb* or *rb* segregants reject them. The animals that rejected the grafts are then used as donors for transplantation onto the A.B parental strain. The grafts from the *bb* segregants are accepted, those from the *rb* animals are rejected.

H-2 haplotype of skin-graft donor: *aa*

H-2 haplotype of segregants: *ab*   *bb*   *rb*

H-2 haplotype of second recipient: *bb*

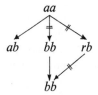

The main drawback of the skin-grafting method is its laboriousness. Furthermore, the grafting, if performed by the classic dorsum-to-dorsum technique, weakens the animals and increases the chance that they might not reproduce. A partial solution to these problems is the use of the tail-to-tail technique of Bailey and Usama (1960); however, the procedure is still more time consuming than serological typing. The advantage of the grafting technique is that it may detect recombinants that are serologically undetectable.

3. Tumor Transplantation

The tumor-transplantation method, although it produced one of the first *H-2* recombinants (Allen 1955a), has not achieved widespread use. The method has recently been used by Shreffler (1971), who challenged mice of an (A × A.B)F$_1$ × A.C outcross with two tumors, one indigenous to A, the other to A.B. The parental-type segregants should have been killed by one of the tumors, the *H-2* recombinants should have rejected both tumors and survived. However, no *H-2* recombinants have been detected. An obvious drawback of the method is that the tumors might overcome the *H-2* barrier of the recombinant and kill the animal.

C. Orthodox Interpretation of H-2 Recombinations

The first known *H-2* recombinant is $H\text{-}2^a$, assumed (but not proved) to have occurred in the early breeding history of strain A when the strain was still segregating for *H-2* haplotypes *d* and *k*. The $H\text{-}2^a$ haplotype received one portion of the *H-2* complex from the *d* haplotype and another portion from the *k* haplotype. As shown in the diagram below, the recombinant divides the *H-2* complex into two regions, *K* coding for antigen H-2.23, and *D* coding for antigen H-2.4:

$$\frac{d}{k} = \frac{(31) \quad\vdots\quad (4)}{(23) \quad\vdots\quad (32)} \searrow a = \frac{(23) \qquad (4)}{} \Bigg\} \quad \text{Regions: } K, D$$

The diagram also shows that antigens H-2.31 and H-2.32 can be indirectly assigned to the *K* and *D* regions, respectively, on the basis of this recombination.

The first three recombinants obtained in a deliberate cross were the $H\text{-}2^i$ $H\text{-}2^h$, and $H\text{-}2^g$ of Gorer and Mikulska (1959). The *i* and *h* recombinants were derived from *a/b* heterozygotes, the *g* recombinant from a *d/b* heterozygote. The *h* recombinant received its *K* region from *a* and its *D* region from *b*; the *i* recombinant received its *K* region from *b* and its *D* region from *a*. When tested with a specific antiserum reacting with antigen H-2.3, the *b* haplotype is negative, whereas the *a* haplotype and both recombinant haplotypes (*h* and *i*) are positive. This result can be interpreted as evidence for the delineation of a third region, *C*, located between the *K* and *D* regions, and coding for antigen 3 (C):

$$\frac{a}{b} = \frac{(23) \quad\vdots\quad (3) \quad\vdots\quad (4)}{(33) \quad\vdots\quad - \quad\vdots\quad (2)} \begin{array}{l} \nearrow i = \dfrac{(33) \quad (3) \quad (4)}{} \\[2em] \searrow h = \dfrac{(23) \quad (3) \quad (2)}{} \end{array} \Bigg\} \quad \text{Regions: } K, C, D$$

(Recombinant *h* separates *C* from *D*, and *i* separates *C* from *K*.)

The third recombinant obtained by Gorer and Mikulska ($H\text{-}2^g$), together with the *i* recombinant, provide evidence for yet another region, *V*, coding for antigen 22 (V). According to Gorer and Mikulska (1959), the anti-H-2.22 antiserum reacted with *b*, *i*, and *g*, but not with *a*:

$$\frac{a}{b} = \frac{(23) \quad - \quad\vdots\quad (3) \quad (4)}{(33) \quad (22) \quad\vdots\quad - \quad (2)} \searrow i = \frac{(33) \quad (22) \quad (3) \quad (4)}{}$$

$$\Bigg\} \quad \text{Regions: } K, V, C, D$$

$$\frac{d}{b} = \frac{(31) \quad\vdots\quad - \quad (3) \quad (4)}{(33) \quad\vdots\quad (22) \quad - \quad (2)} \nearrow g = \frac{(31) \quad (22) \quad - \quad (2)}{}$$

(Recombinant g separates V from K, and recombinant i separates V from C, and thus also from D.)

Evidence for a fifth region, E, coding for antigen H-2.5 (E), is based on recombinants g of Gorer and Mikulska (1959) and $o2$ of Shreffler *et al.* (1966). *H-2* haplotypes b, k, and $o2$ are 5-positive, whereas haplotypes d and g are 5-negative:

$$\frac{d}{b} = \frac{(31) \quad - \quad | \quad - \quad (3) \quad (4)}{(33) \quad (5) \quad |(22) \quad - \quad (2)} \nearrow g = \frac{(31) \quad - \quad (22) \quad - \quad (2)}{}$$

$$\frac{d}{k} = \frac{(31) \quad | \quad - \quad - \quad (3) \quad (4)}{(23) \quad | \quad (5) \quad - \quad (3) \quad (32)} \nearrow o2 = \frac{(31) \quad (5) \quad - \quad (3) \quad (32)}{}$$

$$\left.\begin{array}{r}\\ \\ \\ \\ \end{array}\right\} \text{Regions:} \quad K, E, V, C, D$$

(Recombinant $o2$ separates E from K, and g separates E from V, C, and D.)

The results of the genetic mapping with the determinant for an allotypic serum protein variant, *Slp*, discovered by Passmore and Shreffler (1970), necessitated the postulation of yet another region within the *H-2* complex, the S region. This can be demonstrated on the *o1* and *o2* recombinants of Shreffler and his co-workers (Shreffler *et al.* 1966; Shreffler and David 1972):

$$\frac{d}{k} = \frac{(31)| \; Slp^a \; | \; - \; - \; (3) \quad (4)}{(23)| \; Slp^o \; |(5) \; - \; (3) \; (32)} \nearrow$$

$$o2 = \frac{(31) \; Slp^a \; (5) \; - \; (3) \; (32)}{}$$

$$o1 = \frac{(31) \; Slp^o \; (5) \; - \; (3) \; (32)}{}$$

$$\left.\begin{array}{r}\\ \\ \\ \end{array}\right\} \text{Regions:} \quad K, S, E, V, \quad C, D$$

(Recombinant *o1* separates S from K, and *o2* separates S from E, V, C, and D.)

The *H-2* recombinants *o1* (Shreffler and David 1972) and *i3* (Stimpfling and Richardson 1965) require a seventh region within the *H-2* complex, region A, coding for antigen H-2.1 (A):

$$\frac{a}{b} = \frac{(23) \; (1)| \; Slp^a \; (5) \quad - \quad (3) \; (4)}{(33) \quad - \; | \; Slp^o \; (5) \; (22) \quad - \quad (2)}$$

$$i3 = \frac{(33) \quad - \quad Slp^a \; (5) \quad - \quad (3) \quad (4)}{}$$

$$o1 = \frac{(31) \; (1) \; Slp^o \; (5) \quad - \quad (3) \; (32)}{}$$

$$\left.\begin{array}{r}\\ \\ \\ \\ \end{array}\right\} \text{Regions:} \quad K, A, S, E, \quad V, C, D$$

$$\frac{d}{k} = \frac{(31)| \; - \; Slp^a \; - \quad - \quad (3) \quad (4)}{(32)|(1) \; Slp^o \; (5) \quad - \quad (3) \; (32)}$$

(Recombinant *ol* separates A from K, recombinant *i3* separates A from S, E, V, C, and D.)

Finally, the discovery and mapping of the genes controlling the immune response to synthetic polypeptides (McDevitt *et al.* 1972) led to an eighth region of the *H-2* complex, the *I* region. Recombinants *ol* and *tl* (Shreffler and David 1972) position the *I* region between the K and A regions:

$$\frac{d}{k} = \frac{(31)\; Ir^d\;|\;-\; Slp^a\; -\; -\; (3)\;\;(4)}{(23)\; Ir^k\;|\;(1)\; Slp^o\; (5)\; -\; (3)\; (32)}$$

$$ol = \frac{(31)\; Ir^d\; (1)\; Slp^o\; (5)\; -\; (3)\; (32)}{}$$

$$tl = \frac{(19)\; Ir^a\; (1)\; Slp^o\; (5)\; -\; (3)\;\;(4)}{}$$

Regions:
$K, I, A, S,$
E, V, C, D

$$\frac{al}{s} = \frac{(23)\;|\;Ir^a\; (1)\; Slp^o\; (5)\; -\; (3)\;\;(4)}{(19)\;|\;Ir^s\;\;?\;\; Slp^a\; (5)\; -\; (3)\; (12)}$$

(Recombinant *tl* separates *I* from K, recombinant *ol* separates *I* from A, S, E, V, C, and D.)

Thus, according to the orthodox interpretation, the *H-2* complex consists of no less than eight regions, six (K, A, E, V, C, and D) coding for histocompatibility antigens, one coding for the level of antibody response to certain antigens (I), and one for the production of serum proteins (S). The order of the regions on the genetic map is

$$K \cdots I \cdots A \cdots S \cdots E \cdots V \cdots C \cdots D$$

Serological typing of the *H-2* recombinents for the known H-2 antigens led to the assignment of these antigens to regions, as shown in Fig. 10–1. (Antigens assigned to more than one region are those that could not be positioned more precisely because of a lack of appropriate recombinants.)

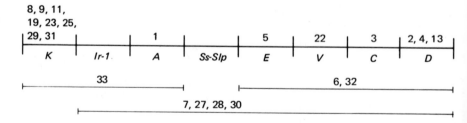

Fig. 10-1. Genetic map of the *H-2* complex according to the multilocus model. Letters designate *H-2* regions, numbers designate H-2 antigens. Antigens that could not be placed into one region are placed on lines extending over several regions.

D. Inconsistencies in the Orthodox Interpretation

The multilocus model of the *H-2* complex, described in the preceding section, is full of internal inconsistencies that make it, in its original form, untenable. The main inconsistencies are the following (Shreffler 1970, 1971; Shreffler *et al.* 1971).

1. *At least three H-2 recombinants contradict the linear order of genetic determinants (genetic map) postulated on the basis of other recombinants.* These recombinants can be fit into the genetic map only if they are assumed to have arisen by triple crossing-over. For example, the simultaneous presence of the H-2.1 antigen and the Slp^a allele in the H-2^{o2} recombinant can be explained by assuming one break between the *I* and *A* regions, another between the *A* and *S* regions, and a third break between the *S* and *E* regions:

$$\frac{d}{k} = \frac{(31)\ Ir^d\ -\ Slp^a\ -\ -\ (3)\ (4)}{(23)\ Ir^k\ (1)\ Slp^o\ (5)\ -\ (3)\ (32)}\ o2 = \frac{(31)\ Ir^d\ (1)\ Slp^a\ (5)\ -\ (3)\ (32)}{}$$

Triple crossing-over must also be postulated for recombinants H-2^a and H-2^{h2}. The occurrence of a triple crossing-over in a relatively short segment of the genetic map is highly unlikely, but not impossible. In the chromosome carrying the *H-2* complex, the frequency of double crossing-over in a segment more than 30 map units long is only about 1 percent (J. Klein and D. Klein 1972); the probability of triple crossing-over in a segment less than one map unit long can, therefore, be expected to be negligible.

2. *All H-2 recombinants derived from F_1 hybrids between H-2.3-positive and H-2.3-negative strains are H-2.3 positive,* while under normal circumstances half of them should be H-2.3-negative. The absence of 3-negative recombinants was first noticed by Stimpfling and Richardson (1965) in crosses involving H-2^a (+3) and H-2^b (−3) haplotypes. Nine *H-2* recombinants have so far been derived from the H-$2^a/H$-2^b heterozygote, and all nine are 3-positive. It has been speculated that the absence of 3-negative recombinants is caused either by asymmetrical pairing accompanied by an unequal crossing-over (Stimpfling and Richardson 1965), or by some sort of interaction between antigen 3 and other H-2 antigens, particularly 4 and 11 (Stimpfling 1965; Shreffler 1970). There is, however, no evidence for either asymmetrical pairing of the *H-2* chromosomes or for an interaction between different H-2 antigens.

3. *Recombinants H-2^{o1} and H-2^{o2}, derived from H-$2^d/H$-2^k (+3/+3) heterozygotes and therefore expected to be 3-positive, have a weak and atypical 3* (Shreffler *et al.* 1966; Shreffler 1970). The H-2.3 in these recombinants is so different from the H-2.3 in the parental *H-2* haplotypes that an anti-3-like antibody can be produced by immunization of the recombinants with parental tissue (see Chapter Five). This too can be explained

by interaction between H-2 antigens (in the presence of 4 and 11, as in *d* and *k*, respectively, a typical 3 is expressed; in the presence of 31 and 32, as in *o2* and *o1*, anatypical "3" appears), however, there is no evidence that such interaction occurs (Shreffler 1970).

4. *Some H-2 antigens controlled by different regions occur on the same molecule in purified preparations.* Presence on the same molecule has been demonstrated for antigens 3 and 4, and 5 and 33 (Cullen *et al.* 1972a), controlled, according to the multilocus model, by regions *C*, *D*, *E*, and *K*, respectively. This discrepancy can be accounted for by postulating an intragenic crossing-over (in the case of 3 and 4) and fusion of the gene products at the post-transcriptional level (in the case of 5 and 33, whose genetic determinants are separated by an intercalated gene, *Slp*, coding for an unrelated antigen).

In summary, serious discrepancies exist in the multilocus model. To resolve them, one must resort to a number of unlikely or rare mechanisms, which are not difficult to accept separately but are totally indefensible when combined together. All this suggests that the entire principle on which the multilocus model has been constructed is, perhaps, false, and that the model as a whole should be abandoned.

E. Unorthodox Interpretation of *H-2* Recombinations

An alternative to the multilocus model has been termed the *two-locus model* because it interprets the *H-2* system as consisting of only two (instead of six) histocompatibility regions, *K* and *D*. A tendency toward the development of a two-locus model has appeared in the recent publications of several investigators (Stimpfling 1971; Snell *et al.* 1971b; Démant *et al.* 1971c), but the idea was most clearly expressed by J. Klein and Shreffler (1971, 1972a).

The assumption underlying the two-locus model is the existence of cross-reactivity between antigens controlled by the *K* and *D* regions. For example, if one assumes that H-2.3-like antigens are controlled by both the *K* and *D* regions, a separate region (*C*) for these antigens is unnecessary, as illustrated through the following example.

Assuming that the *H-2ᵃ* haplotype controls two 3-like antigens, a *K*-region 3 and a *D*-region 3, the two *H-2* recombinants (*h* and *i*) that provided evidence for a separate *C* region can be interpreted as diagrammed below:

$$\frac{a}{b} = \frac{(23, \text{``3''})\ Ir^a\ Slp^a \mid (3, 4)}{(33)\qquad Ir^b\ Slp^o \mid (2)} \quad \longrightarrow h = \frac{(23, \text{``3''})\ Ir^a\ Slp^a \quad (2)}{}$$

$$\frac{a}{b} = \frac{(23, \text{``3''})\ Ir^a\ Slp^a \mid (3, 4)}{(33)\qquad Ir^b\ Slp^o \mid (2)} \quad \longrightarrow i = \frac{(33)\qquad Ir^b\ Slp^o\ (3, 4)}{}$$

Regions: *K*, *D*

The presence of H-2.3 in both the *K* and *D* regions obviates the necessity of a separate *C* region.

In a similar manner, by assuming the existence of a *K*-region 1 and a *D*-region 1 and a *K*-region 5 and a *D*-region 5, the need for separate regions *A* and *E* is also obviated. The *H-2* recombinants can be taken one by one and in all cases the *C*, *E*, and *A* regions disappear once a postulate of *D-K* cross-reactivity is introduced. The *V* region is represented solely by antigen 22; however, as has already been discussed (see Chapter Five), unequivocal evidence for the existence of this antigen is lacking. Antisera specific for antigen 22 are not available, and all attempts to obtain such antisera in combinations supposedly differing in 22 have failed. If antigen 22 does not exist, then there is no need for a separate *V* region.

By deleting *C*, *E*, *A*, and *V* regions from the *H-2* map, only two histocompatibility regions, *K* and *D*, are left, and of course, *I* and *S* regions (Fig. 10–2). The simplified *H-2* map can then be written as follows:

$$K \cdots I \cdots S \cdots D$$

All known H-2 antigens are assumed to be controlled by either the *K* or *D* region (or, in some cases, by both).

The two-locus hypothesis eliminates all the difficulties inherent in the multilocus hypothesis.

In the two-locus model, each *H-2* recombinant, including *a*, *o2*, and *h2*, can be derived from its parental haplotypes by a single crossover event. For example, the *H-2ᵒ²* recombinant, which, in the multilocus model, required the occurrence of a triple crossing-over, can be accounted for in the two-locus model by a single crossing-over in the following way:

$$\frac{d}{k} = \frac{(31, 3) \quad Ir^d \; Slp^a}{(23, 1, 3, 5) \; Ir^k \; Slp^o \, (1, 3, 5, 32)} \blacktriangleright o2 = \frac{(31, 3) \; Ir^d \; Slp^a \, (1, 3, 5, 32)}{}$$

The absence of 3-negative recombinants in crosses involving 3-positive and 3-negative types is expected under the assumption that antigen 3 is a member of

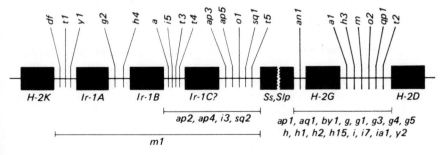

Fig. 10-2. Genetic map of the *H-2* complex according to the two-locus model. Vertical bars indicate position of *H-2* crossovers; individual crossovers are designated by small letters. Order of crossovers in each segment between solid rectangles is arbitrary.

both the *D* and *K* series. No matter what direction the crossing-over takes in the +3/−3 heterozygote, the crossover product will always carry one genetic determinant for this antigen:

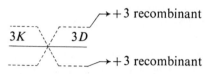

The presence of an atypical H-2.3 in the *o1* and *o2* recombinants can be explained on the assumption that the H-2.3 antigens controlled by different regions and different *H-2* haplotypes are not quite the same (see Chapter Five). Most of the classic anti-3 antisera are directed against the *D*-region 3 of the *H-2^d* haplotype, so it is not surprising that they react (cross-react) only weakly with the *K*-region 3 of *d* and/or the *D*-region 3 of *k* in the *o1* and *o2* recombinants. The difference between the different H-2.3 antigens is apparently great enough to permit production of anti-3 antibodies in combinations in which the donor carries one type and the recipient another type of 3 (e.g., *o2* anti-*k*).

The presence of antigen 3 on the same molecule as antigen 4, and of antigen 5 on the same molecule as antigen 33, constitutes strong evidence in favor of the two-locus model. According to this model, there should be only two types of H-2 molecule in an *H-2* homozygote, one carrying the *K* antigens and the other carrying the *D* antigens.

F. Evidence Supporting the Two-Locus Model

The two-locus model is supported by a number of observations:

1. *Serological cross-reactivity between K and D-region antigens exists.* As discussed previously (see Chapter Five), antisera that react not only with products of the region against which they were produced but also with products of the opposite region have been obtained. However, one might argue that in at least some combinations used for the production of cross-reactive antibodies, the antibodies could have been directed against a product of a chromosomal segment shared by the donor and the test strains.

2. *The central portion of the H-2 complex plays only a minor role, if any, in skin-graft rejection.* Skin grafts exchanged between strain combinations that differ in *A*, *E*, *V*, and/or *C* regions but are compatible in *K* and *D* regions survive indefinitely (Démant *et al.* 1971c; J. Klein and Shreffler 1972a; Démant and Graff 1973; cf. Chapter Eight). A difference in the *K* and/or *D* regions, on the other hand, leads to a rapid graft rejection (J. Klein 1972b; J. Klein *et al.* 1974b). From this it appears that only *K* and *D*, and chromosomal segments closely associated with them, are true histocompatibility regions, and that *A*, *E*, *V*, and *C* regions either have no effect on graft survival or do not exist. (Of course, the *A*, *E*, *V*, and *C* regions could control antigens not expressed on skin cells.)

3. *The private H-2 antigens can be arranged into two mutually exclusive series* presumably controlled by alleles at two genetic loci (Snell *et al.* 1971b). However, because the public antigens do not easily fit into any allelic series, the serological evidence alone does not prove that *K* and *D* are the only histocompatibility regions in the complex (see Chapter Five).

4. *Biochemical analysis has uncovered only two H-2 products,* one carrying *K*-region antigens and the other carrying *D*-region antigens. However, it is possible that, as in the case of immunoglobulin molecules, several *H-2* genes are transcribed into one molecule or that some of the H-2 molecules have a very similar structure and have, therefore, not yet been separated (see Chapter Fifteen).

5. *In the cell membrane, the K-region antigens move independently of the region antigens* (see Chapter Fourteen). However, this has been determined for only a few private antigens; whether the same applies to the public antigens is not known.

In summary, none of the available evidence *alone* provides *definitive* proof that the two-locus model is correct. Objections can be raised to and alternative interpretations found for each single observation listed above. However, taken *all together*, these observations make a strong case in favor of the model. The two-locus model definitely fits the published experimental data much better than the traditional multilocus model and is, at present, the most plausible genetic interpretation of the *H-2* system.

G. Evaluation of the Two-locus Model

The two locus model has been almost generally accepted with a serious dissention coming from only one laboratory (Stimpfling 1973). Although the original proposals of the two-locus model cautioned to leave room for the unexplored aspects in the H-2 studies, this warning was largely ignored, and the model has been uncritically adopted by immunologists outside the H-2 field. As a result important generalizations have been made based on the assumption that the two-locus model is correct. In the meantime, however, evidence has been accumulating suggesting that the two-locus model may be an oversimplification. The two main discrepancies that have been recently discovered are the following.

First, Snell and Cherry (1974) produced an antiserum in a strain combination (B10 × C3H.OH)F_1 anti-B10.D2 (*H-2* haplotype combination *b/o2* anti-*d*) and observed that the antiserum reacted with the *H-2^g* haplotype of strain HTG. Since *o2* is a recombinant that carries the *K* region of *d* and the *D* region of *K*, the antibodies present in the antiserum should be directed against antigens controlled by the *H-2D^d* allele. The *H-2^g* haplotype is a recombinant carrying the *K* region of *d* and the *D* region of *b*, neither of which should cross-react with the anti-*H-2D^d* antibodies. Snell and Cherry tentatively explained the positive reaction with HTG as evidence for a third *H-2* region located between *Ss* and *H-2D*.

Second, Stimpfling (1973) obtained two recombinants from an a/s hetero-zygote, B10.S(7R) and B10.S(9R), both of which derive their K ends from s and D ends from a. According to the two-locus model, the two recombinants should be serologically indistinguishable, as far as classical H-2 antigens are concerned. However, according to Stimpfling (1973) the two recombinants clearly differ in at least one H-2 antigen, antigen H-2.7, the 7R strain being H-2.7 positive, and the 9R strain being H-2.7 negative.

Both of these anomalous results can be explained by postulating a mutation in addition to recombination, in the HTG and 9R strains. Nevertheless, the possibility distinctly exists that they reflect the existence of additional H-2 regions, separable from the K and D regions.

Most recently, additional evidence has been obtained indicating that the H-2.7 antigen is indeed controlled by a region (G) distinct from the K and D regions, and identical with the X region. The evidence for the existence of the G region is discussed on page 208.

However, the existence of additional H-2 regions does not mean a return to the orthodox multilocus interpretation of the H-2 complex. The fact remains that the existence of regions A, C, V, and E, postulated by the orthodox model, cannot be justified. Furthermore, it is clear that loci coding for the classical H-2 antigens, detectable by serological and skin grafting methods, are unevenly and discontinuously distributed over the H-2 map, with the middle portion of the map being either quantitatively or qualitatively dif-ferent from the periphery. In this sense, addition of new regions to the H-2 complex does not negate the two-locus model but rather upgrades it. The upgrading is not an unexpected event in a system undergoing constant re-evaluation.

H. Genetic Location of H-2 Regions, Subregions, and Loci

The chromosomal segment between the K and D regions probably contains a large number of genes that can be grouped into three regions, I, S, and X (G). The genetic evidence for location of these three regions within the H-2 complex is summarized below. A detailed description of the regions will be presented in Part Three of this monograph.

1. Location of the S Region

The S region consists of genes coding for proteins found in the serum of normal mice and detected either by rabbit antimouse xenoantisera (Ss) or by mouse antimouse alloantisera (Slp). The Ss gene (Shreffler and Owen 1963) has two alleles, one (Ss^h) coding for high and the other (Ss^l) for low levels of the Ss antigen. The Slp gene (Passmore and Shreffler 1970) also has two alleles, one (Slp^a) coding for the presence and the other (Slp^o) for the absence of the Slp antigen. The Ss and Slp antigens are closely related, and it is not clear whether they are controlled by one or two genes. A detailed description of the

Ss-Slp trait will be presented in Chapter Sixteen: here, only the genetic location of the *Ss-Slp* determinants will be considered.

The evidence that the *S* region lies within the *H-2* complex can be summarized as follows. Consider two *H-2* haplotypes, *d* and *k*, differing not only in the *K* (31 and 23) and *D* (4 and 32) antigens but also at the *Ss* locus (alleles *h* and *l*, respectively). The *Ss* locus can theoretically be located between *K* and *D* (possibility 1), at the *K* end outside *H-2* (possibility 2), or at the *D* end outside *H-2* (possibility 3). Assuming single crossing-over between the three genes (*H-2K, Ss, H-2D*), the three possible gene orders would produce the following four types of crossover gametes:

Possibility 1:

$$
\frac{d}{k} = \frac{\text{(31)} \quad h \quad \text{(4)}}{\text{(23)} \quad l \quad \text{(32)}}
$$

	I	II	III	IV
I	(31)	*l*	(32)	
II	(23)	*h*	(4)	
III	(31)	*h*	(32)	
IV	(23)	*l*	(4)	

Order: *K–S–D*

Possibility 2:

$$
\frac{d}{k} = \frac{h \quad \text{(31)} \quad \text{(4)}}{l \quad \text{(23)} \quad \text{(32)}}
$$

	I	II	III
I	*h*	(23)	(32)
II	*l*	(31)	(4)
III	*h*	(31)	(32)
IV	*l*	(23)	(4)

Order: *S–K–D*

Possibility 3:

$$
\frac{d}{k} = \frac{\text{(31)} \quad \text{(4)} \quad h}{\text{(23)} \quad \text{(32)} \quad l}
$$

	I	II	III
I	(31)	(32)	*l*
II	(23)	(4)	*h*
III	(31)	(4)	*l*
IV	(23)	(32)	*h*

Order: *K–D–S*

If the *Ss* were located *outside* the *H-2* complex, recombinants between *Ss* and the whole complex should be obtained (gametes I and II under possibility 2, or III and IV under possibility 3). On the other hand, if the *Ss* locus were *inside* the *H-2* complex (possibility 1), such recombinants could arise only by double crossing-over, and so should be extremely rare. In an actual test (Shreffler 1964; Shreffler and David 1972), 3014 segregants from crosses involving *d/k, b/k, k/r, k/q,* and *al/s* heterozygotes were screened for Ss and H-2 antigens, and four recombinants (*a1, a2, o2, t1*) involving *H-2* and *Ss* were found. All four were intra-*H-2* recombinants, and no recombinants between *Ss* and the whole *H-2* complex were found.

Further support for the location of the *Ss* locus in the middle of the *H-2* complex comes from experiments in which a genetic marker (*short tail* or *T*) outside the complex has been employed. In one such experiment in which the positions of four loci (*T*, *H-2K*, *Ss*, *H-2D*) were tested simultaneously (*four-point cross*), the *H-2*^{o1} recombinant was produced in the following manner:

$$\frac{d}{k} = \frac{T\ (31)\ \vert\ Ss^h\ (4)}{+\ (23)\ \vert\ Ss^l\ (32)} \longrightarrow o1 = \frac{T\ (31)\ Ss^l\ (32)}{}$$

This combination of markers can be obtained by a single crossing-over only if the order of these markers on the genetic map is as indicated. If the order is different, double, or even triple crossing-over would be required to produce the *o1* recombinant.

Finally, support for the intra-*H-2* location of the *Ss* locus comes also from *Ss(Slp)* typing of the available *H-2* recombinants. In addition to the four intra-*H-2* recombinants mentioned above, three others (*a*, *m*, and *h3*) were also derived from *Ss*^{h}/*Ss*^{l} heterozygotes, and all three are consistent with positioning the *Ss* locus between *H-2K* and *H-2D*.

The positioning of the *Slp* locus in the middle of the *H-2* complex is based on similar evidence (Passmore and Shreffler 1970). First, in crosses designed to produce recombinants between *H-2* and *Slp*, only intra-*H-2* recombinants were obtained, recombinants separating the whole *H-2* complex from the *Slp* locus never occurred. Second, the results of typing over 36 available *H-2* recombinants derived from *Slp*^{a}/*Slp*^{o} heterozygotes were consistent with the location of *Slp* within the complex.

In cases where the F$_1$ hybrid was heterozygous for both *Ss* and *Slp*, no recombinant between the two loci was detected. This indicates that the *Ss-Slp* loci, if separate, are closely linked and positioned in the same (*S*) region of the *H-2* complex.

The conclusion from the *Ss-Slp* mapping data is unequivocal: the *S* region is located within the *H-2* complex, between the *K* and *D* regions.

2. Location and Division of the I Region

The *I* region, which is located between the *K* and *S* regions, is presently divided into three subregions, *IA*, *IB*, and *IC*, designated according to genes *Ir-1A*, *Ir-1B*, and *Ir-1C*, respectively. Because the first two genes served as genetic markers in the original mapping studies, they will be used to describe the evidence for the location and division of the *I* region. It should be emphasized, however, that both the *IA* and *IB* subregions have been associated with several phenomena that may or may not be controlled by the *Ir-1A* and *Ir-1B* genes. These phenomena, and the evidence for their association with the *I* region, will be discussed in Part Three of this text.

a. The IA Subregion. The level of antibody response to synthetic poly-peptides (T, G)-A- -L, (H, G)-A- -L and (Phe, G)-A- -L is determined by a locus, *Ir-1A*, which has been shown by segregation analysis to be closely linked to the *H-2* complex (McDevitt and Tyan 1968). The response to each of these three polypeptides can be either high or low, but strains that show high response to one polypeptide may show low response to the second or third. For example, strain C57BL is a high responder to (T, G)-A- -L and (Phe, G)-A- -L and a low responder to (H, G)-A- -L. Whether this means that there are actually three loci in the *IA* subregion, one for responsiveness to each of the three polypeptides, is not known.

The mapping of the *Ir-1A* gene was accomplished by the same principle as the mapping of the *S* region loci. In a cross designed to search for crossovers between the *H-2* complex and the *Ir-1A* gene, 484 offspring were tested and two putative recombinants were detected (McDevitt *et al.* 1971, 1972). Further analysis of the two anomalous animals, however, showed that the crossover events occurred not between the *Ir-1A* gene and the *H-2* complex, but *within* the complex. This result suggested that the *Ir-1A* gene is located between the *K* and *D* regions of the complex. The intra-*H-2* location of the *Ir-1A* gene was then confirmed by testing of the available *H-2* recombinants for their *Ir-1A* types (McDevitt *et al.* 1972). Nine of the 11 recombinants tested were shown to carry the same *Ir-1A* type as the donor of the *K* region, implying that the *Ir-1A* subregion is closely associated with this region. Evidence that the *Ir-1A* and *H-2K* were two separate genetic entities came from testing the remaining two of the 11 recombinants, *t1* and *y1*. The *y1* recombinant was obtained in a cross in which the parental *H-2* haplotypes were tagged by outside markers (*T* and *T138*) on both ends of the *H-2* complex (J. Klein *et al.* 1970):

$$\frac{a}{q} = \frac{+\ \ (23)\ \boxed{Ir\text{-}1A^k\ \ Slp^a\ \ (4)\ \ \ \ +}}{T\ \ \ (17)\ \ Ir\text{-}1A^q\ \ Slp^o\ \ (30)\ \ T138} \searrow y1 = \frac{T(17)\ Ir\text{-}1A^k\ Slp^a\ (4)\ \ \ \ +}{}$$

If the *Ir-1A* locus were at the *K* end outside *H-2*, the only other way to obtain the *y1* recombinant would be through a triple crossing-over, an extremely unlikely event. A similar line of reasoning could be applied to the *t1* recombinant. On the basis of these two *H-2* recombinants, it was concluded that the *Ir-1A* locus resides within the *H-2* complex in the region between *H-2K* and *Ss*.

b. The IB Subregion. The level of antibodies produced against myeloma protein MOPC 173 is controlled by gene *Ir-1B*, which has been shown, on the basis of its distribution pattern among the various congenic lines, to be closely linked to the *H-2* complex (R. Lieberman and Humphrey 1972). The assignment of the *Ir-1B* locus to the chromosomal segment between the *Ir-1A* and *Slp* loci is based on the analysis of five *a/b* recombinants of Stimpfling and Richardson (1965). The *h1* and *h2* recombinants carrying the *Ir-1A* and *Slp* loci of *a* and the *H-2D* locus of *b*, respond like *a*; the *i3* and *i5* recombinants, carrying the *Ir-1A* locus of *b* and the *Slp* locus of *a*, respond like *b*; but the *h4* recombinant, carrying the *Ir-1A* locus of *a* and the *Slp* locus of *b*, also responds like *b* (R. Lieberman and Humphrey 1972; R. Lieberman *et al.* 1972). Hence, the *h4* recombinant positions the *Ir-1B* locus to the right of the *Ir-1A* locus on the genetic map, and the *i3* and *i5* recombinants position it to the left of the *Slp* locus.

c. The IC Subregion. The reactivity of antiserum B10.A(4R) anti-B10.A(2R) with *H-2* haplotypes *d* and *p* defines antigen Ia.6, and Ia.6 typing of *H-2* recombinants *i5* and *o1* defines the *IC* subregion in the following way (Shreffler and David 1974):

$$\frac{a}{b} = \frac{K^k\ IA^k\ IB^k\ \overline{\left|Ia.6\ S^d\ D^d\right.}}{K^b\ IA^b\ IB^b\left|\ -\ \ S^b\ D^b\right.} \searrow_{i5} = \frac{K^b\ IA^b\ IB^b\ Ia.6\ S^d\ D^d}{}$$

$$\frac{d}{k} = \frac{K^d\ IA^d\ IB^d\ Ia.6\left|S^d\ D^d\right.}{K^k\ IA^k\ IB^k\ -\ \left|S^k\ D^k\right.}\nearrow^{o1} = \frac{K^d\ IA^d\ IB^d\ Ia.6\ S^k\ D^k}{}$$

The *i5* recombinant places the *Ia.6* determinant to the right of the *IB* subregion, whereas the *o1* recombinant places it to the left of the *S* region, and this location is supported by several other recombinants.

Most recently preliminary evidence has been obtained by Merryman and Maurer (1974) suggesting that the *IC* subregion carries the locus controlling the immune response to antigen GLT^5 (mice carrying *H-2* haplotypes *d*, *i5*, and *o1* are high responders, whereas mice with haplotypes *b* and *k* are low responders). However, since the responsiveness to GLT^5 is quite variable, the assignment of the *Ir-IC* locus to the *IC* subregion must be considered as tentative.

3. Location of the X(G) Region

An easily identifiable marker for the *X* region has been recognized only recently and consequently the knowledge of this region is still rather scanty. Antisera produced in *H-2* haplotype combination *b/a* anti-*p* contain, in addition to antibodies reacting with the private antigen of the *H-2ᵖ* haplotype (antigen H-2.16), an antibody against an antigen originally designated H-2.7. The original finding by Stimpfling (1973) that H-2.7 might be controlled by neither the *K* nor the *D* regions, but rather by a separate region located between *K* and *D* has recently been confirmed by J. Klein *et al.* (1974f) and C. S. David and D. C. Shreffler (*personal communication*). Of the independent *H-2* haplotypes the *b/a* anti-*p* sera react, in addition to *p*, with *f*, *j*, *k*, and *s*. The reaction with *k* is relatively weak and sometimes can be detected only by absorption. The genetic determinant for antigen H-2.7 defined by the above reactivity pattern is placed into the *X* region by *H-2* recombinant haplotypes *t2* and *an1*:

$$\frac{a}{s} = \frac{K^k\ I^k\ S^d\ -\ \left|D^d\right.}{K^s\ I^s\ S^s\ H\text{-}2.7^s\left|D^s\right.}\searrow_{t2} = \frac{K^s\ I^s\ S^s\ H\text{-}2.7^s\ D^d}{}$$

$$\frac{t1}{f} = \frac{K^s\ I^k\ S^k\ \left|H\text{-}2.7^k\ D^d\right.}{K^f\ I^f\ S^f\left|H\text{-}2.7^f\ D^f\right.}\nearrow^{an1} = \frac{K^s\ I^k\ S^k\ H\text{-}2.7^f\ D^f}{}$$

The $H-2^{t2}$ recombinant places the H-2.7 determinant to the left of the D region, and the $H-2^{an1}$ recombinant places it to the right of the S region, i.e., in the X region. This localization is supported by H-2.7 typing of several other $H-2$ recombinants. Since H-2.7 originally was designated G, the designation of the X region should be changed to G, and the $H-2.7$ determinant should be designated $H-2G$, as was suggested by Snell and Cherry (1974). Antigen H-2.7 has so far been detected only on erythrocytes and thus behaves as a typical blood group antigen. However, preliminary results suggest that the G region may contain determinants for weak mixed lymphocyte reaction (Widmer *et al.* 1973c, V. Hauptfeld and J. Klein, *unpublished data*), cell-mediated lymphocytotoxicity (V. Hauptfeld and J. Klein, *unpublished data*), and skin graft rejection (Stimpfling 1973).

I. Genetic Structure of the *H-2* Complex: A Summary

In the two-locus model, the *H-2* complex (Fig. 10–2) is defined as a segment of chromosome 17 delineated by the *H-2K* and *H-2D* loci. It should be emphasized, however, that this delineation is arbitrary, and that in the future it might be necessary to stretch the boundaries of the complex to include genes outside *H-2K* and *H-2D*. The term *complex* corresponds to the old (and improper) term *locus*. The alternative genetic forms of the *H-2* complex are designated *H-2 haplotypes*. An *H-2* haplotype is, then, a particular combination of alleles at the loci comprising the *H-2* complex. This term corresponds to the former improper term *H-2 allele*, and is synonymous with the term *H-2 chromosome*. The individual *H-2* haplotypes are designated $H-2^a$, $H-2^b$, $H-2^d$, and so on.

The *H-2* complex is divided by the *Ss* (*Slp*) locus into two ends, *K* and *D*. The *K* end extends from the *Ss* (*Slp*) locus toward the centromere (to the left on the genetic map in which the centromere is located by convention in the extreme left position); the *D* end extends from the *Ss* (*Slp*) locus toward the telomere (to the right). The complex is comprised of five *regions*, *D*, *I*, *S*, *X* (*G*), and *K*, separated by recombination and consisting of a marker *locus* (*H-2K*, *Ir-1A*, *Ss*, *H-2G*, and *H-2D*, respectively), and possibly a number of other loci.

By assigning at least one locus to each region, it is assumed that the known *H-2* recombinants are inter- rather than intragenic. This assumption is in accordance with current concepts of the recombination process in mammals. The term *region*, in addition to the term *locus*, is necessary because the known regions are associated with several different functions, which may be controlled by genes other than those at the marker loci. The definition of region is deliberately vague, to accommodate possible further subdivision of the *H-2* complex.

The *I* region is divided into three *subregions*, *IA*, *IB*, and *IC*, which are identified by distinct but functionally related marker genes (*Ir-1A*, *Ir-1B*, and *Ir-1C*) and are separated from each other and the other regions by recombination. Division of other regions may follow in the future. For example, it appears likely that, eventually, a recombinant requiring the division of the *S* region into

Table 10-1. Recombinant *H-2* haplotypes (solid vertical bars indicate position of crossing-over; if the precise position of crossing-over is not known, the most probable position is in the area between the two dotted lines of individual haplotypes)

Strain	H-2 haplotype symbol (New)	H-2 haplotype symbol (Old)	Parental H-2 haplotypes	K	IA	IB	IC	S	X(G)	D	Reference
A/Sn, B10.A	a		k/d	k	k	k	d	d	d	d	Snell 1951
A.AL	al	al	k/d	k	k	k	k	k	k	d	Shreffler and David 1972
A.TFR1	an1	te	t1/f	s	k	f	f	f	f	f	Stimpfling *et al.* 1971
B10.M(11R)	ap1	ap	f/a	f	f	f	f	f	f	d	D. C. Shreffler, *personal communication*
A.TFR2	ap2	ta	f/t2	f	f	f	f	s	s	d	D. C. Shreffler, *personal communication*
A.TFR3	ap3	tb	f/t2	f	f	f	f	s	s	d	D. C. Shreffler, *personal communication*
A.TFR4	ap4	tc	f/t2	f	f	f	f	s	s	d	D. C. Shreffler, *personal communication*
A.TFR5	ap5	td	f/t1	f	f	f	f	k	k	d	D. C. Shreffler, *personal communication*
B10.M(17R)	aq1	aq	a/f	k	k	k	d	d	f	f	Stimpfling *et al.* 1971
B10.BYR	by1		y1/b	q	q	k	d	d	⋮	b	J. Klein, *unpublished data*
LG/Ckc	df		d/f?	d	f	f	f	f	f	·	M. Cherry and G. D. Snell, *personal communication*; C. S. David and D. C. Shreffler, *personal communication*
HTG, B10.HTG	g	g-Go, ga	d/b	d	d	d	d	d	⋮	b	Amos *et al.* 1955; Gorer and Mikulska 1959
B10.D2(R101)	g1	g-Eg, gb	d/b	d	d	d	b	d	⋮	b	Vedernikov and Egorov 1973
D2.GD	g2	gd	d/b	d	d	d	b	b	b	b	Lilly and J. Klein 1973
B10.D2(R103)	g3	g-2Eg, gc	da/b	d	d	d	d	d	⋮	b	Vedernikov and Egorov 1973
B10.BDR1	g4	ge	d/b	d	d	d	d	b	⋮	b	H. C. Passmore, *personal communication*
B10.BDR2	g5	gf	d/b	d	d	d	d	d	⋮	b	H. C. Passmore, *personal communication*

												Reference
HTH	h	h-Go, ha	a/b	k	k	k	d	d	d		:	b	Gorer and Mikulska 1959
B10.A(1R)	h1	h-Sg, hb	a/b	k	k	k	d	d	d	:	:	b	Stimpfling and Richardson 1965
B10.A(2R)	h2	h-2Sg, hc	a/b	k	k	k	d	d	d	:	.	b	Stimpfling and Richardson 1965
B10.AM	h3	hg	k/b	k	k	k	k	k	k			b	B. D. Amos, *personal communication*
B10.A(4R)	h4	h-3Sg, hd	a/b	k	k	b	b	b	b			b	Stimpfling and Richardson 1965
B10.A(15R)	h15	h-4Sg, he	a/b	k	k	k	d	d			.	b	Stimpfling et al. 1971
B10.A(18R)	h18	h-5Sg, hf	a/b	k	:	:	b	b	b	:	.	b	J. H. Stimpfling, *personal communication*
HTI	i	i-Go, ia	b/a	b	b	b	b	b	b		:	d	Gorer and Mikulska 1959
B10.A(3R)	i3	i-Sg	b/a	b	b	b	b	.	.	d	:	d	Stimpfling and Richardson 1965
B10.A(5R)	i5	i-2Sg	b/a	b	b	b	d	d	d	d	:	d	Stimpfling and Richardson 1965
B10.D2(R107)	i7	i-Eg	b/d	b	b	b	d	d	b		:	d	Vedernikov and Egorov 1973
B10.D2(R106)	ia1	ia, id	b/da	k	b	b	b	b	b	:	:	da	Vedernikov and Egorov 1973
AKR.M,B10.AKM	m		k/q	k	k	k	k	k	k		k	q	Snell 1958b; J. Klein et al. 1970
B10.QAR	m1		a/q	k	:	:	.	.	:	:	q	q	J. Klein, *unpublished data*
C3H.OL	o1	ol	d/k	d	d	d	d	k	k	k	k	k	Shreffler and David 1972
C3H.OH	o2	oh	d/k	d	d	d	d	d	d	d	:	k	Shreffler et al. 1966
DA	qp1	qs	q/s	q	q	q	q	q	q		s	s	G. D. Snell, *personal communication*
A.QSR1	sq1	ar	s/q	s	s	s	s	:	q	q	q	q	McDevitt et al. 1972
B10.QSR2	sq2	as	s/q	s	s	.	:	:	:	q	q	q	McDevitt et al. 1972
A.TL	t1	tl	s/al	s	k	k	k	k	k	k	k	d	Shreffler and David 1972
B10.S(7R),A.TH	t2	th	s/a	s	s	s	s	s	s	s	s	d	Stimpfling and Reichert 1970
B10.HTT	t3	tt	s/t1	s	s	s	k	k	k	:	k	d	Meo et al. 1973b; J. Klein et al. 1974b
B10.S(9R)	t4	tt	s/a	s	s	s	s	s	s	:	d	d	Stimpfling and Reichert 1970
BSVS	t5		s/a	s	s	s	s	s	s	d	d	d	Shreffler and David 1974
AQR, B10.AQR	y1	y-Klj, ya	q/k	q	k	k	k	d	d	d	d	d	J. Klein et al. 1970
B10.T(6R)	y2	y-Sg, yb	q/k	q	q	q	q	q	q		:	d	Stimpfling and Reichert 1970
B10.S(8R)		Undesignated	a/s	k	:	:	:	:	:	:	:	s	Stimpfling and Reichert 1970
B10.F(13R)		Undesignated	n/b	n	:	:	:	:	:	:	:	b	Stimpfling and Reichert 1970

two subregions (*Ss* and *Slp*) will be found. The *IA* and *IB* subregions themselves may soon be split further into additional subregions corresponding to the various functions of the *I* region (see Chapter Nineteen). The distinction between region and subregion in the *H-2* complex is not very sharp. Regions are either widely separated on the genetic map, or are functionally not conspicuously related (or both); subregions of the same region, on the other hand, are both topographically and functionally related.

In the absence of any better term, the alternative forms of regions and subregions (and, of course, loci) may be called *alleles*[1] and designated by small superscript letters indicating their genetic origin. For example, the *H-2^b* haplotype can be written $H\text{-}2K^b Ir\text{-}1A^b Ir\text{-}1B^b Ir\text{-}1C^b Ss^b H\text{-}2G^b H\text{-}2D^b$ or $K^b IA^b IB^b IC^b S^b G^b D^b$, and, in a table *bbbbbbb*. The recombinant *H-2^a* haplotype can similarly be written $H\text{-}2K^k Ir\text{-}1A^k Ir\text{-}1B^k Ir\text{-}1C^d Ss^d H\text{-}2G^d H\text{-}2D^d$ (abbreviated to $K^k IA^k IB^k IC^d S^d G^d D^d$ or *kkkdddd*), and the *H-2^{y1}* recombinant can be written as $H\text{-}2K^q Ir\text{-}1A^k Ir\text{-}1B^k Ir\text{-}1C^d Ss^d H\text{-}2G^d H\text{-}2D^d$ (abbreviated to $K^q IA^k IB^k IC^d S^d G^d D^d$ or *qkkdddd*). The genotype symbols of the known recombinants are shown in Table 10–1.

J. Natural *H-2* Recombinants

Of the recombinants listed in Table 10–1, six (*a, df, m, qpl, t3,* and *t5*) deserve special comment, as they apparently occurred under conditions that are not precisely known.

H-2^a. The *a* haplotype of strain A appears to be derived from haplotypes *d* and *k*, but it is not known when the derivation occurred and what the source of the *d* and *k* haplotypes was. Strain A originated from a cross, made in 1921 by Strong, between albino mice from Cold Spring Harbor and Bagg albinos (Strong 1936; cf. Table 2–6). The latter mice were also the founders of the BALB/c (*H-2^d*) strain, so they might have been the source of the *d* haplotype in the presumed *H-2^d*/*H-2^k* parent of the original *H-2^a* mouse. The origin of the *H-2^k* haplotype in the *d/k* heterozygote is totally obscure, although here too the Bagg albinos might have been the source. The latter contention is based on the fact that the C3H/St strain carrying the *H-2^k* haplotype was also derived from a cross involving the Bagg albino mice (Strong 1942). It is conceivable that the albinos segregated for both the *d* and *k* haplotypes.

The possibility of the derivation of the *H-2^a* haplotype by recombination from *H-2^d* and *H-2^k* was first raised by Snell (1953) when he demonstrated that the *d/k* heterozygote was susceptible to *a* tumors. Subsequent serological histogenetic and immunological analyses fully supported this possibility.

H-2^{df}. The LG strain was developed from unknown heterogeneous stock by selection for large body size. The strain was separated into two sublines, LG/J and LG/Ckc, the former being *H-2^d* or possibly a minor variant of *H-2^d* (M. Cherry and G. D. Snell, *personal communication*). The LG/Ckc subline

---

[1] The term *allele* is not quite proper as it designates alternate forms of one locus, and regions and subregions may consist of more than one locus.

appears to be a recombinant which carries the K region of $H\text{-}2^d$ and I region of $H\text{-}2^f$ (Shreffler and David 1974). The origin of the D region in LG/Ckc is not clear; according to M. Cherry and G. D. Snell (*personal communication*) it codes for a new private antigen restricted to $H\text{-}2^{df}$.

$H\text{-}2^m$. The m haplotype was discovered by Snell (1958b) in a congenic line, AKR.M, derived from a cross between a noninbred stock, M (carrying coat color genes a a B B Ca Ca, but an unknown $H\text{-}2$ haplotype), and inbred strain AKR ($H\text{-}2^k$). The origin of $H\text{-}2^m$ can be explained by postulating crossing-over between $H\text{-}2^k$ of AKR and $H\text{-}2^q$ of M at some time during the production of the AKR.M line (J. Klein *et al.* 1970; Démant *et al.* 1971c). Unfortunately, stock M is no longer available, and the presumption that it carried the $H\text{-}2^q$ haplotype cannot be tested.

$H\text{-}2^{qp1}$. The $qp1$ haplotype was described by Snell *et al.* (1974) in albino strain DA derived from the so-called Swiss stock. The authors explained the origin of the haplotype as a result of crossing-over between haplotypes q and s, both of which have been extracted from the Swiss stock (strains SWR, SJL, and A.SW).

$H\text{-}2^{t3}$. Shreffler and David (1972) described a recombinant haplotype, $H\text{-}2^{t1}$, derived from a cross, $H\text{-}2^{a1}/H\text{-}2^s \times H\text{-}2^s/H\text{-}2^s$. After its establishment, the $t1$ haplotype was maintained for two generations in a heterozygous state with $H\text{-}2^s$. Two lines, HTT and A.TL, were derived from the heterozygotes, both presumably homozygous for $t1$. However, later testing (Meo *et al.* 1973b; J. Klein *et al.* 1974b) demonstrated that the B10.HTT congenic line derived from the HTT stock carried a slightly different haplotype, denoted $H\text{-}2^{t3}$. The $t3$ haplotype probably resulted from an additional crossing-over between $t1$ and s at the time when the original recombinant stock was maintained in a heterozygous state.

$H\text{-}2^{t5}$. The BSVS strain was derived from a heterogeneous stock maintained at the Rockefeller University in New York. The mice were inbred and selected for susceptibility to salmonella, some encephalitic viruses, and experimental allergic encephalomyelitis. The $H\text{-}2^{t5}$ haplotype of the BSVS strain appears to be a recombinant between $H\text{-}2$ haplotypes s and d (or a; see Shreffler and David 1974).

K. Frequency of *H-2* Recombinations

Published data indicate that 12,629 mice have been screened for $H\text{-}2$ recombinants and 52 recombinants have been detected among them (Table 10–2); of these, 43 were progeny tested and their crossover origin was firmly established. The overall recombination frequency based only on the progeny-tested recombinants is 43/12,629, or 0.34 percent; the overall frequency based on all recombinants is 52/12,629, or 0.41 percent. Some combinations of $H\text{-}2$ haplotypes seem to show higher recombination frequencies than others (Table 10–3). For example, the recombination frequency in the a/b heterozygotes is between 0.51 and 0.58 percent; the frequency in the d/k heterozygotes is only about 0.21

Table 10-2. Intra-*H-2* recombinations in experiments of different investigators

H-2 heterozygous parent	No. of mice screened	No. of recombinants recovered Progeny tested	No. of recombinants recovered Not progeny tested	Reference
a/b	194	2	0	Gorer and Mikulska 1959
a/b	1936	5	2	Stimpfling and Richardson 1965
a/b	256	2	0	Pizarro and Dunn 1970
a/b	339	5	0	Pizarro *et al.* 1961
a/b	197	1	0	Boyse *et al.* 1964b
a/f	284	1	0	Allen 1955a
a/f	617	3	0	Stimpfling *et al.* 1971
a/q	950	1	4	J. Klein *et al.* 1970
a1/f	357	1	1	Shreffler 1970
a1/s	123	1	0	Shreffler and David 1972
b/d	32	1	0	Gorer and Mikulska 1959
b/d	764	2	0	Vedernikov and Egorov 1973
b/d	195	2	0	Passmore (see Shreffler 1970)
b/da	513	2	1	Vedernikov and Egorov 1973
b/f	141	0	0	Stimpfling *et al.* 1971
b/k	839	0	0	Stimpfling and Richardson 1965
b/k	773	0	0	Shreffler 1964, Shreffler and David 1972
b/r	95	0	1	Snell *et al.* 1967b
b/y1	184	1	0	J. Klein *unpublished results*
d/k	1452	3	0	Shreffler 1964, Shreffler and David 1972
f/t1	405	2	0	Shreffler 1970
f/t2	605	5	0	Shreffler 1970
k/q	364	0	0	Shreffler and David 1972
k/r	302	0	0	Shreffler and David 1972
q/s	484	2	0	McDevitt *et al.* 1972
Total	12401	42	9	

percent. In some combinations of *H-2* haplotypes (i.e., *b/f*, *k/q*, and *q/r*), no recombinants have been detected, but the number of progeny tested in these combinations was relatively small and the absence of the *H-2* recombinants could have been caused by chance. In only one combination (*b/k*) was the number of screened animals high enough (1612) to arouse the suspicion that something other than mere chance was responsible for the failure to find any recombinants. In this combination, however, an *H-2* recombinant has recently been found (B. D. Amos, quoted by Shreffler and David 1972).

The recombination frequency seems to be higher in females than in males (Table 10–4). This sex effect is most pronounced in combinations *a/b* and *d/k*, in which a relatively high number of progeny has been tested. In these two combinations, the recombination frequency in males is approximately half that

Table 10-3. Frequency of intra-*H-2* recombination in different *H-2* haplotypes (Summary of Table 10-2)

H-2 heterozygous parent	No. of mice screened	No. of recombinants recovered		Recombination frequency (%)	
		Progeny tested	All recombinants	Conservative estimate*	Nonconservative estimate**
a/b	2922	15	17	0.5133	0.5818
a/f	901	4	4	0.4439	0.4439
a/q	950	1	5	0.1053	0.5263
a1/f	357	1	2	0.2801	0.5602
a1/s	123	1	1	0.8130	0.8130
b/d	991	5	5	0.5045	0.5045
b/da	513	2	3	0.3899	0.5848
b/f	141	0	0	—	—
b/k	1612	0	0	—	—
b/r	95	0	1	1.0526	1.0526
b/y1	184	1	1	0.5435	0.5435
d/k	1452	3	3	0.2066	0.2066
f/t1	405	2	2	0.4938	0.4938
f/t2	605	5	5	0.8264	0.8264
k/q	364	0	0	—	—
k/r	302	0	0	—	—
q/s	484	2	2	0.4132	0.4132
Total	12401	42	51	0.3412	0.4062

* Based on progeny tested recombinants.
** Based on all recombinants, even those that were not progeny tested.

Table 10-4. Frequency of intra-*H-2* recombination in females and males

H-2 heterozygous parent	Females		Males		References
	No. recombinants/ total no. mice	Recombination frequency (%)	No. recombinants/ total no. mice	Recombination frequency (%)	
a/b	7/1119	0.6256	4/1267	0.3157	Gorer and Mikulska 1959, Stimpfling and Richardson 1965, Pizarro and Dunn 1970
a/s	0/71	—	1/52	1.9231	Shreffler and David 1972
b/d	2/764	0.2618	—	—	Vedernikov and Egorov 1973
b/da	3/513	0.5848	—	—	Vedernikov and Egorov 1973
b/k	0/869	—	0/743	—	Shreffler 1964, Stimpfling and Richardson 1965, Shreffler and David 1972
d/k	2/726	0.2755	1/726	0.1377	Shreffler 1964, Shreffler and David 1972
k/r	0/162	—	0/140	—	Shreffler and David 1972
k/q	0/177	—	0/187	—	Shreffler and David 1972
Total	14/4401	0.3181	6/3115	0.1926	

in females. The total recombination frequency in females is 0.32 percent, and in males 0.19 percent.

Recombination frequencies between the individual regions of the *H-2* complex are also different (Table 10–5). The highest incidence of crossing-over is in the chromosomal segment between the *S* and *D* regions (0.19 percent), the lowest between the *K* and *IA* regions (0.02 percent). The *K* end seems to be slightly shorter in terms of genetic distance than the *D* end (0.14 and 0.19 map units, respectively), which indicates that the *Ss* (*Slp*) locus might be located not in the middle of the *H-2* complex but eccentrically (closer to the *K* region).

It should be emphasized, however, that all the frequencies given in Tables 10–2 through 10–5 must be taken with a grain of salt, for several reasons. First, almost all the screening for recombinants was done by serological techniques, which are often unreliable. [The only recombinants detected by transplantation methods were those described by Allen (1955a) and by Vedernikov and Egorov (1973)]. It is likely that some recombinants escaped detection during the serological screening because they mimicked phenotypically the negative parental type of segregants (false negatives). Second, the different combinations of *H-2* haplotypes are not strictly comparable because some antigens are more easily

Table 10-5. Frequency of recombination between different regions and subregions of the *H-2* complex (Based on Table 10-2)

H-2 heterozygous parent	Total number animals tested	K—IA	IA—IB	IB—S	S—D
a/b	2130	0	1	2	4
a/f	617	0	0	0	2
a/q	950	1	0	0	0
al/f	357	0	0	0	1
al/s	123	1	0	0	0
b/d	991	0	0	0	4
b/da	513	0	0	0	2
b/y	184	0	0	0	1
d/k	1452	0	0	1	2
f/t	405	0	0	1	1
f/t2	605	0	0	3	0
q/s	484	0	0	2	0
Total	8811	2	1	9	17

Recombination frequency:

K—IA: 2/8811 = 0.0227 percent
IA—IB: 1/8811 = 0.0113 percent
IB—S: 9/8811 = 0.1021 percent
S—D: 17/8811 = 0.1929 percent
K—S: 12/8811 = 0.1362 percent
K—D: 29/8811 = 0.3291 percent

detected than others, and with the weaker antigens, the probability of false negative results is increased. Third, in some cases the antisera used for screening had a low chance of picking up recombinants. For example, in one experiment (Stimpfling and Richardson 1965), screening for b/k recombinants was carried out with anti-3, anti-8, and anti-11 antisera. Because antigens 8 and 11 belong to the same series (K) and antigen 3 is a member of both K and D series, the absence of recombinants in this particular experiment is not surprising. Fourth, the screening did not always cover the whole *H-2* complex. For instance, the two recombinants detected by Passmore (Shreffler 1970) were found among progeny screened for *Slp* and for the *D*-region antigen 2; no testing for a *K*-region marker was done in this particular cross. For these reasons, the recombination frequency of 0.34 percent is probably an *underestimate*.

In combinations in which sufficient numbers of progeny have been tested, the reciprocal crossover types generally occur with approximately equal frequencies. The only serious exception to this rule is the d/b combination, in which only $K^d D^b$ and no $K^b D^d$ recombinants were found. Recently, however, a $K^b D^d$ recombinant has been described by Vedernikov and Egorov (1973).

The *H-2* recombinants sometimes seem to occur in "clusters." For example, Shreffler and David (1972) described a cross in which 381 animals were tested and two recombinants were found—both in the same litter! Moreover, a third recombinant was found in the immediate progeny of one of the first two. The clustering could be due to chance, to environmental effects, to chromosomal instability, or to a number of other factors (Shreffler and David 1972).

L. How Many Loci are in the *H-2* Complex?

It has been estimated that the diploid nucleus of a mouse cell contains approximately 8.5×10^{-12} g of DNA (Bachman 1972). This corresponds to

$$\frac{(8.5 \times 10^{-12}) \times (6.0234 \times 10^{23})}{327} = 1.565 \times 10^{10} \text{ nucleotides}$$

[(6.0234×10^{23}) is Avogadro's number, and 327 is the average molecular weight of the four nucleotides constituting the DNA molecule.] The number of nucleotide pairs per haploid mouse nucleus is

$$\frac{1.565 \times 10^{10}}{4} = 3.912 \times 10^9$$

Assuming an average cistron length of 600 nucleotide pairs, the number of cistrons in the mouse genome is

$$\frac{3.912 \times 10^9}{600} = 6.5 \times 10^6$$

The average number of chiasmata per mouse meiosis is 25 (Kyslíková and Forejt

1972). Assuming a one-to-one relationship between chiasmata and crossing-over, the total length of the genetic map in the mouse is

$$\frac{25}{2} \times 100 = 1250 \text{ cM}$$

(Of the four chromatids constituting a meiotic chromosome, only two participate in the crossing-over; the total number of chiasmata must, therefore, be divided by 2.) A recombination frequency of 0.4 percent represents

$$\frac{0.4}{1250} = 0.00032 \text{ of the mouse genome}$$

and therefore, the number of cistrons in the *H-2* complex is $0.0003 \times 6.5 \times 10^6$, or approximately 2000.

Such calculations, however, have two main fallacies: they are based on inaccurate figures and on an ignorance of the genetic organization of the mammalian chromosome. The estimates of chiasma frequency vary from 20 to 50 per meiosis, the map length from 1000 to 2500 cM, the amount of DNA from 5 to 9 pg, the average number of nucleotide pairs per cistron from 450 to 1500, and the intra-*H-2* recombination frequency from 0.1 to 1.5 percent. As for the organization of the mouse chromosome, it is not known whether all the DNA is functional, how much of it is reiterated, and whether crossing-over occurs between cistrons as well as within cistrons. Thus, the calculations of the number of *H-2* loci are not very meaningful; all they show is that there is enough space in the *H-2* complex for a great number of genes.

II. Mutation

A. Definitions

A *mutation* is any inheritable alteration of the genetic material not caused by recombination. The alteration can effect a single gene (*gene* or *point mutation*) or a larger segment of a chromosome (*chromosome mutation*). A mutation resulting from a loss of genetic material is a *deletion*; a mutation resulting from a doubling of genetic material is a *duplication*. Mutations may arise in the absence of any definable cause (*spontaneous mutations*), or they may be induced experimentally (*induced mutations*) by various physical or chemical agents (*mutagens*). The probability that a mutation will arise is called the *mutation rate*. The mutation rate in unicellular organisms, such as bacteria, is usually expressed as the probability of a mutation of one gene in a single cell division (one generation), while in more complex organisms, such as the mouse, it is expressed as the probability of a mutation of one gene in a single gamete. The mouse is a diploid organism (each gene is represented twice), so each newly detected mutation represents a change in one of the two gametes that gave rise to the zygote and the individual. Therefore, one mutation found among 1000 mice represents one genetic change per 2000 gametes. Hence, to obtain the mutation rate, the proportion of detected mutations in a given sample of mice must be multiplied by 0.5 (i.e., $1/1000 \times 0.5 = 1/2000$). For the calculation of the mutation rate, only animals whose parents were shown to be free of mutations (i.e., parents that are not *mutation carriers*) must be used. A mutation carrier transmits the mutation into half its progeny and causes the appearance of mutation *clusters* among the tested animals. The inclusion of such clusters into the calculations would result in unnaturally high mutation rates.

Mutations in histocompatibility loci may theoretically result in a *loss*, a *gain*, or both a *loss and gain* of an antigen.

B. Methods of Detection

In theory, screening for mutations affecting *H* loci can be carried out by both serological and transplantation methods. In practice, however, serological screening for *H* mutations is not feasible because it means not only testing each individual with dozens of antisera, but also immunizing with the tissue of the tested animals (to uncover possible gain mutations). In the transplantation method, on the other hand, two grafts on each recipient test for all three mutation types, that is, gains, losses, and losses and gains.

In the grafting system proposed by Bailey and Kohn (1965) for the detection of *H* mutations and known as the *reciprocal circle* (Fig. 10-3a), the mice are divided into groups, each group consisting of eight to ten animals (the number, however, may vary), and grafts are exchanged among the mice in each group

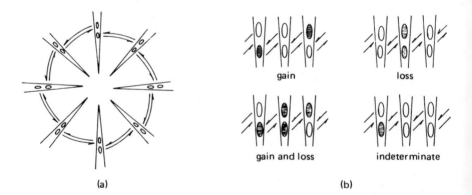

gain   loss

gain and loss   indeterminate

(a)   (b)

Fig. 10-3. (*a*) Reciprocal circle system of skin grafting for detection of *H* mutations. Large V's represent mouse tails, small ovals within the V's represent grafts, and arrows indicate direction of grafting. (*b*) Different patterns of graft rejection expected in segments of the reciprocal circle when *H* mutation occurs. Shaded ovals represent rejected grafts, empty ovals represent permanently accepted grafts. (Reproduced with permission from D. W. Bailey and H. I. Kohn: "Inherited histocompatibility changes in progeny of irradiated and unirradiated inbred mice." *Genetic Research* (Camb.) **6**:330–340. Copyright © 1965 by Cambridge University Press. All rights reserved.)

in such a way that each mouse donates two grafts and receives two grafts. Because the loss-type mutations would not be detectable in *H* homozygotes, the screening is carried out on F_1 hybrids between two standard inbred strains. The three mutation types (gain, loss, loss and gain) can be distinguished by the different pattern of graft rejection found in a segment of the reciprocal circle (Fig. 10–3b). This method should pick up mutations in any of the great number of *H* loci present in inbred mice. To determine whether a mutation has occurred in the *H-2* complex, it must be subjected to a linkage test.

Methods specifically designed to screen for *H-2* mutations have been proposed and used by Egorov. One such method (Egorov and Blandova 1972), a variant of Bailey's reciprocal circle system, is one in which the inbred parents of the F_1 hybrid are replaced by two congenic lines differing in the *H-2* complex. In this case, all the mutations of the loss and loss-and-gain types should be mutations in the *H-2* complex. Loss-type mutations at the non-*H-2* loci are, in this case, undetectable, because the F_1 hybrids are homozygous at all loci except *H-2*; loss-and-gain-type mutations at the non-*H-2* loci would appear as gain-type mutations. Any gain-type mutations occurring in the F_1 hybrid between two *H-2* congenic lines could represent alterations at *H-2* as well as non-*H-2* loci, and the determination of which genes are actually altered must be made by a linkage test.

In the second method proposed by Egorov (1967a), F_1 hybrids between two *H-2* congenic lines, B10 ($H-2^b$) and B10.D2 ($H-2^d$) for example, are challenged with skin grafts from one of the two parental strains (B10.D2). The nonmutant F_1 animals should accept the grafts, the mutants should reject them (provided that the mutation is of a loss or loss-and-gain type). The suspected mutants are then backcrossed to the second parent (B10) and the backcross animals are challenged with two grafts, one from the grandparent (B10.D2) and the other from the mutant F_1 hybrid parent. Animals that reject both grafts are presumed to be the nonmutant *H-2* homozygous segregants (*bb*); animals that reject the graft from the grandparent (B10.D2) but accept the graft from the parent are presumed to be carriers of the mutation:

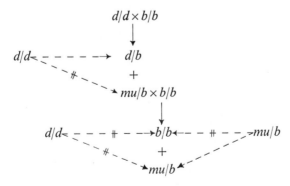

(*mu* = mutant *H-2* haplotype; – – – – – – → = acceptance of a graft from a given donor; – – – ╫ – – → = rejection of a graft from a given donor.)

C. Frequency of *H* mutations

A total of 29,648 mice have been tested for spontaneous *H* mutations by skin grafting (Bailey and Kohn 1965; Bailey 1966; Egorov 1967a; Egorov and Blandova 1972; Kohn 1973; Kohn and Melvold 1974; Melvold and Kohn 1974) and 113, or 0.4 percent, of mutant animals have been found (Table 10–6). However, some of the mutants formed clusters that were probably derived from mutation carriers; for many others the information on mutation carriers could not be extracted from the published data. After exclusion of all these animals, the mutation frequency is 53/28,402, or 0.2 percent, and the mutation rate is 0.93×10^{-3} per gamete (Table 10–7). In other words, approximately one in every 536 mice carries an *H* mutation. This might seem a relatively high figure [in the mouse, the mutation rates of dominant and recessive viable genes are below 10^{-4}, usually below 10^{-5}, and often as low as 10^{-6} (Searle 1972; 1974)], but it must be remembered that this is a mutation rate of a *group* of loci, rather than a single locus. The total number of *H* loci is not known, but the figure is certainly higher than 30 and might be as high as several hundred (see Chapter Eight). To obtain the actual per locus mutation rate, one would have to divide the 0.93×10^{-3} figure by the number of *H* loci.

Similarly, a total of 7132 mice have been tested for induced *H* mutations by the same investigators and 81, or 1.1 percent, of mutant animals have been found (Table 10–6). After exclusion of mutation carriers, the induced mutation frequency is 23/4478, or 0.5 percent, and the mutation rate is 2.57×10^{-3}. As expected, there is considerable variability among the results depending on the type of mutagen used (chemical mutagens seem to be more effective than X-rays)

Table 10-6. Histocompatibility mutations in inbred and F_1 hybrid mice

Strain combination	Treatment of the ♂ parent	No. of mutants found	Total no. tested	Percent of mice with mutation	Reference
$(C57BL/6 \times BALB/c)F_1$	none	68	2609	2.6 ⎫	Bailey and Kohn 1965,
	X-rays	57	3156	1.8 ⎭	Bailey 1966
$(A \times A.CA)F_1$	none	0	204	0.0 ⎫	Egorov and Blandova 1972
	diethylsulphate	1	514	0.2 ⎭	
$(B10.D2 \times C57BL/10)F_1$	none	1	519	0.2 ⎫	Egorov and Blandova 1972
	diethylsulphate	14	864	1.6 ⎭	
$(B10.D2 \times C57BL/10)F_1$	diethylsulphate	1	154	0.6	Egorov 1967a
C57BL/6	none	7	4003	0.2 ⎫	Melvold and Kohn 1974
	triethylenemelamine	0	670	— ⎭	
BALB/c	none	2	4889	0.04 ⎫	Melvold and Kohn 1974
	triethylenemelamine	5	1211	0.4 ⎭	
$(C57BL/6 \times BALB/c)F_1$	none	35	17424	0.2 ⎫	Melvold and Kohn 1974
	triethylenemelamine	3	563	0.5 ⎭	
	Total spontaneous	113	29648	0.4	
	Total induced	81	7132	1.1	

and the dose of the particular mutagen. However, the overall induced mutation rate is significantly higher than the spontaneous rate.

Of the 142 *H* mutations (spontaneous and induced) detected by Bailey and Kohn (1965), Bailey (1966,) Egorov (1967a) and Egorov and Blandova (1972), 134 were of the gain type, 3 of the loss type, and 4 of the loss-and-gain type. In the experiments of Kohn (1973), Kohn and Melvold (1974) and Melvold and Kohn (1974), the distinction between gain and gain-and-loss types of mutations could not always be made; for this reason, the authors grouped together the two types under "gains." Among the 35 independent mutations they found 25 gains and 10 losses (most of the gains that could be analyzed turned out to be of the loss-and-gain type). The preponderance of the gain (or loss-and-gain) type mutations was originally explained by Bailey and Kohn (1965) as an artifact of the method used for the detection of *H* mutations. The two parental strains of the F_1 hybrid carry different alleles at some *H* loci and identical alleles at other *H* loci. In the latter type of *H* loci, only gain-type mutations can be detected, loss mutations at these loci pass undetected. Bailey (1966) also offered an alternative explanation of the preponderance of gain mutations. He speculated that the *H* mutations might actually be the result of incorporation of viral genomes into germinal cells of the parents in a manner paralleling the phenomenon of lysogeny in bacteria. According to Bailey, the incorporation is accompanied by the appearance of new transplantation antigens in the cell membrane of the somatic cells descending from the "infected" germinal cells. In support of this hypothesis, Bailey (1966) cites his observation [later confirmed by Kohn and Melvold (1974)] that the spontaneous mutation rate is significantly influenced by environmental conditions: maintenance of mice in "less-isolated" environments (i.e., more exposed to viral infections) seems to correlate with higher spontaneous *H*

Table 10-7. Mutation rates at histocompatibility loci in inbred and F_1 hybrid mice after exclusion of mutation carriers and/or mutation clusters

Strain combination	Treatment of the ♂ parent	No. mutants found/total no. mice tested	Mutation rate $(\times 10^{-3})$*	Reference
$(C57BL/6 \times BALB/c)F_1$	none	17/1567	5.42	Bailey 1966
$(C57BL/6 \times BALB/c)F_1$	X-rays	4/656	3.05	Bailey 1966
$(B10.D2 \times C57BL/10)F_1$	none	1/519	0.96	Egorov and Blandova 1972
$(B10.D2 \times C57BL/10)F_1$	diethylsulphate	10/864	5.79	Egorov and Blandova 1972
$(A. \times A.CA)F_1$	diethylsulphate	1/514**	0.97	Egorov and Blandova 1972
C57BL/6	none	5/4003	0.62	
	triethylenemelamine	0/670	—	
BALB/c	none	2/4889	0.20	Melvold and Kohn 1974,
	triethylenemelamine	5/1211	2.06	Kohn 1973
$(C57BL/6 \times BALB/c)F_1$	none	28/17424	0.80	
	triethylenemelamine	3/563	3.55	
	Total spontaneous	53/28402	0.93	
	Total induced	23/4478	2.57	

* Per locus per gamete. The calculations are based on the assumption that *H* is a single locus. This assumption is known to be incorrect; the correct figure could be obtained by dividing the calculated rate by the total number of existing *H* loci, but that number is not known.

** The one detected mutation appears to be of spontaneous origin.

mutation rates. The variation in spontaneous mutation rates is a peculiarity of the *H* system; the mutation rates at non-*H* (e.g., coat color) loci are relatively stable under different environmental condition (cf. Searle 1972; 1974).

The frequency of spontaneous mutations at the *H* loci of the *H-2* complex is 14/31,143, or 0.04 percent (i.e., one mutant animal per 2224 mice tested, see Table 10–8). Assuming that there are only three *H* loci in the *H-2* complex, the mutation rate per an *H-2* locus is 7.49×10^{-5}. However, this figure is misleading because there appear to be significant differences in mutability between individual *H-2* loci and *H-2* alleles. The most unstable allele known is *H-2K^b*. Melvold and Kohn (1974) tested an approximately equal number of *H-2^b* and *H-2^d* genes and found nine independent *H-2* mutations among 26,316 screened mice. Eight of the nine mutations turned out to have occurred in the *H-2K^b* gene and only one occurred in the *H-2^d* haplotype. The authors calculated the mutation rate of the *H-2K^b* as being 5.5×10^{-4} per generation, which is by far the highest reported mutation rate for a mammal. This extraordinary mutation rate can be explained in several different ways. The most logical explanation may seem to be that the *H-2K^b* is not a single locus but a cluster of many loci with similar function. Arguing against this explanation is the fact that the eight mutant alleles fail to complement each other (Melvold and Kohn 1974), suggesting that the mutations all occurred at the same locus. Another possibility is that the mutations are regulatory rather than structural. However, all eight mutations are of the loss-and-gain type, and it is difficult to visualize how a regulatory mutation can effect this type of an antigenic change. A third possibility is that *H-2* alleles control products that can tolerate more structural changes than most other proteins (see the discussion of the *H-2* polymorphism in Chapter Twelve). And finally, it is conceivable that the mutations are minor chromosomal aberrations reflecting great evolutionary instability of the *H-2^b* haplotype. Whatever the explanation, it is clear that the *H-2* mutations will provide important clues to understanding of *H-2* genetic structure.

D. *H* Mutations and Divergence of Sublines

Sublines of the commonly used inbred and congenic strains are maintained in many different laboratories and are thus physically separated from each other.

Table 10-8. Mutation rates at the *H-2* complex

Strain combination	*H-2* haplotype	No. mutants found/total no. mice tested	Mutation rate ($\times 10^{-4}$)*	Reference
(C57BL/10 × B10.D2)F₁	b/d	1/154	32.47	Egorov 1967a
(C57BL/6 × BALB/c)F₁	b/d	2/2572	3.89	Bailey and Kohn 1965
(C57BL/10 × B10.D2)F₁	b/d	1/1383	3.61	Egorov and Blandova 1972
(A.CA × A)F₁	f/a	1/718	6.96	Egorov and Blandova 1972
C57BL/6	b/b	3/4003	3.75	Melvold and Kohn 1974
BALB/c	d/d	0/4889	—	Melvold and Kohn 1974
(C57BL/6 × BALB/c)F₁	b/d	6/17424	1.72	Melvold and Kohn 1974
Total		14/31143	2.25	

* Per *H-2* complex per gamete.

This separation can be expected to lead to an accumulation of mutational differences and to a genetic divergence of the sublines. The *H* loci as a group have a high mutation rate, so the different sublines should rapidly become histoincompatible, and histoincompatibilities have, indeed, been detected in independently maintained sublines (Billingham *et al.* 1954; Kindred 1963; Linder 1963; M. Green and Kaufer 1965). There are also, however, several examples of sublines that have been separated for a number of generations and yet remained histocompatible. For instance, sublines CBA/J and CBA/Ca have been separated since 1932, yet in 1965 they permanently accepted mutually exchanged skin grafts (M. Green and Kaufer 1965); sublines C57BL/6J and C57BL/10Sn have been separated at least since 1937 and show only a very minor histoincompatibility (Jeekel *et al.* 1972; McKenzie and Snell 1973). This lack of genetic divergence among the sublines might seem to be at odds with the high mutation rate of the group of *H* loci. However, it must be remembered that not every mutation that occurs is fixed. On the contrary, newly arisen mutations have only a low probability of being transmitted to the next generation, and an even lower probability of becoming homozygous in the pair of mice selected in each generation for propagation of the line.

Histoincompatibilities between sublines can also be caused by factors other than mutations, namely residual heterozygosity at the time of separation of the sublines, or genetic contamination. These two factors, rather than a mutation, are the most likely explanation of cases in which a certain subline suddenly acquires an *H-2* haplotype known to be present in other inbred strains. For example, Borges and Kvedar (1952) developed a new subline of C57BL/10 mice by breeding animals that survived the inoculation of a C57BL/6 (*H-2^b*) strain tumor. The resistant subline was later typed as *H-2^d* (Snell and Borges 1953), and the change from *H-2^b* to *H-2^d* was explained as a mutation. Similar "mutations" were also described in other strains (Borges *et al.* 1954). However, it is highly unlikely that the whole *H-2* complex would mutate as a unit or that it would mutate to a known *H-2* haplotype (Amos *et al.* 1955; Gorer 1956). All the proved *H-2* mutations, as described below, changed the *H-2* chromosome less drastically and always to a new *H-2* haplotype. All the reported instances of "mutations" to known *H-2* haplotypes probably resulted either from residual heterozygosity or from contamination by another line. On the other hand, some minor *H-2* variants (*be*, *ja*, etc.) could be the result of genuine mutational divergence of genetically separated lines and sublines.

E. Description of Known *H-2* Mutations

Seventeen *H-2* mutations have so far been reported in the literature (12 in *H-2^b*, 2 in *H-2^f*, 2 in *H-2^d*, and 1 in *H-2^k*); of these, 10 occurred in the *K* end and 1 in the *D* end (the remaining 6 mutations are unmapped). The 10 *K*-end mutations are detectable only by transplantation methods, the one *D*-end mutation is detectable by both transplantation and serological methods. It is too early to say whether this *K-D* difference is an indication of a general pattern or whether it is simply coincidental. All seventeen mutations effected both gain and loss of antigens. The description of the individual mutations follows.

B6.C—H-2^{ba} This mutation was detected by Bailey and Kohn (1965) and analyzed by Bailey *et al.* (1971). The mutation arose spontaneously in a (C57BL/6 × BALB/c)F$_1$ female and was subsequently placed on the C57BL/6 (B6) background by repeated backcrossing and selection for the mutant phenotype. The resulting congenic line was originally designated B6.C(Hz1), but this was later changed to B6.C-H-2^{ba}. Linkage of the mutation with the *H-2* complex was deduced from the fact that B6 skin grafts were rejected by (B10.D2 × B6.C-H-2^{ba})F$_1$ but not by (B10 × B6.C-H-2^{ba})F$_1$ hybrids. Had the mutation occurred at a locus other than *H-2*, the B6.C-H-2^{ba} congenic line would be expected to carry the *H-2^b* haplotype of the B6 strain and B6 grafts would be accepted by the hybrids. Because the original mutant (B6 × BALB/c)F$_1$ female rejected B6(*H-2^b*) but not BALB/c(*H-2^d*) grafts, Bailey and his co-workers concluded that the mutation occurred in the *H-2^b* haplotype, and the mutant haplotype was designated *H-2^{ba}*. Furthermore, because the *b* grafts were rejected by *ba/h* but not by *ba/i* hybrids, they also concluded that the mutation affected the *K* end of the *H-2* complex, leaving the *D* end intact. This conclusion is based on the principle of genetic complementation:

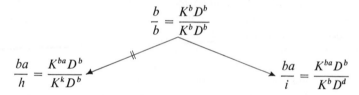

More precise location of the *ba* mutation in the *K* end has not been possible because of a lack of suitable *H-2* recombinants. Most recently, however, data have been obtained that map the mutation at least indirectly. Thus, Nabholz *et al.* (1974b) observed that *H-2^b* lymphocytes sensitized *in vitro* against *H-2^{ba}* cells are cytotoxic not only for *H-2^{ba}* target cells but also to target cells carrying other *H-2* haplotypes, and that this cross-reactivity can be genetically mapped into the *K* region. The observation strongly indicates the *H-2K^b* gene as the site of the *ba* mutation. The rejection of B6.C-H-2^{ba} grafts by B6 recipients (MST of 12.0 days in females and 18.7 days in males) and of the B6 grafts by the B6.C-*H-2^{ba}* recipients (MST of 12.7 days in females and 25.3 days in males) indicates that the mutation affected both a gain and loss of antigens. Attempts to identify the gained and lost antigens with some of the known H-2 antigens or to induce formation of serologically detectable antibodies by cross-immunization of the B6 and B6.C-*H-2^{ba}* strains have been unsuccessful. Although Apt *et al.* (1974) reported that *H-2^{ba}* cells did not absorb antibodies directed against *K^b* region antigens while *H-2^b* cells did, thus suggesting a qualitative serological difference between the two haplotypes, the data of J. Klein *et al.* (1974d) indicate that the difference is merely quantitative. The fact that the mutation affected serologically detectable *K^b* region antigens provides further support for the conclusion that the mutational event occurred in the H-$2K^b$ gene. The mutation can cause, in addition to skin-graft rejection (Bailey *et al.* 1971), stimulation in mixed lymphocyte culture (Widmer *et al.* 1973a), graft-versus-host reaction (J. Klein *et al.* 1974e), and cell-mediated lymphocytotoxicity *in vitro* (Berke and Amos 1973; Widmer *et al.* 1973a). Possibly, the mutation occurred in the carrier portion of the H-2 molecule and left the serologically detectable haptenic portion qualitatively (but not quantitatively) unchanged.

B6.C-H-2^{bb} is another mutation detected by Bailey and Kohn (1965) by skin grafting among (BALB/c × B6)F_1 mice. This mutation was subsequently placed on the B6 background by systematic backcrossing and a new congenic line, B6.C(Hz49), or B6.C-H-2^{bb} was produced. An F_1 test similar to the one used for the *ba* mutation showed that the *bb* mutation occurred in the H-2^b haplotype. The mutant haplotype was designated H-2^{bb}.

B6.M505. In an experiment designed to test the genetic homogeneity of inbred strains maintained at the Stolbovaya animal farm near Moscow, Egorov and Blandova (1968) found a subline of B6 mice that rejected skin grafts from other sublines of the same strain. Subsequent genetic analyses indicated that the rejections were due to segregation of a single H gene and that this gene resided in the H-2^b haplotype. The authors hypothesized that the heterogeneity of the B6 subline was the result of a spontaneous mutation in the H-2 complex, and they designated the postulated mutant haplotype H-2^{bd} (Egorov and Blandova 1971); the congenic line carrying the *bd* haplotype was designated B6.M505. Complementation analysis with the *bd* haplotype (Blandova *et al.* 1972) indicates that the mutation affects the K end of the H-2 complex. This conclusion is based on the fact that B6 grafts are permanently accepted by (B6.M505 × 5R)F_1 hybrids, whereas B6.M505 grafts are rejected by (B6 × 2R)F_1 mice (strains 5R and 2R carry H-2 haplotypes *i5* and *h2*, respectively):

$$\frac{b}{b} = \frac{K^b D^b}{K^b D^b} \rightarrow \frac{bd}{i5} = \frac{K^{bd} D^b}{K^b D^d} \qquad \frac{bd}{bd} = \frac{K^{bd} D^b}{K^{bd} D^b} \Vdash\rightarrow \frac{b}{h2} = \frac{K^b D^b}{K^k D^b}$$

Although the *bd* mutation occurred in the same segment of the H-2^b chromosome as Bailey's *ba* mutation, the two are not identical, because grafts from B6.M505 to B6.C-H-2^{ba} and from B6.C-H-2^{ba} to B6.M505 are rejected in less than 20 days. However, the mutations are not totally different either, because B6 skin grafts are rejected by (B6.C-H-2^{ba} × B6.M505)F_1 hybrids. This latter observation indicates that the *ba* and *bd* types have at least one missing antigen in common. Had there been no overlap between the altered portions of the K^b molecules in *ba* and *bd*, the two mutants should have complemented each other and the grafts should have been accepted.

The H-2^{bd} mutation induces graft-versus-host reaction, and stimulates mixed lymphocyte reaction and cell-mediated lymphocytotoxicity (J. Klein *et al.* 1974e; Forman and J. Klein 1974). Since the H-2^{bd} mutation fails to complement the H-2^{ba}, both mutational sites apparently reside in the same locus, most like the H-$2K$ locus. The localization of the H-2^{bd} mutation in the K region is

supported by the observation that the mutation changed the properties of
H-2.33, an antigen coded for by the *H-2K^b* gene (J. Klein *et al.* 1974d).

M513. The M513 is a mutation found by Egorov and Blandova (1972)
among (B10 × B10.D2)F$_1$ hybrids. The mutation apparently occurred in the
H-2^b haplotype, but the properties of this mutant are still under investigation.

B10.D2(M504). The M504 mutation arose spontaneously in a B10.D2
(*H-2^d*) female mated to a B10 male (Egorov 1967a). The resulting F$_1$ hybrid,
which rejected B10.D2 skin grafts in about 2 weeks, was backcrossed to the B10
strain. All the backcross animals rejected B10.D2 grafts, and about half of
them also rejected grafts from the mutant F$_1$ parent. The latter mice were intercrossed, and a homozygous congenic B10.D2(M504) line carrying the mutant
gene was established. The nature of these transplantation tests was such that it
excluded the detection of any mutations at loci other than *H-2*, and for this
reason it was assumed that the M504 mutation occurred in the *H-2* complex and
led to a new haplotype, *H-2da*. Because grafts from B10.D2 mice were accepted
by [(B10.D2(M504) × B10.A]F$_1$ and [B10.D2(M504) × 5R]F$_1$ hybrids but rejected
by [B10.D2(M504) × HTG]F$_1$ hybrids, Shumova *et al.* (1972) concluded that the
mutation occurred in the *D* end of the *H-2* complex. The principle of the test
leading to this conclusion can be diagrammed as follows:

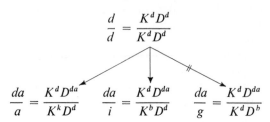

The majority of skin grafts exchanged between the B10.D2 and
B10.D2(M504) congenic lines are rejected in less than 20 days, but some grafts
survive for unusually long periods of time (for more than 60 days and some,
perhaps, indefinitely). The frequency of the "maverick" grafts is relatively high
in cases where the donor or the recipients are *da/−* heterozygotes (Egorov
1967a). This odd phenomenon has yet to be explained, but because the
B10.D2(M504) grafting results in relatively high titers of hemagglutinating
antibodies, mechanisms such as immunological enhancement should be given
serious consideration.

Cross-immunization of the B10.D2 and B10.D2(M504) strains leads to the
production of circulating antibodies (Dishkant *et al.* 1973). The B10.D2 anti-
B10.D2(M504) antisera contain at least one antibody (anti-H-2.50), specific for
the *da* type and its genetic derivative, *ia1*; the B10.D2(M504) anti-B10.D2 antisera contain at least two antibodies, early-appearing strong anti-H-2.40 and late-
appearing weaker anti-H-2.49. The anti-40 antibody reacts with all strains
carrying the *H-2D^d* region, and in this respect, it resembles anti-H-2.4, except
that antigen 4 is present in both *d* and *da*, whereas antigen 40 is present in *d*
but absent in *da*. The anti-49 antibody resembles anti-H-2.3 in its pattern of

reactivity: it reacts with *H-2* haplotypes *a*, *d*, *h*, *i*, *k*, *m*, *o*, *p*, *q*, *r*, *s*, and *u* and does not react with *H-2* haplotypes *b*, *f*, *g*, and *j*. The distinguishing haplotype for the two antigens is *da*, which is 3-positive, 49-negative. The anti-49 antibody can be absorbed from the *da* anti-*d* antisera by any 3-positive, 4-negative cells. Antigen 50 is the private antigen of the *da* haplotype. Because both *d* and *da* also carry antigen 4, they are the only *H-2* haplotypes known to possess three instead of the usual two private antigens (*d* carries private antigens 31, 4, and 40; *da* carries 31, 4, and 50). However, this does not necessarily contradict the general rule of two private antigens per *H-2* haplotype. It is conceivable that the H-2.4 in *da* is not exactly the same as the H-2.4 in *d*. There is no direct evidence supporting this contention as far as the original mutant line is concerned, but serological analysis of an *H-2* recombinant (*ia1*) derived from *da* indicates that this might be so. The $H-2^{ia1}$ haplotype of strain B10.D2(R106) inherited the *D* region from $H-2^{da}$ and the *K* region from $H-2^{b}$. Although the *ia1* haplotype reacts with anti-4 antisera, the reaction is much weaker, particularly in quantitative absorption experiments, than the reaction with other 4-positive cells. Hence, antigen 4 in *ia1* appears to be at least quantitatively different from 4 in *i*, *a*, or *d*.

Serological analysis with known H-2 antibodies did not detect any other serological difference between *d* and *da* except for one antiserum: the antiserum ($h \times q$) anti-*b* reacted with *d* but failed to react with *da*. The antigen responsible for this difference was not identified. Other antigens of the $H-2^d$ haplotype, such as 6, 8, 13, 34, 35, 36, 41, 42, 43, and 44, seem to have remained unimpaired by the *da* mutation.

In summary, the *da* mutation effected a loss of at least two antigens (40 and 49), a gain of at least one antigen (50), and possibly an alteration of one antigen (4). It left intact at least nine antigens of the $H-2^d$ haplotype (3, 6, 13, 35, 36, 41, 42, 43, and 44). It appears, therefore, that the genetic change in the M504 mutant was relatively minor in extent (point mutation). Its effect can perhaps best be depicted as a small alteration of the "shape" of the $H-2D^d$ molecule resulting in a slightly different affinity of the molecule to cross-reactive antibodies. The mutation exposes the fallacy of visualizing the H-2 molecules as arrays of more or less independent antigenic sites in the static picture of the traditional H-2 chart. It clearly shows that the serological dissection of the molecule into separate H-2 antigens is very remote from reality.

The conclusion that the *da* haplotype arose by a point mutation, rather than a deletion affecting several genes, for instance, is supported by the fact that in a cross involving the *da* haplotype, the *H-2* recombination frequency is about the same as in crosses involving the *d* chromosome (Vedernikov and Egorov 1973). More extensive genetic change might be expected to suppress crossing-over in the *H-2* complex. In addition to graft rejection and humoral antibody production, the $H-2^{da}$ mutation also causes stimulation in mixed lymphocyte culture (Rychlíková *et al.* 1972), graft-versus-host reaction (J. Klein and Egorov 1973), and cell-mediated lymphocytotoxicity (Brondz and Goldberg 1970; J. Klein *et al.* 1974e; Forman and J. Klein 1974).

A.CA(M506). The M506 mutant was found by skin grafting among (A.CA × A)F$_1$ mice (Egorov and Blandova 1972). The exceptional female, number 506, was mated to an A.CA male, and an A.506 congenic line was subsequently established. The mutation apparently occurred spontaneously in the *H-2^f* haplotype of A.CA and led to a new haplotype, *H-2^{fa}*. Congenic lines A.CA(*H-2^f*) and A.506(*H-2^{fa}*) reject mutually exchanged skin grafts, indicating a concurrent gain and loss of H antigens in the *fa* haplotype.

Crossimmunization of the A.CA and A.CA(M506) strains produces antibodies that react in both the cytotoxic and hemagglutination tests (Egorov 1974). The A.CA anti-A.CA (M506) serum reacts in the cytotoxic test with *H-2* haplotypes *fa* and *k* and does not react with *b*, *d*, and *f*; the reciprocal antiserum reacts with *f*, *d*, and *k* and is negative with *b* and *fa*.

B10.M—*H-2^{fb}*. This is a spontaneous mutation that arose from *H-2^f* in a [B10.M × B10.RIII(71NS)]F$_1$ male (Mobraaten and Bailey 1973). Congenic lines B10.M(*H-2^f*) and B10.M-*H-2^{fb}* reject mutually exchanged skin grafts.

Unnamed mutations. Melvold and Kohn (1974) reported nine new *H-2* mutations, eight derived from *H-2^b* and one from *H-2^d*. The *H-2^b*-derived mutations fail to complement one another and the *H-2^{ba}* mutation and thus apparently represent genetic changes in the *H-2K* locus. Three mutations are histocompatible with one another despite their independent origin. Grafts exchanged between *H-2^b* and *H-2^{mutant}* congenic lines are rejected in both directions, indicating that the mutations are of the loss-and-gain type. The *H-2^d*-derived mutation is of the loss type.

I. K. Egorov (*personal communication*) obtained a mutation in the *H-2^k* haplotype of strain CBA/HLacSto. The mutant congenic line CBA.M523 rejects CBA skin grafts (and vice versa) and the CBA.M523 cells when injected into CBA mice cause graft-versus-host reaction. F$_1$ tests with skin grafts indicate that the mutation occurred in the *K* end of the *H-2* complex. No serological difference has been detected so far between CBA.M523 and CBA.

Chapter Eleven

Genetics of *H-2*-Linked Loci

I. Cytogenetics of Chromosome 17

In 1904, Darbishire reported that genes *p* (*pink-eye*) and *c* (*albinism*) were associated in segregating populations more often than would be expected under the assumption of independent assortment. However, it was only in 1915 that the meaning of this deviation was understood and the conclusion drawn that genes *p* and *c* were linked (Haldane *et al.* 1915). This was the first group of linked genes discovered in the mouse (or in any other vertebrate), so it was designated *linkage group I* (abbreviated LG I). Twelve years later, Gates (1927) reported that genes *d* (*dilute*) and *se* (*short ear*) were also linked, but segregated independently of the genes in LG I. He therefore concluded that genes *d* and *se* were part of another linkage group, and he designated it linkage group LG II. In subsequent years, additional linkage groups were discovered and designated III, IV, V, and so on. Ninth in the order of discovery was a linkage group consisting of genes for tail anomalies: *T* (*Brachyury*), *Ki* (*Kinky*), and *Fu* (*Fused*) (Dunn and Caspari 1942, 1945). In 1948, Gorer and his co-workers demonstrated that *Fu* and *H-2* were linked, and thus proved that the *H-2* system was part of LG IX. The group has since grown to include more than a dozen loci.

Because each linkage group is carried by one chromosome, there are as many linkage groups as chromosomes in the haploid set (20 in the mouse). Until recently, however, it was not possible to assign linkage groups to their corresponding chromosomes, because the chromosomes were morphologically indistinguishable. In a standard metaphase plate, all mouse chromosomes look alike (Fig. 11–1a) in that all have centromeres at their ends (they are *telocentric*) and they lack any prominent morphological features. Although they are of different lengths, when arranged according to their size, the difference in length between any two neighboring chromosomes is very slight (Levan *et al.* 1962; Crippa 1964; D. Bennett 1965; Stephenson and Stephenson 1970).

The inability to identify specific mouse chromosomes led to a paradoxical situation. Genetically, the mouse was one of the most thoroughly examined mammals, and yet cytogenetically it remained almost totally unexplored. The situation changed about three years ago, when chromosome-banding techniques were developed. It was discovered that treatment of chromosome preparations with SSC (0.3 M sodium chloride and 0.03 M sodium citrate), trypsin, chymotrypsin, and other agents, and staining with Giemsa or quinacrine mustard produces dark and light transverse bands that are reproducible and are characteristic for individual chromosomes. The specific banding patterns can then be used as "identification cards" for the chromosomes. Identified chromosomes are

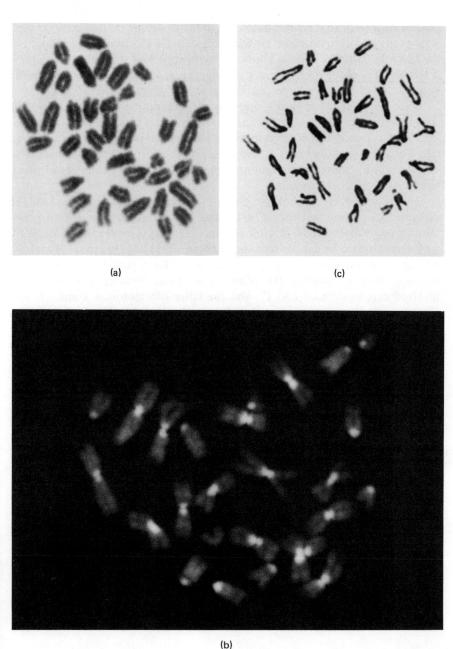

(a)

(c)

(b)

Fig. 11-1. Somatic methaphase chromosomes of *Mus musculus* (a), *Mus poschiavinus* (b), and a mouse carrying two metacentric chromosomes, T(16;17)7Bn (c). Preparations in (a) and (c) stained with standard Giemsa; preparation in (b) stained with benzimidazole and photographed using fluorescence microscope. (b, courtesy of Dr. A. Gropp.)

designated by Arabic numerals according to their position in the *karyotype* (i.e., arrangement of chromosomes on the basis of their morphology, in this case, their length), with the longest chromosome being 1 and the shortest being 19. (Position 20 is occupied by the sex chromosomes, X and Y, with Y being the smallest and X the third largest chromosome in the mouse karyotype.)

Once identified cytologically, the chromosomes can be correlated with their corresponding linkage groups by using chromosomal translocations. A *translocation* is a structural aberration in which a chromosomal segment is transferred into a different position either on the same or on a different chromosome. Most of the known mouse translocations represent reciprocal exchanges between nonhomologous chromosomes.

The principle of the linkage group-to-chromosome assignments will be explained using translocations *T138Ca* and *T190Ca* as examples. Both translocations were discovered by Carter and his colleagues (Carter *et al.* 1955, 1956), who demonstrated by genetic tests that *T138* involved linkage groups II and IX, whereas *T190* involved linkage groups IX and XIII. Cytological investigation of these two translocations (O. Miller *et al.* 1971) revealed that the former involved chromosomes 9 and 17, and the latter chromosomes 1 and 17. The sharing by these two translocations of LG IX and chromosome 17 indicates that LG IX is carried by chromosome 17. Using this approach, it was possible to assign all 19 autosomal linkage groups to their respective chromosomes. (For

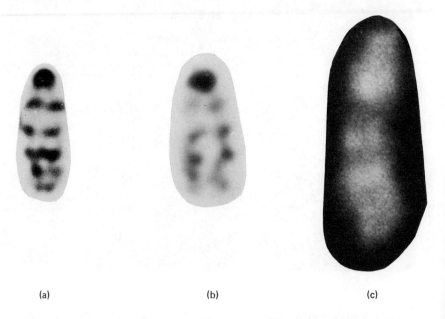

(a)   (b)   (c)

Fig. 11-2. Chromosome 17 showing banding pattern after treatment with trypsin and staining with modified Giemsa (a), after staining with modified Giemsa (b), and staining with quinacrine mustard (c). (a, courtesy of Dr. M. N. Nesbitt; b, c courtesy of Dr. O. J. Miller.)

reviews see D. Miller and O. Miller 1972; Nesbitt and Francke 1973.) The term "linkage group" thus became unnecessary, and it has been recommended that it be dropped (M. Green 1972).

The location of LG IX in chromosome 17 was confirmed by J. Klein (1971b) using a different subspecies of the mouse originally found in a tobacco plant in the Valle di Poschiavo of southeastern Switzerland, the tobacco mouse, *Mus poschiavinus Fatio*. Karyological analysis of the tobacco mouse (Gropp *et al.* 1970) revealed only 26 chromosomes in its karyotype, 14 metacentric and 12 telocentric (Fig. 11–1b). The total number of chromosomal arms is the same (40) in both the tobacco and the house mouse, suggesting that each of the metacentric chromosomes arose by fusion of two telocentric chromosomes at their centromeric ends (*centric fusion* or *Robertsonian translocation*). After it was demonstrated that tobacco mice interbred with laboratory mice and that backcrossing of the hybrids to the laboratory mice led to a gradual and irregular loss of the metacentric chromosomes (Gropp *et al.* 1970, 1971), it was possible to test whether any of the seven pairs of metacentric chromosomes carried LG IX. The testing was done by repeated backcrossing to an inbred strain and simultaneous selection for a particular *H-2* haplotype (J. Klein 1971b). The backcrossings eliminated all the metacentric chromosomes, except one that was shown to carry the *H-2* complex (Fig. 11–1c).

Chromosome 17 (LG IX) is very short, its relative length (expressed as a percentage of the total length of the mitotic haploid complement) being 3.74. (The relative length of the longest mouse chromosome is 7.20, that of the shortest is 2.72; see Nesbitt and Francke 1973). The banding patterns of the chromosome, as revealed by the different banding techniques, are shown in Fig. 11–2 and summarized diagrammatically in Fig. 11–3. The designation of the individual bands in the diagram is based on the nomenclature proposed by Nesbitt and Francke (1973). These authors distinguish two types of band, *major*, which can readily be seen in "minimum information preparations" such as those obtained by quinacrine mustard staining, and *minor*, which can be seen only

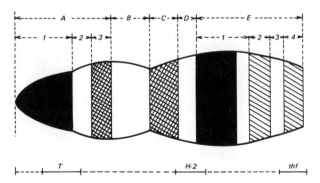

Fig. 11-3. Diagrammatic representation of banding pattern of chromosome 17 (based on Nesbitt and Francke 1973). Postulated positions of three loci (*T*, *H-2*, *thf*) are indicated by horizontal bars.

in excellent preparations of uncontracted chromosomes. The major bands are designated by capital letters in alphabetical order beginning at the centromere; the minor bands are designated by Arabic numerals. Both the major and minor band symbols are preceded by the numerical designation of the chromosome. The bands are either dark or light, causing the chromosome to appear striated. In the best preparations of chromosome 17, five major bands (17A through 17E) can be distinguished, with bands 17A and 17E being further subdivided into three and four minor bands, respectively. The two most prominent features of the chromosome are a darkly stained band, 17A1 (*centromeric heterochromatin*), and a broad, lightly stained band ("space"), 17B, in the first half of the chromosome. According to O. Miller *et al.* (1971), translocation break *T190* lies approximately in the middle of the chromosome, perhaps in band 17C, whereas translocation break *T138* is located more distally, perhaps in band 17E1 or 2. The *H-2* complex is supposedly located between the two breaks, so it can tentatively be assigned to band 17D; the *Brachyury (T)* complex, which is located close to the centromere (C. Hammerberg and J. Klein, *unpublished data*),

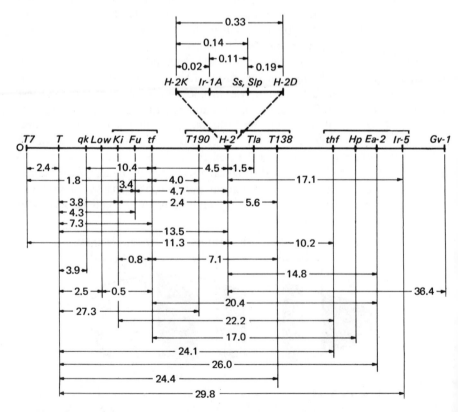

Fig. 11-4. Genetic map of chromosome 17 (LG IX). Centromere is indicated by the circle on the left; brackets indicate that the order of loci is not known; the map distances represent averages for males and females together.

probably lies in band 17A; the *thin fur* (*thf*) locus is probably close to the non-centromeric end of the chromosome because the genetic distance between *T* and *H-2* is approximately the same as the distance between *H-2* and *thf* (J. Klein, *unpublished data*). Inconsistent with this location of *thf* is the position of the *Gv-1* gene, which is believed to be some 36 map units distant from *H-2*; this places the *Gv-1* locus far beyond *thf* at the noncentromeric end. However, there is some doubt as to whether the *Gv-1* locus belongs to LG IX, and until the doubt is dispelled, the genetic relationships in chromosome 17 can be only tentatively interpreted as described above.

In some chromosomal preparations, a constriction can be observed near the centromeric end of chromosome 17 (Dev *et al.* 1971; Nombela and Murcia 1972). Such *secondary constrictions* (the constriction at the centromere being primary) have been proved in other species to be the chromosomal regions coding for ribosomal ribonucleic acid (rRNA). Whether chromosome 17 does carry rRNA genes, as has been suggested by J. Klein and Raška (1968), remains to be determined.

The genetic map of chromosome 17 is shown in Fig. 11-4. The map contains 11 markers outside the *H-2* complex, six or seven between the centromere end *H-2* (*T, qk, Ki, Fu, tf, Low,* and perhaps *Hp*), and three or five on the other side of *H-2* (*Tla, thf, Ea2,* and perhaps *Hp* and *Gv-1*). A summary of the linkage tests that have been performed among the genes in chromosome 17 is shown in Table 11-1 and Fig. 11-5.

The position of the centromere in relation to the loci in chromosome 17 has been determined in at least three different ways.

1. The most direct determination uses the *T7* metacentric chromosome as a

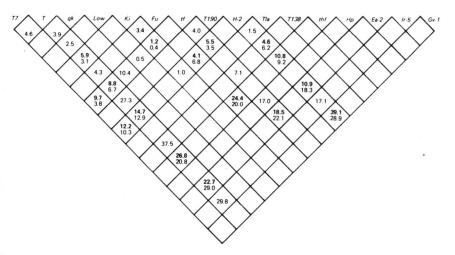

Fig. 11-5. Genetic distances of loci carried by chromosome 17 (LG IX). The boldface figures are for females, lightface figures are for males (or males and females together).

Table 11-1. Recombination of loci in chromosome 17 (LG IX)*

Gene interval	F₁ heterozygote		Recombination		Reference
	Sex	Phase**	Fraction	Frequency ± S.E.	
T-qk	♂	R	4/183	2.2 ± 1.1	E. M. Eicher and J. L. Southard, *personal communication*
	♂	R	6/81	7.4 ± 2.9	M. M. Dickie, *Mouse News Letter* 40:29, 1969
T-Ki	♀	R	16/542	5.9 ± 1.5†	
	♂	R	14/1128	2.5 ± 6.6†	Dunn and Caspari 1945
	♂	C	9/375	4.8 ± 1.5†	
T-Fu	♀	R	0/137	—	Dunn and Caspari 1945
	♂	R	14/657	4.3 ± 1.1†	
T-tf	♀	C	17/220	7.7 ± 1.8	Lyon 1956
	♂	C	13/141	9.2 ± 2.4	
	♀	C	22/261	8.4 ± 1.7	Lyon and Phillips 1959
	♂	C	13/141	9.2 ± 2.4	
	♀	R	36/383	9.4 ± 1.5	
	♀	C	10/116	8.6 ± 2.6	Lyon and Meredith 1964a
	♂	R	27/361	7.5 ± 1.4	
	♂	C	3/136	2.2 ± 1.3	
	♀	C	22/266	8.3 ± 1.7	M. C. Green and J. H. Stimpfling, *Mouse News Letter* 35:32, 1966
	♂	C	19/144	13.2 ± 2.8	
	♂	R	6/169	3.6 ± 1.4	Dunn and Bennett 1968
	♀	C	10/81	12.3 ± 3.7	Pizarro and Dunn 1970
	♂	C	13/312	4.1 ± 1.1	
	♀+♂	C	22/484	4.5 ± 0.9	McDevitt *et al.* 1972
	♀	C	5/119	4.2 ± 1.8	Pizarro and Vergara 1973
	♂	C	11/131	8.4 ± 2.4	
Tc-tf	♀	R	27/282	9.6 ± 1.7	
	♀	C	25/139	18.0 ± 3.3	Searle 1966
	♂	R	28/322	8.7 ± 1.6	
	♂	C	6/136	4.4 ± 1.8	
TF-tf	♀	R	12/115	10.4 ± 2.9	Dunn *et al.* 1962
	♂	R	7/158	4.4 ± 1.6	
Th-tf	♀	R	4/69	5.8 ± 2.8	Lyon 1959
T2J-tf	♂	R	23/183	12.6 ± 2.5	E. M. Eicher and J. L. Southard, *personal communication*
T-H-2	♀	—	1/8	12.5 ± 11.7	Snell 1952
	♂	—	3/73	4.1 ± 2.3	
	♀	—	?	15.4 ± 1.1	Allen 1955a
	♂	—	?	8.3 ± 0.7	
	♀	—	43/266	16.2 ± 2.3	M. C. Green and J. H. Stimpfling, *Mouse News Letter* 35:2, 1966
	♂	—	27/144	18.7 ± 3.3	
	♀+♂	—	9/53	17.0 ± 5.2	Snell *et al.* 1967
	♀	—	13/81	16.0 ± 4.1	Pizarro and Dunn 1970
	♂	—	21/312	6.7 ± 1.4	
	♀+♂	—	57/484	11.8 ± 1.5	McDevitt *et al.* 1972
	♀	—	61/456	13.4 ± 1.6	Shreffler and David 1972
	♂	—	75/452	16.6 ± 1.8	
	♀	—	27/176	15.3 ± 2.7	J. Klein, *unpublished data*
	♂	—	15/109	13.7 ± 3.3	
T-thf	♀	R	96/353	27.2 ± 2.4	Key and Hollander 1972
	♂	R	64/320	20.0 ± 2.2	
	♀	R	46/176	26.1 ± 3.3	J. Klein, *unpublished data*
	♂	R	25/109	22.9 ± 4.0	
T-Low	♂	C	20/?	2.5 ±	Dunn and Bennett 1971a
qk-tf	♂	C	19/183	10.4 ± 2.3	E. M. Eicher and J. L. Southard, *personal communication*
Ki-Fu	♀	R	5/296	3.4† ± 1.1	Dunn and Caspari 1945
	♂	R	0/209	—	
	♀	R	0?/81	—	Dunn and Gluecksohn-Waelsch 1954
	♂	R	0?/904	—	
Ki-tf	♀	R	6/519	1.2 ± 0.5	Dunn *et al.* 1962
	♂	R	2/551	0.4 ± 0.3	
Ki-H-2	?	—	5/95	5.3 ± 2.3	Snell 1952
	♂	—	2/196	1.0 ± 0.7	Allen 1955a
Fu-H-2	?	—	1/18	5.6 ± 5.4	Snell 1952
	♀	—	?	6.9 ± 3.0	Allen 1955a
	♂	—	?	4.1 ± 1.2	
	♀	—	11/268	4.1 ± 1.2	Allen 1955b
	♂	—	5/73	6.8 ± 3.0	

Table 11-1. (*Continued*)

Gene interval	Sex	Phase**	Fraction	Frequency±S.E.	Reference
Fu-thf	♀	R	40/183	21.9± 3.1 ⎱	Key and Hollander 1972
	♂	R	34/196	17.3± 2.7 ⎰	W. F. Hollander, *Mouse News Letter 48*:3, 1973
	♀	C	14/38	36.8± 7.8 ⎱	W. F. Hollander, *Mouse News*
	♂	C	13/39	33.3± 7.6 ⎰	*Letter 48*:3, 1973
Low-tf	♂	C	4/?	0.5± ?	Dunn and Bennett 1971a
tf-H-2	♀	—	21/266	7.9± 1.7	M. C. Green and J. H. Stimpfling
	♂	—	8/144	5.6± 1.9	*Mouse News Letter 35*:32, 1966
	♀	—	3/81	3.7± 2.1 ⎱	
	♂	—	8/312	2.6± 0.9 ⎰	Pizarro and Dunn 1970
	♀+♂	—	19/484	3.9± 0.9	McDevitt et al. 1972
	♀	—	17/398	4.3± 1.0 ⎱	J. Klein, *unpublished data*
	♂	—	3/92	3.3± 1.9 ⎰	
	♀	—	9/119	7.6± 2.4 ⎱	Pizarro and Vergara 1973
	♂	—	5/131	3.8± 1.6 ⎰	
tf-Hp	?	?	?	17.0± 3.0	D. R. Johnson, *Mouse News Letter 17*:52, 1972
H-2-Tla	♀+♂	—	6/397	1.5± 0.9	Boyse et al. 1964b, 1966
H-2-thf	♀	—	19/176	10.8± 2.3 ⎱	J. Klein, *unpublished data*
	♂	—	10/109	9.2± 2.8 ⎰	
Ea-2-H-2	♀	—	13/119	10.9± 2.8 ⎤	
	♂	—	24/131	18.3± 3.3	
Ea-2-tf	♀	—	22/119	18.5± 3.5	Pizarro and Vergara 1973
	♂	—	29/131	22.1± 3.6	
Ea-2-T	♀	—	27/119	22.7± 3.8	
	♂	—	38/131	29.0± 3.9 ⎦	
H-2-Gv-1	♀	—	91/233	39.1± 3.2 ⎱	Stockert et al. 1971
	♂	—	28/94	29.8± 4.7 ⎰	
T7-T	♀+♂	R	4/86	4.6± 2.4	C. Hammerberg and J. Klein, *unpublished data*
T7-tf	♀	R	14/145	9.7± 2.5 ⎱	J. Klein, *unpublished data*
	♂	R	2/53	3.8± 2.6 ⎰	
T7-H-2	♀	—	27/222	12.2± 2.2 ⎱	J. Klein 1971b, and *unpublished data*
	♂	—	22/213	10.3± 2.1 ⎰	
T138-T	♂	R	15/40	37.5± 7.7	Carter et al. 1955
	♀+♂	R	22/93	23.7± 4.4 ⎱	Lyon and Phillips 1959
	?	C	8/30	26.7± 8.1 ⎰	
T138-tf	♀+♂	R	4/56	7.1± 3.4	Lyon and Phillips 1959
T138-H-2	♀	—	2/43	4.6± 3.2 ⎱	J. Klein and D. Klein 1972
	♂	—	4/65	6.2± 3.0 ⎰	
T190-T	♀+♂	C	54/198	27.3± 3.2	M. F. Lyon, *Mouse News Letter 36*: 34, 1967
T190-tf	♀+♂	R	8/198	4.0± 1.4	M. F. Lyon, *Mouse News Letter 36*: 34, 1967

* All estimates of recombination frequencies are based on backcross matings.
** C = coupling, R = repulsion.
† For technical reasons only one crossover class was recovered. The figure represents the frequency of this one crossover class multiplied by 2.

marker for the centromere. Whenever a crossing-over occurs between the centromere and a marker gene (*T* or *H-2*), the marker is transferred from the metacentric to the telocentric chromosome or *vice versa*. The distance between the centromere and brachyury (*T*) has been determined as 2.4 map units (C. Hammerberg and J. Klein, *unpublished data*), and the distance between the centromere and *H-2* as 11.3 map units (J. Klein 1971b, and *unpublished data*). The distance between *T* and *H-2* is known to be 13.5 map units (see Table 11–1), so the *T* locus must be located between the centromere and *H-2*, with the order being

$$centromere \cdots T \cdots H\text{-}2$$

2. Lyon and her co-workers (1968) determined the position of the centromere in chromosome 17 indirectly, using Robertsonian translocation $T(9;19)163H$ [formerly $T(2;12)163H$]. They showed that locus cw is near and locus d far away from the centromere in chromosome 9 (LG II). In translocation $T(9;17)138Ca$, the d locus is on the noncentromeric arm of the translocated chromosome; therefore, the T locus, known to be linked to d in $T138$, must be on the centromeric arm, and the order must be

$$centromere \cdots T \cdots T138\ break$$

3. Cross $T138cw/+cw \times T138+/++$ produces approximately 1 percent cw/cw homozygotes and cross $T138se/+se \times T138+/++$ produces approximately 18 percent se/se homozygotes (J. Klein 1970b; Lyon and Hawker 1970). The production of cw/cw homozygotes from a $cw/+ \times +/+$ cross requires the formation of a gamete carrying two doses of the cw gene and is the result of nondisjunction of the homologous arms in the translocation heterozygote. The same applies to the $se/+ \times +/+$ cross. Nondisjunction of centromeric arms in a translocation heterozygote is a much rarer event than nondisjunction of noncentromeric arms, so the higher frequency of se/se homozygotes over cw/cw homozygotes indicates that the cw gene is located in the centromeric arm and the se gene on the noncentromeric arm in the $T138$ translocation. Because se in $T138$ is linked with T, T must be on the centromeric arm.

Cytological evidence for location of the centromere in chromosome 17 near the T locus has been reported by D. Miller *et al.* (1971). These authors argue that because the $T190$ break is genetically closer to *Brachyury* (T) than the $T138$ break and because the cytological order is $centromere \cdots T190\ break \cdots T138\ break$, the centromere must be close to T. However, the authors' assumption that the $T190$ break is close to T is not supported by any genetic evidence. On the contrary, the $T138$ and $T190$ breaks map at almost exactly the same distance from T. (The length of the $T–T138$ interval is 27.8 cM, and the length of the $T–T190$ interval is 27.3 cM; see Table 11–1.) Moreover, $T138$ and $T190$ are both known to enhance recombination, the former more than the latter. In light of this fact, $T138$ might actually be closer to T than $T190$. It is true that the $t^6–T190$ recombination frequency is very low, but t^6 is known to suppress crossing-over over a long segment of chromosome 17. Furthermore, t^6, as will be shown later, cannot be considered an allele of T. The observations of D. Miller *et al.* (1971), therefore, do not provide any additional evidence for the location of the centromere at the *Brachyury* end in chromosome 17. However, because the results of the three independent determinations quoted above are in full agreement, the order, $centromere \cdots T \cdots H-2$, can be regarded as firmly established.

For some time, there was confusion as to the order of the *H-2K* and *H-2D* loci with respect to the centromere. The confusion stemmed from a determination based on a postulate of a mitotic crossing-over occurring during a selection of tumor variants. Because this will be discussed at length in Chapter Thirteen, it suffices to say here that the postulate led to the order *centromere* · · · *H-2D* · · · *H-2K*. On the basis of this postulate, all *H-2* maps were drawn with *H-2D* on the left (it is an established practice in genetic literature to draw genetic maps with the centromeric end on the left). However, when it was later demonstrated that the centromere was actually located at the *K* end of the *H-2* complex, it became necessary to reverse the order of the *H-2* maps and place the *K* end on the left. Evidence for the positioning of *H-2K* at the centromeric end of chromosome 17 is indirect (a three-point cross with the centromere, *H-2K*, and *H-2D* has not yet been performed) but conclusive. Because the *T* gene is located between the centromere and *H-2* and because the *H-2K* gene is located between *T* and *H-2D*, the *H-2K* gene must be located between the centromere and *H-2D*. Results from three-point crosses involving *T*, *H-2K*, and *H-2D* have been reported by several authors (Allen 1955a; Pizarro and Dunn 1970; J. Klein et al. 1970; McDevitt et al. 1972; Shreffler and David 1972; J. Klein and D. Klein 1972) and all lead to the conclusion that the order is

$$T \cdots H\text{-}2K \cdots H\text{-}2D$$

II. The *Tla* Complex

A. Discovery

Old and his co-workers (1963) produced antisera in C57BL/6 mice by immunization with spontaneous or radiation-induced A or (C57BL/6 × A)F$_1$ leukemias. The antisera were cytotoxic *in vitro* for the cells of several C57BL/6 leukemias but not for normal C57BL/6 tissues. The cytotoxic activity was removed by absorption with C57BL/6 leukemia and A, C58, and (C57BL/6 × A)F$_1$ thymocytes, but not with thymocytes of C57BL/6 and several other strains, nor with normal tissues, other than the thymus, of any strain. These findings were interpreted by the authors as indicating the presence of an antigen shared by C57BL/6 leukemias with normal A and C58 thymocytes. The antigen was designated TL and the locus coding for the antigen, *Tla* (*T*hymus *l*eukemia *a*ntigen) locus.

B. Antigens of the *Tla* System

Boyse et al. (1966, 1968c) demonstrated that TL was not a single antigen but rather a complex consisting of at least four antigens, Tla.1, Tla.2, Tla.3, and Tla.4.[1] The antisera used to define the individual Tla antigens are listed in Table 11–2. Antiserum (BALB/c × C3H)F$_1$ anti-ASL1 (A strain-spontaneous leukemia), absorbed with ERLD (C57BL/6 strain radiation-induced leukemia), and antiserum C57BL/6 anti-ASL1 both react with ASL1. The latter antiserum

---

[1] Originally, strains were classified as TL$^+$ or TL$^-$ according to the presence or absence in their thymocytes of an antigen later designated Tla.1. After the complexity of the TL antigens was recognized, the designation TL$^+$ was used by Boyse's group in reference to cells carrying TL antigen(s) of any specificity.

Table 11-2. Antisera used to define four Tla antigens*

Recipient strain	Donor			Absorption		Expected Tla antibodies	Reaction with thymocytes of strain				Reaction with leukemia of strain			
Strain	Strain	Tissue	Tla type	Strain	Tissue		A	C57BL/6	BALB/c	DBA/2	A	C57BL/6	BALB/c	DBA/2
C57BL/6	A	leukemia ASL1	1, 2, 3, —	A	*in vivo***	1, 2, 3	+	—	±	±	+	+	+	+
(BALB/c× C3H)F₁	A	leukemia ASL1	1, 2, 3, —	—	—	1, 3	+	—	—	—	+	+	+	+
(BALB/c× C3H)F₁	A	leukemia ASL1	1, 2, 3, —	(C57BL/6 × A)F₁†	*in vivo***	3	+	—	—	—	+	—	—	—
129	—	thymus	—, 2, —, —	—	—	2	±	—	±	±	±	+	±	±
C57BL/6 —Tla^a	C57BL/6	leukemia ERLD	1, 2, —, 4	—	—	4	—	—	—	—	—	+	—	+
Postulated antigenic constitution							1, 2, 3, —	—, —, —, —	—, 2, —, —	—, 2, —, —	1, 2, 3, —	1, 2, —, 4	1, 2, —, —	1, 2, —, 4

* Based on Old *et al.* 1968, and Boyse *et al.* 1968b.
** Removes anti-H-2 antibodies; Tla antibodies are not absorbed.
† The F₁ hybrids carried advanced transplants of C57BL/6 leukemia ERLD (Tla 1, 2, —, 4). The leukemia cells absorb out the anti-Tla. 1 antibody.

also reacts with ERLD, whereas the former does not. Apparently, the absorbed (BALB/c × C3H)F$_1$ anti-ASL1 antiserum contains one antibody (anti-Tla.3) that is also present in the C57BL/6 anti-ASL1 antiserum, and the former antiserum contains a second antibody (anti-Tla-1) responsible for the reaction with ERLD. The unabsorbed (BALB/c × C3H)F$_1$ anti-ALS1 antiserum reacts with the ERLD leukemia, indicating that it also contains two antibodies, anti-Tla.1 and anti-Tla.3. The antiserum does not react with thymocytes of strains BALB/c, DBA/2, or 129, indicating that these strains lack antigens Tla.3. A third antiserum, C57BL/6 anti-129 (thymocytes), reacts with 129, BALB/c, and DBA/2 thymocytes; the reaction is attributed to a third antibody, anti-Tla.2. A fourth antiserum, C57BL/6-*Tla^a* anti-ERLD, reacts with C57BL/6 and DBA/2 leukemias. Because antigens Tla.1, Tla.2, and Tla.3 are present in the recipient (strain C57BL/6-*Tla^a* carries the *Tla^a* allele of A on the C57BL/6 background), the antibody in this antiserum must be directed against a fourth antigen, Tla.4 (Boyse *et al.* 1968c).

Anti-Tla.1, Tla.3, and Tla.4 are strong cytotoxic antibodies, whereas anti-Tla.2 is relatively weak.

C. Genetic Control

1. In Normal Cells

Testing with the Tla antisera divides the inbred strains into three groups: strains carrying antigens Tla.1, Tla.2, and Tla.3; strains expressing only Tla.2, and strains failing to express any known Tla antigens (Table 11-3). The determinants coding for these three *Tla* types can be designated *Tla^a*, *Tla^b*, and *Tla^c*, respectively, as they behave as alleles at a single locus (Boyse *et al.* 1964b; Boyse

Table 11-3. Strain distribution of *Tla* haplotypes*

Tla haplotype	Thymocyte phenotype	Prototype strain	Other strains
a	1, 2, 3, −	A/J	A.CA, AKR.K, AKR.M, BDP/J, BUB/BnJ, B10.A, B10.A(5R), B10.AKM, B10.BR, C57BL/6-*Tla^a*, C57BR/cdJ, C58, F/St, HTI, NZB, PL/J, SJL/J, SWR
b	−, −, −, −	C57BL/6	A-*Tla^b*, A.BY, AKR, A.SW, B10.RIII (71NS), CBA/J, C3H/He, C3H/An, C3Hf/Bi, C3H.JK, C57BL/10, C57L, DBA/1, HTG, HTH, I, JK, MA/J, NH, RF/J, ST/bJ
c	−, 2, −, −	BALB/c	B10.D2, B10.129(6M), C57BL/Ks, DBA/2, D1.LP, LP, 129

* Based on Boyse *et al.* 1966; Snell and Cherry 1972; G. D. Snell, *personal communication.*

and Old 1969), the _Tla_ locus, which is closely linked with the _H-2_ complex. The _Tla–H-2_ linkage is supported by the following observations. First, in backcross $(A \times C57BL/6)F_1 \times C57BL/6$, only six of 397 tested animals were recombinants between _H-2_ and _Tla_ (Boyse _et al._ 1964b), indicating a distance between the two loci of about 1.5 map units. Linkage between _H-2_ and _Tla_ was also observed in crosses involving two other Tla^a strains, SJL/J and C58 (Boyse _et al._ 1966). Second, some _H-2_ congenic lines differ from their background strains not only in _H-2_ but also in _Tla_, suggesting that the _Tla_ difference was introduced into the lines from the donor strains along with _H-2_ (Boyse _et al._ 1966; G. D. Snell, _personal communication_). Third, in strains that differ at the _Tla_ locus, intra–_H-2_ recombination is always accompanied by recombination between _H-2_ and _Tla_ (Boyse _et al._ 1966). The _H-2_ recombinants always inherit the _Tla_ type of the _D_-region donor, indicating the location of the _Tla_ locus at the _D_ end of the _H-2_ complex and the order of loci

$$H\text{-}2K \cdots H\text{-}2D \cdots Tla$$

2. In Leukemia Cells

The expression of Tla antigens in leukemia cells is anomalous in two main respects. First, all strains, regardless of whether they express Tla antigens in their thymuses, can give rise to Tla-positive leukemias. Second, the Tla-positive leukemias can be classified, with regard to the Tla antigens they express, into four groups (Table 11–4); however, in only one group (Tla^a) are the Tla phenotypes of the thymus and leukemias the same. In the remaining three groups, leukemia cells express antigens not present on the thymocytes of the strain in which the leukemia arose. Antigens Tla.1 and Tla.2 are present in all Tla-positive lenkemias; Tla.3 and Tla.4 in some but not in others; Tla.3 is expressed in only those leukemias having arisen in strains that carry antigen 3 in their thymocytes, and Tla.4 is present only in leukemia cells and absent in thymocytes of any strain (the antigen is leukemia-specific).

Table 11-4. _Tla_ phenotypes and genotypes*

Prototype strain	Thymocyte Tla phenotype	Leukemia cell phenotype and presumed _Tla_ genotype of mouse
A	1, 2, 3, −	1, 2, 3, −
C57BL/6	−, −, −, −	1, 2, −, 4,
BALB/c	−, 2, −, −	1, 2, −, −
DBA/2	−, 2, −, −	1, 2, −, 4

3. Interpretation

The *Tla* complex can be viewed as consisting of two types of loci: structural, coding for the structure of the Tla molecules; and regulator, determining expression or nonexpression of the structural genes. All strains carry structural genes for antigens Tla.1 and Tla.2 (they all produce Tla.1- and Tla.2-positive leukemias); on the other hand, structural genes for antigens Tla.3 and Tla.4 are present in some strains and absent in others. The *Tla.3* and *Tla.4* determinants may be alleles at the same locus (the two determinants never occur together in a *Tla* homozygote), whereas the *Tla.1* and *Tla.2* can be two separate loci (the Tla.1 and Tla.2 antigens can occur independently of one another). The regulator genes can act by repressing the structural genes in normal thymocytes and derepressing them in leukemia cells. As pointed out by Schlesinger (1970), the *Tla* structural genes need not be in the same chromosome as the regulator genes. Because the *Tla.1* and *Tla.2* structural genes are identical in all strains, it must be the regulator rather than the structural gene that segregates in the backcross $Tla^a/Tla^b \times Tla^b/Tla^b$. Consequently, it is the regulator *Tla* gene that is linked to *H-2*, and the structural gene can be anywhere in the mouse genome.

D. Tissue Distribution

Three of the four known Tla antigens can be detected on normal thymocytes by the cytotoxic test. A majority of the thymocytes (about 80–90 percent) have a high concentration of Tla antigens. These cells are relatively small, dense, rich in Thy-1, Gv-1, and Ly antigens, and contain very few H-2 antigens (Konda *et al.* 1972, 1973). The thymus also contains a minor subpopulation (10–15 percent) of large lymphocytes with low relative density, high H-2 content and a low content of Thy-1 and Ly antigens. These cells contain no Tla antigens detectable by serological methods. The minor subpopulation is identical to cells remaining in the thymus after short-term cortisone treatment and whole-body irradiation (Konda *et al.* 1973).

According to the current dogma, cells from bone marrow migrate continuously into the thymus, differentiate there, and then leave the thymus to become T lymphocytes. Neither B nor mature T cells react with anti-Tla antibodies in the presence of the complement, indicating that if they contain Tla antigens at all, the quantity of these antigens must be considerably lower than that of the thymocytes. The restriction of Tla antigens to thymocytes leads to the conclusion that the expression of Tla regulator genes requires the thymic environment. This conclusion is supported by the findings of Schlesinger and his co-workers (1965), who lethally irradiated A (*Tla^a*) or C57BL/6 (*Tla^b*) mice, protected them with bone marrow cells from A or C57BL/6 donors, and then tested the thymocytes of the chimeras for Tla antigens. They found that bone marrow cells from *Tla^a* donors repopulate thymuses of *Tla^b* recipients with *Tla^a* lymphocytes, whereas cells from *Tla^b* donors supply *Tla^a* hosts with *Tla^b* thymocytes. In other words, the Tla phenotype of a chimera is determined by the *Tla* genotype of the donor, not by the genotype of the host. An alternative explanation of these results is the selection of a small population of *Tla* precursor cells. However, such an explanation is unlikely, because exposure of the A strain bone marrow cells to Tla antibodies and complement, either *in vitro* (Schlesinger *et al.* 1965) or *in vivo* (Boyse *et al.* 1966), does not affect the ability of these cells to repopulate the thymus of C57BL/6 mice with *Tla^a* lymphocytes.

Recent reports indicate that inoculation of spleen, lymph node, or bone marrow cells from *Tla^a* donors into *Tla^b* recipients results in formation of Tla antibodies (Komuro *et al.* 1973). This observation can be explained by assuming either that a small population of *Tla^a* cells preexists in the inoculum, or that the *Tla^b* cells in the inoculum mature into *Tla^a* cells under the influence of the host's thymus. The latter explanation is supported by the finding that thymectomized mice produce Tla antibodies when immunized with thymocytes (mature *Tla^a* cells) but not when immunized with lymphocytes from bone marrow, spleen, or lymph nodes. It is possible, however, that the thymus is needed not only for the *Tla^b* → *Tla^a* transformation, but also for the continuous expression of the *Tla* genes in the extrathymic lymphocytes. The *Tla^a* cells in the inoculum might, therefore, revert to *Tla^b* cells when they find themselves in a thymus-deprived environment.

E. Is *Tla* a Histocompatibility Locus?

Boyse and his co-workers developed two pairs of *Tla* congenic lines by transferring the *Tla^b* chromosome of strain C57BL/6 onto the A strain background, and the *Tla^a* chromosome of strain A onto the C57BL/6 background. The C57BL/6-*Tla^a* and A-*Tla^b* lines were produced by 15 and 26 backcrossing generations, respectively, and should therefore have been histocompatible with their inbred partners. However, this was not the case. Both skin grafts and leukemia grafts exchanged between the *Tla* congenic lines were rejected (Boyse *et al.* 1972).

After so many backcross generations, it is unlikely that the lines differ in anything other than a short chromosomal segment adjacent to the *Tla* complex, so the hypothetical histocompatibility gene responsible for these rejections has tentatively been assigned to the *Tla* region. Skin-graft rejections ascribable to the *Tla* region have also been reported by Snell *et al.* (1971d), Démant and Graff (1973), and Flaherty and D. Bennett (1973). The *Tla*-associated histoincompatibilities are peculiar in two ways. First, skin grafts exchanged among female mice are rejected rapidly (usually between 14 and 25 days), whereas those exchanged among males survive much longer and sometimes permanently. Second, mice that reject first grafts often permanently accept second grafts from the same donor. Theoretically, the rejections can be caused either by an *H* locus closely linked to, but separate from *Tla*, or by the *Tla* complex itself. The former possibility is supported by the following observations (L. Flaherty, *personal communication*). First, C57BL/6 mice do not reject *Tla* positive leukemia ERLD, although they are fully capable of making antibody to Tla antigens.

Thus, the *Tla* locus itself does not appear to be a histocompatibility locus. Second, the tissue distribution of the *Tla* and *H(Tla)* antigens is different. *Tla* is only expressed on thymus and leukemia cells, whereas *H(Tla)* is expressed on skin, leukemias, melanomas, and fibroblasts. Third, *H(Tla)* is genetically complex and at least some of the *H(Tla)* loci are separable from *Tla* by recombination. Two *H(Tla)* loci have been identified so far, *H(Tla-1)* and *H(Tla-2)*, with the *H(Tla-1)* locus closely linked to *Tla*, and the *H(Tla-2)* locus separable from both *H(Tla-1)* and *Tla*. Fourth, the *H(Tla-1)* genotype does not depend on the *Tla* genotype. Mice have been typed as $H(Tla-1)^c Tla^b$ as well as $H(Tla-1)^b Tla^b$.

F. Antigenic Modulation

Mice immunized against Tla antigens and containing high titers of cytotoxic Tla anbitodies might be expected to resist syngeneic *Tla*-positive leukemias. Paradoxically, not only do such mice succumb to the tumors, but the tumors (recovered after their outgrowth in the immunized mice) lose their sensitivity to Tla antisera *in vitro* and their ability to absorb cytotoxic Tla antibodies (Boyse *et al.* 1963). The loss is only temporary, because a single passage of the tumors in untreated syngeneic hosts leads to a complete reappearance of the Tla antigens. The phenomenon of temporary loss of Tla antigens after exposure to Tla antibodies has been termed *antigenic modulation*. Subsequent studies (Boyse *et al.* 1967) have shown that antigenic modulation has the following five characteristics.

First, it can be accomplished by passive transfer of Tla antisera into unimmunized tumor-bearing mice. Second, it occurs in leukemias induced in *Tla*-negative as well as *Tla*-positive mice. Third, it occurs in normal *Tla*-positive thymocytes *in vivo* after passive administration of Tla antibodies. Fourth, it can be induced in thymuses of young mice suckling on mothers immune to Tla antigens. Fifth, it occurs *in vitro* after exposure of the cells to Tla antibodies. (Leukemia cells modulate readily, usually in less than 90 min; thymocytes modulate little, even after several hours of exposure to Tla antisera.)

Antigenic modulation can be induced by homologous as well as nonhomologous antibodies (Old *et al.* 1968; Table 11–5). For example, anti-Tla.3 modulates not only antigen Tla.3, but also antigens Tla.1 and Tla.2. The only exception is that the modulation of Tla.2 occurs after exposure to anti-Tla.1 or anti-Tla.3, in the absence of Tla.2 antibodies, but not after exposure to anti-Tla.2. The Tla.2 antibodies are not only unable to modulate any Tla antigen, but they actually hinder antigenic modulation by other Tla antibodies. (Antisera containing anti-Tla.2 are less effective in causing modulation than antisera from which the anti-Tla.2 has been removed.) This inhibition of modulation can be explained by the closeness of Tla.2 to Tla.1 and Tla.3 sites on the cell surface and mutual interference among the respective antibodies (Boyse *et al.* 1968a). The failure of anti-Tla.2 to modulate indicates that the precise site of attachment of a Tla antibody is critical in determining whether modulation will ensue (Boyse *et al.* 1968c). The comodulation phenomenon (modulation by nonhomologous antibodies) can be explained by a supposition that the Tla antigens are carried by one molecule or membrane fragment. Such a supposition, however, contradicts the multiple gene hypothesis of the *Tla* complex.

Antigenic modulation is an active metabolic process (Old *et al.* 1968) influenced by temperature (it proceeds best at 37°C, slows down at 22°C, and stops at 0°C) and by metabolic inhibitors (it is arrested by exposure to actinomycin D or iodoacetamide).

Antigenic modulation cannot be attributed to blocking of the antigenic sites by Tla antibodies for four reasons (Boyse *et al.* 1967). First, modulated cells do not stain with fluorescein-labeled antiglobulin sera. Second, the loss of Tla antigenicity in modulated cells is accompanied by an increase in H-2 antigenicity (see below). Third, at 0°C, the cells bind Tla antibodies but do not modulate. Fourth, modulation of Tla.3 with anti-Tla.3 also modulates Tla.1, but blocking of Tla.3 does not block Tla.1.

Antigenic modulation is not the result of the selection of Tla-negative variants from the cell population as it occurs

1. rapidly (*in vitro* it can be demonstrated within an hour after exposure to Tla antibodies; Boyse *et al.* 1967);
2. in the absence of lytic complement at dilutions of antibodies higher than those showing cytotoxic effect in the presence of complement (Boyse *et al.* 1967);
3. after exposure to F(ab) fragments that do not bind complement (Lamm *et al.* 1968).

Biochemical studies (Yu and Cohen 1974a, b) indicate that in tissue culture Tla antigens prelabeled with radioisotopes disappear more rapidly from cells undergoing antigenic modulation than from control nonmodulating cells.

Table 11-5. Capability of Tla antibodies to modulate Tla antigens*

Tla antibody	Modulation of Tla antigen**			
	1	2	3	4
1	+	+	?	+ ?
2	−	−	−	−
3	+	+	+	?
4	+	+	?	+

* Reproduced with permission from L. J. Old, E. Stockert, E. A. Boyse, and J. H. Kim: "Antigenic modulation. Loss of TL antigen from cells exposed to TL antibody. Study of the phenomenon *in vitro*. *Journal of Experimental Medicine 127*:523–539. Copyright © 1968 by The Rockefeller University Press. All rights reserved; E. A. Boyse, E. Stockert, and L. J. Old: Properties of four antigens specified by the Tla locus. Similarities and differences. In *International Convocation on Immunology*, pp. 353–357. Copyright © 1968c by S. Karger, Basel. All rights reserved.

** +(−) = antigen is (is not) modulated by indicated antibody.

However, the antigens are released into the tissue culture medium from both modulating and nonmodulating cells, and the total quantity of the Tla antigens recovered from the medium is the same in both groups. Also, the synthesis of the Tla antigens in modulating and nonmodulating cells is the same. All this indicates that the modulating cells either degrade the Tla antigens more readily than nonmodulating cells or that the antigens are removed from the cell surface by pinocytosis. In this respect antigenic modulation resembles antibody-induced antigen redistribution (capping, cf. Chapter Fourteen). However, it appears that pinocytosis of Tla antigens does not require "cap" formation because: (1) staining with fluorescent antibodies of modulated cells does not reveal significant numbers of caps; (2) monovalent F(ab) antibody fragments can induce modulation but not capping.

G. Interaction of Tla Antigens in the Cell Membrane

Studies on quantitative expression of Tla antigens in normal thymocytes led to the following conclusions (Boyse *et al.* 1968b; Table 11–6). First, heterozygotes Tla^a/Tla^b express half the quantity of Tla.1 and Tla.3 present in Tla^a/Tla^a homozygotes. Second, heterozygotes Tla^a/Tla^c express the full quantity of Tla.1 and Tla.3 (in contrast to Tla^a/Tla^b heterozygotes) but a reduced quantity of Tla.2. Third, homozygotes Tla^a/Tla^a express a higher quantity of Tla.2 than homozygotes Tla^c/Tla^c, even though both homozygotes contain the same amount of genetic information coding for antigen Tla.2. Fourth, heterozygotes Tla^b/Tla^c express half the quantity of Tla.2 present in Tla^c/Tla^c homozygotes.

It is tempting to explain the 50 percent reduction of antigens Tla.1 and Tla.3 in the Tla^a/Tla^b heterozygotes by the effect of dosage: in the homozygote, two alleles of the same kind produce two doses of the same antigen, while in the heterozygote two different alleles at the same locus produce two different antigens, each in a single dose. Such an explanation, however, requires an

Table 11-6. Quantitative representation of Tla antigens on thymocytes of different genotypes*

Tla haplotype	*Tla* genotype	Tla antigen**		
		1	2	3
a/a	1, 2, 3, − / 1, 2, 3, −	100 (s)	100 (s)	100 (s)
a/b	1, 2, 3, − /−, −, −, −	50	·	50
a/c	1, 2, 3, − /−, 2, −, −	100	80	50
c/c	−, 2, −, − /−, 2, −, −	0	60	0
b/c	−, −, −, − /−, 2, −, −	0	30	0

* Based on Boyse *et al.* 1968b.
** s = standard; all other values expressed as percent standard. · = information not available.

expression of *Tla.1* and *Tla.3* structural genes in the *Tla^b* chromosome, a possibility contradicted by the fact that no Tla.1 and Tla.3 antigens can be found in normal *Tla^b/Tla^b* thymocytes. It is equally unlikely that the *Tla.1* and *Tla.3* structural loci in the *Tla^b* chromosome carry different, as yet unrecognized alleles. If this were the case, *Tla^b* leukemias would not be expected to express antigen Tla.1, which they do. Boyse and his co-workers (1968b) explain the reduced *Tla^a* antigenicity in *Tla^a/Tla^b* heterozygotes as resulting from interaction of the *Tla* locus with the *H-2* complex (see below).

H. Interaction Between Tla and H-2 Antigens

Quantitative determination of H-2 antigens in the thymocytes of strains carrying different *Tla* alleles provided the following information about *Tla–H-2* interaction (Boyse *et al.* 1967, 1968b; Table 11-7).

First, antigens controlled by the *K* region are not influenced by the Tla phenotype. Second, thymocytes of *Tla^a/Tla^a* or *Tla^c/Tla^c* homozygotes have a reduced quantity of H-2D antigens compared to *Tla^b/Tla^b* thymocytes. This reduction occurs regardless of the *H-2* haplotype (it has been observed in *H-2^a*, *H-2^b*, and *H-2^k* thymocytes). Third, the two known Tla-positive phenotypes of the thymus (1, 2, 3, − and −, 2, −, −) reduce the surface representation of the H-2D antigens equally. Fourth, the reduction of H-2 antigens in *Tla^a/Tla^b* thymocytes is half that occurring in *Tla^a/Tla^a* thymocytes. Fifth, in *H-2* heterozygotes, the reduction equally affects the products of both *H-2* haplotypes. Finally, the reduction of H-2 antigens occurs regardless of whether the *Tla* and *H-2D* complexes are in *cis-* or *trans*-relation.

An inverse relationship between the expression of Tla and H-2D antigens is also observed *in vitro* in cells undergoing antigenic modulation. Cells exposed to Tla antibodies in the absence of complement show an increase of H-2D antigenicity concurrently with the decrease of Tla antigenicity (Boyse *et al.* 1967; Old *et al.* 1968). This observation indicates that it is the Tla phenotype rather than the genotype that is responsible for the fluctuation of H-2D antigenicity.

Table 11-7. Effect of Tla phenotype on the expression of H-2 antigens*

			Relative content of antigens controlled by**			
H-2 haplotype	*Tla* haplotype	*Tla* genotype	*H-2D^a*	*H-2D^b*	*H-2K^a*	*H-2K^b*
b/b	b/b	−, −, −, −/−, −, −, −	−	100 (s)	−	100 (s)
b/b	a/a	1, 2, 3, −/ 1, 2, 3, −	−	58	−	101
a/a	b/b	−, −, −, −/−, −, −, −	100 (s)	−	100 (s)	−
a/a	a/a	1, 2, 3, −/ 1 2, 3, −	47–77	−	100	−
a/b	b/b	−, −, −, −/−, −, −, −	100 (s)	100 (s)	·	·
a/b	a/b	1, 2, 3, −/−, −, −, −	72	66	100 (s)	100 (s)
a/b	b/a	−, −, −, −/ 1, 2, 3, −	74	64	98	102
a/b	a/a	1, 2, 3, −/ 1, 2, 3, −	52	34	·	·

* Based on Boyse *et al.* 1968b.
** (s) = standard; all other values expressed as percent of standard; · = information not available; − = absence of antigen.

The mechanism of *Tla–H-2* interaction remains unexplained. It may involve steric masking of the H-2 sites by Tla, competition for a common precursor, or competition for space in the cell membrane.

I. Biochemistry

Membrane fragments containing Tla activity are separable from those containing H-2 activity (D. Davies *et al.* 1967, 1969; Vitetta *et al.* 1972b; Muramatsu *et al.* 1973; Yu and Cohen 1974a), indicating that the Tla and H-2 antigens probably reside on different molecules. The Tla fragments are glycoproteins with molecular weights of 40,000–50,000 daltons, which is approximately the same as the molecular weight of H-2 fragments. The carbohydrate chain of the Tla glycoprotein is larger than that of the H-2 glycoprotein: the former has a molecular weight of 4500 and the latter a molecular weight of 3500 (Muramatsu *et al.* 1973). Attempts to separate individual Tla antigens biochemically have failed.

III. The *T-t* Complex

The *T-t* system consists of two series of factors, dominant (*T*) and recessive (*t*). (For reviews, see Grüneberg 1952; Dunn 1964; Dunn *et al.* 1962; D. Bennett 1964; Gluecksohn-Waelsch and Erickson 1970.) The expression of these factors is pleiotropic, with syndromes ranging from mere shortening of the tail to embryonic lethality. The shortening of the tail is one effect shared by different *T-t* factors, and it is chiefly because of this effect, and because the factors all seem to map in the same chromosomal region, that they are considered members of the same system. Apart from these similarities, however, they form a heterogeneous group that almost certainly encompasses more than one locus. Because of a striking difference between the dominant and the recessive series, the two will be discussed separately.

A. The T Factors

The first member of the *T* series was described by Dobrovolskaia-Zavadskaia in 1927 and named *Brachyury* (*Short-tail*, *T*). The short-tailed mouse was discovered in an experiment involving X-irradiation, but it does not appear that the *T* mutation was induced by the X-rays. Most of the presently maintained *T* stocks are descendants of the original brachyury mouse of Dobrovolskaia-Zavadskaia. In addition, six other *T* factors have also been discovered: *T* (Carter and Phillips 1950), T^h (Lyon 1959), T^{hg} (Kuminek 1959), T^c (Searle 1966), T^J (K. P. Hummel, *personal communication*), and T^{2J} (D. W. Bailey, *personal communication*). However, it is not certain whether all these mutations occurred independently of the original *T* and, if they did, whether they occurred at the same locus. Phenotypically, different *T* factors are indistinguishable from one another.

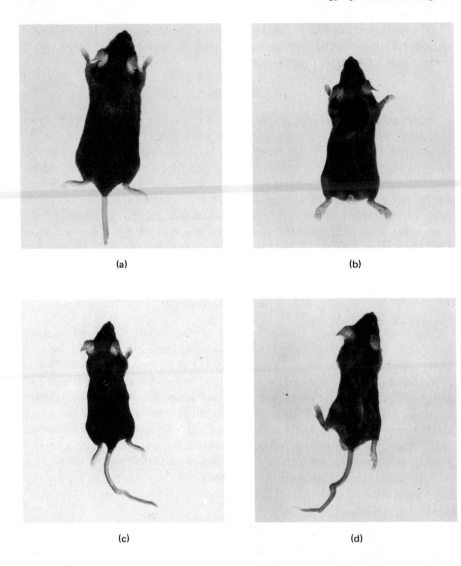

(a)   (b)

(c)   (d)

Fig. 11-6. Mutant genes in chromosome 17. (a) *Short tail* (*T*), (b) *tailless* (*t*), (c) *Fused* (*Fu*), (d) *Kinky* (*Ki*), (e) *Hair-pin Tail* (*Hp*), (f) *tufted* (*tf*) (dorsal view), (g) *tufted* (*tf*) (abdominal view), (h) *thin fur* (thf).

Phenotypic expression of the *T* gene in a heterozygous state is extremely variable and depends to a great extent on the genetic background. In some inbred strains (e.g., C3H), the tails of the *T*/+ heterozygotes have almost normal lengths with only a few terminal vertebrae missing (the tail is blunt, rather than pointed). Some animals of such strains do not express the *T* factor at all, even though it is possible to demonstrate by a progeny test that they carry the factor. Such animals are known as *normal overlaps*. In other strains (e.g., C57BL/10),

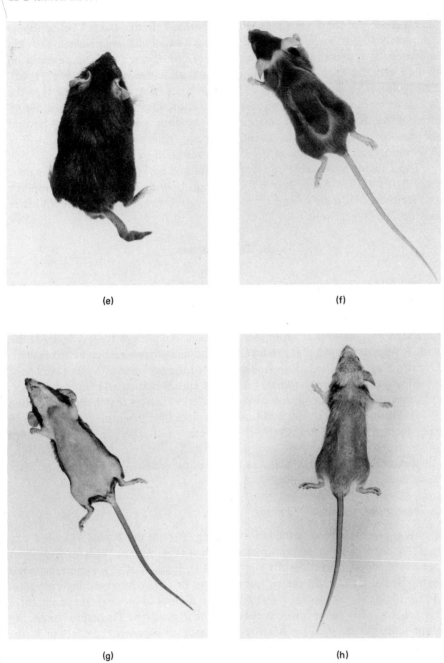

(e)

(f)

(g)

(h)

Fig. 11-6

the expression of the T gene may reach the other extreme, the tail being almost completely absent. Such mice usually possess a small filament consisting of skin and connective tissue, but no tail vertebrae. In most cases, however, expression of the T gene causes the tail to be shortened to half its normal length (Fig. 11–6a). Embryological studies of the $T/+$ heterozygotes have demonstrated that the tail is normal until the eleventh day of gestation. On the eleventh day, a constriction develops at varying positions and the distal portion of the tail beyond the constriction degenerates, eventually being resorbed (Chesley 1935). The T/T homozygotes die at about $10\frac{1}{2}$ days of gestation (see below).

The T factor is available on several noninbred backgrounds and in congenic lines B10.T (G. D. Snell, *personal communication*) and B10.T(6R) (Stimpfling and Reichert 1970); the T^J and T^{2J} mutants are present in congenic line BALB.T^J and B6.T^{2J}, respectively.

B. The t Factors

1. Discovery

The first member of the recessive t series was discovered by Dobrovolskaia-Zavadskaia and Kobozieff (1932) in an outcross of the brachyury stock to an unrelated normal mouse. From the outcross, three lines of tailless mice, A, 29, and 19, were developed that produced only tailless offspring when mated *inter se*. Genetic analysis of the tailless stocks revealed the presence of a recessive factor which was called *anury* (*tailless, t*). Lines 19 and 29 carried an identical t factor, t^1 (Dunn 1939), whereas line A carried a different factor, t^0 (Chesley and Dunn 1936). Since then, over 100 additional t factors have been described, some in mice from wild populations (t^{w1}, t^{w2}, t^{w3}, etc.), and others in laboratory mice (t^1, t^2, t^3, etc.).

The recessive t factors display a number of unusual characteristics, which are described below.

2. Interaction with the T Factor

Most t factors enhance the tail-modifying effect of the T gene in such a way that T/t heterozygotes are completely tailless (Fig. 11–6b). This property has been used for the detection of t factors in a population. The $t/+$ heterozygotes have normal tails, as do the t/t homozygotes or t^x/t^y compound heterozygotes if they happen to be viable (t^x and t^y are two different t factors). However, there are t factors that either have no effect on the T gene (the T/t heterozygotes are short-tailed just as the $T/+$ heterozygotes are), or suppress the effect of T (the T/t heterozygotes have normal tails). It is possible that because T has been used as a diagnostic marker for finding new t factors, a selection for the enhancing factors has unknowingly been effected, and it may be that in natural populations, the T-suppressing factors are as frequent as the T-enhancing factors. Specific examples of the different genotypes and corresponding phenotypes are provided in Table 11–8.

3. Lethality

The viability of the t/t homozygotes divides the t factors into three groups: lethal, semiviable, and viable. The lethal group contains factors that kill the t/t homozygotes before or shortly after birth. In the semiviable group, some of the t/t homozygotes die during embryonic development, while others may live long after birth. In the viable group, the t/t homozygotes demonstrate normal, or close to normal, viability. The lethal factors can further be divided into five complementation groups, the factors of different groups complementing each other genetically and those of the same group failing to do so (c.f. Table 11-9). A lethal factor t^n is considered different from lethal factor t^x if viable, normal-tailed offspring are obtained in cross $T/t^n \times T/t^x$ and these offspring prove to be t^n/t^x (Dunn 1956). The complementarity of two different factors, t^n and t^x, is explained by assuming that t^n has a defect in one region of the chromosome and t^x in another region, and that the defective regions have unaffected, normally functioning counterparts in the homologous chromosomes. The proportion of normal-tailed offspring produced by cross $T/t^n \times T/t^x$ is usually lower than the proportion that would be expected had the t^n/t^x heterozygotes had the same viability as their T/t^n or T/t^x sibs. The proportion of normal-tailed animals can be as low as 13 percent with some t factors, and approach the expected number with other t factors. The five complementation groups are listed in Table 11-9. Each complementation group is characterized by a uniform time of death of t/t embryos and characteristic syndromes preceding the death. In the following paragraphs, the embryonic effects of the t factors are described and fit into the

Table 11-8. Phenotypic expressions of various t factors

Genotype*	Phenotype
$+/+$	normal tail
$T/+$	short tail
T/T	embryonic lethal
T/t^0 (T/t^1 or T/t^3)	tailless
$+/t^0$ ($+/t^1$ or $+/t^3$)	normal tail
t^0/t^0 (t^1/t^1, t^{h7}/t^{h7}, or t^{h18}/t^{h18})	embryonic lethal
t^3/t^3	viable; normal tail
t^{AE5}/t^{AE5}	viable; short tail
t^0/t^1	viable; normal tail
t^0/t^3 (or t^1/t^3)	viable; normal tail
T/t^{h7}	normal tail
T/t^{h18}	short tail

* Factor t^3 was derived from T/t^1 heterozygotes (Dunn and Gluecksohn-Schoenheimer 1950); factors t^{h7} and t^{h18} from T/t^6 heterozygotes (Lyon and Meredith 1964a); h7 and h18 are seventh and eighteenth t factors discovered at the Radiological Research unit at Harwell, England; t^{AE5} is the fifth t factor discovered at the Albert Einstein College of Medicine, Bronx, New York (Glucksohn-Waelsch and Erickson 1970).

framework of normal development. (Fig. 11–7 and Table 11–10). [Detailed accounts of mouse embryology are provided by Snell and Stevens (1966), Rugh (1968), and Theiler (1972).]

The mouse egg is fertilized in the ampulla, the uppermost portion of the oviduct, and the first cleavage division, which results in two cells of equal size (*blastomeres*), is completed near the exit of the ampulla within 24 hr. At 2 days, the egg, while still in the oviduct, has advanced to the 16-cell stage (the *morula*). It enters the uterus on the third day, at which time it begins to develop a small, excentrically located cavity, the *blastocoel*. At 4 days, the enlargement of the blastocoel leads to the development of a ball-like, fluid-filled structure, the *blastocyst*. At one pole of the blastocyst the cells aggregate into a knob (the *inner cell mass*), while the rest of the blastocyst forms a single layer of flat cells, the *trophectoderm*.

The earliest t factor (and the earliest lethal factor known in mammals), t^{12}, affects the transition from the morula to the blastocyst. In the t^{12}/t^{12} homozygotes, development is arrested at the morula stage, causing degeneration of the cells and resorption of the embryo (Smith 1956). A prominent sign of morula degeneration is a change in the morphology of the nucleolus. In normal embryos, the round and smooth nucleoli of the morula become elongated and rough in the blastocyst, while in t^{12}/t^{12} morulae, the nucleoli remain spherical and smooth. The degenerative morphological changes are accompanied by biochemical defects. While in normal development the transition from a morula to a blastocyst is marked by a sharp increase in RNA synthesis, no such increase occurs in the t^{12}/t^{12} embryos (Mintz 1964; Hillman 1972). Ultrastructural studies of the t^{12}/t^{12} morulae reveal the presence of lipid droplets, of fibrillo-granular bodies resembling nucleoli, large numbers of free ribosomes, and contraction of nucleolonema (Calarco and Brown 1968), all features absent in the $+/+$ morulae. Which of these changes represents a cause and which an effect is not known. It has been suggested, but not proved, that the t^{12} factor might represent the deletion of a nucleolar organizer coding for ribosomal RNA (J. Klein and Raška 1968). Death of the t^{12}/t^{12} homozygotes occurs at $3\frac{1}{2}$ days.

Table 11-9. Complementation groups of t factors

Complementation group	Other members of the group
t^{12}	t^{w32}
t^{0}	$t^{1}, t^{2}, t^{6}, t^{w4}, t^{30}$
t^{w5}	$t^{w6}, t^{w10}, t^{w11}, t^{w13}, t^{w14}, t^{w15}, t^{w16}, t^{w17}, t^{w37},$ $t^{w38}, t^{w39}, t^{w41}, t^{w46}, t^{w47}, t^{w74}, t^{w75}$
t^{4}	$t^{9}, t^{w18}, t^{w30}, t^{w32}, t^{w52}$
t^{w1}	$t^{w3}, t^{w12}, t^{w20}, t^{w21}, t^{w22}, t^{w71}, t^{w72}$

Implantation of the normal embryo begins at $4\frac{1}{2}$ days, when the uterine wall is invaded by the *ectoplacental cone*, an outgrowth of the inner cell mass. Almost simultaneously, the inner cell mass enlarges and bulges into the blastocoel, to produce a conelike protrusion, the *egg cylinder*. The layer of cells on the blastocoelic surface of the developing egg cylinder differentiates morphologically and functionally from the rest of the embryo and becomes the *endoderm*. The endoderm layer is eventually found on the entire inner surface of the blastocoel (now called the *yolk cavity*), outside the egg cylinder. The endoderm lining the egg cylinder is called *proximal*, while the endoderm lining the trophectoderm is called *distal*. The ectoderm of the elongating egg cylinder divides the cylinder into two regions, *embryonic* and *extraembryonic*, separated by a shallow furrow.

It is approximately at this stage that the t^0 factor exerts its effect on the embryo. In the t^0/t^0 homozygotes, the inner cell mass fails to differentiate into the two types of ectoderm, the endoderm lifts off the undifferentiated ectoderm, the cells of the embryo become pycnotic, and the whole embryo degenerates and is resorbed (Gluecksohn-Schoenheimer 1940). The t^0/t^0 embryos can first be distinguished from normal embryos at the age of about $5\frac{1}{4}$ days; they die within the following 40 hr, and their resorption begins about 7 days after fertilization. The t^0 factor appears to affect primarily the differentiation process that leads to the formation of the definitive ectoderm (D. Bennett 1964).

In normal embryos, the egg cylinder continues to elongate and to protrude more deeply into the yolk cavity. At about 6 days of gestation, a small cavity appears in the cylinder, first in the embryonic and later also in the extraembryonic ectoderm; the two cavities later coalesce into one, forming the *proamniotic cavity*.

Table 11-10. Time table of early development of the mouse embryo*

Stage of development	Days	Hours	Stage of development	Days	Hours
Fertilization	0	0	Exocoelom	7	
2 cells		24–38	Head process	7	
4 cells		38–50	Amnion, chorion	7	6
5–8 cells		50–64	Allantois	7	6
9–16 cells		60–70	Yolk sac	7	6
Blastocyst		74–82	Neural groove	7	6
Egg cylinder	4		Notochord	7	6
Implantation	4	12	Foregut pocket	7	12
Embryonic and extra-			First somites	7	12
embryonic ectoderm	4	12	Hindgut pocket	7	18
Proamniotic cavity	5		Turning of the embryo	8	
Ectoplacental cone	5		4 somites	8	8
Primitive streak	6	12	10 somites	8	12
Mesoderm	6	12	Closing of midgut	8	18
Amniotic fold	6	12			

* Based on Snell and Stevens 1966; and Rugh 1968.

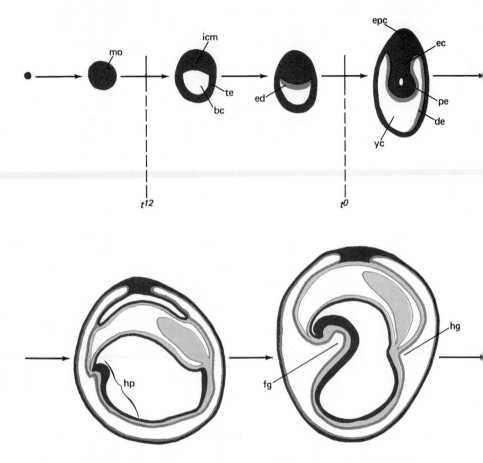

Fig. 11-7. Diagrammatic representation of the early embryological development of the mouse embryo. The individual *t* factors act at indicated stages. aca = amniotic cavity; af = amniotic fold; al = allantois; am = amnion; bc = blastocoel; ch = chorion; de = distal endoderm; ec = egg cylinder; eca = ectoplacental cavity; ed = endoderm; ee = embryonic ectoderm; eee = extraembryonic ectoderm; epc = ectoplacental cone; exc = exocoelom; fg = foregut; hg = hindgut; hp = head process; icm = inner cell mass; m = mesoderm; mg = midgut; mo = morula; pac = proamniotic cavity; pe = proximal endoderm; ps = primitive streak; te = trophectoderm; yc = yolk cavity; ys = yolk sac.

In embryos homozygous for the t^{w5} factor, the differentiation proceeds no further (D. Bennett and Dunn 1958). In embryos reaching the egg-cylinder stage, the cells of the embryonic ectoderm begin to degenerate and are gradually resorbed while the rest of the embryo remains unaffected and may continue to develop for another 2 or 3 days. The localization of the defect to a small area

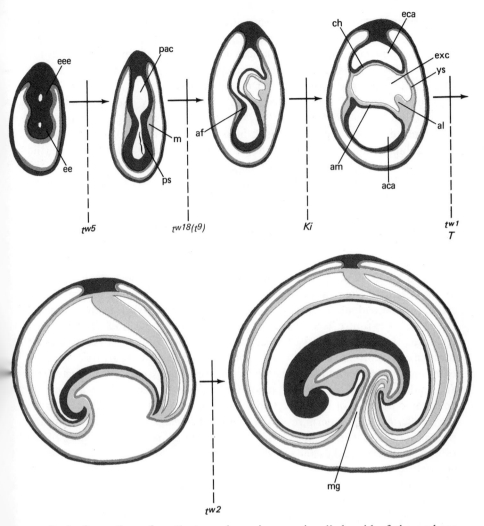

results in formation of an "extraembryonic organism," devoid of the embryo proper but containing all the embryonic membranes. The t^{w5}/t^{w5} embryos are first recognized as abnormal at $6\frac{1}{2}$–7 days; they die after 8–10 days of gestation. The major effect of the t^{w5} factor appears to be on the differentiation of the embryonic ectoderm.

In normal mice, the embryo proper develops from the embryonic ectoderm and endoderm. Prior to 6 days of gestation, however, this portion of the embryo is merely a cone lacking any indication of the future location of the embryo's main axis. At 6 days, the longitudinal (anterioposterior) axis of the embryo is first established by a thickening of the embryonic ectoderm into a narrow strip, called the *primitive streak*. The streak extends from the junction of the embryonic and extraembryonic ectoderms (from the area where the tail of the future embryo will be located) to about halfway to the tip of the egg cylinder. Although after this point most of the growth activity in the embryo originates from the primitive streak, the streak itself later disappears. It seems to represent merely an organizational and growth center of the embryo.

The formation of the primitive streak is affected by the t^{w18} factor (D. Bennett and Dunn 1960). In the t^{w18}/t^{w18} embryos the streak grows more than in normal embryos and bulges as a high crest into the proamniotic cavity, causing duplication of portions of the embryo, particularly the neural tube (the crest pushes through the midline of the neural tube and splits it in half). The first morphologically recognizable abnormality in the t^{w18}/t^{w18} embryos appears at 7 days, and the embryos die between 8 and 11 days after fertilization. A similar effect has been described for factors t^9 and t^4 (Moser and Glueksohn-Waelsch 1967), which belong to the same complementation group as t^{w18}.

In normal embryos, the growth activity of the primitive streak results in the formation of a third germinal layer, the *mesoderm*. The first mesodermal cells appear at about $6\frac{1}{2}$ days by delamination from the caudal (posterior) end of the primitive streak. The mesoderm grows as a sheet pushing between the embryonic ectoderm and endoderm on both sides of the primitive streak from the caudal end toward the future head of the embryo. By 7 days, the mesoderm has all but separated the ectoderm and endoderm layers in the embryo proper except for the area of the primitive streak. Some mesoderm cells also depart from the area of the embryo proper and force themselves between the extraembryonic ectoderm and endoderm. At the line of junction between the embryonic and extra-embryonic portions of the egg cylinder, the insertion of the mesoderm between the ectoderm and endoderm results in a ridge, the *amniotic fold*, bulging into the proamniotic cavity, and later constricting the egg cylinder. The bulging of the ridge is most rapid at the caudal end of the primitive streak, where the mesoderm entered the extraembryonic portion of the egg cylinder. In this region, the first fold is soon followed by a second, and each fold becomes hollow as cavities develop in it. The cavities eventually coalesce into one, forming the *exocoelom*. Closing of the constriction divides the proamniotic cavity into three cavities: the *amniotic* cavity lined with embryonic ectoderm, the exocoelom lined with mesoderm, and the *ectoplacental* cavity lined with extraembryonic ectoderm. The cavities are separated by two membranes: *amnion*, between the amniotic cavity and the exocoelom, and *chorion*, between the exocoelom and the ecto-placental cavity. The membranes consist of the ectoderm and mesoderm, whereas the lateral walls of the exocoelom (*splanchnopleura* or *yolk sac*) consist of endoderm and mesoderm. Shortly after the exocoelom becomes established, the mesoderm at the caudal end of the primitive streak sends a saclike protrusion (the *allantois*) into it. The allantois grows toward the ectoplacental cone and eventually fuses with the chorion, forming a wall in which vessels connecting the embryo to the maternal circulation develop. Prior to the seventh day, the growth from the primitive streak is limited to the caudal portion of the embryo and to both sides of the streak. At the seventh day, however, growth begins from the opposite (cephalic) end of the streak and produces a wedgelike structure between the ectoderm and the mesoderm, with the tip of the wedge pointing toward the head of the future embryo proper. The wedgelike *head process* sends out a thin sheet between the ectoderm and the mesoderm in the entire cephalic portion of the egg cylinder. When the front of the head process meets the front of the mesoderm, the two cell layers overlap with the head process adjacent to the endoderm and the mesoderm adjacent to the ectoderm. Simultaneously, the embryonic ectoderm develops a shallow trough in the axis of the primitive streak. The trough, the beginning of the *neural groove*, extends from the cephalic end of the primitive streak, toward the embryonic and extraembryonic junction. The neural groove gradually deepens and later closes at the top to form the *neural tube*. Concurrently with the development of the neural groove, the head process beneath the groove thickens into the *notochord*. The origin of the notochord is questionable, but most embryologists agree that it is derived from the endoderm.

The development of the neural tube is affected by the t^{wl} factor (D. Bennett *et al.* 1959). In t^{wl}/t^{wl} homozygotes, the first abnormalities observed are pycnosis and degeneration of the ventral portion of the neural tube in the hindbrain area, from which the degenerative process spreads along the longitudinal axis of the embryo in both directions, affecting the head first and tail last. The process begins at about 9 days and reaches its peak at about 11 days, when approximately half the embryos are severely affected and die. Damage in the other half of the embryos is less extensive, consisting of reduced size, edema, hydrocephaly, and microcephaly, and the embryos may even live until birth.

The primary target of the T factor is probably the notochord (Chesley 1935; Gluecksohn-Schoenheimer 1940; Grüneberg 1958), because in most T/T embryos the notochord is either completely missing or is greatly reduced in size. T/T homozygotes are first distinguishable at about $8\frac{1}{2}$ days of gestation by the presence of mysterious blebs and vesicles on either side of the longitudinal axis and by irregularities in the neural tube, mainly lateral deviations of the tube from the main axis. The blebs disappear 1 day later, but the irregularities of the neural tube persist and grow larger, particularly in the posterior end of the embryo. Reduction of the whole posterior region of the body follows, with the embryos failing to develop allantoic connection with the mother and dying at about $10\frac{3}{4}$ days after fertilization.

The notochord seems also to be affected by the Ki gene (Gluecksohn-Schoenheimer 1949), because the main abnormalities of Ki/Ki embryos are the development of more than one longitudinal embryonic axis and hyperplasia of embryonic tissues, particularly of neural ectoderm and mesoderm. The multiplication (most commonly duplication) of the embryonic axis could lead to completely separate twins or to single embryos with two hearts, double allantois, or two heads. The uncontrolled growth of embryonic tissue produces masses of ball-shaped, unorganized tissues (*Bauchstücks*). The formation of embryonic membranes is also highly disturbed, and the embryos are often found outside them. The *Ki/Ki* embryos die between 8 and 10 days after fertilization.

In normal embryos, beginning at $7\frac{3}{4}$ days, the portion of mesoderm parallel to the notochord differentiates into paired segmental structures (*somites*). The first pair of somites appears anteriorly to the caudal portion of the primitive streak. Formation of over 60 additional somites then follows in more or less regular intervals, and this regularity provides a convenient means for estimating the embryo's age. Approximately 7 days after fertilization, a small invagination (the *foregut*) develops in the endoderm of the embryo's cephalic portion; a similar invagination develops later in the caudal portion of the embryo (the *hindgut*), giving the embryo an S-shaped appearance. At about $8\frac{1}{2}$ days, the embryo begins to rotate along its longitudinal axis, the head in one direction and the tail in the opposite direction. The rotation changes the flexure of the dorsum from concave to convex and the shape of the embryo from "S" to "C." The rotation also joins the walls of the exocoelom (the splanchnopleures) at the ventral side of the embryo and connects the foregut and hindgut pockets with a *midgut* groove. The splanchnopleures eventually fuse together into a single tube and the foregut and hindgut break through to the outside, giving rise to the mouth and anus. After the main features of the embryo are formed, the organogenesis begins and birth occurs 21 days after fertilization.

The last-acting t factors belong to the semiviable group [t^{w2}, t^{w8}, t^{w36}, t^{w40}, and others (D. Bennett and Dunn 1969)]. These factors are similar in their properties, but it is not clear whether they are all identical. The embryological abnormalities caused by the semiviable factors are recognizable at 14 days of gestation, perhaps even earlier (D. Bennett and Dunn 1969). The organ most severely affected in the t^{sv}/t^{sv} homozygotes (t^{sv} = semiviable t factor) is the brain, particularly the forebrain region. The embryos display various degrees of otocephaly, with the most extreme otocephalics totally lacking the forebrain; anopthalmia and micropthalmia are observed in less extreme cases. Most of the affected embryos are also small in size and retarded in their development. The viability of the t^{sv}/t^{sv} homozygotes ranges from 51 percent for t^{w2} to 1.7 percent for t^{w49}, and the death of the abnormal embryos is also spread over a relatively long period of time. The semiviable t factors seem to act during the stage of neural ectoderm differentiation into brainstem and forebrain.

In summary, several generalizations can be made about the embryological effect of the various t factors. First, the t factors act over almost the entire span of embryological differentiation, each group of factors acting at a specific time and in a specific manner. Second, the earlier a particular t factor acts, the more severe is its effect, with the latest-acting factors permitting survival of some embryos. Third, most t factors seem to affect ectodermal, and more specifically, neuroectodermal derivatives. Fourth, the different groups of t factors seem to act on different switch points of neuroectodermal differentiation, as is illustrated below (D. Bennett *et al.* 1972a):

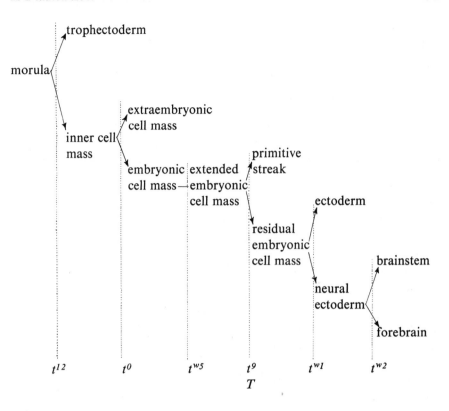

t^{12} t^0 t^{w5} t^9 t^{w1} t^{w2}

T

4. Segregation Distortion

A mating $T/t♀ × +/+♂$ produces an equal proportion of $T/+$ (short-tailed) and $+/t$ (normal-tailed) progeny, as expected for a system following simple Mendelian principles of gene segregation. In the reciprocal mating, $+/+ ♀ × T/t ♂$, however, the proportion of t factors transmitted to the progeny departs markedly from the expected value of 0.5 (Kobozieff 1935; Chesley and Dunn 1936). The departure (*segregation distortion*) can be either toward a *high transmission ratio* (proportion of t factors among the progeny > 0.50, and often as high as 0.99) or toward a *low transmission ratio* (proportion of t factors < 0.50 and sometimes as low as 0.1). Transmission ratios (TR) of the more common t factors are listed in Table 11-11. These ratios represent averages obtained by testing several different males, each characterized by his own transmission ratio, which may differ from the average ratio (*between-male heterogeneity*; see Dunn 1943, 1960; Braden 1960; Braden and Weiler 1964). In addition, heterogeneity in transmission ratios appears to exist between litters sired by a single male (*within-male heterogeneity*; see Dunn 1943; Yanagisawa et al. 1961; Braden and Weiler 1964). Within-male heterogeneity is superimposed on the normal variability caused by small sample size (Braden and Weiler 1964), as can be demonstrated by special statistical treatment of the segregation data.

Table 11-11. Transmission ratios of the more common t factors

Lethal factor	TR	Reference	Semiviable factor	TR	Reference	Viable factor	TR	Reference
t^{12}	0.90	Dunn 1960	t^{w2}	0.95	Dunn 1960; D. Bennett and Dunn 1969	t^3	0.43	L. C. Dunn, *personal communication*
t^0	0.73	Dunn 1960	t^{w8}	0.76	D. Bennett and Dunn 1969	t^8	0.49	L. C. Dunn, *personal communication*
t^{w5}	0.73	Dunn 1960	t^{w36}	0.97	D. Bennett and Dunn 1969	t^{13}	0.35	L. C. Dunn, *personal communication*
t^9	0.45	Dunn 1960	t^{w49}	0.95	D. Bennett and Dunn 1969	t^{25}	0.50	L. C. Dunn, *personal communication*
t^{w18}	0.59	Dunn 1960				t^{28}	0.27	L. C. Dunn, *personal communication*
t^{w1}	0.89	Dunn 1960				t^{34}	0.23	L. C. Dunn, *personal communication*
t^6	0.61	Erickson 1973				t^{38}	0.17	L. C. Dunn, *personal communication*
t^{w12}	0.96	Dunn 1960				t^{w19}	0.38	L. C. Dunn, *personal communication*

The heterogeneity leads to the appearance of "clusters" of offspring with either the t or the T factors in great excess among individual litters from a T/t male (Dunn 1960). Such clusters are not found among the offspring of males with an undisturbed transmission ratio. The causes of within-male heterogeneity may lie in physiological and environmental conditions existing at the time of mating. The T factor is irrelevant to the segregation distortion in T/t males, because the same distortion also occurs with $+/t$ males.

An effect of the female's T-t genotype on the male transmission ratios has been postulated by Bateman (1960a, b) and by Braden (1960). According to Bateman (1960a, b) spermatozoa carrying a t^e factor (t-Edinburgh) unite more frequently with $+$ than with T eggs and more frequently with T than with t eggs; according to Braden (1960), spermatozoa carrying t^0, t^3, t^9, or t^{12} factors unite more frequently with t than with $+$ eggs. However, Braden's more recent results (1972) with the same t factors indicate no preference of the t-bearing sperm for t or $+$ eggs. A similar conclusion can be drawn from a large body of data published by Dunn and Gluecksohn-Schoenheimer (1939, 1953). It is therefore doubtful that the T-t effect of the eggs is real; in fact, Braden (1972) is now inclined to attribute the effect to within-male heterogeneity.

When and where the actual distortion takes place is not known. It is known, however, that at the time of meiosis the two chromosomes (t and $+$) segregate normally in a 1:1 ratio. Evidence for this comes from metaphase II counts in experiments in which the $+$-bearing chromosome was marked by the $T(19;17)7Bn$ translocation (C. Hammerberg and J. Klein, *unpublished data*). It is also known that the litter size in mating $T/t \, \male \times +/+ \, \female$ is the same as in reciprocal mating $T/t \, \female \times +/+ \, \male$. Because the former mating shows segregation distortion and the latter does not, it follows that the distortion is not due to the death of $T/+$ zygotes or embryos. Finally, it has recently been demonstrated that male gametes may function in the complete absence of the T-t complex; spermatozoa in which the T-t complex has been deleted can still fertilize eggs and give rise to zygotes (Lyon *et al.* 1972). These findings can be taken as evidence that the actual distortion occurs after meiosis and before fertilization, even though the biochemical event leading to the distortion may take place before meiosis.

There is some evidence that the degree of segregation distortion can be influenced by conditions in the female reproductive system. One example of this evidence comes from the observation that late mating may change the male transmission ratios. In normal mice, coitus usually takes place 1–5 hr before ovulation, although the female will accept the male for up to 8 hr after ovulation. In females copulating prior to ovulation, an additional several hours elapse before the egg is fertilized. The average interval between coitus and penetration of the egg by the spermatozoon is about 8 hr. By manipulating the time of copulation in relation to the time of ovulation, it is possible to shorten this interval to about 3 hr (*late mating*). According to Braden (1958), late mating significantly lowers the transmission ratio of t, in some cases to an almost normal ratio of 0.5. This finding was interpreted by Braden as evidence that the t and T

sperm are produced in normal proportions and that the distortion is caused by physiological effects exerted on the sperm in the interval between ejaculation and fertilization. However, it was later demonstrated that the effect of late mating can be observed only with some t factors and not with others (Yanagisawa *et al.* 1961); furthermore, the effect is not always reproducible, even with a factor known to be influenced by late mating (D. Bennett and Dunn 1971). In a recent study, Braden (1972) examined six different t factors and found a significant reduction in transmission ratios after late mating in 13 of the 20 T/t males and three of the eight $t/+$ males tested. A total of 56 males have been tested by various investigators (Braden 1958, 1972; Yanagisawa *et al.* 1961), and 42 have been demonstrated to have their transmission ratios lowered after late mating by > 0.03; only two males had nonsignificantly higher ratios after late mating than after normal mating.

Some maternal effect on t spermatozoa is also suggested by the experiments of Olds (1971a), who observed that spermatozoa from T/t males, when injected into the ovarian bursa of ovulating females, penetrated the eggs significantly later than spermatozoa from $+/+$ males or spermatozoa from T/t males mated to $+/+$ females.

Two t factors with different transmission ratios interact in a t^x/t^y heterozygote to produce a new transmission ratio for each factor (D. Bennett and Dunn 1971). The interaction can be illustrated using the following example. Lethal factor t^1 has a TR of 0.87 in T/t^1 males; viable factor t^{26} has a TR of 0.55 in T/t^{26} males. When the two factors are combined in a single t^1/t^{26} male, one of two things can happen, theoretically. First, the high TR factor t^1 will be "dominant" over the lower TR factor t^{26} and the ratio will be $0.87t^1$ to $0.13t^{26}$. (Or, the t^{26} factor could be dominant and the ratio could be $0.45t^1$ to $0.55t^{26}$.) Second, the high TR factor t^1 will be transmitted in the same relative ratio from T/t^1 and from t^1/t^{26} males, so that

$$0.87:0.5 = x:0.55$$
$$x = 0.95$$

where x is the expected new TR of the t^1 factor. The observed ratio of t^1 in t^1/t^{26} males is 0.99, which is close to the expected ratio on the basis of the second possibility. A similar phenomenon was observed in several additional combinations of t factors.

Attempts to differentiate the t and T spermatozoa have been made by several authors. Bryson (1944) compared the sperm motility of normal males with that of T/t^0 or T/t^1 heterozygotes and found no difference. He also compared the frequency of gross abnormalities in the three types of sperm and again found no difference. There are, however, two reports describing a higher frequency of ultrastructural abnormalities (disorganized, duplicated, or missing organelles) in T/t spermatozoa as compared to $+/+$ spermatozoa (Yanagisawa 1965c; Olds 1971b). Difference in viability between t- and T-bearing spermatozoa has been postulated by Yanagisawa (1965a), who obtained living sperm from T/t and $+/+$ males, incubated them for several hours at room temperature, and determined their viability by counting at regular intervals. The curves of declining viability for T/t and $+/+$ sperm differed in that the T/t samples always showed a sudden drop in viability after the first 1 or 2 hr, whereas the viability of the $+/+$ sperm declined gradually over a longer time span. The sudden drop of viability in the T/t sperm was interpreted by Yanagisawa as evidence for the presence of two populations of spermatozoa, with the t spermatozoa being more viable. Yanagisawa (1965b) also attempted to demonstrate a similar viability difference *in vivo* by ligating the epididymis of T/t males and mating the animals to normal females 7–10 days later. During the time after ligation, the spermatozoa already stored in the epididymis should gradually have degenerated and if the degeneration rates of T and t spermatozoa differed, the ligated males should, according to Yanagisawa, have shown altered transmission ratios; but no alteration was observed. It seems, however, that there is no *a priori* reason to expect an alteration; if the T spermatozoa degenerate more rapidly, they should do so in ligated as well as in normal males, and the transmission ratio should remain the same.

It has recently become possible to differentiate not only among $+$, t, and T spermatozoa, but also among sperm bearing various t factors. An antigen specific for T spermatozoa has been identified by D. Bennett *et al.* (1972b) with two antisera: $+/+\ \male$ anti-T/t^{w2} sperm and BALB $\male$ anti-BALB-T^J sperm, both absorbed with testicular tissue to remove sperm autoantibodies. The absorbed antisera killed (in the presence of complement) a maximum of 60 percent of sperm from males carrying the T or T^J factors; they did not react with any other tissue tested. The low percentage of killing was interpreted by the authors as an indication that the T antigen is present only on a subpopulation of spermatozoa. The fact that the antisera did not distinguish between T and T^J is interesting, because the two factors are supposed to be of independent origin and one would therefore expect that they would differ antigenically.

Yanagisawa *et al.* (1974a) produced antisera by immunizing $+/+$ recipients with sperm from T/t^0, T/t^{w1}, T/t^{w5}, or T/t^{w32} males. After sperm autoantibodies were removed by absorption with sperm of the recipient type, each antiserum reacted in the cytotoxic test with sperm from males carrying one or both immunizing $T(t)$ factors. Cytotoxicity was highest when both immunizing factors were present and lower when only one was present. For example, serum $+/+$ anti-T/t^{w1} gave high cytotoxicity with T/t^{w1} sperm, lower cytotoxicity with $+/t^{w1}$ or $T/+$ sperm, and only background cytotoxicity with $+/+$, $+/t^0$, or t/t^{w32} sperm. When tested immediately after extraction from the epididymis, the percentage of sperm killed by the anti-T/t^{w1} serum was the same for sperm donors of the genotypes $T/+$ and $+/t^{w1}$. However, during incubation *in vitro*, the cytotoxicity of the $+/t^{w1}$ sperm tested with the anti-T/t^{w1} serum gradually *increased* from the initial value to a maximum at about 5 hr, after which no further specific cytotoxicity could be assayed (Yanagisawa *et al.* 1974b). When an antiserum specific for the wild-type allele $(+)$ was substituted for the anti-T/t^{w1} serum, the cytotoxicity of the $+/t^{w1}$ sperm *decreased* from the initial value to a minimum at about 5–6 hr. When the two antisera were tested against $T/+$

sperm, no change in the percentage of cytotoxicity was observed during the 5-hr incubation period. Yanagisawa and his co-workers (1974b) interpret these results as evidence for selective elimination of viable $+$-bearing spermatozoa from the $+/t$ sperm population. They postulate that initially the two sperm types ($+$ and t) are produced in equal proportions, but that during the waiting period before fertilization the $+$-bearing spermatozoa die off in greater numbers than the t-bearing spermatozoa, so that at the time of fertilization the ratio of t to non-t is shifted in favor of the t spermatozoa. This hypothesis could explain the success, as well as occasional failure, of late mating to alter the transmission ratios, because the alteration would depend on how far the shift in the t:non-t proportion has progressed in each individual case. It is conceivable that the rapidity of the shift depends on a particular t factor as well as on particular microenvironmental conditions at the time of mating.

The observations described above lead to the conclusion that the segregation distortion occurs between the end of spermiogenesis and the beginning of fertilization, either in the male genital tract (after spermiogenesis, before ejaculation) or in the female genital tract (after copulation, before fertilization).

The t segregation distorter resembles a similar system in *Drosophila* (Braden *et al.* 1972), but the two systems differ in that the latter has been associated with degeneration of spermatozoa during spermiogenesis. (For a review, see Peacock and Miklos 1973.) The observation of Yanagisawa *et al.* (1974b), if confirmed, would indicate that, in the mouse, the degeneration of $+$-bearing spermatozoa in the presence of t spermatozoa occurs only after spermiogenesis is completed.

The actual mechanism of the interaction between the two types of spermatozoa remains obscure. One possibility, suggested by Gluecksohn-Waelsch and Erickson (1970), is that the t spermatozoa secrete products that "poison" the $+$ or T spermatozoa; another possibility is that the t and $+$ spermatozoa display different surface properties that allow them to react differently to the microenvironment of the female genital tract.

The occurrence of the distortion in the postmeiotic interval provides strong evidence for gene expression during the haploid phase of male gametogenesis, although it can still be argued that the observed shift in sperm proportion is a delayed consequence of an event that occurred in the diploid phase before meiosis.

5. Male Sterility

Males carrying two t factors, identical or different, frequently display reduced fertility, with the degree of reduction varying from complete sterility to nearly complete fertility, depending on the t factors involved. Females with two t factors are always fully fertile. The fertility effects of the different types of t factors are summarized in Table 11–12.

Males heterozygous for two different (complementing) lethal t factors (t^{l1}/t^{l2}) and males homozygous for a semiviable t factor (t^{sv1}/t^{sv1}) are completely sterile, but the cause of the sterility in these two cases is different (Bryson

1944; Braden and Gluecksohn-Waelsch 1958; Dunn and D. Bennett 1969; P. Johnson 1968). The t^{11}/t^{12} males produce normal numbers of sperm, but the spermatozoa are incapable of reaching the site of fertilization (Braden and Gluecksohn-Waelsch 1958; D. Bennett and Dunn 1967; Olds 1970), a fact for which several explanations have been suggested. First, the spermatozoa are morphologically abnormal and, as such, they are unable to traverse the uterotubal junction (Braden and Gluecksohn-Waelsch 1958). Morphological abnormalities, both gross (Bryson 1944) and ultrastructural (Olds 1971b), as well as reduced motility (Bryson 1944; Braden and Gluecksohn-Waelsch 1958) have indeed been described in spermatozoa from sterile males. Second, the semen from the sterile males contains factors that cause the uterotubal junction to close (Olds 1970). Third, semen of sterile males coagulates in the uterus, and the coagulate traps the spermatozoa (Olds 1970). Fourth, the spermatozoa reach the ampulla, but are unable to remain there because of impaired motility, and are swept out at the fimbrial end (D. Bennett and Dunn 1967).

The t^{sv1}/t^{sv1} males have virtually no spermotozoa in their ejaculates (Johnson 1968; D. Bennett and Dunn 1971), and their testes weight is about half that of normal mice. The absence of spermatozoa is due to a breakdown in meiosis (the cells reach the zygotene stage but fail to differentiate; cf. D. Bennett and Dunn 1971). The primary cause of these defects is unknown.

6. Suppression of Recombination

The presence of a lethal t factor suppresses crossing-over in the vicinity of T, a fact first demonstrated for the interval between T and Fu (Dunn and Caspari 1945), and later also for the interval between T and tf (Lyon and Phillips 1959). There is at least one unpublished report (M. C. Green and G. D. Snell, *Mouse News Letter* 40:29, 1969) that the suppression of the lethal factor, t^6, extends

Table 11-12. Fertility effects of different t factors*

Genotype**	Male fertility	Defect
t^{sv1}/t^{sv1}	complete sterility	no sperm present; breakdown of meiosis and of spermatid differentiation
t^{11}/t^{12}	complete sterility	normal numbers of sperm present; spermatozoa have impaired motility
t^1/t^{sv}	complete sterility	normal numbers of sperm present; spermatozoa have impaired motility
t^{sv1}/t^{sv2}	complete sterility	? ?
t^v/t^l or t^v/t^{sv}	variable; range from near sterility to near fertility	? ?
t^{v1}/t^{v1}	complete(?) fertility	

* Based on D. Bennett and Dunn 1971.
** l = lethal; sv = semiviable; v = viable; 1, 2 = different t factors.

beyond *tf* toward *H-2*, and reduces the recombination frequency between *tf* and *H-2* from 0.071 to 0.006. Similar reduction of recombination frequency in the *tf-H-2* interval has been recently observed in crosses involving factors t^{w1}, t^6, and t^{12}; in these crosses, the recombination suppression effect does not seem to extend beyond the *H-2* complex (C. Hammerberg and J. Klein, *unpublished data.*)

7. Recombination Within the *t* Complex

The lethal *t* factors are maintained by a balanced lethal system in which T/t^x heterozygotes are intercrossed to produce only T/t^x heterozygotes (the homozygotes die prenatally):

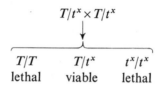

The offspring of this cross are all tailless, but occasionally normal-tailed exceptions carrying a new *t* factor (t^n) in combination with the original one (t^x/t^n heterozygotes) are found. The change from t^x to t^n was originally explained as mutation (Dunn and Gluecksohn-Schoenheimer 1950), but when it was later demonstrated that the appearance of new *t* factors was always accompanied by recombination of linked loci (Lyon and Phillips 1959), the mutation hypothesis was abandoned. Instead, it was postulated that new *t* factors arose by crossing-over within the *t* complex. The frequency of the intra-*t* crossing-over is approximately 2×10^{-3} (i.e., approximately one in every 500 animals is a normal-tailed exception). The new t^n factors differ from the original t^x factor in that they are usually viable in a homozygous state.

A thorough recombinational analysis of the *t* complex has been performed by Lyon and Meredith (1964a, b, c), who obtained 11 new *t* factors from lethal factor t^6, and five additional *t* factors from one of the 11 t^6 derivatives (t^{h7}). The properties of the 16 factors are summarized in Table 11–13. Lyon and Meredith offer the following interpretation of their results (Fig. 11–8). The t^6 factor represents an altered segment of chromosome 17 between *T* and *tf* and perhaps even beyond these two markers. The altered segment contains at least two separate genetic elements, the lethality factor, *Lf*, and the tail-enhancing factor, *T(ef)*, responsible for the *t* syndrome. *Lf* is located close to the *tf* gene, and *T(ef)* in the vicinity of the *T* gene. The new *t* factors shown in Table 11–13 were derived from t^6 by recombination between *T(ef)* and *Lf*, each recombinant receiving one or the other of the two elements, *Lf* or *T(ef)*. The t^{h7} factor was derived by unequal crossing-over between sister chromatids, resulting in a duplication of the *T(ef)* element. The double dose of the *T(ef)* element on one chromosome causes suppression rather than enhancement of *T* on the homologous chromosome, so the T/t^{h7} mice are normal-tailed. In two of the five recombinants derived from t^{h7} (t^{h14} and t^{h16}), the crossing-over is postulated to have occurred between the duplicated *T(ef)* elements, restoring the single dose of $T(ef)$ and, consequently, the typical tail-enhancing effect. In two other recombinants (t^{h13} and t^{h18}), the mutant $T(ef)$ element was replaced by a normal allele that has no effect on T (T/t^{h13} and T/t^{h18} animals have short tails).

The other two characteristics of the t syndrome, segregation distortion and crossing-over suppression, do not map in any particular point of the t^6 segment, but instead they seem to be governed by a relatively long chromosomal region. The t recombinants that display the two abnormal properties seem to have retained a large segment of the t^6 region, whereas those showing normal segregation and permitting crossing-over carry only a small portion of the altered region.

As for the nature of the alteration in the t^6 region, Lyon and Meredith speculate that the lethality factor is probably a deletion, whereas the rest of the t^6 region represents heterochromatinization (i.e., a change from an active

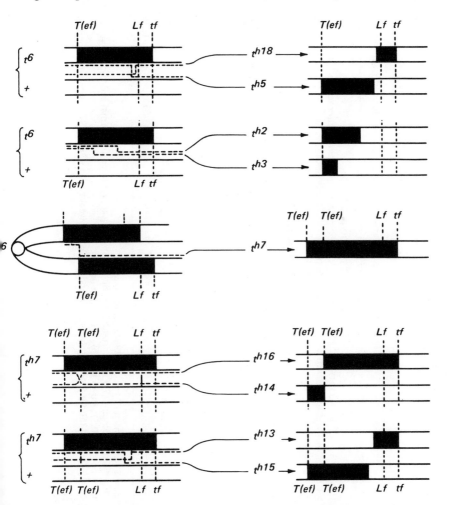

Fig. 11-8. Postulated origin of t factors in the experiment of Lyon and Meredith (1964 a, b, c). $T(ef)$ = tail-enhancing factor; Lf = lethal factor; tf = tufted. Direction of crossing-over is indicated by interrupted lines. Explanation in text.

Table 11-13. Properties of recombinant t factors derived from t^6*

Prototype t factors	Other factors of the same group	Origin of prototype t factor		Interaction with T**	Homozygous effect	Transmission ratio†	Crossing-over‡
		Genotype of parents	Genotype of offspring				
t^6	t^0, t^1, t^2, etc.	$Ttf/t^6 +$	—	En	lethal	Hi	Ss
t^{h2}	t^{h6}, t^{h8}, t^{h9}		$Ttf/t^{h2}tf$	En	viable	Lo	Ws
t^{h3}	t^{h4}, t^{h10}, t^{h11}		$t^6 +/t^{h3}tf$	En	viable	O	Nor
t^{h5}	—	$× \quad Ttf/t^6 +$	$t^6 +/t^{h5}tf$	En	viable	Lo	Ss
t^{h7}	—		$Ttf/t^{h7} +$	Su	lethal	O	Ss
t^{h18}	—	$+tf/t^6 + × Ttf/+tf$	$Ttf/+(t^{h18})+$	No	lethal	O	Nor
t^{h13}	—	$Ttf/t^{h7} + ×$	$T(t^{h13})+/+tf$	No	lethal	O	Nor
t^{h14}	—	$+tf/t^{h7} + × Ttf/+tf$	$+tf/t^{h14}tf$	En	viable	O	Nor
t^{h15}	—	$+tf/t^{h7} + × Ttf/+tf$	$Ttf/t^{h15}tf$	En	viable	Lo	Nor
t^{h16}	—	$Ttf/t^{h7} + × Ttf/t^{h7} +$	$Ttf/t^{h16}+$	En	lethal	Hi	Ss

* Based on Lyon and Meredith 1964a, b, c.
** En = enhancement (T/t mice are tailless); Su = suppression (T/t mice are normal-tailed); No = no effect (T/t mice are short-tailed).
† O = normal (0.5); Lo = (<0.5); Hi = high (>0.5).
‡ Nor = normal (about 8 percent between T and tf); Ws = weakly suppressed; Ss = strongly suppressed.

euchromatin into inactive heterochromatin). Cytological evidence for the presence of structural aberrations in *t*-bearing chromosomes has been reported by Geyer-Duszynska (1964).

The balanced lethal system, the most frequent source of *t* recombinants, is not at all ideal for recombinational analysis of the *t* complex because it permits detection of only a small fraction of the crossovers. From the cross

$$\frac{T \quad +}{T(ef)\ Lf} \times \frac{T \quad +}{T(ef)\ Lf}$$

four recombinant classes can theoretically arise:

$\dfrac{T\ Lf}{T\ +}$	$\dfrac{T \quad Lf}{T(ef)\ Lf}$	$\dfrac{T(ef)\ +}{T \quad +}$	$\dfrac{T(ef)\ +}{T(ef)\ Lf}$
lethal	lethal	viable, tailless	viable, normal-tailed?

Of these, the first two classes will die prenatally, the third class will be indistinguishable from the parental types, and only the fourth class might be detectable. It would be more efficient to study *t* recombination using a cross such as

$$\frac{T\ tf\ H\text{-}2^x}{t\ +\ H\text{-}2^y} \times \frac{+\ tf\ H\text{-}2^z}{+\ tf\ H\text{-}2^z}$$

in which all recombinant classes can be identified.

8. High Frequency of t Factors in Wild Populations

Almost all thoroughly studied wild populations of the house mouse have been found to carry recessive *t* factors, sometimes with a frequency as high as 40 percent. This feature of *t* factors will be discussed in detail in Chapter Twelve.

9. Interpretation

The interpretation of the *t* complex described below is based primarily on the work of Lyon and Meredith (1964a, b, c).

Chromosome 17 is extremely unstable and easily subject to alterations—both structural (deletions, duplications, inversions, etc.) and functional (oscillation between enchromatin and heterochromatin). The alterations occur frequently when chromosomes from unrelated populations are brought together into a single cell. The chromosomal instability is phenotypically expressed as a series of characteristics that are somewhat artificially assembled under the name of the *t* system. The present view of the *t* system is biased by the limitations of the techniques used in its study; broadening of the techniques will probably lessen the contrasting nature of the features of the system and produce a continuum of highly variable properties. Because it is clear that the *t* system is not a single locus and that it is not allelic with the *T* gene, the terms "*t* locus" and "*t* alleles" should be abandoned.

Different *t* properties appear to be governed by different regions of chromosome 17. The lethality factors appear to be structural aberrations (perhaps deletions), which are probably located in different positions on the chromosome, depending on the particular *t* factor. Each lethal factor is presumed to alter—perhaps only functionally—chromosomal segments of different length, as shown in Fig. 11–9. Consequently, some of the *t* regions are longer, others are shorter; a long region can produce a shorter region by crossing-over, but the reverse cannot occur. The tail-enhancing effect seems to be caused by a relatively short chromosomal segment, perhaps by only one locus. The segregation distortion and the crossing-over suppression effects, on the other hand, appear to be caused by changes in large segments of the chromosome. It has recently been shown that the centromeric region of each mouse chromosome contains a large bulk of heterochromatin containing reiterated DNA. Because the *T* factor is located close to the centromere (J. Klein 1971b), it can be speculated that the centromeric heterochromatin is somehow involved in the distribution of chromosomes during cell division, and that change in the heterochromatin leads to abnormal transmissions.

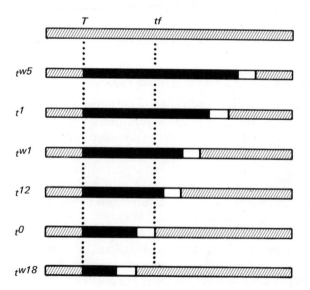

Fig. 11-9. Speculative interpretation of the more common *t* factors. *T* = *Brachyury;* *tf* = *tufted.* Solid bars indicate inactivation, open bars deletion of chromosomal regions. (Based on M. F. Lyon and R. Meredith. "Investigations of the nature of *t*-alleles in the mouse. III. Short tests of some further mutant alleles". *Heredity* **19**:327–330, 1964c).

IV. *T*-Related Traits

A. *Low*

This mutation was discovered in a single male heterozygous for the Brachyury (*T*) factor (Dunn and D. Bennett 1968, 1971a; D. Bennett and Dunn 1971). This male, when mated to normal females, produced 44 offspring, of which only two were short-tailed (22 short-tailed animals were expected). The ability to distort the transmission ratio of *T* was later demonstrated to be controlled by what appeared to be a single gene. The gene was originally designated *Lr* (*low ratio*), but this was later changed to *Low* because the *Lr* symbol had previously been used for another gene. Heterozygous males *T Low/+ +* (or *T+/+Low*) transmit the *T* factor to only about 12 percent of their offspring (instead of the expected 50 percent), with individual males showing a variation within a range of ± 8 percent. There is also a considerable within-male heterogeneity in the transmission ratio. The heterozygous *TLow/+ +* females transmit the *T* factor in a normal 1:1 ratio. The *Low/Low* homozygotes are viable and fertile, and show no effect on either male or female transmission ratios. The *Low* factor is located between *T* and *tf*, with map distances of approximately 2.5 cM between *T* and *Low* and 0.5 cM between *Low* and *tf*. Recombination frequencies between *T* and *tf* in the presence of *Low* are 0.03 in males and 0.065 in females, compared to normal frequencies (no *Low* gene present) of 0.072 in males and 0.096 in females. The reduced recombination frequencies indicate that the *Low* factor weakly suppresses crossing-over in the *T-tf* interval. This suppression, however, occurs only in *Low/+* heterozygotes; recombination in the homozygotes is normal. It appears that the *Low* factor influences the transmission after recombination has occurred, that is, when it becomes associated with a "new" centromere. The *Low* effect is not caused by depletion of the brachyury offspring before birth, and it is affected by late mating. The *Low* factor interacts with *t* factors in a way that restores normal *t*-transmission ratios in *T Low/t^{high}* and *T Low/t^{low}* heterozygotes (t^{high} and $t^{low} = t$ factors with high and low transmission ratios, respectively), but it lowers *t*-transmission ratios in *T Low/t^{normal}* heterozygotes. The fertility of the *T Low/t* heterozygotes is normal. The mechanism of the *Low* factor action is not known, but there is no reason to suspect that it differs greatly from other segregation distorters in the *t* complex. Actually, the *Low* factor might represent a rudiment of the complex derived by intra-*t* recombination. Supporting this contention is the fact that the *Low* factor occurred in a male derived from the *T190* stock that once carried the t^6 factor (Dunn 1967).

B. *Fused* (*Fu*)

Fused is a dominant mutation affecting the tail vertebrae and thus the morphology of the tail (Reed 1937). Even in highly inbred strains, its expression is extremely variable, ranging from an absence of any visible morphological abnormality (*normal overlaps*) to a lack of the whole or part of the tail, absence of several ribs, and extreme twisting or even bifurcation of the tail (Fig. 11–6c). Some *Fu* animals are anemic at birth, and may show circling behavior, deafness, and reduction or absence of kidneys. The frequency of normal overlaps is usually higher among the offspring of a female (rather than a male) *Fu*/+ heterozygote (the *Reed phenomenon*), indicating that the intrauterine environment of the female is unfavorable for the expression of the *Fu* gene. The *Fu*/*Fu* homozygotes are viable, but the viability is low, especially in males, and depends to a great extent on the genetic background, with certain backgrounds causing the death of the embryos *in utero* (*conditioned lethal*). Developmental abnormalities of the *Fu*/*Fu* embryos are first detected on the ninth day of gestation and are characterized by hypertrophy of neural tissue and duplication of the neural tube (Theiler and Gluecksohn-Waelsch 1956).

The *Fu* locus is located between *T* and *H-2*, in the vicinity of *tf*; the order of the *Fu* and *tf* loci has not yet been determined. The *Fu*/*T* heterozygotes are viable and display the same abnormalities as either *T*/+ or *Fu*/+ heterozygotes, indicating that the *T* and *Fu* genes do not interact.

C. Kinky (*Ki*)

Kinky is a dominant mutation, lethal in homozygous condition (Caspari and David 1940). The *Ki*/+ heterozygotes are viable, with their tails showing a characteristic flexure that may vary from a barely perceptible crook to multiple twists (Fig. 11–6d). The tail kinks are caused by fusion of vertebrae, insertion of small bones between the vertebrae, and ankylosis. A reduced number of vertebrae shortens the tail to as little as half its normal length. The abnormalities sometimes extend to sacral, lumbar, and thoracic vertebrae, causing fusion of the corresponding ribs. Some of the *Ki*/+ animals are deaf and display circling behavior.

The *Ki* gene has an incomplete penetrance with frequent normal overlaps (*Ki*/+ heterozygotes appearing phenotypically normal). The gene maps between *T* and *tf*, in the same general area as *Fu*. The *Ki* and *Fu* genes closely resemble each other in their phenotypic manifestations, the main differences between them being that *Ki*/*Ki* homozygotes are lethal, whereas *Fu*/*Fu* homozygotes are viable, and that *Ki* displays a higher penetrance (close to 100 percent) than *Fu*. Recombinants between *Fu* and *Ki* were reported by Dunn and Caspari (1945), but these were questioned by Dunn and Gluecksohn-Waelsch (1954), who found no evidence of crossing-over between the two genes. The latter authors considered the *Ki* gene an allele of *Fused* and referred to it as *Fu^{Ki}*. Heterozygotes *Fu*/*Ki* are viable and display the same abnormalities as either *Ki*/+ or *Fu*/+ heterozygotes.

V. Other Genes in Chromosome 17

A. Quaking (*qk*)

Quaking is a recessive, spontaneous mutation characterized by a disorder in myelin formation (Sidman *et al.* 1964). The *qk*/*qk* homozygotes show a rapid tremor during their motor activity and are subject to occasional tonic seizures in which they maintain motionless posture for many seconds. The tremor is most pronounced in the caudal part of the trunk and in the hindlimbs, so that the mice appear to be bouncing on their haunches. It disappears when the mice are at rest and their bodies are in contact with the bedding. The abnormal motor behavior is first recognizable when the mouse is 10–12 days old and reaches its full expression about 3 weeks after birth. The life span of the homozygotes is at least several months. The *qk*/+ heterozygotes appear to be normal; *qk*/*qk* males are infertile (W. Bennett *et al.* 1971), the infertility being caused by a defect in the postmeiotic period of spermatogenesis and being the result of an abnormal development of the nuclear membrane in the spermatids. Because of this condition, the *qk* gene must be maintained by mating *qk*/*qk* females with *qk*/+ males. It is not known how a single gene mutation can influence such widely different cell types as neurons and spermatids, but it has been speculated that the membrane defect is the common denominator of the pleiotropism.

The *qk* mutation, which arose in the DBA/2 strain, is available in a congenic line, C57BL/6-*qk*. The *qk* gene maps between *T* and *tf*, in the vicinity of *Fu*, *Ki*, and *Low*, but the order of these latter three genes in relation to *qk* is not known.

B. Hair-pin Tail (*Hp*)

Hair-pin tail arose as a spontaneous mutation in strain AKR/J (Dickie *et al.* 1965). The *Hp*/+ heterozygotes have short kinky tails (Fig. 11–6e) and various skeletal abnormalities (fused vertebrae, scoliosis of lower and upper lumbar vertebrae, and a reduced number of lumbar and caudal vertebrae). The phenotype of the heterozygote appears to depend upon the source of the *Hp* gene; if the gene is inherited via the egg, many of the heterozygous embryos die *in utero*; if the gene is supplied by the sperm, the heterozygotes live and are far less affected morphologically (D. Johnson 1972). The *Hp*/*Hp* homozygotes are probably inviable. The gene has been mapped 17 ± 3 units from *tufted* (*tf*), but its position with respect to other genes in the map is not known. In Fig. 11–4 it is arbitrarily placed near *thf*.[2]

C. Tufted (*tf*)

Tufted is a recessive mutation characterized by repeated loss and regrowth of

---

[2]According to the most recent data of D. R. Johnson (*Genetics 76:* 795–805, 1974) the *Hp* gene is an allele at the *T* locus; as such it is designated *T^hp*.

hair (Lyon 1956). The tufted phenotype of the *tf*/*tf* homozygotes is first detectable at about 4 weeks of age, when the animals begin to lose their baby coats. At this time, a wave of hair loss followed closely by a wave of hair growth begins on their heads and proceeds toward their tails (Fig. 11–6f). The first loss-regrowth wave is followed by a second, then by a third, and so on. The first wave passes from the head to the tail in about 1 week, the second in about 3 weeks, the third and all subsequent waves in about 1 month. In young adult mice, the tufted individuals are sometimes difficult to distinguish from normal mice; in older mice, the succession of several waves of hair loss causes easily recognizable baldness of whole areas of the body, particularly of the abdomen (Fig. 11–6g). Expression of the *tf* gene may be under hormonal control, because the cyclic hair loss and growth stops during pregnancy and lactation and is renewed at the end of the lactation period. The *tf*/*tf* homozygotes are fully viable, and the *tf* gene is 100 percent penetrant; the expression of the mutant allele does not appear to be influenced by different genetic backgrounds. The *tf*/+ heterozygotes are indistinguishable from the +/+ homozygotes.

The *tf* allele is present in congenic lines B10.T(6R) and B10.G (Stimpfling and Reichert 1970), B10.A-*tf* (J. Klein, *unpublished data*), and several noninbred strains. The *tf* locus maps between *T* and *H-2*; estimates of the recombination frequency between *H-2* and *tf* range from 2.6 to 7.9 percent, with a mean of 5.5 percent for heterozygous females and 3.5 percent for heterozygous males (Table 11–1).

D. Thin Fur (*thf*)

Thin fur is a recessive mutation affecting hair growth (Key and Hollander 1972). The *thf*/*thf* homozygotes are first recognizable when they are 4–6 weeks old by an absence of underfur, which gives the impression of balding (Fig. 11–6h). The expression of the *thf* gene appears to be somewhat influenced by the genetic background. The *thf*/*thf* homozygotes are fully viable, and the penetrance of the *thf* gene is complete; the *thf*/+ heterozygotes are indistinguishable from the +/+ homozygotes. The *thf* locus is one of few markers located on the noncentromeric side of *H-2*, the distance between *H-2* and *thf* being 9–10 map units (J. Klein, *unpublished data*).

The *thf* mutation arose spontaneously in a strain heterozygous for the chromosome translocation *T(5;8)Sn* and is presently maintained on a semiinbred background. Congenic line B10-*thf* is in preparation (J. Klein, *unpublished data*).

E. Gross Virus Antigen Locus-1 (*Gv-1*)

Inoculation of Gross virus into newborn rats of strain W/Fu results in a leukemia that, when transplanted to (W/Fu × BN)F$_1$ rats, stimulates production of antibodies cytotoxic for murine lymphoid cells (Stockert *et al.* 1971). One of these antibodies is directed against an antigen, designated G$_{IX}$, which is present in some inbred strains of mice and absent in others. Strains tested

Table 11-14. Quantitative representation of G_{IX} antigen on thymocytes of various mouse strains*, **

$G_{IX}3$	129, CE/J
$G_{IX}2$	C58, AKR, AKR.K, AKR-*H-2ᵇ*, A, A-*Tlaᵇ*, A-*Thy-1ᵃ*, I, C3H/He
$G_{IX}1$	SJL/J, DBA/2, C3H/An, 101
$G_{IX}-$	C57BL/6, C57BL/6-*H-2ᵏ*, C57BL/6-*Tlaᵃ*, C57BL/6-*Ly-1ᵃ*, C57BL/6-*Ly-2ᵃ*, C57BL/10J, B10.129(5M), B10.129(9M), B10.129(10M), B10.129(12M), B10.129(13M), BALB/c, BALB/c-*Tʲ*, CBA/J, CBA-T6, RF/J, DBA/2J, MA/J, SWR, HTH, HTI, HTG, C57BR/J, C3Hf/Bi (when young)

* Convention of expressing the representation of G_{IX}:

$G_{IX}3$	highest quantity (129 and CE only)
$G_{IX}2$	approximately two-thirds of 129 quantity
$G_{IX}1$	approximately one-third of 129 quantity
$G_{IX}-$	no demonstrable antigen

** Reproduced with permission from E. Stockert, L. J. Old, and E. A. Boyse: "The G_{IX} system. A cell surface a-llo-antigen associated with murine leukemia virus: implications regarding chromosomal integration of the viral genome". *Journal of Experimental Medicine* *133*:1334–1335. Copyright © 1971 by The Rockefeller University Press. All rights reserved.

with the G_{IX} antiserum fall into one of four categories (Table 11–14): strains with high ($G_{IX}3$), intermediate ($G_{IX}2$), or low ($G_{IX}1$) content of the antigen on thymocytes, and strains lacking the antigen completely ($G_{IX}-$). The differences between the three categories of G_{IX}-positive strains are quantitative rather than qualitative, because each G_{IX}-positive strain absorbs all cytotoxic activity for all other G_{IX}-positive strains. In normal mice, G_{IX} is present only on lymphoid cells. The distribution of G_{IX} among the different lymphoid tissues depends on the presence of another Gross virus-associated antigen, GCSA (Gross cell surface antigen). In strains that are G_{IX}-positive and GCSA-positive (prototype AKR), the G_{IX} is demonstrable in all lymphoid tissues at any age; in strains that are G_{IX}-positive and GCSA-negative (prototype 129), G_{IX} is demonstrable only on thymocytes. In one strain (C3Hf/Bi), a conversion occurs with aging from G_{IX}-negative and GCSA-positive to G_{IX}-positive and GCSA-positive in all lymphoid tissues. The G_{IX} antigen can, however, appear in leukemias of both G_{IX}-positive and G_{IX}-negative strains, thus resembling the *Tla* system.

The genetic control of the G_{IX} antigen is complex. The G_{IX} typing of $[(129 \times C57BL/6)F_1 \times C57BL/6]BC$, $[(129 \times C57BL/6)F_1 \times 129]BC$ and $(129 \times C57BL/6)F_2$ generations indicate segregation of two unlinked genes, *Gv-1* and *Gv-2*, each with two alleles, *a* and *b* (Table 11–15). At the *Gv-1* locus, expression of G_{IX} is semidominant (the *Gv-1ᵃ*/*Gv-1ᵇ* heterozygotes express half the quantity of G_{IX} present in the homozygotes); at the *Gv-2* locus, the expression of G_{IX} is fully dominant (the *Gv-2ᵃ*/*Gv-2ᵇ* heterozygotes express the same amount of G_{IX} as the homozygotes). In both cases, however, the second gene must also be taken into account. The relationship between the *Gv* genotypes and the G_{IX} phenotypes is summarized in Table 11–16.

Table 11-15. Segregation of loci *Gv-1* and *Gv-2* determining antigen G_{IX} in backcrosses between strains 129 and C57BL/6*,**

	Genotype		Phenotype	
Backcross	*Gv-1*	*Gv-2*	(percent G_{IX} expression)	Expected proportion
(129 × C57BL/6)F₁ × 129	*aa* *aa*	*aa* *ab* }	100	$\frac{1}{2}$
	ab *ab*	*aa* *ab* }	50	$\frac{1}{2}$
(129 × C57BL/6)F₁ × C57BL/6	*ab*	*ab*	50	$\frac{1}{4}$
	bb *ab* *bb*	*ab* *bb* *bb* }	0	$\frac{3}{4}$

* 129: *Gv-1ᵃ Gv-1ᵃ Gv-2ᵃ Gv-2ᵃ*; C57BL/6: *Gv-1ᵇ Gv-1ᵇ Gv-2ᵇ Gv-2ᵇ*.
** From Stockert *et al.* 1971.

Simultaneous testing of the segregating populations for G_{IX} and H-2 anti-gens revealed a linkage of the semidominant *Gv-1* gene with the *H-2* complex (hence, the designation G_{IX} = Gross antigen controlled by a gene in linkage group IX). The map distance between *H-2* and *Gv-1* was estimated at 36.4 ± 2.7 map units, and a three-point cross with *T*, *H-2*, and *Gv-1* placed the *Gv-1* locus at the noncentromeric end of *H-2*. The *Gv-2* gene was later located in chromosome 7 (LG I; cf. Stockert *et al.* 1972). The location of *Gv-1* in chromosome 17 is contradicted by the finding that in crosses involving the AKR strain (instead of 129), the semidominant gene maps in chromosome 4 (LG VIII; cf. Ikeda *et al.* 1973). Two explanations have been offered for this discrepancy. First, the same gene (*Gv-1*) occupies two different sites in strains 129 and AKR, being located in chromosome 17 in the former and in chromosome 4 in the latter. This may seem heretical from the viewpoint of classical genetics, but if one assumes, as has been suggested by Stockert *et al.* (1971), that the *Gv-1* gene represents a viral genome incorporated into the mouse chromosome, one may as well postulate that incorporation into different chromosomes occurs in different strains. Second, the association of G_{IX} with *H-2* in the backcrosses involving the 129 strain is an example of pseudolinkage. The recombination frequency between *Gv-1* and *H-2* is relatively high (approximately 37 percent), so such an explanation is not at all unlikely. The location of *Gv-1* in chromosome 17 must therefore be considered tentative.

F. Erythrocyte Alloantigen Locus-2 (*Ea-2*)

See Chapter Eight.

G. Immune Response Locus-5 (*Ir-5*)

See Chapter Seventeen.

Table 11-16. Relationship between the Gv-1Gv-2 genotypes and the G_{IX} phenotype*

Genotype				Phenotype
Gv-1	*Gv-1*	*Gv-2*	*Gv-2*	(percent G_{IX} expression)
a	*a*	*a*	*a*	100
a	*b*	*a*	*a*	50
a	*a*	*a*	*b*	100
a	*b*	*a*	*b*	50
a	*a*	*b*	*b*	0
b	*b*	*a*	*a*	0
b	*b*	*a*	*b*	0
a	*b*	*b*	*b*	0
b	*b*	*b*	*b*	0

* Reproduced with permission from E. Stockert, L. J. Old, and E. A. Boyse: "The G_{IX} system. A cell surface allo-antigen associated with murine leukemia virus; implications regarding chromosomal integration of the viral genome". *Journal of Experimental Medicine* *133*:1334–1335. Copyright © 1971 by The Rockefeller University Press. All rights reserved.

VI. Translocations Involving Chromosome 17

A. Principle of Translocation Analysis

Translocations can serve as useful markers in cytological as well as genetic analyses. In genetic mapping, the presence of a translocation in a heterozygous state can be detected either by progeny testing or by cytological analysis.

1. *Progeny testing.* Translocation heterozygotes produce a certain proportion of unbalanced gametes (gametes with gene duplications and deletions), which can fuse and result in zygotes (embryos) that die *in utero*. Consequently, the size of the litters born to such heterozygotes is reduced, and the heterozygotes appear to be "semisterile." The semisterility can be measured either by counting the dead and live embryos in the pregnant female or by counting the progeny after birth. The degree of semisterility can vary in different translocations according to the length of the chromosomal segments involved in the exchange and according to the centromere position.

2. *Cytological detection of a translocation.* A translocation heterozygote contains four chromosomes partially homologous to one another. At meiosis these four chromosomes form a single, cross-shaped element (a *quadrivalent*), the presence of which indicates the presence of a translocation. The shape of the quadrivalent and its relative frequency depend primarily on the frequency of chiasmata in the translocated chromosomal segments. Preparations of female meiosis are not easily attainable, so the cytological detection of translocations is limited to males. Translocation homozygotes show neither semisterility nor quadrivalents in their

meiosis; to prove that they carry a translocation, they must be crossed to normal mice and the progeny diagnosed as translocation heterozygotes. In genetic tests, the translocation break behaves as a single Mendelian marker whose position in the map can be determined by regular mapping.

Chromosome 17 is known to have been involved in three translocations: *T(9;17)138Ca*, *T(1;17)190Ca* and *T(16;17)7Bn*.

B. *T(9;17)138Ca*

In an experiment designed to produce chromosomal inversions, Carter and his co-workers (1955, 1956) X-irradiated males of heterogeneous stock CWX and mated them to normal females of the CBA strain. Instead of inversions, they obtained a series of translocations between different chromosomes. The chromosomes involved in these translocations were identified by testing for linkage between the translocation breaks (semisterility) and nine marker genes. One of the two translocations (serial number 138) showed linkage with two genes, *dilute* (*d*) in LG II (chromosome 9), and *Brachyury* (*T*) in LG IX (chromosome 17). The recombination frequencies were

$$d\text{--}T138 \cdots 19.0 \text{ percent}$$
$$T\text{--}T138 \cdots 37.5 \text{ percent}$$
$$d(se)\text{--}T \cdots 40.1 \text{ percent}$$

These results were later confirmed by Lyon and Phillips (1959), who located the translocation break between *d* and *tf* and determined the distance between *T138* and *tf* as approximately 10.7 map units. They also noted that the presence of the *T138* translocation enhanced the recombination in chromosome 17; in the presence of the translocation, the recombination frequency in the *T–tf* interval is 16 percent; in the absence of the translocation, the frequency is 7 percent. Introduction of the t^6 factor into the translocation heterozygote reduces the recombination frequency between *T138* and *T* to 14.7 percent and that between *d* and *T* to 27.3 percent (22.2 percent in females and 32.4 percent in males). The translocation break is located on the noncentromeric side of *H-2*, the distance between *T138* and *H-2* being some 6 map units (J. Klein *et al.* 1970; J. Klein and D. Klein 1972). The *T138* marker is available as a translocation homozygote in a noninbred stock of the same name. A B10.T138 congenic line is being developed (J. Klein, *unpublished data*).

C. *T(1;17)190Ca*

The *T190* translocation was obtained by Carter *et al.* (1955, 1956) in the same experiment which produced *T138*. It arose in a stock carrying the t^6 factor, and it was a linkage with this factor that suggested involvement of chromosome 17 in the genetic exchange. The recombination frequency between *T190* and t^6 was estimated at 5.5 percent. Additional genetic tests revealed that the t^6

marker in the T190 stock was linked with *ln*, and perhaps also with *fz* in chromosome 1 (LG XIII). The recombination frequencies for the t^6-*ln*-*fz* intervals are

$$t^6-ln \cdots 27.3 \text{ percent}$$
$$t^6-fz \cdots 49.9 \text{ percent}$$
$$ln-fz \cdots 38.4 \text{ percent}$$

The position of the *T190* break with respect to *tf* was determined by Lyon (1967), who arrived at the order *T*-*tf*-*T190* with recombination frequencies of 19 percent between *T* and *tf* and four percent between *tf* and *T190*. The 19 percent recombination is higher than that obtained in the absence of *T190* (7 percent), indicating that *T190* enhances recombination; whether the enhancing effect extends to the *tf*-*T190* interval is not known. The *T190* break is probably located between *tf* and *H-2*.

The original *T190* chromosome carried the t^6 factor, but Lyon and Phillips (1959) later obtained a recombinant that lost at least some of the properties of the t^6 syndrome. The presently available T190 stock was derived from this recombinant; however, the stock might still carry the lethal factor of the original t^6 chromosome, which would explain why attempts to obtain *T190/T190* homozygotes have failed.

D. *T(16;17)7Bn*

As mentioned earlier, the *T(16;17)7Bn* translocation was found in the tobacco mouse, *M. poschiavinus*, and has been interpreted as being the result of a centric fusion between chromosomes 16 and 17. Both heretozygotes *T7/+* and homozygotes *T7/T7* are available on the C57BL/10Sn background.

Chapter Twelve

Population Genetics of the *t* and *H-2* Systems

I. Basic Concepts of Population Genetics

A. Definitions

A *population* is an assembly of individuals sharing a common *gene pool*, that is, the group of genes from which those of the next generation are chosen. Genetic constitution of a population is defined by the gene and genotype frequencies calculated from the corresponding phenotype frequencies. *Phenotype (genotype, gene) frequencies* are obtained by counting the individuals carrying the particular phenotype (genotype, gene) and dividing the sums by the number of individuals in the population. The frequencies are expressed as percentages (0–100 percent) or fractions, ranging from 0 to 1. All phenotype frequencies and the genotype frequencies for dominant genes are obtained by direct counting; genotype frequencies for recessive genes are computed using special statistical methods. Gene frequencies are calculated from genotype frequencies as illustrated by the following example. Take two genes, A_1 and A_2 and their frequencies, p and q, respectively, where $p+q = 1$. Consider three genotypes, A_1A_1, A_1A_2, and A_2A_2, and their respective frequencies P, H, and

Q, where $P+H+Q = 1$. The relationship between gene and genotype frequencies is then expressed by the equations

$$p = P+\tfrac{1}{2}H$$
$$q = Q+\tfrac{1}{2}H$$

B. Infinite Populations

The simplest population is one that:

1. contains genes inherited in classic Mendelian fashion,
2. is infinitely large,
3. contains randomly mating individuals (i.e., any one individual in the population has an equal probability of mating with any individual of the opposite sex; such an ideal status is sometimes called *panmixia*, and the population *panmictic*),
4. has no new genes introduced into it and no existing genes lost from it (e.g., by mutation or migration),
5. has no alleles preferred over others (i.e., by selection).

Such a simple Mendelian population is in a state of *genetic equilibrium* in which both gene frequencies and genotype frequencies are constant from generation to generation. The equilibrium is defined by the *Hardy-Weinberg law*, expressed by the formula

$$(p+q)^2 = p^2+2pq+q^2$$

where p and q are gene frequencies of A_1 and A_2, respectively. The law makes two important predictions. First, after one generation the genotypes for a single locus with two alleles (A_1 and A_2) will be present in frequencies $p^2A_1A_1$: $2pqA_1A_2:q^2A_2A_2$. Second, these frequencies will not change in subsequent generations, and the population will remain in equilibrium. Both predictions apply to any gene considered independently of other genes in the population. However, if two genes are considered jointly, the situation becomes more complex. Take, for instance, two genes, each with two alleles, A_1 and A_2 and B_1 and B_2, and consider their frequencies as p and q, and r and s, respectively, where $p+q+r+s = 1$. The genes can be arranged into four gametic combinations: A_1B_1, A_1B_2, A_2B_1, and A_2B_2, with frequencies x_1, x_2, x_3 and x_4, respectively, where $x_1+x_2+x_3+x_4 = 1$, $p = x_1+x_2$, $q = x_3+x_4$, $r = x_1+x_3$ and $s = x_2+x_4$. The population will be in equilibrium with respect to the A and B genes when $x_2x_3 = x_1x_4$ or $x_2x_3-x_1x_4 = 0$. If the latter product is not equal to zero, but instead to some value, D (which can be positive if $x_2x_3 > x_1x_4$ or negative if $x_2x_3 < x_1x_4$), the population is in a momentary *disequilibrium*. Given enough time, it eventually approaches equilibrium by gradually decreasing the value of D. How rapidly this occurs depends on the initial value of D and on the relationship between the two loci in consideration. If the two loci are not linked, D is halved in each generation and asymptotically approaches 0; if the two loci are linked, it is the value rD (where r is the recombination frequency between A and B) that is halved in each generation. The gametic frequencies in each generation can be calculated by adding the halved value of D (unlinked loci) or rD (linked loci) to the frequencies of the previous generation. A practical example of this calculation is shown in Tables 12–1 and 12–2. How quickly the two linked loci reach equilibrium depends on the strength of the linkage: the closer the linkage, the longer the process toward equilibrium. With closely linked loci, the approach to equilibrium is slow and the population remains in disequilibrium for many generations. However, all loci should eventually attain equilibrium no matter how close the linkage between them. At equilibrium, there is a fundamental difference between the behavior of closely linked loci in a genetic cross and in a population. In a cross, the loci show association by linkage, while in a population they show no association at all. Existence of

Table 12-1. Calculation of D and the equilibrium frequencies of gametes for a population in which the frequencies of two separate gene pairs Aa and Bb are $A = B = 0.6$ and $a = b = 0.4$, and the initial genotypic frequencies are $AABB = AAbb = aaBB = 0.30$ and $aabb = 0.10*$

		Gametes	
Initial population	Type	Initial frequency	Equilibrium frequency
30% $AABB$	AB	0.3	$0.3 + D$
30% $AAbb$	Ab	0.3	$0.3 - D$
30% $aaBB$	aB	0.3	$0.3 - D$
10% $aabb$	ab	0.1	$0.1 + D$

$$D = (Ab)(aB) - (AB)(ab) = (0.3)(0.3) - (0.3)(0.1) = 0.06$$

Attainment of equilibrium

Generation	Amount added (AB, ab) or subtracted (Ab, aB)	Gametes			
		AB	Ab	aB	ab
1		0.3	0.3	0.3	0.1
2	$0.5D$	0.33	0.27	0.27	0.13
3	$0.75D$	0.345	0.255	0.255	0.145
4	$0.875D$	0.3525	0.2475	0.2475	0.1525
5	$0.9375D$	0.35625	0.24375	0.24375	0.15625
.					
.					
.					
equilibrium	D	0.36	0.24	0.24	0.16

disequilibrium in a population may mean either that a particular combination of genes has recently been introduced into the population and there has not been adequate time for equilibrium to be reached, or that a particular combination of alleles has a selective advantage. If the latter condition exists, selection will hold the favored alleles together and a stable state will ensue with nonrandom distribution of gene combinations.

C. Small Populations

The criteria of the ideal Mendelian population are rarely, if ever, met. Natural populations are not infinitely large, the mating pattern is not always random, genes are lost and gained through mutation and migration, and selection operates on some of the alleles. All these factors can change gene and genotype frequencies.

The first factor to be considered is population size. Natural populations are often divided into smaller groups, which may be governed by laws different from those for an infinite population. In an infinite population, the gametes represent the whole parental gene pool, whereas in a small subpopulation, the gametes represent only a *sample* of the pool and are therefore subject to a sampling error that leads to random fluctuation of gene frequencies from one generation to another (*genetic drift*). The drift may result in the *loss* of one allele from a population and *fixation* of another allele at the same locus. The effect of random drift can be likened to drawing black and white marbles from a bag. Imagine a bag containing five black and five white marbles. Draw one marble, record its color, and then put it back in the bag; draw another marble, record its color, and again return it to the bag. Repeat the process ten times and then count

Table 12-2. Attainment of the difference between initial and equilibrium value (D) under different degrees of recombination*

| Generation | Recombination (%) | | | | |
	50 (independent assortment)	40	30	20	10
1	$0.5D$	$0.4D$	$0.3D$	$0.2D$	$0.1D$
2	$0.75D$	$0.64D$	$0.51D$	$0.36D$	$0.19D$
3	$0.875D$	$0.784D$	$0.657D$	$0.488D$	$0.271D$
4	$0.9375D$	$0.8704D$	$0.7599D$	$0.5904D$	$0.298D$
5					
.					
.					
.					
equilibrium	D	D	D	D	D

the ratio of black to white marbles drawn. If the drawing is completely random, the drawn sample can theoretically contain any ratio of black to white marbles, and the probability of a given ratio will be determined by the rules of binomial distribution. A one-to-one ratio has a high probability of occurrence, a one-to-zero ratio has a very small probability. Assume that the first ten drawings yield six black and four white marbles. Take another bag with six black and four white marbles and proceed with ten more drawings, always recording the color and returning the marble to the bag. The second sample may again contain any ratio of black to white marbles, although the most probable ratio is 6:4. Assume that the actual ratio is 8:2; then, in the next series of ten drawings from a bag containing eight black and two white marbles, there is a high probability that the outcome will be all white or all black marbles. If this happens, one color is "lost" and the other is "fixed," bringing the drawings to an end. Now, replace marbles with alleles, and drawings with the random selection of gametes, and a simplified picture of what happens to genes in a small population emerges. The gene frequencies fluctuate at random, and the fluctuation results in fixation of one or the other allele. The number of generations necessary for fixation of an allele depends on the population size and on the initial frequency of the two alleles: the larger the population, the longer it takes to achieve fixation. The effect of the initial gene frequencies on the fixation rate is best illustrated through a metaphor provided by Falconer:

> To visualize the process (of the dispersion of gene frequencies) one might think of a pile of dry sand in a narrow trough open at the two ends. Agitation of the trough will cause the pile to spread out along the trough, till eventually it is evenly spread along its length. Toward the end of the spreading out some of the sand will have fallen off the ends of the trough, and this represents fixation and loss. Continued agitation after the sand is evenly spread will cause it to fall off the ends at a steady rate, and the depth of sand left in the trough will be continually reduced at a steady rate until in the end none is left. The initial gene frequency is represented by the position of the initial pile of sand. If it is near one end of the trough, much of the sand will have fallen off that end before any reaches the other end, and the total amount falling off each end will be in proportion to the relative distance of the initial pile from the two ends (Falconer 1960, pp. 55–56).

The position along the trough can be likened to the gene frequency, and the depth of the sand to the probability of a population having a particular gene frequency. The fixation of genes in a small population is counterbalanced, or at least retarded, by selection, migration, and mutation.

Random sampling procedures similar to the marble drawing described above are used by population geneticists to simulate *stochastic* processes occurring in natural populations. The simulation is carried out with a computer, which speeds the procedure immensely.

D. Selection, Migration, and Mutation

In contrast to random drift (which is always unpredictable in its direction and thus represents a *dispersive process*), selection, migration, and mutation are *systematic processes* that tend to change gene frequencies in a manner predictable in both amount and direction.

1. Selection

In contrast to the individuals of an ideal population, all of which are expected to contribute equally to the next generation, individuals in a natural population differ in their *fertility* (the rate at which they produce progeny) and *viability* (the probability that the progeny survive to maturity), and therefore contribute different numbers of offspring to the next generation. The viability and fertility of a particular individual (or a genotype) compared to the viability and fertility of a standard individual (genotype) is called biological *fitness* (adaptive or selective value). The simplest way of measuring fitness is by counting the number of progeny produced by one genotype and comparing it to the progeny produced by a standard genotype. For example, if individuals of standard genotype N produce an average of 100 offspring that survive to maturity, and individuals of mutant genotype M produce only 80 offspring, the fitness of $M(W_M)$ is $80/100 = 0.8$ [the fitness of $N(W_N)$ is always taken to be equal to 1]. By this definition, fitness can have values ranging from 0 to 1.

The process responsible for the differential fitness of a genotype is *selection*; the quantitative measure of the selection's intensity is the *selection coefficient* (s), defined as the proportional reduction in the gametic contribution of a particular genotype compared with a standard genotype $(s = 1 - W)$. In the above example, $s = 0$ for N, and $s = 0.2$ for M.

2. Migration

Small populations are rarely completely isolated from one another; in the absence of physical barriers, some movement (*migration*) of individuals from one population to another always occurs, and results in the addition of new alleles (*gene flow*) to a particular gene pool. The proportion of immigrants per population is the *migration rate*. The effect of migration on gene frequencies depends on the particular *migration model*. In the simplest case, the subpopulations can be portrayed as separate islands among which only an occasional interchange of migrants takes place (*island model*). In a more complex model, the population is visualized as more or less continuous, distance being the major factor determining migration (*isolation by distance*). In the latter model, the migration is assumed to be highest between neighboring subpopulations (*neighborhood model*).

3. Mutation

The effect of mutations on gene frequencies depends primarily on the mutation rate and on the recurrence versus nonrecurrence of mutations. Recurrent mutations (those arising repeatedly) develop a *mutation pressure*, which tends to increase the frequency of a particular allele in the gene pool.

E. Genetic Polymorphism

On the basis of their selective value, mutations can be divided into two categories, neutral and nonneutral. A neutral mutation is one that has the same effect on the fitness of its carrier as does the wild-type allele. The number of neutral mutations maintained in a population is determined by the balance between the mutation rate and the rate of random extinction through genetic drift. If, in a population consisting of N individuals and $2N$ genes, the rate of neutral mutations per generation per gene is μ, the number of newly arisen neutral mutations in each generation is $2N\mu$. Of the $2N$ genes, some are transmitted to the next generation, while others become extinct. Ultimately, in one of the subsequent generations, all genes in the population are derived from one of the original $2N$ genes. Because all genes in each generation (including the mutant genes) have the same chance of being transmitted to the next generation (or conversely, of becoming extinct), the probability of the establishment in future generations of any of the $2N$ genes is $1/2N$. The number of new mutations established in each generation is $2N\mu \times 1/2N = \mu$, a constant. Hence, it can be expected that a population will always contain a certain number of mutant alleles coexisting with the wild-type alleles. Presence in the same population of two or more alleles, each with appreciable frequency, at one locus is called *genetic polymorphism*. The definition of the "appreciable frequency" is arbitrary; for human populations it is considered to be 1 percent (Cavalli-Sforza and Bodmer 1971). According to the neutral mutation hypothesis, most known polymorphisms are consequences of the mutations' neutrality.

An alternative to the neutral hypothesis of genetic polymorphisms is the selective hypothesis, which assumes that most mutations are either deleterious or advantageous. Because deleterious mutations impose a selective disadvantage on the carriers by lowering their fitness, they are selected against and eliminated from the population. Advantageous mutations, on the other hand, increase the fitness of an individual and are therefore favored by selection. The resulting selection pressure opposes the elimination of the advantageous mutation from the population and leads to establishment of a genetic polymorphism. The selective forces most frequently held responsible for maintaining a polymorphism in natural populations are heterozygous advantage, frequency-dependent selection, time- and place-dependent selection, and selection acting in opposite directions in gametes and zygotes.

1. *Heterozygous advantage.* If, at any locus, heterozygote *Aa* is more fit than both *AA* and *aa* homozygotes, a stable polymorphism will result. A classic example of heterozygous advantage is the relationship between sickle-cell anemia and malaria in man. The sickle-cell polymorphism is maintained at a relatively high frequency because the heterozygous

sickle-cell hemoglobin carriers are more resistant to malaria than normal homozygotes (the mutant homozygotes develop anemia, which is often fatal before the reproductive age).

2. *Frequency-dependent selection.* If a mutant allele has the advantage of rarity, it will increase in frequency when introduced into a population carrying the standard allele. For example, if a virus or bacteria is adapted to attack individuals carrying a more common allele, the rare allele will be favored by selection and a stable polymorphism at some intermediate gene frequency will develop.

3. *Selection varying in direction with time or place.* A stable polymorphism can also result if allele A is favored in one generation and allele a in the next generation, or if A is favored in one geographical region and a in another.

4. *Selection acting in opposite directions in gametes and zygotes.* This type of selective force is exemplified by the t system, in which the t factors are selected for in gametes (through high t transmission ratios of $t/+$ males) and selected against in zygotes (the t/t homozygotes are either lethal or male sterile). The balance of the two opposing forces results in a stable polymorphism.

It was originally believed that the proportion of polymorphic genes in a population was exceedingly low, and that all polymorphisms could be accounted for in selective terms. In the last 10 or 15 years, however, through use of electrophoretic and immunological methods, a large number of polymorphic loci has been discovered. In the mouse, the average population is polymorphic in at least 26 percent of its loci, and the average individual is heterozygous in at least 8.5 percent of its loci (Selander 1970). In other species, estimates of polymorphic loci are even higher. The unexpectedly high frequency of polymorphisms in natural populations have led some geneticists to a more critical examination of the selectionist interpretation and to investigation of the role played by neutral mutations. Currently, there are two conflicting interpretations of genetic polymorphism; selectionists believe that most, if not all polymorphisms are maintained by selection, whereas neutralists claim that most polymorphisms arise because so many mutations are neutral. Most likely, however, the true interpretation will be found between these two extremes.

II. Structure of Mouse Populations

Information on the population structure of commensal mice, the most intensively studied wild mice, has been drawn from three major sources: first, from direct observation of free-living mice in their natural habitats (H. Young *et al.* 1950; R. Brown 1953; Crowcroft 1955, 1966; Southwick 1958; Crowcroft and Rowe 1963; Rowe *et al.* 1963; Kaczmarzyk 1964; Adamczyk and Ryszkowski 1965;) second, from observations of confined populations (Strecker and

Emlen 1953; Crowcroft and Rowe 1957, 1958; Southwick 1955a, 1955b; Andrzejewski *et al.* 1959; Petrusewicz 1959; Crowcroft and Jeffers 1961; Reimer and Petras 1967, 1968); third, from studies of genetic variation (Weber 1950; Deol 1958; Lewontin and Dunn 1960; Anderson 1964, 1966, 1970; Petras 1967a, b, c, d; Selander 1970; Selander *et al.* 1969a, b; Selander and Yang 1969; Iványi and Démant 1970; J. Klein 1970a, 1973a; J. Klein and Bailey 1971; Wheeler 1972; Wheeler and Selander 1972; Micková and Iványi 1972).

These sources revealed that the mouse population is divided into small subpopulations or *demes* (breeding units, family units, tribes, colonies), each with a rigid social structure. Each deme occupies a small territory probably not larger than a few square meters. Demarcation of the territory is behavioral rather than physical, because the territories are established even in a single room with no physical barriers. A territory is vigorously defended from intrusion, primarily by one male. The rate of immigration into established demes is thus negligible, with the demes behaving as isolates open in one direction (out) and virtually closed in the opposite direction (in).

An average deme consists of 7–12 adult mice (3–5 males and 4–7 females), and is ruled by a *dominant male* who fights to achieve and maintain his superior position. All other males present in the deme are *subordinate* and probably do not sire any progeny. On the other hand, the females in the deme seem to be equal socially. Each pregnant female builds a separate nest in which she bears and rears her young. The average litter size is 6–8, with each female bearing 3–5 litters per year. Reproductive activity of wild mice is highest in prevernal and autumn seasons, the population density being maximal around April and November and minimal around January and June. Most of the young leave the deme after reaching maturity, settle in unoccupied territories, and establish new demes; if no new territories are available in the buildings, they move into fields surrounding the buildings and establish transitory feral populations. The pressure to leave the deme is higher for males than for females, and consequently more males are found among the feral mice in the vicinity of human dwellings. As the weather becomes colder and the food supply more limited, the feral mice attempt to move back into buildings; those unable to return usually perish. Dwindling of the food supply also leads to decimation of the indoor populations, with the subordinate males dying first and the dominant males last. During extremely cold winters a large proportion of indoor mice vanishes (the population is said to go through a *bottleneck phase*). When the weather improves, the few survivors start new demes, and a new population cycle begins.

The dynamics of the mouse population are influenced by such factors as climatic conditions, physical setting of the locality, predation, and availability of food and cover. However, although these factors may alter the population parameters to some extent, they usually do not influence the main characteristics of commensal mouse populations, which are small population size, isolation of the demes, rigid social order within the demes, and rapid changes from population minima to population maxima. To what degree these characteristics also apply to the populations of feral and aboriginal mice has not been determined.

III. Population Genetics of t Factors

One of the most astonishing features of t factors is their ubiquity (Table 12–3), the factors being present in wild populations all over the world; North America, Europe, Australia, and Asia (Dunn and Morgan 1953; Dunn 1955; Komai 1955; Dunn et al. 1960; Lewontin and Dunn 1960; Dunn 1964; Braden and Weiler 1964; Petras 1967b; Dunn and D. Bennett 1971b). On the North American continent they are found from Canada to Texas and from New York to Cali-

Table 12-3. Frequency of t factors in wild populations

Location	Year of sampling	No. of $+/t$ total no. mice	$f(+t)$	(ft)	Reference
Mystic, Connecticut, U.S.A.	<1953	1/3	0.333	0.167	Dunn and
Norwich, Vermont, U.S.A.	<1953	0/4	0.000	0.000	Morgan
Madison, Wisconsin, U.S.A.	<1953	0/14	0.000	0.000	1953
Rumford, Virginia, U.S.A.	1955	1/8 ⎫ 9/22	0.125 ⎫ 0.409	0.062 ⎫ 0.204	
	1959	8/14 ⎭	0.571 ⎭	0.286 ⎭	Lewontin
Storrs, Connecticut, U.S.A.		5/7	0.714	0.357	and Dunn
Clinton, Montana, U.S.A.	1957	0/11	0.000	0.000	1960
	1958	3/3	1.00	0.500	
Sarasota, Florida, U.S.A.		1/4	0.250	0.125	
Austin, Texas, U.S.A.		3/10	0.300	0.150	
Tucson, Arizona, U.S.A.		1/4	0.250	0.125	
Norwich, Vermont, U.S.A.		2/9	0.222	0.111	
Lawrence, Kansas, U.S.A.		1/6	0.167	0.083	
El Paso, Texas, U.S.A.		3/3	1.000	0.500	
Corte Madera, California, U.S.A.		1/1	1.000	0.500	
Clark Fork River, Montana, U.S.A.		1/20	0.05	0.02	
Tieman Pl., New York, U.S.A.		1/1	1.00	0.500	
Madison, Wisconsin, U.S.A.		1/6	0.167	0.083	
Rumford, Virginia, U.S.A.		2/11	0.182	0.090	
Chester, Nova Scotia, Canada		0/1	—	—	
Lewiston, Maine, U.S.A.		0/2	—	—	
Lewiston, Maine, U.S.A.		0/3	—	—	
So. Strafford, Vermont, U.S.A.	Prior to	0/3	—	—	Dunn et al.
So. Strafford, Vermont, U.S.A.	1960	0/2	—	—	1960
Norwich E., Vermont, U.S.A.		0/12	—	—	
Hanover, New Hampshire, U.S.A.		0/4	—	—	
Hanover, New Hampshire, U.S.A.		0/3	—	—	
Mansfield, Connecticut, U.S.A.		0/2	—	—	
Mansfield, Connecticut, U.S.A.		0/7	—	—	
Riverhead, L.I., New York, U.S.A.		0/1	—	—	
Riverhead, L.I., New York, U.S.A.		0/3	—	—	
Great Gull Island, New York, U.S.A.		0/3	—	—	
Great Gull Island, New York, U.S.A.		0/37	—	—	
West Side, New York, U.S.A.		0/4	—	—	
Raleigh, N. Carolina, U.S.A.		0/2	—	—	
Brookings, S. Dakota, U.S.A.		0/1	—	—	
Clinton, Montana, U.S.A.		0/2	—	—	
Adin, California, U.S.A.		0/11	—	—	
Calgary, Alberta, Canada	1962	13/34 ⎫ 42/176	0.382 ⎫ 0/239	0.191 ⎫ 0.119	Anderson
	1963	29/142 ⎭	0.204 ⎭	0.102 ⎭	1964
Ann Arbor, Michigan, U.S.A.	1959	10/18 ⎫	0.555 ⎫	0.278 ⎫	
	1960	19/66 ⎪ 57/182	0.287 ⎪ 0.313	0.144 ⎪ 0.156	Petras
	1961	16/51 ⎪	0.313 ⎪	0.157 ⎪	1967b
	1962	12/47 ⎭	0.255 ⎭	0.128 ⎭	
Jutland Peninsula, Denmark, South	1969	1/20 ⎫ 7/43	0.050 ⎫ 0.163	0.025 ⎫ 0.081	Dunn and
North	1969	6/23 ⎭	0.261 ⎭	0.130 ⎭	D. Bennett 1971b
Total		141/643	0.219	0.109	

fornia (Dunn *et al.* 1960). All thoroughly studied wild populations (except that of Great Gull Island, a small, uninhabited island off the New York coast) have been shown to carry *t* factors. Repeated samplings of the Great Gull Island population has revealed a complete absence of *t* factors, a fact of considerable importance to the interpretation of the *t* system. The frequency of *t* factors may vary from locality to locality and from year to year (Table 12–3). The overall frequency calculated from samples collected at widely different geographic areas and localities is 0.11, indicating that approximately 22 percent of mice in any given population are *t*/+ heterozygotes.

All *t* factors found in wild populations are either homozygous lethals or homozygous semiviables (male sterile) with high male transmission ratios.

The high frequencies of lethal and sterile *t* factors in natural populations represent a challenging problem for population geneticists. The models proposed to explain the high frequencies are of two groups, deterministic and stochastic.

The deterministic models assume that mice live in an ideal Mendelian population (infinite size and random mating). The first deterministic solution of the *t* population problem was proposed by Prout (1953), but his equations depended upon the occurrence of segregation distortion in both sexes. Because it is known that segregation distortion occurs only in males, the model was abandoned. A deterministic solution assuming homozygous lethality and segregation distortion in males only was proposed by Bruck (1957):

$$q_l = \frac{1}{2} - \frac{\sqrt{m(1-m)}}{2m}$$

where q_l = equilibrium frequency of lethal *t* factors and m = male transmission ratio. A corresponding equation for homozygous semiviable (sterile) *t* factors was derived by Dunn and Levene (1961):

$$q_s = 2m - 1$$

where q_s = equilibrium frequency of sterile *t* factors. The two equations predict that the mouse population is in a genetic equilibrium in which the frequency of *t* factors is determined by their transmission ratios. For example, a lethal *t* factor with a transmission ratio of 0.95 should, according to Bruck's model, have an equilibrium frequency of 0.385. However, the observed frequencies of *t* factors in natural populations do not correspond to those predicted by the deterministic model. The observed frequencies are generally less than half the predicted values, indicating that the deterministic model is incorrect.

Stochastic models for the behavior of lethal and semiviable *t* factors have been proposed by Lewontin and Dunn (1960) and by Lewontin (1962). The basic assumption of the stochastic models is that mice live in small, relatively isolated, endogamous family units (demes). Because of the small size, the general trend in the demes is toward fixation of wild (+) factors and elimination of *t* factors by random genetic drift. This process is slowed by segregation distortion, but the direction of the trend is clearly pronounced.

A given geographical population can therefore be expected to consist of two deme types, one having the wild allele already fixed, the other approaching fixation. The average frequency of *t* factors for a specific locality is determined largely by the proportion between the two types of demes. The rate of *t* factor loss in the demes depends on the degree of segregation distortion; the lower the *t* transmission ratio, the faster the *t* factor elimination. Only factors with very high transmission ratios remain in the population for appreciable periods. A population that has lost a *t* factor can easily be "infected" by a new *t* factor if this factor is introduced into the deme by a heterozygous male. According to this model, *t* polymorphism is in a continual state of decay and is subject to violent oscillations. The *t* factors tend to pass through the demes, running the risk of extinction in each, but tending to spread in the population as a whole.

The stochastic model has been tested by a computer simulation (Lewontin and Dunn 1960; Lewontin 1962) and by ecological studies involving free-living mouse populations (Anderson *et al.* 1964). The simulation was based on a computer program in which an analogue of a real population conforming to genetic rules of meiosis, fertilization, and selection was developed and the chance element provided by a Monte Carlo sampling. Because of the chance factor, no two runs of the program gave identical results even if the initial parameters (population size and transmission ratio) were the same. Each run therefore represented a separate experiment on an independent population. By varying the input parameters of the program, it was possible to determine the effect of these parameters on the behavior of *t* factors in successive generations (100 or more). The frequencies of *t* factors obtained by Lewontin and Dunn (1960) and by Lewontin (1962) in the simulated populations were much closer to the observed frequencies than those obtained in the deterministic models.

Some predictions made on the basis of simulated populations were verified experimentally by Anderson and his colleagues (1964), who released mice heterozygous for lethal factor t^{w11} into an isolated mouse population believed to be free of *t* factors. In the years following the release, the population was periodically sampled and tested for the presence of t^{w11}. The experiment demonstrated that lethal *t* factors can be introduced successfully into the population within a relatively short time, despite the selection against homozygotes. However, in the absence of repeated "infection" with new *t* factors, the introduced factors were eventually eliminated.

The original model of Lewontin and Dunn (1960) was reexamined by Levin *et al.* (1969), who demonstrated that random drift has an important effect on *t* factor frequencies only if the demes are totally isolated and composed of fewer than 12 mice; allowing for a 1 percent migration between the demes, the effective population size of the deme would have to be fewer than eight, with a 3 percent migration rate fewer than four, and so on. It thus appears that the random drift alone does not fully explain *t* polymorphism, and that other factors, such as systematic inbreeding within demes, must be considered.

An important fact is that all the simulations have been based on non-overlapping generations and have completely ignored the social organization of the demes. A more realistic simulation taking these latter factors into account might bring the observed and predicted *t* frequencies to a point of complete agreement.

The stochastic model does not explain the ultimate origin of the "infecting" *t* factors that are necessary to maintain the observed frequencies. One possible source of new *t* factors could be a chromosomal imbalance resulting from inter-mixing of unrelated mice. After the population bottleneck, when mice from different demes mingle and establish new demes, the chromosomal complements of their progeny pass through a period of temporary imbalance, which is out-wardly expressed as the *t* syndrome. A similar imbalance occurs after crossing wild mice with inbred strains. The imbalance primarily affects chromosome 17, which appears to be unstable. The imbalance hypothesis can be verified experi-mentally by demonstrating that wild mice express *t*-like effects only when mated to unrelated individuals (mice from different demes, inbred mice) but not when mated to members of the same deme.

IV. Population Genetics of the *H-2* System

A. Extent of *H-2* Polymorphism

Population analysis of the *H-2* system has long been among the most neglected areas of H-2 studies. The first attempt to type noninbred mice was made by Rubinstein and Ferrebee (1964), who used the hemagglutination assay to test red cells of some 50 randomly bred Swiss-Webster animals against 14 H-2 antisera. The typing suggested that there are probably many more *H-2* haplotypes and H-2 antigens than those known to exist in the inbred strains. Serological analysis of mice captured in the wild has recently begun in the laboratories of P. Iványi (Iványi *et al.* 1969; Iványi and Démant 1970; Micková and Iványi 1971; Iványi and Micková 1972) and J. Klein (1970a, 1971a, 1972a, 1973a). In the latter laboratory, a long-term multiphasic program is in progress to obtain information regarding *H-2* population behavior.

In the first phase of this program (J. Klein 1970a, 1971a), operationally monospecific antisera prepared by cross-immunization of inbred strains were applied to panels of wild mice sampled from different localities of a single geo-graphic area (Ann Arbor, Michigan). The typing done by the direct PVP hemagglutination test, and complemented in a few instances by an absorption analysis, demonstrated that the public antigens of inbred strains are widely distributed among wild mice, whereas the inbred private H-2 antigens occur rarely, if at all, in wild populations. For example, public antigen H-2.5 was found in 95 percent of wild mice trapped in the Ann Arbor area, while private antigens H-2.4, H-2.23, and others were not present in a sample of over 2000 mice. Some wild mice did not react with *any* inbred-derived H-2 antisera, a result interpreted as being caused by the absence of all known H-2 antigens ("null *H-2* haplotypes"). However, direct typing was obscured by nonspecific reactions and cross-reactions.

Nonspecific reactions can be illustrated by mice captured at the KE farm in the Ann Arbor area (J. Klein 1970a). The mice, when tested with a monospecific anti-H-2.16, were all positive, and this result was confirmed by several retypings. However, after some of the mice were mated to an inbred strain and the hybrids tested again with the same antiserum, the antigen disappeared. This observation can be explained by assuming a polygenetically controlled nonspecific reactivity in KE mice. The cell membrane relief in KE mice could be such that it binds the anti-H-2.16 antibodies nonspecifically; the reactivity is lost by the outcrossing because the segregation breaks up the particular constellation of loci and, consequently, the particular conformation of the membrane responsible for the nonspecific reaction.

An example of the complications caused by cross-reactions is provided by mice from the KP farm in Ann Arbor. These mice reacted with a monospecific anti-H-2.17 antiserum in the PVP hemagglutination test, and the reaction was highly reproducible on repeated testing. The reactivity was inheritable, because semicongenic B10.KP mice were also positive with the H-2.17 antiserum. However, *in vivo* absorption tests gave peculiar results. Absorption of the antiserum in B10.KP mice removed the anti-B10.KP activity but did not change the activity against the inbred donor strain (C3H.Q). The antiserum behaved as a monospecific anti-H-2.17 before and after absorption in B10.KP mice; yet the absorption apparently removed some factor from the antiserum, because the absorbed serum lost its capacity to react with B10.KP cells. A similar phenomenon was described by Iványi and Micková (1972). The cross-reactive factor removable by B10.KP absorption could be a broadly reactive fraction of the H-2.17 antibody spectrum or an antibody directed against one subcomponent of the H-2.17 complex.

In general, the typing of wild mice with inbred-derived antisera provides only limited information about population behavior of the *H-2* system. The inbred private antigens are too rare and the public antigens too common among wild mice to be useful for differentiation of wild *H-2* haplotypes. For this reason, in the second phase of population studies, an attempt to produce antisera identifying wild-specific H-2 antigens is being made. The simplest way to obtain anti-H-2^{wild} reagents might seem to be immunization of inbred strains with tissues from wild mice. Such immunization, however, is complicated by several factors: antisera must be tested against mice other than the donor (the donor is sacrificed), the immunizing tissue is in short supply, and the same antiserum cannot be reproduced at will. Furthermore, antisera produced by immunization with wild mice as donors are usually complex, containing not only multiple H-2 but also numerous non-H-2 antibodies. In view of these difficulties, an alternative method of producing anti-*H-2*^{wild} antisera has been designed. The *H-2* haplotypes of wild mice are first transferred onto a defined genetic background of strain C57BL/10 and the ensuing B10.W congenic or semicongenic lines become tissue donors for immunization. Currently, more than 50 B10.W lines are being developed in this writer's laboratory, many nearing their completion. The lines are produced by repeated backcrossing to the B10 strain, using one of the two systems described in Chapter Two (i.e., either the system with Ss as a marker for $H\text{-}2^{wild}$ haplotypes or the system based on alternative matings to two B10 congenic lines). Upon completion, the B10.W lines are cross-immunized with each other as well as with inbred strains and the antisera produced are serologically analyzed, using panels of inbred strains and B10.W lines. The second phase is expected to accomplish two major goals: to characterize serologically $H\text{-}2$ haplotypes of B10.W lines and to provide operationally monospecific anti-$H\text{-}2^{wild}$ antisera, which can then be used in the next phase.

In phase three, the battery of anti-$H\text{-}2^{wild}$ antisera will be employed for direct typing of wild mice to determine such parameters as population frequencies of $H\text{-}2^{wild}$ antigens and $H\text{-}2^{wild}$ haplotypes, the extent of $H\text{-}2$ polymorphism, and the relationship of $H\text{-}2$ polymorphism to the population structure.

In phase four, the information garnered in phase three will be used to obtain an insight into the mechanisms maintaining $H\text{-}2$ polymorphism in natural populations.

The feasibility of the multiphasic approach has been demonstrated on a small scale, and some information pertinent to the extent of $H\text{-}2$ polymorphism has already been obtained (J. Klein 1972a, 1973a). So far, antisera against some congenic B10.W lines (i.e., lines that underwent backcrossings to the B10 background) have been produced and tested against a panel of inbred and B10.W strains. In 12 of these antisera, a prominent component is an antibody directed against private antigens of the B10.W donor. These 12 antisera react either with only the B10.W donor and no other cells in the panel, or with cells of a few other B10.W lines, usually those derived from the same locality as that of the donor. The remaining 18 antisera contain a mixture of antibodies directed against public H-2 antigens, and in a few instances, also against non-H-2 antigens. These antisera react not only with a number of B10.W lines, but also with several inbred strains. The reaction patterns of the anti-H-2 public antisera are sufficiently diverse to permit a tentative conclusion that the $H\text{-}2$ haplotypes of their respective B10.W donors are probably all different. In five instances, the $H\text{-}2^{wild}$ haplotypes have been analyzed with all available antisera and their antigenic configuration determined. The new $H\text{-}2$ haplotypes were originally designated $H\text{-}2^{wa}$ through $H\text{-}2^{we}$, but this was later changed to $H\text{-}2^{w1}$ through $H\text{-}2^{w5}$.

Each $H\text{-}2^{wild}$ haplotype is characterized by the presence of a particular array of public H-2 antigens, although the assignments of public antigens to the individual $H\text{-}2^{wild}$ haplotypes are questionable because of the problems encountered during the serological analysis. For example, it is quite common to obtain a strong reaction of a particular $H\text{-}2^{wild}$ haplotype with one anti-H-2.1 antiserum and no reaction with another anti-H-2.1 antiserum. The typing of $H\text{-}2^{wild}$ haplotypes for the H-2 public antigens therefore has a dubious value. Because the private antigens sufficiently characterize a given $H\text{-}2$ haplotype, it may become necessary to limit H-2 typing of wild mice to the determination of private antigens (or, more generally, to less cross-reactive antigens). Each of the 12 B10.W lines possesses only one private H-2 antigen, but the absence of a second private antigen is almost certainly caused by the unavailability of *H-2* recombinants, permitting separation of private K and D antibodies.

Altogether, some 40 different *H-2* haplotypes are now known, 30 derived from wild and 10 from laboratory mice (not counting the recombinant *H-2* haplotypes). The indications are that many more new *H-2* haplotypes exist among the 50 B10.W lines maintained in this writer's laboratory, and when haplotypes that are presently being identified in Dr. Iványi's laboratory are taken into account, the number of known *H-2* haplotypes can safely be estimated at at least 100. The actual number of existing *H-2* haplotypes is difficult to predict, the minimal estimate being several hundred. *H-2* polymorphism already far exceeds any other known polymorphism in the mouse; if the number of different *H-2* haplotypes does indeed run into the hundreds, the *H-2* complex will become the most polymorphic system known.

Preliminary data have also been obtained regarding the relationship between *H-2* polymorphism and the population structure of the mouse. Typing with both anti-*H-2*^{inbred} (J. Klein 1970a, 1971a) and anti-*H-2*^{wild} (J. Klein 1972a) antisera indicates *H-2* similarity among mice from the same locality and *H-2* diversity among mice from different localities. These findings have been interpreted as evidence for the deme structure of the mouse population. In a highly polymorphic system such as *H-2*, the population's subdivisions into small isolated colonies almost certainly must result in genetic homogeneity within each deme and genetic heterogeneity among the demes. However, there is no evidence so far that mice with similar *H-2* haplotypes come from the same deme and mice with different *H-2* haplotypes from different demes. An interesting case of *H-2* homogeneity in a large feral mouse population has recently been reported by Micková and Iványi (1971), who tested 100 mice captured at Great Gull Island and found only three *H-2* haplotypes among them. Because the island is completely isolated, its mouse population represents a closed colony in which a high degree of genetic homogeneity has apparently been attained.

The postulate of genetic homogeneity within each locality (deme) is supported by skin-graft analysis of hybrids between wild and laboratory mice (Iványi *et al.* 1969; Iványi and Démant 1970; J. Klein and Bailey 1971; Micková and Iványi 1972). It has been shown (J. Klein and Bailey 1971; Micková and Iványi 1972) that skin grafts exchanged between mice sired by males from the same locality have relatively long mean survival times, broad rejection ranges, and some survive permanently. In contrast, grafts exchanged between mice sired by males from different localities have short mean survival times, narrow rejection ranges, and none survive permanently. Apparently, mice from the same locality have a more similar histocompatibility endowment than mice from different localities. The percentage of permanently surviving grafts in the former group has been used to calculate the effective number of alleles per locus and the effective number of segregating histocompatibility loci. The estimates range from two to nine heterozygous *H* loci per mouse (J. Klein and Bailey 1971; Micková and Iványi 1972), depending on the particular locality, the particular inbred strain used to produce the hybrids, sex of the recipient, and other factors.

The H heterozygosity of wild mice is thus considerably lower than that of an F_1 hybrid between two inbred strains of the laboratory mouse (see Chapter Eight).

B. Biological Significance of *H-2* Polymorphism

The immensity of *H-2* polymorphism poses the question as to whether there is any adaptive value associated with this antigenic variability. Because this question is closely linked to the problem of the *H-2* function, which will not be considered until the last section of this monograph, it will be necessary to limit this discussion to a few specific questions.

1. Does H-2 Polymorphism Actually Exist?

Is it possible that serological methods detect more differences than actually exist, or that the K and D regions consist of large groups of loci, each locus having only a few alleles? The first possibility is unlikely because the estimates of the extent of *H-2* polymorphism are based on the variability of private *H-2* antigens; were the estimates based on public antigens, which may be serological artifacts, this hypothesis could be considered more seriously. The second possibility, that *H-2* polymorphism might be a genetic illusion, is more realistic. If both K and D regions contained several loci, with each locus having only two alleles, the allelic combinations of these loci could produce numerous *H-2* haplotypes. If this were true, a postulation of an allelic exclusion similar to that known in immunoglobulin loci would be necessary; of the series of K (or D) loci, only one would have to be expressed genetically in each individual (a different one in each individual), because only one K (or D) private antigen can be detected in an *H-2* homozygote. In contrast to the allelic exclusion of immuno-globulin loci, which occurs at the cellular level, allelic exclusion of *H-2* loci would have to occur at the organism level. As there is no experimental evidence supporting such a highly unorthodox view of the *H-2* system, we must assume that *H-2* polymorphism exists both serologically and genetically.

2. Is H-2 Polymorphism Exceptional?

Could it be that polymorphism at loci other than *H-2* has not yet been dis-covered because methods for detecting multiple allelism are not available? Arguing against this possibility is the fact that among the 500 or so known loci in the mouse, a number have been discovered by serological techniques similar to those used in detecting *H-2*, and yet none is even remotely so polymorphic as the *H-2* complex. In addition, electrophoretic methods, which are probably as powerful as serological methods used in the study of the *H-2* system, have not led to the discovery of a high degree of polymorphism at other loci.

3. Does H-2 Polymorphism Have Any Adaptive Value?

As mentioned earlier, the tenet that every polymorphism must have an adaptive value has recently been shaken by the discovery that many more polymorphisms than were expected exist in natural populations. It has been postulated that some of these polymorphisms have no adaptive value and that the variants present in the populations are selectively neutral. Is it possible that such neutrality also exists in the *H-2* system? Because of the vastness of *H-2* variability, the idea of *H-2* neutrality might seem shocking, but closer examination reveals that it is not an unreasonable possibility. The H-2 glycoprotein may differ from other proteins, and particularly enzymes, in that it has a high degree of tolerance to mutational changes. In an enzyme, almost any mutation affecting binding with a substrate and thus causing partial or complete loss of enzymatic activity is harmful, and is therefore selected against. On the other hand, in H-2 molecules, which are, perhaps, relatively inert biologically in that they do not display any enzymatic or similar activities, there is greater tolerance of genetic variability. Many mutations that would be deleterious to most enzymes may have no effect on the function of the H-2 glycoprotein. Supporting this hypothesis is the observation that the mutation rate of *H-2* loci is higher than that of other loci in the mouse. It may be that this seemingly increased rate is not caused by higher mutability of *H-2* loci, but rather by the fact that more *H-2* mutants survive.

4. What Might Be the Adaptive Value of H-2 Polymorphism?

If the neutrality hypothesis does not hold, several adaptive values for *H-2* polymorphism can be suggested.

a. Variability as a Requirement for H-2 function. One possibility is that H-2 participate in cell-to-cell interaction, and that the interaction is dependent upon the diversity of the interacting molecules. (For details, see Chapter Twenty.)

b. Protection Against Outgrowth of Somatic Variant Clones (1) *Protection against contagious tumors.* Gorer (1960) suggested that "were it not for the antigenic diversity of most species and the existence of a mechanism to react against the antigens, contagious tumors would be relatively common." According to this hypothesis, the function of *H-2* loci (and *H* loci in general) is to create diversity among individuals of the same species so that tumor cells of a diseased animal encounter a nontraversible barrier when accidentally transmitted to another individual. There are, however, at least three arguments against the contagious tumor hypothesis. First, when contagious tumors occurred (in dogs and hamsters, for example) they overcame histocompatibility barriers. Second, contagious tumors are unknown in histocompatible inbred strains. Third, tumor cells are not parasitic organisms in the strictest sense, and therefore are not adapted to infectivity.

(2) *Immune surveillance.* According to the surveillance hypothesis, the function of the immune system is to guard against somatic (tumor) variants arising constantly in different tissues of the body (see Chapter Twenty). The surveillance would be facilitated by the existence of loci that are vast in number, widely spread throughout the genome, and have a tendency to produce new antigens whenever they mutate. The *H* loci fulfill all three requirements in that they

are numerous, are present in different chromosomes, and code for antigenic molecules. The somatic accidents leading to the appearance of variant cells or clones are likely to involve one of the many *H* loci and thus result in the appearance of a new histocompatibility antigen. The antigen is then recognized as foreign by the immune system and the variant cell or clone is liquidated. The existence of a highly variable *H* locus, such as the *H-2* complex, could thus have an adaptive value even if the polymorphism itself were nonadaptive; the numerous alleles could arise because the *H-2* loci are highly variable (and this variability is advantageous), and could be maintained because they are selectively neutral. However, it is difficult to accept the idea that nature would maintain hundreds of loci, the only function of which is to await involvement in a somatic accident, and hundreds of alleles with no function at all.

   c. Resistance to Pathogens. Three mechanisms of *H-2* involvement in resistance to pathogens were proposed by Snell (1968) and mathematically analyzed by Hull (1970).

   (1) *Molecular mimicry.* The first mechanism assumes molecular mimicry, a sharing of cross-reacting antigens between the pathogen (virus or bacteria) and the host. The sharing lowers the immunological resistance of the host and thus renders it more susceptible to the pathogen. The existence of heterophile antigens (antigens shared by two unrelated species) has long been an established fact; there is even evidence that heterophile antigens may participate in transplantation immunity (for a review, see Rapaport 1972), but there is no evidence that H-2-like antigens are synthesized by viruses or bacteria.

   (2) *Passenger antigens.* The second mechanism assumes incorporation of host cell membrane fragments into the external coat of a virus particle, leading to a possible acquisition of some host antigens (including H-2) by the virus. A host of a different *H-2* haplotype may then resist the virus by reacting against the "passenger" antigens of the virus particle. Presence of H-2 antigens in mammary tumor viruses was postulated by Nandi (1967; cf. Chapter Sixteen).

   (3) *Virus receptor.* The third mechanism assumes that the initial step in virus infection is the attachment of the infectious particle to a specific receptor site on the cell membrane of the host, and that the receptor may, in some cases, be the H-2 molecule.

   Because in all three mechanisms the *H-2* heterozygote is expected to be susceptible to the pathogen, *H-2* polymorphism would have to be maintained by frequency-dependent selection rather than heterozygote advantage. The polymorphism would be a continuous effort by the host to escape infection by the constant formation of new antigens to which the pathogens are not adapted.

   Association of the *H-2* system with virus susceptibility has definitely been established (cf. Chapter Sixteen), yet it is unlikely that any of the three mechanisms mentioned above plays a significant role in this susceptibility. The current consensus is that the susceptibility is governed not by *H-2K* or *H-2D*, but by the region between these two loci, specifically the *I* region.

   d. Fetal-Maternal Interactions. Hull (1964a) observed that reciprocal matings $a/a^t \times a^t/a^t$ (where a and a^t are coat-color genes—nonagouti and black and tan, respectively) produced a significant deviation from the expected one-to-one ratio of offspring:

Mating	Relative frequency of offspring	
	a/a^t	a^t/a^t
$a/a^t♀ \times a^t/a^t♂$	0.411	0.589
$a^t/a^t♀ \times a/a^t♂$	0.576	0.424

The deviation was the number of offspring having the same genotype as their mother being reduced. The effect could not be attributed to a lower fitness of a particular genotype (the a/a^t offspring were reduced in one cross, the a^t/a^t in the reciprocal cross), and was, instead, explained by Hull as caused by a specific interaction between mother and fetus. Since the mean litter sizes in the two matings were not significantly different, the selective elimination apparently took place in the uterus at an early time when an excess of embryos was available. (It is estimated that approximately one-third of the embryos in normal mice are eliminated before birth.) A theoretical examination of the evolutionary significance of fetal-maternal incompatibility (Hull 1964b, 1966; Clarke and Kirby 1966) led to the conclusion that the incompatibility could result in a stable genetic polymorphism at the locus involved. Clarke and Kirby (1966) suggested that the reduction of offspring in Hull's crosses could be explained by the effect of closely linked H loci rather than the a (agouti) locus itself. The suggestion was tested by Hull, who demonstrated that fetal-maternal incompatibility is indeed associated with *H-3* and *H-13* loci located in the same chromosome as the a locus (Hull 1969), and that the two strains involved in the original cross in which the incompatibility was first noted (C3Hf/HeHa and Hg/Hu) differ in the *H-3* and *H-13* loci (Hull 1971)[1]. The effect of the a region on gene frequencies was demonstrated in closed populations derived from a cross between C3Hf/HeHa and Hg/Hu strains (Hull 1972). In these populations the a^t allele was slowly replaced by the a allele at the rate of about 1 percent/generation. The observed changes were similar to those expected with fetal-maternal incompatibility at the a locus or at H loci closely linked to a.

A possible clue to the physiological basis for the effect of fetal-maternal incompatibility on offspring viability was suggested by the finding that the incompatibility leads to an increase in the size of the placenta (Billington 1964; James, 1965, 1967; McLaren 1965), a property believed to be favorable for the development of the fetus. The increase can be enhanced by immunization of the mother against paternal antigens and diminished by rendering the mother tolerant to these antigens (James 1967). This and the observation that a similar increase occurs when homozygous blastocysts are transferred into the uteri of an

---

[1] However, Hetherington (1973) recently failed to observe any increase in decidual or placental weight in a series of matings between congenic lines differing at the *H-3* locus.

allogeneic strain (Billington 1964) demonstrated that the increase is due to antigenic dissimilarity rather than heterosis. One possible hitch to this explanation is that the selective reduction in the number of compatible embryos apparently occurs before the placenta reaches an appreciable size.

In spite of its seeming attractiveness, the fetal-maternal incompatibility hypothesis is an unlikely explanation of *H-2* polymorphism. First, an attempt to demonstrate influence of the *H-2* complex on placental or decidual size failed (Finkel and Lilly 1971; Hetherington 1973). Second, mathematical analyses demonstrated that the hypothesis is not easily applicable to polymorphisms involving more than three alleles at a given locus (Hull 1966; Clarke and Kirby 1966), although Warburton (1968) showed that a balanced polymorphism with an indefinitely large number of alleles can be maintained if it benefits a fetus to elicit an immunological reaction from its mother. Third, the conditions existing in wild mouse populations are probably not favorable for the occurrence of fetal-maternal incompatibilities, as the *H* heterozygosity in the demes is relatively low.

e. Selection at Closely Linked Loci. One possibility worth considering is that the selection does not occur at the *H-2K* or *H-2D* loci themselves but at some other loci in chromosome 17, and that *H-2* polymorphism is merely a consequence of a "piggybacking" mechanism. The two most likely candidates for the piggybacking function are the *Ir* genes and the *t* factors.

The *Ir* genes are located between the *H-2K* and *H-2D* loci and are concerned with immune response to a wide spectrum of antigens, including antigens of viruses and other pathogens. It is believed that, in a broader sense, the *Ir* genes are involved in resistance to diseases, that is, in a function of great evolutionary significance for the organism (cf. Chapter Seventeen). The close linkage between the *H-2* and *Ir* loci may lead to a polymorphism at the *H-2* loci even if they themselves are selectively neutral.

The *t* complex is physically located at some distance from the *H-2* complex, but genetically the two can be assumed to be closely linked because of the strong crossing-over suppressing effect of *t*. The *t* complex is acted upon by a strong selective force, the high male transmission ratio. As first pointed out by Snell (1968), the crossing-over suppressing effect and the high male transmission ratios provide favorable conditions for fixation of *H-2* mutations in natural populations. The conditions become even more favorable when the peculiar structure of the mouse population is taken into account. It is easy to imagine how an *H-2* mutation carried by a dominant male in an association with a *t* factor rapidly spreads through a deme and how this event leads to *H-2* diversification of the demes.

f. Conclusion. It is unlikely that a complex phenomenon such as *H-2* polymorphism has a single cause; the polymorphism is probably maintained by a combination of factors, including low frequency of deleterious *H-2* mutations, requirement of variability for the *H-2* function, linkage to loci of great evolutionary significance, and conditions favorable for rapid spreading of new *H-2* mutations (linkage with the *t* complex, and peculiar population structure).

Chapter Thirteen

The *H-2* Complex and Somatic Cell Genetics

For more than half a century, mammalian genetics has been concerned almost exclusively with the mechanisms by which genetic information is transmitted through *germ cells*; an inquiry into the principles governing the expression of genetic information in *somatic cells* has only recently begun. The *genetics of somatic cells* is aimed at understanding such phenomena as differentiation, antibody formation, neoplasia, and cell-virus interaction. The existence of somatic cell genetics is dependent upon the ability to detect variant forms (*variants*) of somatic cells, that is, rare deviations from the norm, which can then be used as markers in genetic analysis. The markers must fulfill two major criteria: they must be expressed in an easily detectable form in the somatic cells, and they must provide ways of selecting a new variant from a population of normal cells. The antigens controlled by the *H-2* complex meet both these criteria: they can be detected in all, or almost all normal and neoplastic tissues using a variety of relatively simple serological tests, and they can be subjected to a strong selection pressure in the form of an immune reaction. It is therefore not surprising that H-2 antigens have frequently been used in somatic cell genetics and have contributed considerably to the development of this field. Only one example of this contribution—the variant formation (both specific and nonspecific) in tumor cells—will be considered here.

I. Specific *H-2* Variants

A. Principle of *H-2* Variant Selection

The system used in the detection of H-2 antigenic variant cells is ingeniously simple (Lederberg 1956; cf. Fig. 13–1). A tumor induced in a $(P_1 \times P_2)F_1$ hybrid (where P_1 and P_2 are two congenic lines differing at the *H-2* complex) should express H-2 antigens of both parents, because the antigens are inherited codominantly. Such a tumor should not encounter any resistance when propagated in syngeneic F_1 hybrids; when transplanted to the P_1 parental strain, the tumor should elicit an allograft reaction directed against H-2 antigens inherited from the P_2 strain, and should be rejected. Similarly, the tumor should also be rejected when transplanted to the P_2 strain, because of the reaction against

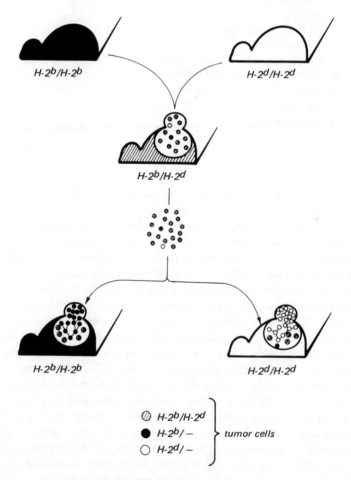

Fig. 13-1. Selection of parental tumor variants from an *H-2* heterozygous tumor.

P_1-derived H-2 antigens. However, if genetic variation occurs in somatic cells of the F_1 tumor, variant cells that have lost the H-2 antigens of one parent and retained those of the other parent might arise. Such alloantigenic variant cells should still be able to grow in the F_1 mice, but, in addition, they would also grow in one parental strain (the strain whose H-2 antigens they retained). The allograft reaction would therefore provide a selection pressure that would eliminate all nonvariant cells, retaining only the variants.

The sensitivity of the allograft selection system was demonstrated by G. Klein and E. Klein (1956), who mixed $(A \times A.SW)F_1$ and A tumor cells ($H-2^a/$ $H-2^s$ and $H-2^a/H-2^a$, respectively) in different proportions, inoculated the mixture into A strain recipients, and inspected the inoculated animals for tumor growth. The recipients should have reacted against the $H-2^s$ component of the $H-2^a/H-2^s$ tumor and all the F_1 cells in the mixture should have been destroyed. The homozygous $H-2^a/H-2^a$ cells, on the other hand, were compatible with the recipient and should therefore have developed into tumors that would eventually kill the recipient. The experiments proved that even in cases where compatible cells composed only a small fraction of the mixture (less than 4×10^{-7} compatible cells admixed with more than 5×10^7 incompatible cells), they were able to develop into progressively growing tumors. The authors therefore concluded that the allograft reaction is very sensitive and apparently has the capacity to select out, under the right conditions, a single variant cell from a large population of nonvariant cells.

Experiments performed in a number of laboratories demonstrated that tumors induced in F_1 hybrids between two CR lines display one of three patterns of behavior (specific, nonspecific, and semispecific) when transplanted into foreign hosts. The *specific tumors* are restricted in their growth to the F_1 genotype of origin; they do not take in the two parental strains or, for that matter, in any other foreign genotypes. The *nonspecific tumors* are on just the opposite end of the specificity scale; they grow progressively not only in both parental strains but also in many completely unrelated allogeneic strains. The *semispecific tumors* grow progressively in the syngeneic F_1 hybrids and throw off *variants* in the parental strains; they do not grow in any other foreign genotypes.

An example of a semispecific tumor is shown in Fig. 13–2. The tumor was induced in a $(B10 \times B10.D2)F_1$ hybrid by subcutaneous injection of 3-methylcholanthrene (J. Klein 1965b, 1966b). In each passage the tumor (BD24) was inoculated into the syngeneic F_1 hybrids and both parental strains; it grew in 100 per cent of the F_1 hybrids (117 mice), in approximately 4 percent of the B10 animals (3 mice out of 77 inoculated) and in 12 percent of the B10.D2 mice (10 out of 80 inoculated). Of the three tumors that took in the B10 strain, one turned out to be a *false positive*, that is, it died out in the subsequent passage, and the remaining two were established as separate sublines. Only one of the two sublines (BD24D) is shown in Fig. 13–2; it grew in 100 percent of the B10 mice (68 animals). Thus, a variant of the original F_1 hybrid tumor was established with host range specifically broadened from the F_1 hybrid to one of the two parental strains (*parental tumor variant*). The transplantation behavior of the subline seemed to indicate that the H-2 antigens of the B10.D2 parent were either lost or reduced in quantity. If reduction of H-2 antigens were responsible for the broadening of the host range, the subline should have failed to grow in B10 mice preimmunized against B10.D2 antigens, because preimmunization is usually an efficient method of eliciting rejection of weakly antigenic tumors. However, as shown in Fig. 13-2, the subline grew in preimmunized B10 recipients as well as in unimmunized mice.

B. Properties of Specific Tumor Variants

1. The Predilection Phenomenon

The tumor shown in Fig. 13-2 threw off variants in both parental strains, but the frequency of variants in one strain (B10.D2) was slightly higher than in the other (B10). Tumors with a very strong predilection toward one parental strain were described by G. Klein and E. Klein (1958), who observed that sarcomas induced in (A♂ × A.SW♀)F$_1$ hybrids gave rise to variants in the

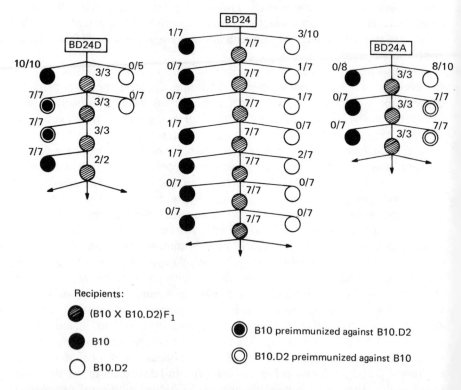

Recipients:

- (B10 × B10.D2)F$_1$
- B10
- B10.D2
- B10 preimmunized against B10.D2
- B10.D2 preimmunized against B10

Fig. 13-2. Transplantation history of tumor BD24 derived from a (B10 × B10.D2)F$_1$ hybrid. Fractions indicate number of animals that died from the tumor/number of animals inoculated with the tumor. Explanation in text.

maternal A.SW strain, but never in the paternal A strain. Variants compatible with the A strain were not obtained even after temporary growth of the F_1 tumor was achieved through passive enhancement [injection of A anti-$(A \times A.SW)F_1$ serum into the A recipients]; the enhanced tumors regressed as soon as they were transferred to untreated A mice (Bayreuther and E. Klein 1958). In the $(A\male \times A.CA\female)F_1$ hybrids, variants appeared in both parental strains but were more frequent in the maternal A.CA strain. Preference for the maternal strain was also indicated by tumors of $(A\male \times A.BY\female)F_1$ and $(A.SW\male \times A.CA\female)F_1$ hybrids; altogether, 23 tumors of five different F_1 hybrids displayed a predilection toward the maternal strain. It was therefore postulated that the unidirectionality of variant formation was caused by an undetermined maternal effect. However, the maternal effect hypothesis had to be abandoned when it was demonstrated that A.SW remained the favored strain of variant formation even in the reciprocal $(A\female \times A.SW\male)F_1$ hybrids (G. Klein and E. Klein 1959; E. Klein *et al.* 1960).

Three alternative explanations of the predilection phenomenon were then suggested (G. Klein and E. Klein 1958). First, some cytogenetic peculiarity that makes one change more likely to occur than the other is involved. Second, the lines are not fully congenic and differ from the background strain (A) in more than one *H* locus; the additional differences produce a barrier between A and $(A \times A.SW)F_1$ stronger than that between A.SW and $(A \times A.SW)F_1$. Third, the different H-2 antigens themselves present barriers of different strength. The explanation based on residual heterozygosity of the congenic lines seems the most likely, since it was demonstrated that the A strain CR lines used by the Kleins' group were not fully congenic or even homozygous (Linder and Klein 1960). In similar experiments performed using lines that are known to be truly congenic (CR lines on B10 background), the predilection phenomenon was either completely absent (Dhaliwal 1964a) or expressed only in much milder form (J. Klein 1965b, 1966b). In the latter case, the predilection varied from tumor to tumor, one tumor having preference for one parental strain and another tumor having preference for the second.

2. The Effect of Genetic Background and H-2 Zygosity

Since the phenomenon of variant formation has been observed in lines with completely different backgrounds (strains A and B10), it is obviously not restricted to one particular genotype. It does not seem to be limited even to congenic lines, as was demonstrated by K. Hellström (1960), who was able to extract variants compatible with either DBA/2 or C3H strains from $(DBA/2 \times C3H)F_1$ lymphomas. Parental variants from tumors induced in $(B10 \times DBA/2)F_1$ hybrids were obtained by E. Klein *et al.* (1960).

However, all attempts to isolate variants from tumors induced in homozygous inbred strains have invariably failed. Thus, E. Klein *et al.* (1957) were unable to force an A strain tumor to grow in A.SW recipients. G. Klein and E. Klein (1959) tested 16 homozygous tumors produced in strains A, A.SW, or

A.CA for takes in their congenic partners; of the few takes obtained, all proved to be either false positives or caused by nonspecific forms. Similarly, K. Hellström (1960), working with C3H or DBA/2 lymphomas, and Dhaliwal (1964a), working with B10 sarcomas, were unable to obtain variants specifically compatible with any particular foreign genotype. Apparently, specific variants can be obtained from *H-2* heterozygous, but not from *H-2* homozygous tumors.

3. Tissue of Origin

The tissue of origin of the tumor does not seem to play any significant role in variant formation. Specific variants were obtained from methylcholanthrene-induced sarcomas and carcinomas (E. Klein *et al.* 1957; Dhaliwal 1961, 1964a; J. Klein 1965a, b), spontaneous mammary carcinomas (Mitchison 1956; E. Klein *et al.* 1960; E. Klein 1961), spontaneous lymphomas (K. Hellström 1960), radiation-induced lymphomas (Dhaliwal 1964a; Boyse *et al.* 1970), estrogen-induced lymphomas (Bjaring and G. Klein 1968), and estrogen-induced testicular tumors (G. Klein and Hellström 1962). An attempt was also made by Dhaliwal (1964b) to isolate variants from normal embryonic cells by subcutaneously inoculating tissue from 10 to 13-day-old embryos into syngeneic adult recipients. The tissue was vascularized, grew actively for 2 or 3 weeks, and differentiated into cartilage and muscles, surviving for at least 2 months. When a mixture of compatible and incompatible embryonic cells was inoculated into the adult recipients, growth was observed with only 10^4 or more compatible cells present in the mixture. With this great a number of compatible cells required for growth, the chances of detecting a variant cell or cell clone from a heterozygous embryo are negligible. Accordingly, no variants were found when $(B10 \times B10.D2)F_1$ embryonic tissue was inoculated in either of the parental strains; the tissue regressed completely within 10 days.

4. Stability

The variants are usually very stable, although the tumor may undergo a period of temporary instability during the first few passages in the new host. E. Klein and E. Möller (1963) described a case in which a variant that seemed to be specific for the A.CA strain was selected from an $(A \times A.CA)F_1$ tumor; after four passages of the variant through the A.CA host and five subsequent passages through the F_1 host, the same tumor became specifically compatible with the opposite parental strain (strain A). The authors explained these results by postulating that the first four passages in A.CA mice did not provide a sufficiently strong selection pressure to eliminate all *H-2* heterozygous cells from the population; some F_1 cells apparently survived in the allogeneic A.CA hosts, multiplied in the syngeneic F_1 host, and became a source for selection of a new variant, this time compatible with strain A. However, such behavior of the variants is only an exception; the majority of the variants are "true-breeding"; once established in one of the two parental strains, they are strictly specific for that strain.

A variant specifically compatible with parental strain P_1 cannot be altered to form a variant specifically compatible with parental strain P_2, even after prolonged passage in newborn and/or irradiated P_2 mice (K. Hellström 1960; E. Klein *et al.* 1960; Bjaring and G. Klein 1968). If any change results from the switching attempts, it is toward general nonspecificity.

Variants returned from their selective hosts to the original F_1 hybrid and carried in the nonselective F_1 environment for 10–15 serial passages, do not lose their specificity; that is, they remain fully compatible with one parental strain and will not grow in any other foreign genotypes (G. Klein and E. Klein 1959; E. Klein *et al.* 1960; Dhaliwal 1964a). In a sense, the variants are more specific than the original F_1 tumor because, in contrast to the tumor, they lack the ability to broaden their host range. In this respect, their behavior resembles that of a homozygous tumor.

5. Evidence for Antigen Loss

The transplantation behavior of the specific variants suggests that the variants lost the H-2 antigens of the opposite parent. This suggestion is supported by findings obtained using a variety of immunological methods: immunization of P_2 mice with P_1 variants and testing for induction of hemagglutinins and cytotoxins (E. Klein *et al.* 1957; Bayreuther and E. Klein 1958; E. Klein 1959; J. Klein 1965b); absorption of H-2 antibodies with tumor cells (E. Klein *et al.* 1957; J. Klein 1965b); direct cytotoxic test with variant lymphomas (K. Hellström 1960); indirect immunofluorescence test (Bjaring and G. Klein 1968; Ozer *et al.* 1966), and induction of second-set allograft reaction to skin transplants with tumor cells (J. Klein 1965b). The results of these tests point to the same conclusion: while the original F_1 tumor carries H-2 antigens of both parents, in the variant tumor only H-2 antigens of the compatible parent can be detected.

6. D-K Asymmetry

In a situation in which an F_1 tumor is transplanted to the P_1 strain, the selection pressure is directed against the entire *H-2* complex of the P_2 strain. However, experimental systems can be designed in which the selection pressure is directed against only a portion of the *H-2* complex. This can be achieved, for instance, by transplanting the F_1 tumor to another F_1 hybrid that shares some H-2 antigens with the tumor donor and differs in others. Experiments of this type were described by Bayreuther and E. Klein (1958), G. Klein and E. Klein (1959), E. Klein (1961), and K. Hellström (1961), who transplanted $(A \times A.SW)F_1$ tumors into $(DBA/2 \times A.SW)F_1$ and $(C3H \times A.SW)F_1$ recipients and obtained variants specifically compatible with one or the other selective host (Fig. 13-3). Because the $H-2^a$ haplotype of strain A is probably the result of crossing-over between haplotypes $H-2^d$ (present in DBA/2) and $H-2^k$ (present in C3H), strains DBA/2 and C3H differ from strain A in only one of the two peripheral *H-2* loci: DBA/2 shares with A the same allele at the *H-2D* locus, and C3H shares with A the same allele at the *H-2K* locus. Hence, in the

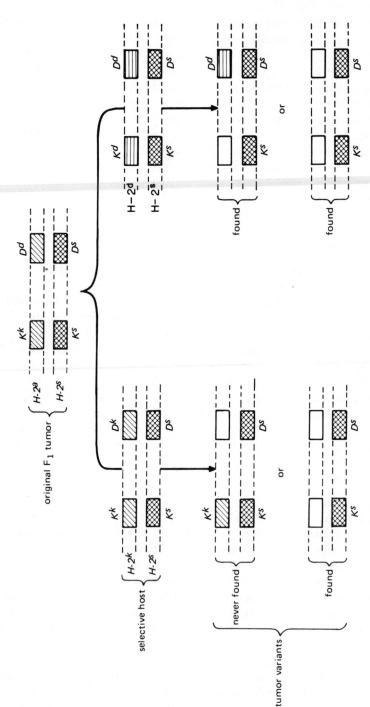

Fig. 13-3. Asymmetry observed by G. Klein's group in selection of variants from $H\text{-}2^k/H\text{-}2^s$ heterozygous tumors.

(DBA/2 × A.SW)F$_1$ hybrid challenged with an (A × A.SW)F$_1$ tumor, the selection pressure is directed against the *H-2^k* allele, and a variant that has lost this allele and retained the *H-2D^d* allele of the *H-2^a* haplotype is compatible with the new host. However, a variant that has lost not only the *H-2K^k* but also the *H-2D^d* allele, against which there is no selection pressure, will also be compatible with the (DBA/2 × C3H)F$_1$ host. Similarly, in the (C3H × A.SW)F$_1$ hybrid, a variant that has lost either *H-2D^d* alone or *H-2D^d* together with *H-2K^k* will be compatible with this selective host. The loss (or inactivation) of *H-2D^d* or *H-2K^k* is signaled by the absence of the private (or semiprivate) antigens determined by these two alleles, H-2.4 and H-2.11, respectively.

In spite of the fact that A and DBA/2 or C3H differ in many non-*H-2* loci, variant sublines compatible with (DBA × A.SW)F$_1$ or (C3H × A.SW)F$_1$ can be obtained from the (A × A.SW)F$_1$ tumor. As expected, the variants compatible with the (DBA/2 × A.SW)F$_1$ hybrid are either +4, −11, or −4, −11. Surprisingly, however, the variants compatible with the (C3H × A.SW)F$_1$ hybrid are always −4, −11; the second class of the expected variants, −4, +11, is never found. Similar results are also obtained with (A × A.CA)F$_1$ and (A × A.BY)F$_1$ hybrid tumors. Here again, only −4, −11 variants are recovered in the (C3H × A.CA)F$_1$ and (C3H × A.BY)F$_1$ selective hosts, and the class of −4, +11 variants is completely missing.

The situation changes, however, when the *H-2K^k* and *H-2D^d* alleles occur in *trans*-position (on different *H-2* chromosomes) rather than in *cis*-position (on the same *H-2* chromosome, as in *H-2^a* of strain A). The *trans*-position can be obtained, for instance, by using (DBA/2 × C3H)F$_1$ hybrids, which are *H-2^d/H-2^k* (or *H-2K^{d}H-2D^d/H-2K^{k}H-2D^k*) heterozygotes. E. Klein and G. Klein (1964) demonstrated that a (DBA/2 × C3H)F$_1$ tumor transplanted onto a C3H (*H-2^k/H-2^k*) host throws off variant sublines selectively compatible with strain C3H. Quantitative absorption with the variant tumor cells indicates that the cells have lost the H-2.4 antigen controlled by the *H-2D^d* allele and retained the H-2.11 antigen controlled by the *H-2K^k* allele. Thus, with the *H-2D^d* and *H-2K^k* alleles in *trans*-position, the −4, +11 variants can be obtained.

7. Behavior of Individual H-2 Antigens

Ozer *et al.* (1966) carried the analysis of tumor sublines derived from (A × A.SW)F$_1$ lymphomas somewhat further, and attempted to discover what happened to the other H-2 antigens in variants that lost H-2.4 or H-2.11, or both. They found that H-2 antigens determined by the *H-2^s* haplotype alone (antigens 7 and 19), or by both the *H-2^s* and *H-2^a* haplotypes (antigens 3 and 5) were retained, as expected, in all variants selected in *H-2^d/H-2^s*, *H-2^k/H-2^s*, or *H-2^s/H-2^s* hosts. Unexpected results were obtained in tests involving antigen H-2.8, which, like antigens H-2.4 and 11, is controlled by the *H-2^a* chromosome alone. The factor controlling antigen H-2.8 is located at the *K* end of the *H-2* map and, according to the two-locus hypothesis, the antigen should be controlled by the *H-2K^k* allele, the same allele that controls antigen H-2.11. One would, therefore, expect that antigen H-2.8 would be absent in all variants having lost antigen H-2.11. However, this is not the case. Of the five +4, −11 variants tested by Ozer and his co-workers, only one was also −8. The authors interpreted this result as indicating that genetic factors for antigens H-2.4, 8, and 11 are separate entities and that, in the genetic map, the factor for antigen H-2.8 is positioned between factors for antigen H-2.4 and H-2.11. This is not necessarily the only possible interpretation. The "segregation" of H-2.8 in the variants can also be explained as being the result of the complexity of the antisera used for detection of this antigen. Antigen H-2.8 is poorly defined, it is broadly cross-reactive, and all anti-H-2.8 sera always contain more than one antibody. The anti-H-2.8 sera used by Ozer and his co-workers could have contained several additional antibodies, some of them reacting with the *H-2D* product of the *H-2ᵃ* haplotype. Another possibility is that antigen H-2.8 is controlled—like many other public H-2 antigens—by both the *H-2K* and *H-2D* loci. Also, when working with antibodies against public *H-2* antigens, it is difficult to distinguish between the loss of an antigen and the mere decrease in antigen concentration below the detectable level.

This latter difficulty is best illustrated by the work of Bjaring and G. Klein (1968). These authors induced a lymphoma in $(A \times A.CA)F_1$ hybrids and selected a variant from this tumor in a $(DBA/2 \times A.CA)F_1$ hybrid. The variant, when tested by direct cytotoxic and indirect fluorescence tests, seemed to be of the following phenotype: −3, +4, −5, −11, +9. Thus, in addition to antigen H-2.11, it seemed to have also lost public antigens H-2.3 and 5, controlled by the *H-2ᵃ* haplotype. However, when the variant subline was subjected to further selection, first in $(C3H \times A.CA)F_1$ hybrids and then in strain A, it remained H-2.11 negative, it lost antigen H-2.9 (controlled by the *H-2ᶠ* haplotype), but *it regained antigens H-2.3 and 5.*

In the *H-2ᵃ* haplotype, antigen H-2.3 seems to be present on products of both the *H-2Kᵏ* and *H-2Dᵈ* alleles; it is therefore possible that with the disappearance of the *H-2Kᵏ* product from variants isolated in $(DBA/2 \times A.CA)F_1$ hybrids, the concentration of the H-2.3 antigen on the cell surface dropped below the level detectable by the methods employed. Later, compensation for the missing product could have taken place and the vacant space could have been taken over by the product of the *H-2Dᵈ* allele. Because the *H-2Dᵈ* allele also controls antigen H-2.3, the compensation process again increased the quantity of this antigen to a detectable level.

Partial loss of H-2 antigens in somatic cell variants was also described by Dhaliwal (1966) and J. Klein (1966b). Dhaliwal isolated B10 (*H-2ᵇ*)- and B10.D2 (*H-2ᵈ*)-compatible variants from a $(B10 \times B10.D2)F_1$ lymphoma and tested them, by absorption of hemagglutinins, for the presence or absence of several antigens determined by the two parental *H-2* haplotypes. He found that the B10 variants lost H-2 antigens 3, 4, 8, and 13, all determined by the *H-2ᵈ* haplotype, and retained H-2 antigens 2, 5, and 33, determined by the *H-2ᵇ* haplotype. These results were fully consistent with the transplantation behavior of the variants. Somewhat unexpected was the finding that the B10 variants seemed to lack antigen H-2.6, which is controlled by both parental *H-2* haplotypes (*H-2^b* and *H-2^d*). Dhaliwal explained the absence of H-2.6 as being the result of mutation. Another possibility is that the disappearance was actually only a decrease in antigen concentration on the cell surface. This possibility is supported by the fact that the antisera used by Dhaliwal for detection of antigen H-2.6 was relatively weak and of a low titer.

The B10.D2 variant in Dhaliwal's experiment lost antigens H-2.2 of the *H-2^b* complex and H-2.3 and 8 of the *H-2^d* complex; it retained antigens H-2.5 and 33 of the *H-2^b* complex and H-2.4 and 13 of the *H-2^d* complex. It seemed, therefore, that this variant lost the *H-2D^b* allele and retained the *H-2K^b* allele of the *H-2^b* haplotype, and at the same time lost the *H-2K^d* allele and retained the *H-2D^d* allele of the *H-2^d* haplotype. If this were indeed the case, the attribution of the event to a reciprocal genetic exchange (crossing-over) between the two parental *H-2* haplotypes is very tempting. However, how the variant managed to grow progressively in B10.D2 mice (and even in B10.D2 mice preimmunized against B10 tissue) even with part of the *H-2^b* complex expressed remains a mystery.

J. Klein (1966b) obtained variants by transplanting a (B10 × B10.D2)F$_1$ sarcoma to (B10 × CBA)F$_1$ hybrids. The selection pressure in this case was directed against H-2 antigens 4, 13, and 31, which are determined by the *H-2^d* haplotype, but not against antigens H-2.3 and 8, shared by the *H-2^d* haplotype of the tumor and the *H-2^k* haplotype of the selective host. Yet, the latter two antigens were absent in the (B10 × CBA)F$_1$-compatible variants, as indicated by the ability of these variants to grow progressively in the B10 host, and also by quantitative absorption tests. The author interpreted the results as indicating that selection against the extreme ends of the *H-2* complex also leads to a loss of the middle portion of the complex, by which antigens H-2.3 and 8 were thought to be controlled. However, the finding is also fully consistent with the two-locus hypothesis of the *H-2* complex, which requires a concurrent loss of all public H-2 antigens controlled by a given allele if the private antigens are lost.

8. Mechanism of Variant Formation

The mechanism of variant formation remains unknown. Although in some cases variants can be obtained directly from a preimmunized parental strain (*one-step variants*), multiple-step variant formation seems to be more frequent (G. Klein and E. Klein 1959). The *multiple-step variants* first grow in all un-immunized mice of one parental strain but do not grow in preimmmunized mice. Only after several passages in the unimmunized hosts do the variants become compatible with preimmunized hosts as well. Variants that have accomplished the first step (characterized by growth in untreated selective hosts and lack of growth in preimmunized hosts) remain in this stage if the selection pressure is removed by returning the variants to the original F$_1$ environment (G. Klein and E. Klein 1959; E. Klein *et al.* 1960). The requirement for the variants to progress beyond the first step could have been due, however, to non-*H-2* loci segregating in the CR lines. According to this explanation, the first step in variant formation would be overcoming the residual non-*H-2* barrier. This is probably true in the case of the A strain congenic lines, but the variants arising in the *truly* congenic B10 lines should be all one-step, because there are no non-*H-2* barriers to be overcome.

Variants arising from the same tumor could represent repeated selection from a single clone preexisting in the F_1 tumor, or could appear repeatedly in a series of independent events. Certain evidence seems to be pointing to the latter possibility. First, cytological examination of different variant sublines derived from the same tumor reveals a remarkable individuality of their karyotypes (Bayreuther and E. Klein 1958); if all the sublines were derived from the same clone, one would expect their karyotypes to be similar. Second, the frequency of variants formed from an $(A \times A.SW)F_1$ tumor in the unimmunized A.SW host is 24 percent, whereas that in the host preimmunized against A tissue is only 2 percent (Bayreuther and E. Klein 1958); the frequency should be the same in unimmunized and immunized hosts if the variants had preexisted in the form of a small clone. Third, according to Bayreuther and E. Klein (1958) and K. Hellström (1960), there is no correlation between the number of the tumor cells and the frequency of variant formation; that is, an inoculum with fewer cells throws off the same percentage of variants as an inoculum with many cells. If variants preexist as a minority in the population, they should have a greater chance of being eliminated by the use of an inoculum with fewer cells. [This last piece of evidence is not so simple as it seems: even with variants arising independently, one would expect that some correlation with sample size would emerge; such correlation has indeed been found by Dhaliwal (1964a).] Fourth, attempts to select a minor preexisting clone of variant cells by treatment of the F_1 tumor *in vitro* with antibodies against H-2 antigens of one parent, in the presence of complement, have failed (E. Klein *et al.* 1960; K. Hellström 1960). Although the treatment kills 50–90 percent of the tumor cells, it does not significantly increase the frequency of parental variants.

Consistent with the idea of *de novo* formation of variants are observations indicating that the frequency of parental variants can be increased by prolonging the period of the tumor's "background growth," during which the allograft reaction is either completely absent or greatly reduced in intensity. Background growth can be achieved by passaging the F_1 tumor via newborn mice of the P_1 or P_2 strain (Mitchison 1956; K. Hellström 1960).

Differences that occur in the period of background growth and are caused by an unequal strength of H-2 antigens can also explain at least some cases of the variants' predilection toward one parental strain. E. Klein and E. Möller (1963) obtained a methylcholanthrene-induced $(A \times A.CA)F_1$ sarcoma that threw off twice as many variants in A.CA ($H-2^f$) as in A ($H-2^a$) parental strains. Quantitative absorption analysis of the original F_1 tumor revealed that the tumor cells had a significantly higher concentration of $H-2^f$ than $H-2^a$ antigens. Yet, after immunization with the F_1 tumor, anti-$H-2^a$ antibodies appeared earlier and in higher titers than anti-$H-2^f$ antibodies. The authors explained these seemingly paradoxical findings by postulating enhancement of tumor growth across the weaker barrier. Because the F_1 tumor had a low concentration of H-2^a antigens, it was relatively resistant to the allograft reaction when transplanted into A.CA mice. Prolonged presence of the tumor cells in the A.CA hosts elicited an early humoral response to the H-2^a antigens, and the anti-H-2^a antibodies, in turn, induced a state of immunological enhancement of the tumor cells. The enhancement further prolonged the period of the F_1 tumor's proliferation in the allogeneic host and thus provided more time for the variants to arise and become established. J. Klein (1965b) observed a similar situation with a $(B10 \times B10.D2)F_1$ sarcoma, which threw off variants more frequently in the B10.D2 (H-2^d) than in the B10 (H-2^b) strain. Immunization with the F_1 tumor elicited anti-H-2^d hemagglutinins more rapidly and in higher titers than anti-H-2^b hemagglutinins.

a. **Immunological Enhancement.** The above observations cause one to consider whether immunological enhancement could be the actual mechanism of variant formation. Immunological enhancement resembles the phenomenon of variant formation in that it too leads to broadening of a tumor's host range. However, there are important differences between the two phenomena. First, when an enhanced tumor progressively growing in a foreign host is transplanted to a preimmunized host, it is rejected (Kaliss 1958); specific tumor variants, on the other hand, grow even in preimmunized hosts. Second, the change in the host range of an enhanced tumor is temporary, the property being lost after few passages in untreated allogeneic recipients (Kaliss 1958); antigenic variants, on the other hand, are permanently changed and can be passaged in the new host for an apparently indefinite period of time. Third, immunological enhancement can be achieved with H-2 homozygous tumors, whereas variants are never obtained from such tumors. Direct evidence against enhancement as a mechanism of variant formation was obtained by E. Klein and her co-workers (1960), who pretreated P_1 recipients with either P_1 anti-P_2 antiserum or with an extract obtained from a $(P_1 \times P_2)F_1$ tumor, and then inoculated the pretreated mice with the F_1 tumor. They observed that, although the frequency of takes of the tumor in the pretreated P_1 mice increased significantly, the increase was caused by a larger number of false positive takes; the frequency of specific variants remained unchanged. Thus, intentional induction of enhancement did not seem to facilitate variant formation. It is therefore unlikely that immunological enhancement is actually responsible for broadening of the variants' host range; its role in variant formation is probably only secondary in that it prolongs the background growth of the F_1 tumor in the parental strains.

b. **Antigen suppression.** Variant formation is always associated with the disappearance of H-2 antigens that are selected against. One possible explanation for the disappearance is that the genes for the missing antigens are still present in the variant cells and that the antigens are merely suppressed phenotypically. Such *antigen suppression* is known, for example, in the case of immunoglobulin allotypes. The phenomenon was discovered in rabbits by Dray (1962) and later shown to be operating also in mice (Herzenberg *et al.* 1967). Dray immunized female rabbits homozygous for one allotype against the allotype of the male with whom the immune female was mated. The production of the paternal allotype in the offspring of this mating was greatly suppressed, and the suppression lasted for months or even years. However, the gene for the paternal allotype was not lost, as indicated by the fact that suppressed animals were eventually able to produce the missing immunoglobulins. Although allotype suppression resembles variant formation in some characteristics, the resemblance between the two phenomena is only superficial, the basic differences between them being that allotype suppression is mediated by humoral antibodies, while variant formation is not (K. Hellström 1960; E. Klein *et al.* 1960), and that the disappearance of the suppressed allotype is only temporary, while the disappearance of H-2 antigens in tumor variants is permanent.

The permanence of the change in tumor variants and the stability and irreversibility of the variants strongly suggest that a genetic mechanism is involved. Among the mechanisms worth considering are point mutation, transfer of genetic material between somatic cells, genetic inactivation, deletion, and mitotic crossing-over.

c. **Point mutation.** Point mutation is a rather unlikely mechanism of variant formation, the main argument against it being that the change producing variants always involves loss, never gain, of H-2 antigens. The absence of gain-type variants was demonstrated by E. Klein and her co-workers (1960), who transplanted an $(A \times A.SW)F_1$ tumor in $(A \times A.BY)F_1$ recipients and obtained variants compatible with the new host. Theoretically, the variants could have been of two types: one in which the $H-2^s$ complex of the A.SW strain was lost (loss-type change), and another in which the $H-2^s$ complex was changed into a new $H-2$ haplotype, for example, $H-2^b$ carried by strain A.BY (gain-type change). Both types should have been compatible with the $(A \times A.BY)F_1$ hybrid, but only the former (loss type) was also compatible with strain A $(H-2^a)$. If both types of variants actually had arisen, some of the variants should have been rejected when transferred to A strain mice. However, this did not happen; all variants compatible with the $(A \times A.BY)F_1$ host were also compatible with A hosts. The weakness of this experiment was the inherent expectation that all of the possibly hundreds of genes in the entire $H-2$ complex could mutate in the same direction.

Dhaliwal (1964b) attempted to detect $H-2$ mutations in tumor cells by using immunological enhancement. He found that a $(B10 \times B10.M)F_1$ tumor could be enhanced to grow progressively in DBA/1 recipients by pretreating the recipients with antisera against both parental $H-2$ haplotypes; the use of an antiserum against only one parental haplotype was ineffective in enhancing the hybrid tumor, but did enhance the homozygous parental tumor. Therefore, if DBA/1 recipients were treated with anti-B10 $(H-2^b)$ serum and then challenged with a $(B10 \times B10.M)F_1$ tumor, for example, the tumor would be enhanced only if the $H-2^f$ haplotype of the B10.M strain mutated to the $H-2^b$ haplotype of strain B10. However, no takes of the hybrid tumor in recipients conditioned with one antiserum were observed.

Attempts to increase the frequency of variant formation by treatment of the F_1 tumor cells with various mutagens provided inconsistent results. An increase was reported after X-irradiation by E. Klein *et al.* (1957) and after X-irradiation and treatment with triethylenemelamine by Dhaliwal (1961). No effect was reported after X-irradiation and treatment with methylcholanthrene by E. Klein *et al.* (1960), or after irradiation and treatment with nitrogen mustard by J. Klein (1965b, 1966b). Because of the variability in variant frequency from one transplant generation to another, a meaningful test of a small mutagenic effect would have to be performed on an extremely large number of animals, which was not the case in any of the experiments cited above.

d. Transfer of genetic material. Transfer of genetic material between the host and the tumor cells can theoretically occur in the form of transduction (i.e., transfer of genetic information from one cell to another by a virus) or fusion of somatic cells. Experimental evidence against involvement of such mechanisms in variant formation was obtained by E. Klein *et al.* (1960) and by K. Hellström (1960). E. Klein and her co-workers (1960) mixed $(A \times A.SW)F_1$ and $(A.BY \times A.CA)F_1$ tumor cells in equal proportions and inoculated the mixtures into newborn DBA/2 or C3H mice, removed the developing tumors, and transplanted them into $(A \times A.BY)F_1$, $(A \times A.CA)F_1$, $(A.SW \times A.BY)F_1$, and $(A.SW \times A.CA)F_1$ adult mice. If an exchange of genetic material had occurred between the tumor cells in the mixture, variants specifically compatible with some of the four test hybrids should have been obtained; however, no such variants were observed.

e. Genetic inactivation. Renwick and Pontecorvo (quoted by E. Klein and G. Klein 1964) suggested that the *H-2* complex may behave as an operon[1] subject to repression and derepression as is an operon in viruses or bacteria. However, such an explanation is unlikely. First of all, operons are still restricted to the realm of microbial genetics, and their existence in higher organisms is purely hypothetical; second, available experimental data argue strongly against operon-type inactivation. Boyse *et al.* (1970) obtained a $(C57BL/6 \times A)F_1$ leukemia that was genotypically $H-2^bTla.2, 4/H-2^aTla.2, 3$ and by passaging the tumor in $(C57BL/6 \times A.SW)F_1$ mice they selected a specific variant that behaved as if it had lost the $H-2^a$ antigens. The loss was confirmed by quantitative absorption of cytotoxic antibodies. The absorption tests also demonstrated an absence of antigen Tla.3 and suggested that, along with the $H-2^a$ complex, the adjacent *Tla* locus was also lost in the process of variant formation, and that this happened in the absence of immunoselection against the Tla.3 antigen. The loss was permanent and occurred in hosts that were not producing Tla antibodies, thus indicating that it was not caused by antigenic modulation. Because *H-2* and *Tla* loci can be repressed and derepressed under very different physio-

---

[1] An *operon* is a series of adjacent genes that behave as a unit of genetic transcription (code for single messenger RNA molecules) and of genetic regulation.

logical conditions, it is highly improbable that they all belong to the same operon; yet in the process of variant formation the whole chromosomal segment, including the *Tla* locus, is affected as a unit.

f. Deletion.   One of the more plausible hypotheses of variant formation is genetic deletion, involving either the whole chromosome 17 or just the *H-2* complex. Cytological analysis of the variant tumors does not provide evidence either in favor of or against the deletion hypothesis. Most of the variants studied by Bayreuther and E. Klein (1958) were characterized by new chromosome modal numbers as well as new chromosomal markers, indicating that "structural remodeling has taken place during the origin and/or the subsequent development of the variant karyotypes." Dhaliwal (1961, 1964a) also found the karyotypes of the variants to be different from the karyotypes of the original F_1 tumors; while the original sarcomas or lymphomas had chromosome modal numbers almost exactly diploid, the variants showed a tendency toward hyperdiploidy and triploidy. In contrast to these findings, K. Hellström (1960), working with lymphomas, found no substantial chromosomal difference between the original F_1 tumors and the variants; all the lymphomas had a predominant cell type containing 41 chromosomes and no typical marker. In none of these studies was it possible to identify the chromosome carrying the *H-2* complex. A first step toward such identification was made by Bjaring *et al.* (1970), who used the *T190* translocation, consisting of one extralong and one extrashort chromosome. However, in (A.CA × T190)F_1 lymphomas, the two *T190* markers always segregated together and thus precluded the possibility of determining whether the *H-2* complex was located on the short or on the long chromosome. Variants from the (A.CA × T190)F_1 tumors have not yet been reported.

g. Mitotic crossing-over.   The asymmetrical behavior of H-2 antigens 4 and 11, described earlier in this chapter, led E. Klein (1961) and K. Hellström (1961) to propose a hypothesis of variant formation based on the assumption of mitotic crossing-over. According to this hypothesis, crossing-over, which is normally restricted to germ cells undergoing meiosis, can occasionally occur in somatic cells during mitosis. As shown in Fig. 13–4, the consequences of such *mitotic crossing-over* depend on the position of the genetic exchange and on the distribution of the centromeres during cell division. Mitotic crossing-over has been demonstrated in *Drosophila* and in certain fungi, but its occurrence in mammalian cells is questionable. To explain why the variants can lose antigen 11 alone or together with antigen 4, but cannot lose antigen 4 alone without losing antigen 11, one has to postulate that the genetic determinant for antigen 4 is closer to the centromere than the determinant for antigen 11 (Fig. 13–4). On this basis, it was believed for some time that the order of markers in chromosome 17 was *centromere* $\cdots$ *H-2D*(4) $\cdots$ *H-2K*(11). However, it was later convincingly demonstrated that the actual order is *centromere* $\cdots$ *H-2K*(11) $\cdots$ *H-2D*(4) (see Chapter Eleven), dealing the mitotic crossing-over hypothesis a serious blow. The hypothesis can be salvaged by making additional assumptions (J. Klein 1972b), such as the existence of a histocompatibility locus outside the *H-2* complex.

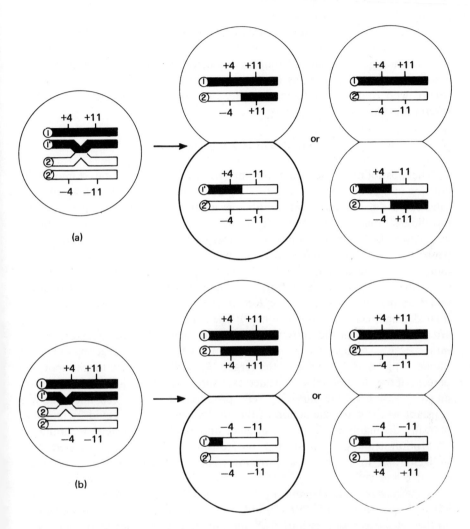

Fig. 13-4. Interpretation of the *K-D* asymmetry in production of tumor variants on the basis of mitotic crossing-over. Numbers in circles represent centromeres; ±4, ±11 represent H-2 antigens. The hypothesis incorrectly postulates that the locus coding for antigen H-2.4 is closer to the centromere than the locus coding for antigen H-2.11. If, in the somatic cell, crossing-over occurs within the *H-2* complex (a), of the four possible products of the mitosis, three are phenotypically +4, +11, and only one (marked by boldface line) is +4, −11. In selective hosts that are either of +4, −11 or −4, +11 genotype, only the +4, −11 variant can survive. If the mitotic crossing-over occurs between the centromere and the *H-2* complex (b), of the four mitotic products, three are again phenotypically +4, +11 and one is −4, −11 (marked by boldface line). In the selective hosts only the −4, −11 variants survive. Thus the mitotic crossing-over can produce +4, −11 and −4, −11, but not −4, +11 variants.

Evidence allegedly supporting the mitotic crossing-over hypothesis of variant formation was reported by K. Hellström (1960) and K. Hellström and Bjaring (1966), who observed an almost twofold increase in the concentration of H-2 antigens in the variants compared to the original F_1 tumor, and attributed the increase to a conversion from an *H-2* heterozygous to an *H-2* homozygous state. Homozygosity at the *H-2* complex would be expected if the variants arose by mitotic crossing-over. The observation was disputed, however, by Boyse *et al.* (1970), who found no difference in the quantity of H-2 antigens between a variant and the original F_1 tumor.

C. Selection of H-2 Variants *in Vitro*

The possibility of selecting variants from *H-2* heterozygous tumor cells growing in tissue culture was explored by Cann and Herzenberg (1963a, b), who substituted the treatment with antibodies in the presence of complement for the allograft reaction as the vehicle of selection. The efficiency of this treatment was demonstrated by Cann and Herzenberg (1963b), using homozygous *H-2^d* lymphoma ML–388 (subline 2B-2), grown in tissue cultures continuously for more than 6 years. When 2B-2 cells were exposed to a polyvalent anti-*H-2^d* serum and guinea pig complement, more than 99 percent of the cells were killed under optimal conditions. (The cytotoxic effect was assessed by an inability of treated single cells to form colonies.) The killing began almost immediately after treatment with the antiserum, and no further killing occurred after 5–15 min at 37°C. An oligospecific antiserum, C3H.SW anti-C3H, reacting only with public antigens H-2.3 and 8 of the target *H-2^d* cells, was able to kill about 80 percent of the cultured cells. Repeated exposure (14 times) to anti-*H-2^d* antiserum and cultivation of the surviving cells produced a variant cell line that was resistant to the cytotoxic action of the *H-2^d* antibodies and could be morphologically distinguished from the original anti-*H-2^d*-sensitive line. Quantitative absorption studies revealed that the resistant subline still possessed *H-2^d* antigens, but in a lower concentration than had been found in cells of the sensitive line.

Papermaster and Herzenberg (1966) obtained a cell line from (C3H × DBA/2)F_1 lymphoma (*H-2^k/H-2^d*) and demonstrated that the line was susceptible to the cytotoxic action of anti-*H-2^d* and anti-*H-2^k* antibodies (although during the course of the experiment, spontaneous development of resistance to alloimmune cytotoxicity was observed on two occasions approximately 6 months apart). Exposure of the line to B10 anti-B10.D2 antibodies (anti-*H-2^d*) produced a variant subline that was genetically resistant to the action of anti-*H-2^d* antibodies. (A similar treatment with normal serum and complement produced a temporary resistance that faded in subsequent passages.) The variant subline retained its resistance even after 1 year of continuous cultivation in the absence of selecting antisera. Quantitative absorption analysis of the subline indicated that it had lost antigen H-2.4 of *H-2^d* and retained antigens H-2.11 and 5 of *H-2^k*; the quantity of antigen H-2.8 determined by both *H-2^d* and *H-2^k* seemed to be significantly reduced. The results with anti-H-2.3 serum were inconclusive; both the original and the variant subline slightly reduced the titer of this antiserum, indicating that perhaps both lines contained this antigen in approximately the same quantity. On the basis of these data, the resistant subline could be viewed as lacking either the H-$2D^d$ products or products of the whole H-2^d complex. (Because antigen H-2.31, controlled by the H-$2K^d$ allele, was not tested by the authors, the distinction between partial and complete loss was not possible.) Attempts to isolate permanently resistant variants after treatment of the original line with anti-H-2^k sera failed; only temporary resistance, similar to that observed after treatment with normal serum, was obtained.

D. Conclusions

Although much work has been done on the problem of H-2 variation in tumor cells, mainly by the Kleins' group in Stockholm, the basic question—whether the variation is of genetic nature—remains unanswered. Experimental evidence supporting the genetic explanation is available, but direct proof is still missing. Conclusive proof that a genetic change is indeed involved would require the study of genetic segregation in somatic cells, and this can currently be done only in very special situations. In the meantime, one can apply a substitute approach that takes advantage of the revolutionary discoveries in mouse cytogenetics that provide means of identifying individual mouse chromosomes. The chromosome bearing the H-2 complex can now be distinguished by the Giemsa banding technique (Buckland *et al.* 1971), as well as morphologically (J. Klein 1971b). These techniques, when applied to the study of variant formation, could test whether antigenic variation is a consequence of such gross chromosomal abnormalities as the complete loss of chromosome 17.

The asymmetry of the H-2 antigenic losses is perhaps the most fascinating discovery produced by the study of variant formation. Its importance, however, is somewhat diminished by the fact that the asymmetry has been demonstrated so far in only one H-2 haplotype, H-2^a. The availability of additional, well-defined H-2 recombinant haplotypes now makes feasible the extension of the analysis to other combinations and the testing of whether the asymmetry phenomenon is universal or whether it represents just a curiosity of one particular antigen combination.

The definition of individual H-2 antigens has progressed a great deal since the time the first studies on alloantigenic variation began. It is now possible to prepare antisera containing a limited number of H-2 antibodies; such antisera could now provide a much better picture of the serological events accompanying variant formation.

The *in vitro* approach to H-2 antigen variation, too, has much broader prospects now, and therefore much better chances of success than it had a few years ago. New techniques based on cell-mediated cytotoxicity have become available that could provide a much more effective immunoselection system than humoral cytotoxicity.

The recent work on the role of the central segment of the *H-2* complex in MLR and in immune response (see Chapter Eighteen) also brings a fresh stimulus to the study of variant formation. One would particularly like to know to what extent the *Lad* and *Ir* loci are involved in variant selection, and how they themselves are affected by the selection. Using the right type of tumor and slightly modifying the currently available techniques, both these questions can now be approached experimentally.

II. Nonspecific *H-2* Variants

Nonspecific tumors differ from specific variants in four main characteristics (K. Hellström 1960). First, nonspecific sublines can be derived in foreign genotypes from both *H-2* homozygous and heterozygous tumors. Second, once established in one foreign host, the nonspecific sublines can usually grow in several other genotypically unrelated hosts. Third, the growth of nonspecific sublines in foreign hosts can usually be prevented by preimmunization. Fourth, the formation of nonspecific sublines is usually not accompanied by a loss of H-2 antigens; the antigens can still be demonstrated by serological techniques.

Nonspecific broadening of a tumor's host range can occur spontaneously, especially after prolonged serial transplantation, or it can be induced. Induction of nonspecificity can be achieved by passage of strain-specific tumors through newborn mice, lethally irradiated mice treated with bone marrow of a different genotype, or mice preconditioned for immunological enhancement (E. Möller 1964, 1965). In all three instances, the immunological unresponsiveness of the hosts is only temporary, and the tumors therefore enjoy a short period of unresisted growth before they encounter the allograft reaction. The change toward nonspecificity seems to proceed in a stepwise fashion (E. Möller, 1964). During the initial phase (usually the first three passages in the foreign host), the nonspecific sublines can still be reverted to strain specificity by retransplantation into the original host. After three or more passages in the foreign host, nonspecificity becomes irreversibly fixed. The stepwise progression in the direction of nonspecificity suggests that the resistant tumors develop from a small fraction of variant cells in the population. This contention is supported by the observation (E. Möller 1964) that in mice injected with enhancing antisera and then treated with strain-specific allogeneic tumors, tumors first develop into palpable masses, then completely regress, and after about 30 days start to reappear. When the enhanced tumors are removed from the antiserum-treated recipients before this 30-day interval and transplanted to allogeneic untreated mice, they regress; tumors that grew for more than 30 days in the primary foreign host are usually able to grow progressively in untreated, adult *H-2*-incompatible recipients; that is, they become nonspecific. Apparently, the conversion of a tumor from specific to nonspecific requires a certain period of background growth, which might be necessary for selection of the nonspecific variant cells.

The nonspecifically growing tumors stimulate H-2 antibody production in the foreign host (E. Möller 1965), with the titers fluctuating parallel to the growth of the tumor, increased tumor growth being accompanied by increased antibody production. Splenectomy, which is known to decrease the production of humoral antibodies without diminishing the efficiency of the allograft reaction, inhibits the growth of nonspecific tumors (again parallel to the inhibition of H-2 antibody production). This finding indicates that the nonspecific growth of a tumor may be facilitated by a process of self-enhancement (E. Möller 1965).

The fact that nonspecific tumors can induce H-2 antibody production indicates that they must contain at least some H-2 antigens; however, several studies indicate that the quantity of H-2 antigens in nonspecific tumor cells is substantially reduced (Amos 1956; Hauschka *et al.* 1956; Hoecker and Hauschka 1956; E. Klein and E. Möller 1963; E. Möller 1964, 1965). In contrast, Forman and Ketchel (1972) could not find any difference in the concentration of antigens H-2.3 and 4 between specific and nonspecific sublines of a DBA/2 (*H-2^d*) leukemia.

E. Möller (1964, 1965) explains the conversion of a specific tumor to a nonspecific one in the following way. Each tumor population contains a small fraction of variant cells with a drastically reduced concentration of H-2 antigens on their cell surfaces. In a syngeneic host these cells are usually at a selective disadvantage; however, if a tumor is transplanted to an *H-2* allogeneic host and allowed to grow for a certain period of time, the disadvantage changes into advantage. With the onset of allograft reaction, the nonvariant cells are eliminated, whereas the variant cells, which are relatively resistant to the allograft reaction because of the low content of H-2 antigens, survive and elicit synthesis of humoral H-2 antibodies. The circulating antibodies then block the antigenic receptors for cellular immunity and thus contribute further to the progressive growth of the tumor and to a gradual selection of cells with increased resistance to the allograft reaction.

This, however, is probably not the full explanation of nonspecific tumor growth, as indicated, for instance, by the finding that the nonspecific tumor lines contain normal levels of H-2 antigens, at least in some cases (Forman and Ketchel 1972). The mechanism allowing nonspecific growth is probably much more complicated and probably involves afferent as well as efferent inhibition of the allograft reaction. Möller's hypothesis also leaves unanswered the question of how the variants with reduced concentration of H-2 antigens arise in the first place. One possibility originally suggested by Gorer (1948) is that the genic imbalance in tumor cells leads to displacement or "crowding out" of the H-2 antigens by inactive substitutes. The genic imbalance could be primarily a consequence of accidental shifts in chromosome number. This explanation is in agreement with the repeatedly observed reduced specificity of heteroploid cells: whenever diploid and heteroploid sublines of the same tumor were available, the former was usually specific and contained a normal level of H-2 antigens, whereas the latter was nonspecific and contained reduced levels of H-2 antigens (Hauschka 1952; Hauschka and Levan 1953; Hauschka and Schultz 1954;

Hoecker and Hauschka 1956; Hauschka *et al.* 1956; Amos 1956; Hauschka and Amos 1957; Hauschka 1957).

A specific example of crowding out has recently been provided by Haywood and McKhann (1971) and by Ting and Herberman (1971). The former authors compared five methylcholanthrene-induced sarcomas for their capacity to absorb monospecific H-2 antisera, and to induce tumor-specific transplantation immunity in syngeneic mice, and found an inverse relationship between the two characteristics: tumors with a high concentration of H-2 antigens had a low content of tumor-specific transplantation antigens, and vice versa. Ting and Herberman (1971) observed a similar relationship between tumor-specific cell surface antigens and the H-2 antigens in cells transformed by polyoma virus. Although appearance of a tumor-specific transplantation antigen is insufficient to explain the transplantation behavior of the nonspecific tumors, the above two observations demonstrate that the expression of H-2 antigens can be influenced by changes occurring in the cell membrane during neoplastic transformation.

Section Four

Biochemistry

Chapter Fourteen

Cellular and Subcellular Distribution of H-2 Antigens

I. Tissue Distribution

A. Methods of Study

The presence or absence of H-2 antigens on various tissues and organs of the body can be determined by transplantation and serological methods. Using transplantation methods, the antigens can be detected in three basic ways. One way is to transplant a tissue across the *H-2* barrier in a congenic line; rejection indicates that H-2 antigens are present in that tissue. Another way is to inject cells or cell extracts from the tested tissue into a mouse, and then challenge the same recipient with an indicator graft; accelerated rejection of the graft signals the presence of H antigens in the sensitizing tissue. The third way is to use the tested tissue for induction of immunological tolerance in newborn animals and to determine the presence of tolerance by transplantation of adult animals with indicator grafts; prolonged survival of the grafts indicates their sharing of H antigens with the tolerance-inducing tissue.

With serological methods, the presence of H-2 antigens is established either by immunization with the tested tissue to produce humoral antibodies or by demonstration of the tested tissue's capacity to remove (absorb) or bind H-2 antibodies from a serum.

The transplantation methods are more sensitive, but are not as quantitative as the serological methods. Both methods probably detect antigens that are on the cell surface and exposed to the external milieu; antigens inside the cell or those masked by other cell surface structures may escape detection. Regardless of the method used, the results of H-2 antigen determination must be interpreted with caution, because almost any organ or tissue can be contaminated by elements of the blood, particularly erythrocytes and lymphocytes.

B. H-2 Antigenicity of Various Tissues

1. Lymphoid Organs and Liver

The results obtained using different methods of H-2 antigen determination on various tissues (Table 14–1) lead to two main conclusions. First, H-2 antigens are present in most, if not all tissues that have been tested; and second, the quantity of H-2 antigens in different tissues varies considerably (Fig. 14-1).

Table 14-1. Content of H-2 antigens in adult tissues according to different authors*, **

Tissues	Pizzaro et al. 1961	Amos et al. 1963b	Schlesinger 1964	Basch and Stetson 1962	Heberman and Stetson 1965	Graziano and Edidin 1971
lymph node	—	—	—	—	0.50	0.77
spleen	1.00	1.00	1.00–0.50	1.00	1.00	1.00
liver	1.00	0.50	0.50	0.50	0.67	0.20
thymus	—	—	0.25	0.25	—	0.78
lung	—	0.25	0.50	0.25	0.25	—
adrenal	—	—	—	0.25	—	—
gut	—	0.25	—	—	—	—
kidney	0.12	0.12	< 0.25	0.12	0.20	0.05
submaxillary salivary gland	—	—	—	—	—	0.10
red cells	—	0.12	—	0.00	0.02	0.01
testis	> 0.00	0.00	—	—	—	—
heart	—	—	0.06	0.06	—	—
skeletal muscle	> 0.00	0.00	—	0.00	0.02	> 0.00
brain	—	0.12	—	0.00	> 0.00	?
feces	—	0.12	—	—	—	—

** All values normalized to activity of spleen.

The organ with the highest H-2 antigenicity is the spleen, followed by other lymphoid organs, lymph nodes, bone marrow, and thymus. Among the different cell types in the lymphoid tissues, the highest concentration of H-2 antigens is found in lymphocytes. A relatively high concentration of H-2 antigens is also present in the liver, but liver homogenates contain a factor capable of suppressing the *in vivo* sensitizing ability of this as well as of other tissues (Mandel *et al.* 1965; Palm and Manson 1965; Hilgert and Krištofová 1966). The suppression factor, which seems to reside in lysosomes (Manson *et al.* 1968), does not have any pronounced effect on the *in vitro* absorbing capacity of the tissue extracts. The H-2 activity in the liver is primarily associated with Kupfer cells and, to a much lesser degree, with parenchymal cells (Basch and Stetson 1962; Edidin 1972b).

Of the other tissues tested, the H-2 antigenicity of epidermis, lung, kidney, heart, muscle, and red cells has never been questioned; nervous tissues, spermatozoa, ova, and trophoblasts are more controversial.

2. Nervous Tissue

Hemagglutination (Pizarro *et al.* 1961, 1963) and cytotoxicity (Basch and

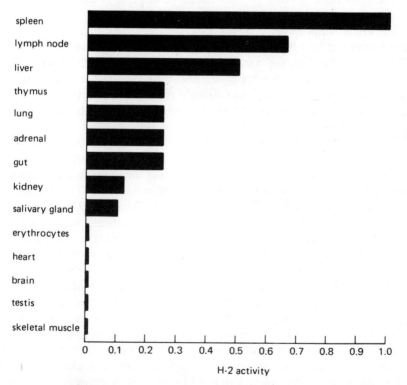

Fig. 14-1. Quantity of H-2 antigens in various tissues (summary of Table 14-1).

Stetson 1962) inhibition studies have suggested that the brain is practically devoid of H-2 antigens. However, brain tissue is capable of inducing transplantation immunity (Barnes 1964), and of staining in the indirect fluorescent antibody assay (Gervais 1968, 1970). The bright, specific fluorescence is restricted to the neurons, while the staining of the glial tissue is much less intense. The strongly positive cells occur with relatively low frequency, explaining why nervous tissue has such a low absorptive capacity.

3. Sperm

The detection of H-2 antigens on spermatozoa is hampered by three main factors. First, sperm is difficult to work with, particularly when viable cell suspension is required for the experiment; even in the best preparations, about 20–30 percent of the sperm are usually dead at the onset of the experiment; in some strains (e.g., C57BL), the proportion of dead sperm can increase to 50 or 60 percent. Second, sperm contain strong tissue-specific antigens to which the mouse, because of the anatomical isolation of the testes, is not tolerant; immunization with sperm, therefore, induces strong sperm-specific antibodies that must be absorbed from the antiserum. Third, most normal mouse sera, as well as sera from other species, contain natural antisperm antibodies that, again, must be removed prior to any tests.

The first attempt to detect alloantigens on sperm was made by Snell (1944), who immunized BALB/c females with spermatozoa from strains C57, P, and $(C57 \times P)F_1$, absorbed the antisera with BALB/c sperm to remove sperm-specific antibodies, and then tested the absorbed antisera for their capacity to agglutinate sperm from the immunizing donor. He found that the BALB/c anti-C57 serum agglutinated C57 and P sperm, but was unable to identify the antigens involved in this reaction.

Tests aimed specifically at the detection of H-2 antigens on sperm resulted in conflicting reports when performed by different investigators. The controversy revolves around the use of the indirect immunofluorescent antibody technique. Using this technique, two groups of investigators (Vojtíšková et al. 1969; Vojtíšková and Pokorná 1971, 1972a, b; Erickson 1972) were able to demonstrate H-2 antigens on sperm, while three other groups (Barth and Russell 1964; Gervais 1972b; M. Johnson and Edidin 1972) failed. The staining observed by Vojtíšková and her co-workers was restricted to the acrosome; Erickson (1972), on the other hand, observed staining over the entire surface of the head and midpiece. Both staining patterns have been observed by other investigators, but were attributed to the presence of natural, nonspecific, rather than to H-2-specific antibodies. The discrepancy is even more curious in view of the fact that Vojtíšková and her co-workers used unabsorbed antisera.

Other techniques used for demonstration of H-2 antigens on sperm produced slightly less controversial results. Vojtíšková and her co-workers (1969) were able to demonstrate that sperm can presensitize mice to subsequent skin grafts, although the objection can be raised that the presensitization was caused by epithelial cells present in the sperm suspension. The same objection applies to experiments demonstrating the capacity of sperm to absorb H-2 hemagglutinins and cytotoxins (Vojtíšková 1969; Vojtíšková and Pokorná 1971, 1972a, b), although in this case great care was taken to conduct the experiment so as to rule out the possibility that the observed absorption was caused by the contaminating cells.

The best evidence so far for the presence of H-2 antigens on sperm comes from the use of the dye-exclusion cytotoxic test (Goldberg *et al.* 1970; M. Johnson and Edidin 1972) and an antiglobulin technique utilizing ^{125}I-rabbit-antimouse γ globulin (Erickson 1972). Using the former test, an attempt has also been made to determine whether there is a haploid expression of the *H-2* loci in sperm. Haploid expression requires the existence of two sperm populations in an *H-2* heterozygote, one expressing H-2 antigens of one parent and the other those of the second parent. Fellous and Dausset (1970) observed that only about 50 percent of the sperm from *HL-A* (and *H-2*) heterozygotes was lysed by antibodies against antigens determined by one of the parental haplotypes, while a mixture of antibodies against both parental haplotypes lysed 70–80 percent of the sperm. The authors interpreted these results as evidence for haploid expression of HL-A and H-2 antigens. However, Goldberg and her co-workers (1970) reported that although a greater percentage of cells is lysed in sperm from *H-2* homozygotes than in sperm from *H-2* heterozygotes, the percentage of cells lysed in sperm from an F_1 hybrid by an antibody against one parental haplotype is often higher than 50. The slight difference in lysis between the *H-2* homozygotes and heterozygotes can probably be explained as being the result of the gene dosage effect (*H-2* heterozygous spermatozoa have fewer sites of one kind and are therefore more resistant to lysis than *H-2* homozygous spermatozoa). Moreover, since the cytotoxic test with sperm is notorious for high backgrounds, its quantitation is subject to gross errors. Hence, at present, haploid expression of H-2 antigens on sperm must be considered a hypothesis with very little experimental support.

The question of whether H-2 antigens exist at all in sperm can best be answered at this time as follows: "H-2 antigens may be present on mouse spermatozoa but probably at very low levels or with highly restrictive distribution. Selection and location of the antigens by other more sensitive tests is highly desirable and the influence of naturally occurring antispermatozoal antibodies requires careful examination" (M. Johnson and Edidin 1972).

4. Ova

Although H-2 antigens apparently are present on unfertilized eggs (Edidin 1972b), their presence on fertilized eggs is difficult to demonstrate. Olds (1968) observed a positive mixed hemagglutination reaction with two-cell zygotes, but the antiserum that she used (C3H anti-BALB/c) could have contained non-H-2 antibodies. Palm and her co-workers (1971) failed to demonstrate H-2 antigens on two-cell eggs using the indirect fluorescent antibody technique, although they were able to obtain positive fluorescence with anti-Ea-6 and anti-H-3, H-13 antisera. Heyner *et al.* (1969) observed killing, in the presence of complement, of eight-cell embryos incubated with DBA/2 anti-C3H serum but not with A.SW anti-A serum, again suggesting that the positive reaction was due primarily to non-H-2 antibodies.

Nor have transplantation tests resolved the controversy. Simmons and Russell (1962) found no difference between syngeneic and allogeneic (CBA and A) two- to eight-cell ova transplanted to the kidney capsule. However, the same authors later reported that in another strain combination (C3H and C57BL/6), differentiation of two- to eight-cell eggs was inhibited in allogeneic hosts (Simmons and Russell 1965, 1966). A similar conclusion was reached by Kirby *et al.* (1966) and by Tyan and Cole (1962). In all these reports, however, the positive result could have been caused by non-H-2 antigens.

The presence of H-2 antigens on fertilized eggs must therefore be considered uncertain. The solution will have to come through the use of more sensitive techniques and better defined experimental systems.

5. Trophoblast and Placenta

The trophoblastic tissue is the only tissue which consistently behaves, in serological (Schlesinger 1964) as well as in transplantation tests (Simmons and Russell 1962; Kirby *et al.* 1966; Simmons and Ozerkis 1967), as if it lacked H-2 antigens. Whether the failure to detect H-2 antigens on the trophoblast is due to an actual absence or merely a masking of these antigens remains to be resolved. Because the trophoblast separates the embryo from the mother, the absence of H-2 antigens in this tissue is probably of great functional significance, and is probably one of the factors contributing to protecting the fetus from being destroyed by the mother's immunological system.

The placenta appears to be weakly antigenic in transplantation tests (Uhr and Anderson 1962; Hašková 1963), but it has not been determined whether the antigenicity is caused by *H-2* or other *H* loci.

6. Cell Lines in Culture and Neoplastic Tissue

Cell lines in tissue culture demonstrate a remarkable stability in their H-2 antigen phenotypes, as documented by several reports. Cann and Herzenberg (1963a, b) detected H-2 antigens by hemagglutinin absorption in a line of DBA/2($H\text{-}2^d$) lymphoma cells grown in culture for 6 years, and in two fibroblastic lines of C57BL/Ka($H\text{-}2^b$) and (B10.D2 × B10)F_1($H\text{-}2^d/H\text{-}2^b$) origin grown in culture for 1 year. Spencer *et al* (1964) studied three established cell lines of C3H and Swiss mouse origin, and five somatic hybrid lines derived by cell fusion *in vitro*, and found persistence of alloantigens in the parental lines and full antigenic codominance in the hybrid lines. Manson *et al.* (1960b, 1962) were able to induce transplantation immunity with DBA/2 lymphoma cells (or with lipoprotein fractions prepared from these cells) maintained in tissue culture for several years. Gangal *et al.* (1966) and Drysdale *et al.* (1967) detected six antigens controlled by the H-2^k haplotype on cell line L–M derived from a C3H (H-2^k) mouse and maintained in tissue culture for over 29 years! Barth *et al.* (1967 demonstrated H-2 antigens by mixed hemadsorption on cells maintained in continuous culture for periods ranging from 3 to 30 months. And finally, D. Klein and her co-workers (1970) found no evidence of any H-2 variation during the cultivation of lines NCTC3814 and NCTC3815, which were in culture for over a year.

Transplantable tumors, in general, also display an extraordinary stability in their H-2 phenotypes. However, this stability is not absolute, because several instances of H-2 variation in tumor cells have been described and well documented. (These were discussed in Chapter Eleven.)

II. Ontogenetic Development

The presence of H-2 antigens on embryonic tissues during various stages of development has been the subject of numerous investigations using a variety of methods. The results of these investigations can be summarized by saying that H-2 antigens are *probably* present on early embryos and are *definitely* present on midterm and late embryos, and that the quantity of the H-2 antigens gradually increases during embryonic and early postnatal development, until it reaches the level of an adult organism at the end of the third postnatal week.

The question of H-2 antigen expression in early embryos (in the first week of gestation) remains somewhat controversial. Reports are about equally divided between those indicating a presence and those indicating an absence of H-2 antigens.

The presence of H-2 antigens on early embryos is suggested by at least three observations. First, mice that received intrarenal transplants of allogeneic blastocysts show prolonged survival of skin grafts from the donor strain (Kirby 1968, 1969), suggesting a sharing of H antigens between blastocysts and skin. Second, allogeneic blastocysts transferred to kidneys of hyperimmune hosts fail to produce trophoblasts, an indication of the embryo's failure to develop (Kirby *et al.* 1966). Third, blastocysts treated with anti-*H-2* serum and complement fail to grow after a transfer to the kidney of an allogeneic host (James 1969).

Absence of H-2 antigens in early embryos is suggested by at least two observations. Palm and her co-workers (1971), using an indirect immunofluorescence assay, were unable to detect H-2 antigens on blastocysts. And Patthey (cited by Edidin 1972b) failed to observe early lymphocytic infiltration of 6-day-old embryos transplanted to allogeneic preimmunized recipients, while 7-day-old embryos were infiltrated at 2 days after grafting. However, neither Palm and her co-workers nor Patthey actually disprove the presence of H-2 antigens in early embryos. The immunofluorescence technique might not be sensitive enough to detect a low concentration of these antigens, while in Patthey's experiments, the infiltration observed at 4 days and attributed by him to maturation of the transplant could actually have been caused by delayed stimulation due to a low concentration of antigens in the 6-day-old embryo.

In summary, because no conclusive evidence for the absence of H-2 antigens in early embryos has been provided, and because, on the contrary, some evidence suggesting the presence of these antigens is available, it seems more likely than not that a low level of H-2 antigens exists in embryos prior to the seventh day of gestation.

The presence of H-2 antigens in older embryos (seventh day and on) is far less controversial. Although here, too, negative results were reported by some investigators, these were almost certainly caused by insensitivity of the methods used; whenever more sensitive techniques were applied, the antigens were detected. Transplantation techniques such as grafting of embryos into untreated or preimmunized allogeneic recipients combined with observation of histological changes in the transplants (Simmons and Russell 1962, 1966; Edidin 1964), presensitization with embryonic tissues of recipients to subsequent skin (Billingham *et al.* 1956; Chutná and Hašková 1959; Hašková 1959; G. Möller and E. Möller 1962b; J. Klein 1965d) or bone marrow grafts (Doria 1963), or induction of immunological tolerance with embryonic cells (Billingham and Silvers, quoted by Medawar 1959), revealed the presence of H-2 antigens in 7-day-old or older embryos. Serological methods, on the other hand, can detect H-2 antigens only in later stages of embryonic development.

The application of serological methods to the study of H-2 antigens in ontogenesis provides a good example of how the conclusions about the antigenicity of tissues are influenced by sensitivity of the techniques employed. The first investigator to notice that H-2 antigens are subject to a maturation process was Gorer (1938), who observed that erythrocytes from newborn A strain mice were not agglutinated by the anti-II sera in saline, although the same sera agglutinated erythrocytes from adult mice. The erythrocytes developed full agglutinability at 6 weeks after birth. Using a slightly more sensitive human serum technique, Mitchison (1953) was able to demonstrate agglutinability of mouse erythrocytes with anti-H-2 sera at 8–12 days after birth. Pizarro *et al.* (1961), using a still more sensitive human serum-dextran agglutination technique, demonstrated H-2-mediated hemagglutination at 3 days after birth. When cytotoxicity and immunofluorescence tests were substituted for hemagglutination techniques, the threshold of detection shifted even further, down to the sixteenth day of gestation (G. Möller 1961b, 1963; G. Möller and E. Möller 1962b; E. Möller 1963). Finally, techniques such as induction of hemagglutinins (G. Möller and E. Möller 1962b; J. Klein 1965d), induction of enhancing antibodies (J. Klein 1965d), and absorption of hemagglutinins (Schlesinger 1964; Edidin 1964; J. Klein 1965d) allowed detection of H-2 antigens in 14- or even $10\frac{1}{2}$-day-old embryos. This movement toward earlier detection of H-2 antigens with the employment of more sensitive techniques indicates in itself that negative results cannot be taken as evidence for the absence of H-2 antigens in embryonic tissues.

Most of the experiments described above are open to two criticisms. First, the mouse strains employed by some authors were not congenic, and so the possibility that non-H-2, rather than H-2 antigens were involved was not precluded. Second, the transplanted embryonic tissues could have continued their development in the host, and the H-2 antigens might have matured after grafting. However, these two criticisms do not apply to the experiments of the Möllers and J. Klein, who used *H-2* congenic lines and lethally irradiated embryonic cells. Also, the criticisms do not apply to the *in vitro* tests, which deal mostly with H-2 antigens and which are too short to allow a significant maturation of these antigens.

Evidence for the continuing maturation of H-2 antigens in explanted tissues was obtained by J. Klein (1965d), who cultured liver cells from 15- to 16-day-old embryos and observed an *in vitro* increase in antigenicity parallel to that observed *in vivo*. Hence, the embryonic cells seem to be preprogrammed to a certain timetable of H-2 antigen maturation.

Genetic control of the maturation process was suggested by G. Möller and E. Möller (1962b), who observed that the rate of H-2 antigen development is strain dependent. Erythrocytes of strains C57BL and C57L($H-2^b$) are agglutinated with H-2 antisera at birth, while C3H($H-2^k$) and A($H-2^a$) erythrocytes become agglutinable only 3 days later. Red blood cells from $(A \times C57BL)F_1$ hybrids are agglutinated at birth by A anti-C57BL sera, and at 3 days by C57BL anti-A sera. These results were confirmed and extended by Boubelík and Lengerová (1971), who also observed that $H-2^a$ antigens of B10.A and $H-2^b$ antigens of A.BY mature early. To explain the latter finding, the authors postulated that the gene controlling the expression of H-2 antigens is linked to *H-2* but is not a part of the *H-2* complex. According to the authors, the B10.A strain received, during congenization, the allele for early expression from B10, while the A.BY strain did not receive the allele for late expression from A. Because B10.A(2R) and B10.A(5R) are early and late agglutinators, respectively, the authors speculated that the controlling locus is at the *D* end of the *H-2* complex.

The antisera used in most serological studies of H-2 antigen development were polyspecific. Pizarro and her co-workers (1961) were the only investigators who used oligospecific antisera. They were able to conclude that the development of individual H-2 antigens (they tested antigens 4, 5, and 11) proceeds at the same rate, suggesting a coordinate expression of the *H-2* genes during ontogenesis.

III. Subcellular Distribution

The distribution of H-2 antigens among the various cell organelles has been studied by immunolabeling and cell fractionation. The immunolabeling approach is based on the attachment of a tag, visible either by light microscopy (immuno-fluorescence methods) or by electron microscopy (ferritin-labeling methods; see Chapter Fourteen) to the antibodies, and observation of the tag's distribution following binding of the antibodies to cells. The cell fractionation methods consist of disrupting the cells, purifying fractions containing different cell organelles, and testing each fraction for H-2 antigenicity through its capacity either to inhibit serological reaction or to provoke immune response (antibody formation or presensitization to subsequent skin grafts). A major drawback of the fractionation methods is that it is almost impossible to obtain a pure fraction of any one organelle. The fractions are always contaminated, particularly with membrane fragments, and this contamination makes interpretation of the results of this method difficult. The fractionation methods can therefore only suggest an approximate subcellular distribution of antigens; they cannot prove it. The proof must come from the immunolabeling methods. A serious limitation of current immunolabeling methods is that they work only for intact cells; methods for labeling the cell interior have not been developed.

The general concensus from the numerous reports on the subcellular distribution of H-2 antigens is that the antigens are present in a high concentration in the cell (plasma) membrane. This conclusion is supported by several observations: the involvement of H-2 antigens in membrane-mediated serological reactions (agglutination, cytolysis, and binding of fluorescent-, ferritin-, or otherwise labeled antibodies); the removal of 60 percent of H-2 antigenicity by treatment of tumor cells with papain under conditions permitting no cell lysis (Schwartz and Nathenson 1971b), and the presence of H-2 activity in partially purified membrane fractions (Billingham *et al.* 1956, 1958; Kandutsch and Reiner-Wenck 1957; Kandutsch 1960; Herzenberg and Herzenberg 1961; D. Davies 1962b; Manson *et al.* 1962, 1963; Hilgert *et al.* 1964; Dumonde *et al.* 1963; Monaco *et al.* 1965; Basch and Stetson 1963; Herberman and Stetson 1965; Moreno 1966).

Whether H-2 antigens are also present inside the cell is still a much-debated question. There are those who believe that most, if not all H-2 activity is restricted to the cell surface (Haughton 1966), and there are others who maintain that the interior of the cell can be as good a source of H-2 antigens as the exterior (Manson *et al.* 1968). The strongest evidence for the restriction of H-2 antigens to the cell surface comes from the observation that cell rupture is not accompanied by the appearance of new *H-2* sites (Haughton 1966). If H-2 antigens were present both outside and inside the cell, one would expect a large increase in H-2 antibody binding activity following the breakage of the cell. However, tests with various cell types, including carcinomas, lymphomas, and normal lymphocytes, indicate that at least 80 percent of the total H-2 binding activity displayed by intact cells is present at the cell surface. One possible objection to this type of experiment is that cell rupture may inactivate some H-2 sites in the membrane, and the lost activity can then be compensated for by intracellularly located sites.

There is no agreement among those who believe that H-2 antigens are also located inside the cell on the precise location of these antigens. Almost every major organelle in the cell has been implicated: nuclei (Billingham *et al.* 1956, 1958; Oth and Castermans 1959; Albert and D. Davies 1973), mitochondria

(L. Mann *et al.* 1962), microsomes (Dumonde *et al.* 1963; Palm and Manson 1965; Herberman and Stetson 1965; Ozer and Wallach 1967; Manson *et al.* 1968), lysosomes (Basch and Stetson 1963; Herberman and Stetson 1965), and cytoplasm (Ozer and Wallach 1967).

The conclusions regarding the intracellular location of H-2 antigens are based solely on cell fractionation studies. In a typical experiment, the cells are broken up by one of many available treatments (mechanical disruption in a homogenizer, lysis in distilled water, ultrasonic disintegration, or nitrogen decompression), the particulate and the soluble fractions are separated by centrifugation, and the particulate fraction is further divided by a series of washings and centrifugations into subfractions, each subfraction containing predominantly one cellular organelle. The degree of the subfractions' purity varies considerably, according to the cell source and the fractionation method. The most common contaminant of the fractions are small membrane fragments —hence, the difficulty in interpreting the results.

One interesting observation made in cell fractionation studies is that individual H-2 antigens may be present in different fractions. Thus, Ozer and Wallach (1967) found H-2 antigens 3, 8, and 19 in the cell membrane fraction, 5 in the soluble fraction, 4 in the microsomes, and 23 in cell membranes and endoplasmic reticulum. Differential distribution of H-2 antigens was also reported by D. Davies (1966), Monaco *et al.* (1965), Moreno (1966), Oth and Castermans (1959), Palm and Manson (1965), Rubinstein (1964), and others. The most peculiar among these observations is the presence of H-2.5 in the cytoplasmic fraction. An odd, unexplained behavior of antigen 5 was also reported by Pizarro *et al.* (1963), Rubinstein (1964), Kandutsch and Stimpfling (1963), and Moreno (1966).

IV. Topography of Cell Surface H-2 Antigens

A. Methods

The spatial arrangement of H-2 antigens on the cell surface can be studied by antibody blocking and immunolabeling (immunofluorescence and immuno-ferritin) methods. In blocking assays, cells are incubated with an H-2 antibody in the absence of complement, and when they show no further capacity to absorb this antibody they are washed and incubated with another H-2 antibody. Following the second incubation, the antiserum is removed and tested for residual anti-H-2 activity. If the cells fail to absorb the second antiserum in spite of the fact that they are known to carry the relevant antigens, it is concluded that the antigens are blocked by the first serum. To explain blocking, it is postulated that antigens reacting with the first and second antisera are located very closely on the cell surface, and that attachment of antibodies to the former antigens leaves no room for attachments of antibodies to the latter. Information about the spatial interrelationships of H-2 antigens can also be obtained by

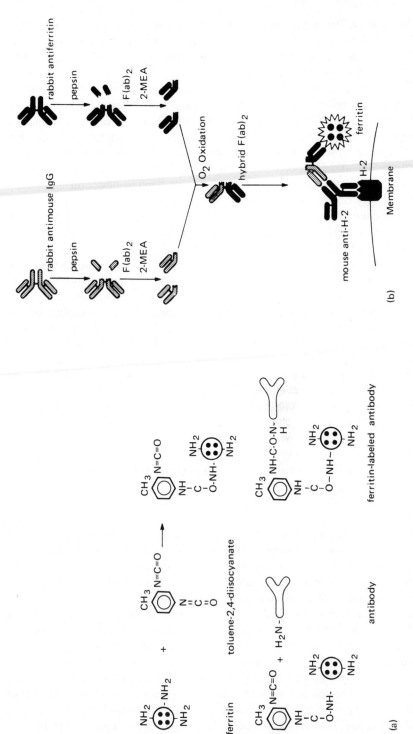

Fig. 14-2. (a) Principle of the direct ferritin-labeling technique. (b) Principle of the hybrid antibody technique of ferritin labeling.

mixed kinetics experiments, in which cells are lysed with a mixture of two noncross-reacting alloantisera, and the lytic rate of the mixture is compared with that of the two antisera acting independently (Cresswell and Sanderson 1968). If the former is found to be less than the sum of the rates of the two antisera taken separately, the conclusion is drawn that mutual inhibition of the two antisera occurred on the cell surface.

With ferritin-labeling methods, the antibodies are tagged by an attachment of ferritin, which can then be visualized in the electron microscope.[1] The attachment of the ferritin molecules to antibodies can be achieved either chemically or immunologically. The chemical attachment in *direct ferritin-labeling techniques* proceeds in two steps (Fig. 14–2a). In the first step, ferritin molecules are reacted with a coupling agent such as toluene-2,4-diisocyanate, and in the second step the resulting complex is conjugated with H-2 antibody molecules (W. Davis and Silverman 1968). The ferritin-labeled antibodies are then applied directly to the cells and the specimens are prepared for electron microscopy. Alternatively, in the *indirect ferritin-labeling method,* ferritin may be coupled to rabbit antimouse IgG antibodies, which are then reacted with anti-H-2 antibodies bound to H-2 antigens on the cell surface (Aoki *et al.* 1968). The indirect method has the advantage that a single labeled antiserum can be used to tag more than one antigen.

The major disadvantages of ferritin-labeling methods are nonspecific staining, loss of antibody activity because of chemical manipulations during the conjugation, and heterogeneity of the conjugate due to binding of ferritin to proteins other than the specific antibodies.

The immunological attachment in the *hybrid antibody technique* (U. Hämmerling *et al.* 1968) is achieved through the use of antiferritin antibodies (Fig. 14–2b). In this procedure, antibodies are produced in rabbits by ferritin immunization, the antibody molecules are enzymatically split into Fab fragments, and the fragments reconstituted into hybrid $F(ab)_2$ molecules by oxidation with Fab fragments obtained from rabbit antimouse IgG molecules. [Each $F(ab)_2$ molecule consists of one rabbit antiferritin and one rabbit antimouse IgG fragment.] The cells to be examined are first exposed to H-2 allo-antibodies (mouse IgG), then to the hybrid $F(ab)_2$ reagent, and finally to ferritin. Each hybrid $F(ab)_2$ molecule binds through its one combining site with the H-2 antibody on the cell surface, and through its second combining site with the ferritin molecule (Fig. 14–3).

The hybrid antibody method obviates the loss of antibody activity caused by the chemical coupling and permits the use of markers other than ferritin, for example, plant viruses or bacteriophages (U. Hämmerling *et al.* 1969a).

Two new methods allowing simultaneous labeling of the same cell with two distinct markers have recently been described by Lamm *et al.* (1972). In the

---

[1] Ferritin is a protein consisting of about 20 percent iron in the form of a ferric hydroxide-phosphate complex. Each ferritin molecule has a protein shell enveloping an inner core of four iron micelles. The high electron-scattering capacity of the micelle makes the ferritin molecules easily identifiable in electron-microscope preparations.

hybrid antibody bridge method, a hapten (e.g., benzylpenicilloyl) is chemically coupled to the H-2 alloantibody, which is allowed to bind to cells. The cell-bound antibodies are then bridged to a marker (ferritin or virus) by a hybrid $F(ab)_2$ antibody containing one combining site for the hapten and another for the marker. In the *untreated antihapten antibody bridge method*, the hapten is chemically coupled to both the H-2 alloantibody and the marker (ferritin, virus). Cells are then coated with the hapten-coupled H-2 alloantibodies, which are bridged to the hapten-coupled marker by rabbit antihapten antibody.

The electron microscopy of the ferritin-labeled cells can be carried out

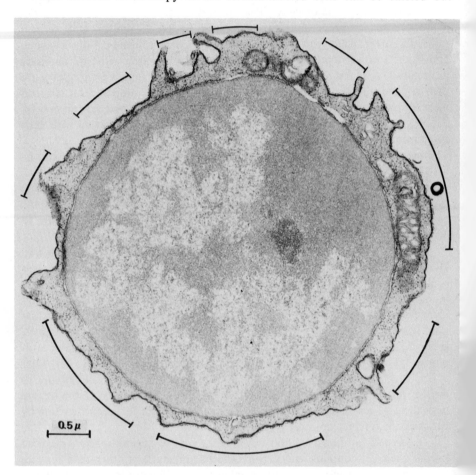

Fig. 14-3. A thin section of a mouse lymph node lymphocyte labeled for H-2 by reacting sequentially with mouse anti-H-2 serum, hybrid antibody (rabbit antimouse IgG-rabbit antiferritin), and ferritin. The distribution of ferritin, marked by brackets, is in discontinuous sectors. × 30,000. (Reproduced with permission from U. Hämmerling, C. W. Stackpole, and G. Koo: "Hybrid antibodies for labeling cell surface antigens." *Methods in Cancer Research* **9**:255–282. Copyright © 1973 Academic Press. All rights reserved.)

essentially in two ways. One way is to embed the specimen, section it, and observe the essentially one-dimensional distribution of the tag on the cell surface (W. Davis and Silverman 1968; Aoki *et al.* 1968; U. Hämmerling *et al.* 1968). Two or three-dimensional pictures can be obtained by serially sectioning single cells and constructing models from the serial electron micrograph (Stackpole *et al* 1971). Another way, used recently by Nicolson *et al.* (1971), is to lyse the cells at an air-water interface. The membrane spreads out flat on the interface and can then be picked up on an electron microscopic grid, the ferritin-labeled antibody can be applied to it, and the grid can be examined by direct-transmission electron microscopy.

B. Blocking Studies

The blocking studies are based on the assumption that when two antigens are in close proximity, the absorption of antibodies by one of them interferes with the absorption of antibodies by the other. The studies can produce three types of result: absence of blocking, reciprocal blocking, and nonreciprocal blocking. Absence of blocking indicates that two antigens are relatively far apart on the membrane; reciprocal blocking (i.e., A anti-B reduces the absorbing capacity of C anti-D, and vice versa) indicates that two antigens are relatively close to one another, and nonreciprocal blocking (i.e., A anti-B inhibits C anti-D, but C anti-D does not inhibit A anti-B) indicates "that two antigens are close to one another but that there is a substantial difference in their disposition" (Boyse *et al.* 1968a).

Blocking studies with H-2 antisera were reported by three groups of investigators, Boyse *et al.* (1968a), Cresswell and Sanderson (1968), and Krištofová *et al.* (1970). Boyse and his co-workers worked with thymocytes and antisera against antigens of five different genetic systems: *H-2, Tla, Thy-1, Ly-1* and *Ly-2.* They were able to demonstrate that, in instances wherein reciprocal blocking was observed, the antigens could be divided into two groups—one comprised of the antigens controlled by the *H-2D, Tla* and *Ly-2* loci, the other comprised of *H-2K* and *Ly-1* antigens. No blocking was observed between the antigens of the first and the second groups, whereas members of the same group were within the blocking range of some, but not other members of that group. Antisera against Thy-1 antigens blocked antisera against all other tested antigens except H-2 and Tla.3, but were not blocked by any of these other antisera. The authors interpreted these results as reflecting the following relative position of antigens in the cell membrane (Boyse *et al.* 1968a):

$$
\begin{array}{cccccc}
\textit{Thy-1} & \textit{Thy-1} & \textit{Thy-1} & \textit{Thy-1} & & \textit{Thy-1} \\
\downarrow & \downarrow & \downarrow & \downarrow & & \downarrow \\
\textit{Tla.3} \rightleftarrows \textit{Tla.2} & \rightleftarrows \textit{Tla.1} & \rightleftarrows \textit{H-2D} & \rightleftarrows \textit{Ly-2} & \textit{Ly-1} & \rightleftarrows \textit{H-2K}
\end{array}
$$

(The arrows indicate the direction of blocking: antibody against antigen at the arrowhead blocks absorption of antibody against antigen at the arrowtail.)

According to this view, the H-2K and H-2D antigens are located relatively far apart in the membrane.

Cresswell and Sanderson (1968) studied the spatial distribution of H-2 antigens by blocking and mixed kinetics tests and found reciprocal inhibition with one pair of antisera and nonreciprocal inhibition with another pair. The $H\text{-}2^a$ anti-$H\text{-}2^b$ serum inhibited the absorption of $H\text{-}2^b$ anti-$H\text{-}2^a$ serum by $H\text{-}2^a/H\text{-}2^b$ cells, and vice versa. In contrast, $H\text{-}2^d$ anti-$H\text{-}2^k$ serum inhibited the absorption of $H\text{-}2^k$ anti-$H\text{-}2^d$ serum by $H\text{-}2^a/H\text{-}2^a$ or $H\text{-}2^d/H\text{-}2^k$ cells but $H\text{-}2^k$ anti-$H\text{-}2^d$ serum did not inhibit the absorption of $H\text{-}2^k$ anti-$H\text{-}2^d$ serum by the same cells. The authors explain these findings by postulating that there are more sites specific for the $H\text{-}2^d$ anti-$H\text{-}2^k$ antibody than sites specific for the $H\text{-}2^k$ anti-$H\text{-}2^d$ antibodies. An alternative explanation is that the $H\text{-}2^d$ anti-$H\text{-}2^k$ serum coated the K-end sites on the $H\text{-}2^a$ cells, and the only antibodies that could then react with the coated cells were those directed against the D-end antigens (particularly antigen 4). Because anti-H-2.4 is usually a relatively poor cytotoxin, its poor reactivity might have been mistaken for blocking.

Krištofová and her co-workers (1970) observed that coating of $H\text{-}2^k$ cells with anti-H-2.5 antibodies strongly blocked (up to 67 percent) subsequent absorption of anti-H-2.11 antibodies, and vice versa. Since 5 and 11 are both believed to be K-series antigens, presumably carried by the same molecule, the result is not unexpected. In other combinations, where the target antigens of the coating and test antisera belonged to different series ($H\text{-}2^a$ cells coated with anti-4 and tested for absorption of anti-11 or anti-5 antibodies, and vice versa), the authors observed only a moderate blocking (23–29 percent). In only one combination, where the target antigens were in different series and their genetic determinants were in *trans*-position ($H\text{-}2^b/H\text{-}2^d$ cells coated with anti-33 and tested for absorption of anti-4, and vice versa), did Krištofová and her co-workers observe almost no blocking.

The blocking studies can be criticized on several grounds. First, coating with the first antibody may cause redistribution of the antigenic sites in the membrane, producing relationships among the antigens that do not exist in untreated cells. Second, two of the three studies were performed with poly-specific antisera containing an unspecified number of unidentified antibodies with unknown absorptive and cytotoxic potencies. Only Krištofová and her co-workers used oligospecific antisera. Third, the existence of cross-reactivity between the antigens of the K and D series may obscure the results, as the same antibodies may apparently become attached to different antigenic sites. The main objection to these studies, however, is that they have provided very little positive information, because the three groups obtained discrepant results from which no firm conclusions can be drawn.

C. Immunofluorescence and Ferritin-Labeling Studies

Cerrotini and Brunner (1967), using a high-resolution indirect fluorescent antibody technique on fixed cells, were among the first to demonstrate that, under certain conditions, H-2 antigens are not distributed uniformly over the cell surface. They observed that the fluorescent label occurred in patches or flecks, the arrangement of which varied according to the cell type. Mastocytoma and lymphoma cells maintained in a tissue culture either bore small patches distributed evenly on the cell surface or displayed crescentlike staining at one pole while the rest of the cell remained unstained. In lymph nodes, the majority of lymphocytes bore large patches of fluorescence separated by narrow unstained areas. In bone marrow, about half of the cells displayed numerous, intensely fluorescent areas, while the other half of the cells bore only a few small, faintly fluorescent flecks. In the thymus, two similar types of cell occurred with a frequency of 15 and 85 percent, respectively. Erythrocytes stained with only a few faint flecks.

A similar patchy distribution of H-2 antigens was also observed using indirect and hybrid antibody ferritin-labeling techniques (Aoki *et al.* 1969; U. Hämmerling *et al.* 1969a). On electron micrographs, the highest concentration of H-2 antigens was observed in reticular cells from thymus, lymph nodes, and spleen, and a slightly lower concentration in lymphocytes from lymph nodes and spleen, plasma cells, and eosinophils. In all these cell types, the H-2 antigens occupied the majority of the cell surface (Fig. 14–3). Considerably fewer H-2 antigens were found in thymocytes and erythrocytes, and very few in peritoneal macrophages. Thymocytes and erythrocytes bore several small sectors of ferritin labeling widely separated from one another. Macrophages were usually completely devoid of H-2 antigens on the cell surface, but their phagocytic vacuoles were often lined with ferritin. This finding was surprising, because macrophages and reticular cells were believed to be closely related.

Labeling for antigens other than H-2 showed the confinement of Tla to small sectors on thymocytes, and of Thy-1 to large sectors in thymocytes and small sectors in some lymph node and spleen lymphocytes.

Three-dimensional models constructed from serial sections of single cells (Stackpole *et al.* 1971) showed the occurrence of H-2 antigens in small, isolated areas on the surfaces of thymocytes, and large, interconnected areas on the surfaces of lymphocytes. Most of the protrusions and microvilli of the lymphocytes were H-2-negative. The H-2-positive areas were studded with H-2-negative regions, which were often the sites of surface protrusions. According to Aoki and his co-workers (1970), the H-2-negative areas are the sites at which maturation and budding of viruses, such as the Gross virus, takes place.

A patchy distribution of H-2 antigens was also observed by Nicolson *et al.* (1971), who used two-dimensional ferritin labeling of erythrocyte membranes flattened out by lysis on air-water interfaces. The authors observed that H-2 antigens were restricted to patches containing clusters of ferritin grains. Each patch consisted of one to ten clusters (mean of three), and each cluster of two to eight grains. By analogy from their work on the distribution of the Rh antigens in human erythrocytes, the authors calculated that each cluster corresponded to one antigenic site. The distribution of the patches was highly irregular.

The authenticity of the patchy distribution was questioned by W. C. Davis (Davis and Silverman 1968; Davis *et al.* 1971; Davis 1972). Davis and Silverman

(1968), using the direct immunoferritin-labeling method, observed an essentially continuous distribution of the ferritin label on the surface of lymphocytes, polymorphonuclear leukocytes, eosinophils, platelets, and erythrocytes, with the lymphocytes displaying the highest concentration of H-2 antigens. There were no large areas of unlabeled membrane in the lymphocytes, and antigens were present even on the surface of the protrusions.

The discrepancy between the findings of Davis and his co-workers and those of Aoki and Hämmerling can probably be attributed to the difference in the techniques used by these investigators. A comparison of the direct and indirect immunoferritin techniques by Davis *et al.* (1971) demonstrated that the former produced continuous and the latter patchy distribution of H-2 antigens. Hence, the question arises as to which of the two techniques produces a more authentic picture of H-2 cell surface topography. Davis (1972) believes that patchy distribution is an artifact caused by antiglobulin-induced redistribution of H-2 antigens in the indirect techniques. His view is supported by recent findings indicating that the natural distribution of H-2 antigens on cells fixed with paraformaldehyde is random (Parr and Oei 1973).

D. Studies Indicating Membrane Fluidity

In blocking studies, and in most immunolabeling studies, H-2 antigens were regarded as rigidly fixed to specific locations in the membrane, and the membrane itself was regarded as a solid or semisolid wall. The plausibility of this view has recently been undermined by several findings, all of which suggest a considerable fluidity of the cell membrane and mobility of its components, including H-2 antigens.

1. Membrane Mixing in Fused Cells

The first indication that H-2 antigens can move freely in the membrane plane was provided by Frye and Edidin (1970), who fused cells from established tissue culture lines of mouse and human origin and produced heterokaryons[2] bearing both mouse (H-2) and human (species-specific) surface antigens. They made the antigens visible through treatment of the heterokaryons, first with a mixture of mouse antimouse H-2 sera and rabbit antihuman cell line sera, and then with a mixture of fluorescein-labeled goat antimouse IgG and tetramethylrhodamine-labeled goat antirabbit IgG sera. Using proper filters on the fluorescence microscope, the authors identified the H-2 and human antigens on the cell surface through their green and red fluorescence, respectively. They observed that, at the time of cell fusion, the heterokaryons displayed unmixed staining, with half of each cell stained green and the other half red. However, within 40 min at 37°C, total mixing of the mouse and human antigens occurred in 90 percent of the heterokaryons, as indicated by the simultaneous green and red

---

[2] Heterokaryon is a product of cell fusion containing genetically different nuclei in common cytoplasm.

circumferential fluorescence of each cell. From this observation, the authors concluded that the parental antigens in the fused cells diffused freely through the membrane until they became completely intermixed. The human antigens appeared to diffuse faster than the mouse antigens, because many cells assumed red circumferential fluorescence earlier than green. The speed with which the intermixing occurred and the fact that the treatment of the parental cells with a variety of metabolic inhibitors did not strongly influence antigen spreading suggested that "the cell surface of heterokaryons is not a rigid structure, but is 'fluid' enough to allow free 'diffusion' of surface antigens resulting in their intermingling within minutes after the initiation of fusion" (Frye and Edidin 1970). This conclusion was further strengthened by the observation that lowering of the temperature (and, hence, lowering of the membrane's viscosity) slowed down or arrested completely the antigen intermixing.

2. Antibody-Induced Redistribution of Membrane Antigens

Strong support for the concept of a fluid membrane was provided by the discovery that the spatial distribution of antigens in the membrane can be modified by antibodies.

Although investigators using indirect fluorescence methods repeatedly observed occasional polar distribution of the stain, resulting in the appearance of crescentlike or caplike cells, it was not until 1971 that two groups of investigators (R. Taylor and Dufus, Raff and dePetris), working independently, recognized the significance of this phenomenon. Careful examination of the conditions leading to the appearance of capped cells demonstrated that the formation of caps represented antibody-induced redistribution of antigen molecules in the cell membrane (Taylor *et al.* 1971). The redistribution can occur in three forms: patch formation, cap formation, and pinocytosis, often following one another in that order (Raff and dePetris 1973).

Patch formation is the aggregation of diffusely and randomly distributed antigens into clusters following the addition of a bivalent antibody. The phenomenon is temperature dependent, being high at 37°C, low (although significant) at 0°C, and arrested at −7°C (Raff and dePetris 1973); it can occur in the presence of metabolic inhibitors. One explanation of patch formation is that it occurs through two-dimensional lattices formed by the interaction of bivalent antibodies with multiple determinants of mobile antigenic molecules in the cell membrane. (Monovalent Fab fragments fail to induce it.) The process is probably based on passive diffusion, requiring very little metabolic energy.

Cap formation (capping) is the movement of the patches toward, and their aggregation at one pole of the cell, invariably the pole with the Golgi apparatus. During capping, the original round cell often elongates into a tail process or uropod. Capping can be blocked by the addition of metabolic inhibitors, but not by inhibitors of protein or RNA synthesis (Taylor *et al.* 1971; Edidin and Weiss 1972). Blocking by inhibitors of cell motility, such as cytochalasin B, has been reported by some (Taylor *et al.* 1971; Edidin and Weiss 1972), but questioned by others (Karnovsky and Unanue 1973). Capping is rapid at 37°C, considerably slower at room temperature, and stops completely at 0°C. While some antigens form caps after the addition of a single antibody layer, others require the addition of a second (antiglobulin) layer. DePetris and Raff (1973) explain cap formation as being an immobilization of the antigen molecule in the membrane by antibody-mediated cross-linking, followed by a sweeping of the antigen aggregates to the uropod. As a part of normal cell movement, the free membrane components flow forward, whereas the aggregates move actively backward and accumulate over the tail of the cell. The backward movement may involve interaction of the aggregates with the underlying cytoplasmic contractile system.

Capping may be followed by *pinocytosis* (endocytosis) of the aggregates: after a relatively short incubation time, the aggregates begin to disappear from the cell surface and to appear in vesicles inside the cell (Taylor *et al.* 1971). However, capping and pinocytosis are not interdependent: pinocytosis can occur without capping, and capping is not always followed by pinocytosis. Karnovsky and Unanue (1973) even suggest that with some antigens the caps are exfoliated (shed off), rather than pinocytosed. Thus, the stimuli for capping and pinocytosis seem to be different.

Although most of the work on antibody-induced antigen redistribution was done using B lymphocytes and antibodies against Ig receptors, the phenomenon was also observed with other cell types (e.g., cultured fibroblasts, cf., Edidin and Weiss 1972), and with a variety of antigens (Thy-1, Tla, concanavalin A, phytohemagglutinin, and others). The phenomenon has also been described with regard to H-2 antigens, but two main controversies in this area remain to be solved. First, according to Raff and dePetris (1973) and W. C. Davis (1972), patch formation can be induced after the addition of antiglobulin serum, but not by H-2 antibody alone; according to Edidin and Weiss (1972), the anti-globulin serum is not necessary. Second, according to Karnovsky and Unanue (1973), H-2 antigens cap only to a limited extent, even after the addition of antiglobulin serum; on the other hand, good capping was reported by Edidin and Weiss (1972), Raff and dePetris (1973) and Neauport-Sautes *et al.* (1973).

However, the major unsettled question is whether the true distribution of H-2 antigens is diffuse or patchy. There are those who believe that the patchiness is an artifact induced by cross-linking with antibodies (W. Davis 1972; Raff and dePetris 1973), and those who maintain, in spite of the new developments, that patchy distribution of the H-2 antigens is real (Karnovsky and Unanue 1973). Although no firm conclusion can be drawn in this regard, one is never-theless tempted to side with the former group for the simple reason that no data have yet been published that demonstrate patchy distribution after direct coating with a single layer of H-2 antibodies.

3. Redistribution of H-2K and H-2D Antigens

The capping phenomenon was used by Neauport-Sautes and her co-workers (1973) to obtain information about the molecular relationship between antigens controlled by different *H-2* regions. The question the authors asked was simple: can antigens controlled by the *K* region cap independently of the antigens controlled by the *D* region?

The authors incubated *H-2*^{b} lymph node lymphocytes with tetramethyl-rhodamine isocyanate-conjugated anti-H-2.33 for 30 min at 37°C, washed the cells, and then incubated them for additional 45 min at 37°C to induce redistribution of the antibody-coated H-2 antigens. At the end of the incubation period they cooled the cells to 0°C, incubated them for 30 min at 0°C with fluorescein isothiocyanate-conjugated anti-H-2.2 antibodies, and, after washing in the cold to minimize the redistribution of the H-2.2 antigens, examined the cells for red and green fluorescence. They found that the red fluorescence corresponding to antigen 33 was accumulated in a cap at one pole of the cells, whereas the green fluorescence remained diffuse, clearly separated from the red cap. Apparently, the capping of *K*-region antigen 33 occurred independently of *D*-region antigen 2, suggesting that the two antigens are carried by separate molecules. The authors also obtained similar results for antigens 23 and 32 of the *H-2*^{k} cells, and for all four private antigens present in *H-2*^{b}/*H-2*^{k} hetero-zygous cells, both in *cis*- and *trans*-position. All the data indicate that the H-2K and H-2D antigens migrate independently at the cell surface. Independent redistribution of H-2K and H-2D antigens was also observed by Davis (1973), using ferritin-labeled antibodies.

4. Antigen Modulation

Although the relationship between capping and pinocytosis is not yet totally understood, it is clear that the former is frequently followed by the latter, and that this sequence of events can result in a temporary absence of antigens from the cell surface. Taylor and his colleagues (1971) speculate that this stripping of the cell membrane could be the mechanism of the antigen modulation phenomenon.

Antigen modulation is defined as the disappearance of antigens from the cell surface after exposure to specific antibodies. The phenomenon was first discovered by Boyse and his colleagues (1967) during their studies on the effect of anti-Tla antibodies on the expression of Tla antigens (cf. Chapter Eleven). Although the original attempt to demonstrate modulation of H-2 antigens failed (Lamm *et al.* 1968), several investigators have recently been able to induce H-2 modulation, either by the addition of antiglobulin serum to the cells coated with alloantibodies (Takahashi 1971; Lengerová *et al.* 1972), or with H-2 alloantibodies alone (Schlesinger and Chaouat 1972). A phenomenon resembling H-2 antigen modulation was also described by Amos *et al.* (1970). The above authors observed that peritoneal, leukemia, or bone marrow cells, when incu-bated at 37°C with H-2 alloantibodies, or with anti-H-2 and antiglobulin antibodies, became resistant to lysis after subsequent exposure to complement. The resistance was not induced when the cells were incubated at 0°C. Lengerová *et al.* (1972) were able to correlate the degree of modulation with the frequency of capped cells detectable by immunofluorescence and with the occurrence of pinocytic vesicles lined with labeled antigen. The authors suggest that the absence of H-2 antigens on the surface of peritoneal macrophages observed by Aoki *et al.* (1969) might also have been caused by antigen modulation. Lengerová and her co-workers also demonstrated that H-$2^a/H$-2^b bone marrow cells, modulated with anti-H-2^a serum and inoculated into H-$2^b/H$-2^b mice, displayed an improved capacity (compared to untreated cells) to form colonies in the spleen.

Schlesinger and Chaouat (1972, 1973) demonstrated that H-2 modulation can be abrogated by exposing the cell to metabolic inhibitors and that, in H-$2^b/H$-2^k heterozygous cells, H-2^b antigens can modulate independently of H-2^k antigens and vice versa. When modulated cells were transferred to an antibody-free medium, they recovered their H-2 antigenicity within 2 hr.

All of the above observations indicate that there is a great similarity between capping (and pinocytosis) and antigen modulation, and that the former might indeed be the mechanism of the latter. As pointed out by Lengerová *et al.* (1972), to what degree the differences in tissue distribution of H-2 antigens can be attributed to the cell's capacity to modulate remains to be seen.

Chapter Fifteen

Biochemical Aspects of H-2 Antigens

I. Architecture of the Plasma Membrane

A. Chemistry

Plasma membranes are composed primarily of three constituents: lipids (and cholesterol), proteins, and water, their proportions varying from one cell to another.

The membrane *lipids* fall into two categories, phosphoglycerides and sphingolipids. The *phosphoglycerides* are derived from glycerol by replacing two hydroxyl groups with long-chain fatty acids, and the third group with phosphoric acid (Fig. 15–1). Diversity of phosphoglycerides is achieved through variation in the fatty acids and through the attachment of additional groups to the phosphate. In lecithins and cephalins, the two most common classes of phosphoglycerides, the phosphate group is linked with choline and ethanolamine, respectively. The two fatty acid chains are believed to project from the three-carbon glycerol base in a direction opposite that of the phosphate group. The structure of the phosphoglyceride molecule can be likened to a tuning fork, the fatty acid chains constituting the "prongs" and the phosphate group the

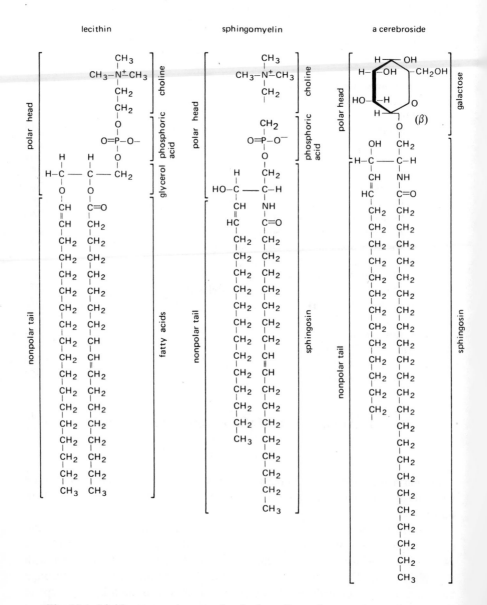

Fig. 15-1. Lipids commonly occurring in the cell membrane.

"handle."[1] When separated, the prongs and handle demonstrate different properties. The prongs are soluble in organic solvents such as ether or chloroform but are insoluble in water; the handle, on the other hand, is not soluble in organic solvents, but dissolves readily in water. The difference in solubility is explained by the electrical properties of the two fragments. In the phosphate groups, the negatively charged electrons are asymmetrically distributed in relation to the positively charged nuclei, so that the whole group is *polar*—one portion carries a considerable negative charge while the other portion is positively charged. Because water molecules are also strongly polarized, they are attracted to the polar phosphate groups (the groups are *hydrophilic*). In the fatty acid chains the electrons are symmetrically distributed around the nuclei so that the chains are *nonpolar* and repel water molecules (they are *hydrophobic*). A molecule having one end hydrophilic and the other hydrophobic is called *amphipathic*.

The *sphingolipids* are based on the sphingosine molecule, which is an unsaturated aminoglycol having two hydroxyl groups and one amino group. The molecule is organized into a tuning-fork structure similar to that of the phosphoglycerides, but with one prong of the fork (15-carbon fatty acid) always constant and the second prong variable; the latter can be one of several fatty acids attached to the sphingosine base through the amino group. The handle of the sphingolipid molecule may be phosphate and cholin (sphingomyelin), a simple hydroxyl (ceramides), a simple sugar (cerebrosides), or a complex polysaccharide (gangliosides).

The membrane proteins can be divided into two categories, integral and peripheral. The *integral proteins* are usually amphipathic, with their hydrophobic portions penetrating deeply into the hydrophobic part of the lipid layer. The proteins, therefore, can be liberated from the membrane by reagents that disrupt hydrophobic interactions. The hydrophilic portion of an integral protein usually protrudes into the aqueous medium surrounding the membrane. The *peripheral proteins* do not penetrate the membrane, but are held at the membrane surface by predominantly electrostatic interactions. They can be removed from the membrane by reagents that disrupt electrostatic interactions, and once liberated they are soluble in aqueous solutions.

B. Structure

Electron micrographs of membrane cross sections show two densely stained parallel lines separated by a faintly stained inner core. The double line is interpreted as representing a bimolecular lipid layer arranged in an orderly fashion. The lipid molecules are believed to lie side by side in sheets, with the hydrophilic polar handles pointing in one direction and the hydrophobic nonpolar prongs pointing in the opposite direction. Each membrane is composed of at least two such sheets, with the nonpolar prongs facing each other inside the membrane,

[1] D. Chapman, Lipid dynamics in cell membranes, *Hospital Practice*, pp. 79–88, February 1973.

and the polar handles on the outer and inner surfaces (Fig. 15–2). In electron microscopic preparations, the polar groups in the lipid bilayers combine easily with heavy, strongly electron-scattering metal atoms of the fixative and produce the characteristic densely stained double line.

C. Membrane Models

While the organization of membrane lipids into the bilayer described above is almost universally accepted, organization of membrane proteins is still controversial. Several models of membrane structure have been proposed, but only two or three have attained widespread attention. Until recently, the most favored has been the *Davson-Danielli-Robertson model*, in which the proteins were believed to be in a stretched form (β-conformation) and simply to lie on top of the lipid bilayer (Fig. 15–2). However, the model ran into serious difficulties when it was discovered that the majority of membrane proteins were in globular (α-helical) form, and that the membrane was in a dynamic state, with at least some proteins highly mobile (see Chapter Fourteen). The new data on membrane structure have been accommodated by the *fluid mosaic model* (S. Singer and Nicolson 1972). In this model, the membrane is visualized as a "sea" of lipid in which the integral proteins float as "icebergs" (Fig. 15–3), with their hydrophobic portions submerged and their hydrophilic portions exposed.

However, even the fluid mosaic model is far from being generally accepted. Its details have been challenged, and it is opposed by models in which some restrictions, based on the assumption of protein-protein interactions and

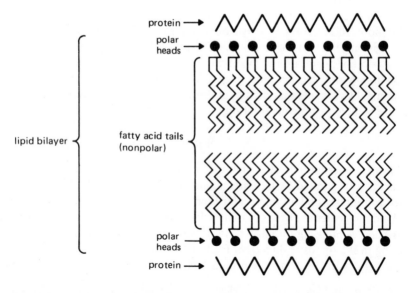

Fig. 15-2. Davson-Danielli-Robertson model of the plasma membrane.

organization of the protein complexes into lattices and domains, are placed on protein mobility (Capaldi and Green 1972; Wallach 1972).

II. Biochemistry of H-2 Antigens

Biochemistry is one area of H-2 studies in which the quantity of available information is not proportional to the number of publications. Although more than a dozen papers on H-2 biochemistry appeared each year for almost three decades, biochemists were not able in all that time to establish with certainty even such a basic fact as the chemical identity of H-2 antigens. Progress toward defining H-2 biochemistry has been slow for two principal reasons (Kandutsch 1961). First, assays for the detection of H-2 antigenicity have long been laborious, time consuming, and semiquantitative at best, and have required relatively large amounts of material. Second, H-2 antigens are associated with a complex organelle (the cell membrane) from which they are released only with difficulty.

A. Methods

The general approach to biochemical analysis of H-2 antigens consists of three steps: solubilization, purification, and characterization. Each step requires a special, often complicated methodology as well as assays for monitoring H-2 antigens.

1. Solubilization

Solubilization consists of releasing H-2 macromolecules from the membrane into solution. An H-2 preparation is considered solubilized when it is optically

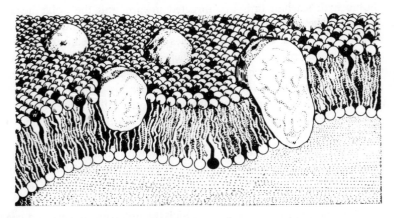

Fig. 15-3. Fluid mosaic model of the plasma membrane. In the bilayer sea of lipids (shaded) and cholesterol (solid), the globular and amphipathic proteins float as icebergs, with their hydrophilic ends protruding from the membrane and their hydrophobic ends embedded in the bilayer. (Reproduced with permission from S. J. Singer: "Architecture and Topography of Biologic Membranes." *Hospital Practice* 8:31–90. Copyright © 1973 by Hospital Practice Co. All rights reserved.)

clear and does not sediment at high-speed centrifugation (10^7g). However, this definition is not meant to imply that the H-2 molecules are actually dissolved in solution in the same way as, for instance, a salt crystal is dissolved in water. Both criteria (optical clarity and failure to sediment) can be met by a mere dispersion of the membrane into fine particles without reducing the proteins and lipids to their fundamental molecular size. The criteria indicate only a considerable reduction in particle size.

The source of material for solubilization can be transplantable tumors (Kandutsch and Reinert-Wenck 1957; Kandutsch and Stimpfling 1963), normal lymphoid tissues (Billingham *et al.* 1958; Oth and Castermans 1959; Manson *et al.* 1960b), liver (Herzenberg and Herzenberg 1961; Ozer and Herzenberg 1962), embryonic tissues (Edidin 1966), and lymphoid cells in a long-term tissue culture (Manson and Palm 1968).

The membrane components are believed to be held together by coulombic, van der Waals, hydrophobic, and hydrogen bonds; covalent lipid-protein bonds and interchain disulfide linkages do not seem to contribute significantly to stabilization of the membrane architecture. It is therefore not surprising that among the agents used to disperse membrane components, those that disrupt electrostatic and hydrophobic interactions are prominent. The agents used for solubilization of H-2 antigens are detergents, organic solvents, proleotytic enzymes, chaotropic and chelating agents, and low- or high-frequency sound.

a. **Detergents.** A detergent is a substance that gives cleansing properties to a liquid when dissolved in it. Detergents resemble such lipids as phosphoglycerides in that they too have strong polar regions and long-chain hydrocarbon nonpolar tails. The introduction of a detergent into water results in the formation of *micelles*, that is, small, usually spherical aggregates in which the hydrophobic hydrocarbon tails are directed inward and the polar heads are oriented toward the aqueous environment (Fig. 15–4). When a detergent comes into contact with a lipid, the lipid molecules are incorporated into the micelles by a mechanism, the precise nature of which is dependent on the properties of the lipid. If the lipid is relatively polar, its molecules are simply integrated with those of the detergent; if, on the other hand, the lipid is nonpolar, its molecules are engulfed by the micelle and incorporated into the tail portions of the detergent molecules (Fig. 15–4). Because the detergent is dissolved in water (in the form of micelles), the incorporation into the micelles solubilizes the lipid. Solubilization of the cell membrane by the detergent is believed to occur on the same principle, namely by incorporation of the membrane lipids into the micelles and release of the membrane proteins into the solution.

Detergents can be classified, on the basis of the nature of their polar groups, into three major categories: *anionic*, in which the polar group carries a negative electric charge, *cationic*, with positively charged polar groups, and *nonionic*, in which the whole molecule carries no electric charge and produces electrically neutral micelles in solution.

The detergents used for H-2 antigen solubilization are Triton X-100 (Kandutsch and Reinert-Wenck 1957), Triton X-114 (Hilgert *et al.* 1969), deoxycholate (Moreno 1966), sodium dodecyl sulfate (Manson and Palm 1968), potassium cholate (Hilgert *et al.* 1969) and Nonidet P-40 (Schwartz and Nathenson 1971a; Vitetta *et al.* 1972a).

The Triton series is a group of commercially developed nonionic detergents, effective at concentrations from 0.1 to 10 percent. The H-2 preparations obtained after *Triton X-100*, treatment are homogeneous by electrophoretic and ultra-centrifugal analysis in the presence of the detergent; removal of the detergent by dialysis against water causes aggregation and precipitation of the anti-genically active fraction (Kandutsch and Stimpfling 1963). The water-insoluble material can be solubilized by digestion with snake venom, specifically with the enzyme phospholipase A, which is present in the venom (Kandutsch *et al.* 1965). The enzyme apparently acts by removing one of the fatty acids of the lecithin

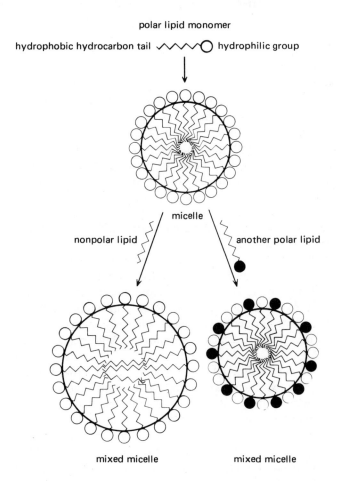

Fig. 15-4. Formation of micelles in the presence of a detergent. (Reproduced with permission from E. J. Masoro: *Physiological Chemistry of Lipids in Mammals.* Copyright © 1968 by W. B. Saunders Co. All rights reserved.)

(or cephalin) and producing lysolecithin, which then inhibits aggregation of the antigenically active material. *Triton X-114* appears to be more efficient in solubilizing H-2 antigens than Triton X-100; the former requires a shorter extraction period (30 min compared to 10 days of Triton X-100 treatment) and a lower concentration of detergent (Hilgert *et al.* 1969).

Nonidet P-40 (NP-40) is a commercially developed nonionic detergent, probably the best H-2 solubilizing agent currently available. Its efficiency is estimated to be close to 100 percent, it solubilizes plasma membranes but not nuclear membranes, it acts in a low concentration (0.5 percent), and it interferes with neither antigen-antibody nor enzymatic reactions (Schwartz and Nathenson 1971a).

Cholates are salts of bile (cholic) acid, a steroid produced by degradation of cholesterol (deoxycholates are similarly derived from deoxycholic acid). They act as strong anionic detergents, disrupting the cell membrane into fine lipoprotein particles.

Sodium dodecyl sulfate (SDS) is an anionic detergent widely used in membrane chemistry. Brief incubation of cells with saturating levels of SDS often fully dissociates membrane proteins from each other and from membrane lipids, and transforms them into protein-SDS and lipid-SDS complexes, bearing the charge of the detergent. The protein-SDS complexes exist in the form of detergent monomers rather than micelles. In the complexes, the proteins apparently always assume the same conformation, one in which the polypeptide chain is folded into a hairpinlike structure stabilized by an envelope of bound SDS. A successful use of SDS for solubilization of H-2 antigens is briefly mentioned by Manson and Palm (1968), who were able to maintain the antigens in solution even after removal of the detergent. More recently, U. Hämmerling *et al.* (1971) employed SDS in combination with starch stearate (SST), a derivative of fatty acid that is present in starch.

In general, detergents have an advantage over other solubilizing agents in that they probably release the H-2 macromolecules in a state that is very close to that in the cell membrane. They act in very low concentrations, often stoichiometrically related to the amount of protein, and are therefore believed to be substituting for lipids formerly associated with H-2 molecules. Their main disadvantage is that they are difficult to remove without reaggregating the H-2 preparation.

b. Organic solvents. Although lipids contain polar groups, the enormous physical mass of the two nonpolar hydrocarbon chains causes them to behave essentially as nonpolar molecules. Consequently, they can easily intermingle with other nonpolar molecules such as molecules of nonpolar (organic) solvents (the lipid and solvent molecules do not significantly attract each other, and thus can intermix). Upon extraction of membrane fragments with butanol, the lipids enter the butanol phase, the proteins separate into the water phase, and small amounts of insoluble protein collect at the interphase.

c. Proteolytic Enzymes. Proteolytic enzymes (proteases) catalyze the hydrolysis of the peptide bond between two amino acids in a polypeptide chain.

Because it is assumed that the bulk of H-2 antigenicity resides in protein, and because the enzymes often attack a specific peptide bond in the polypeptide chain, it should be possible, theoretically, to find a protease that would attack the bond close to the H-2 molecule's membrane anchoring site and thus release a major fragment of this molecule from the membrane. Enzymes that have been used for H-2 antigen extraction include ficin (Nathenson and D. Davies 1966b), trypsin (Edidin 1966, 1967), papain (Nathenson and Shimada 1968), bromelin (Summerell and D. Davies 1969), and chymotrypsin, subtilisin, and thermolysin (Cherry *et al.* 1970).

Papain, an enzyme isolated from the latex of *Carica papaya*, has a rather broad specificity, although it does show some preference for peptide bonds involving the amino acids arginin and lysin. Maximum proteolytic activity of this enzyme is achieved in the presence of cysteine and ethylenediamine tetra-acetate (EDTA). Other plant proteases, such as ficin and bromelin, appear to act in a way similar to that of papain.

Trypsin is a protease, derived from mammalian pancreas, which catalyzes the hydrolysis of the peptide bond involving the amino acids arginin and lysin. *Chymotrypsin* splits peptide bonds involving aromatic amino acids.

Proteolytic action is also presumed to be the major factor in solubilization of H-2 antigens by *autolysis* (Nathenson and D. Davies 1966a), a method in which cell homogenates are suspended in Tris-buffered saline and incubated at physiological pH and a temperature of 37°C. In this case, the enzymes are supplied by the cells themselves. The main drawback of the autolysis method is its lack of reproductibility. An obvious disadvantage of the enzymatic methods in general is their fragmentation of H-2 molecules, which makes interpretation of results at the molecular level difficult. In addition, the methods usually suffer from relatively small yields, with losses of H-2 activity as high as 98 percent.

d. Chaotropic agents. The nonpolar groups of membrane components are insoluble in water because first, they carry no charge and therefore have no strong attraction for water molecules, and second, water molecules have a relatively strong attraction for each other and therefore do not permit simple mixing with nonpolar molecules. It follows that any agent that disorganizes the structure of water and reduces the attraction among water molecules, should, theoretically, facilitate the entry of nonpolar molecules into the aqueous phase. Such facilitation has been demonstrated for *chaotropic agents*, which are inorganic ions with a disorganizing effect on water structure. Of the numerous chaotropic agents that have been applied to solubilization of membrane proteins, only the Cl^- anion in the form of 3 M KCl has been used for solubilization of H-2 antigens (Götze *et al.* 1972; Götze and Reisfeld 1974; Ahmed *et al.* 1973; Ranney *et al.* 1973). However, according to D. Mann (1972), the antigens released during the KCl solubilization procedure are not the result of chaotropic action of the Cl^- anions, but are, rather, the products of digestion by intracellular enzymes.

e. Chelating agents. Chelating agents are ligands[2] capable of attachment to

---

[2] Ligands are molecules, atoms, or ions capable of donating electrons to an acceptor.

a metal atom or ion at more than one point. Treatment with those chelating agents that bind divalent cations has been found to dissociate a variety of tissues of both embryos and adult animals. The release of H-2 antigens upon treatment of embryonic tissues with ethylenediaminetetraacetic acid (EDTA or Versene) was reported by Edidin (1966). The mechanism of EDTA action in solubilization of H-2 antigens is not known.

f. Sonication. The introduction of ultrasound into a cell suspension sets into motion several complex phenomena, the most prominent of which is *cavitation.* As the sound wave passes through the liquid, the succession of positive and negative pressures produces cavities, which become filled with any gas dissolved in the liquid. The cavities expand and then violently collapse and thus produce surface changes that result in cell destruction and dispersion of the membrane components. The degree of destruction depends on the intensity of the ultrasound: the greater the intensity, the more pronounced are the changes. Low-intensity sounds cause primarily simple mechanical fragmentation, whereas high-intensity sonication is accompanied by more complex chemical alterations such as peptide bond breakage, disulfide interchange reactions, and denaturation of proteins.

High-intensity sonication was first used as a method of H-2 antigen solubilization by Billingham *et al.* (1956); it produced very poor yields and proved harmful to antigenic activity of the solubilized preparations (Haughton 1966). The use of low-intensity sonication for solubilization of H-2 antigens was reported by Kahan (1965).

The main drawback of sonication methods is that the treatment shears membranes into particles that may not reflect the native state of membrane constituents and their organization. H-2 molecules in these particles may also be noncovalently attached to a number of other membrane proteins.

g. Miscellanea. Other solubilization procedures include hypotonic salt, extraction (Haughton and D. Davies 1962; Pizarro *et al.* 1963; Haughton 1964, 1965; D. Davies 1966), differential centrifugal flotation (Manson *et al.* 1964), hydrolysis with HCl at pH 2 (Vranken-Paris *et al.* 1962), and treatment with citraconic anhydride (DiPadua *et al.* 1973).

Naturally occurring, extramembraneous H-2 antigens have been reported in cell-free ascitic fluid induced by tumor cells (Hašková and Hilgert 1961; D. Davies 1962a, b); however, it is probable that the antigens were associated with cell fragments present in the fluid, which were not originally sedimented under the relatively mild centrifugal conditions used. Such fragments are probably generated by cytolysis.

2. Purification

Solubilization procedures release other components along with H-2 macromolecules from the membrane, and so they result in a heterogeneous mixture from which the antigens must be separated (*purified*). The separation of a specific class of components from a mixture takes advantage of specific physicochemical properties of that component (i.e., its size, density, charge and chemical affinity). Because no single procedure fully separates H-2 antigens from the contaminants, purification usually consists of a series of steps involving different separation techniques. The techniques most frequently used are salt fractionation, centrifugation, chromatography, and radioimmunoprecipitation.

a. Salt fractionation. The addition of a high concentration of neutral salts to an aqueous protein solution changes the properties of water molecules and lowers their interaction with the polar groups of proteins. The interaction between neighboring protein molecules then becomes more favorable than that between protein and water molecules, and the proteins precipitate from the solution (*salting-out effect*). The salts commonly used for salt fractionation are ammonium sulfate and sodium sulfate. Salt fractionation is a simple and convenient technique, but it suffers from a very low resolution power.

b. Centrifugal fractionation. The behavior of a particle during centrifugation depends on its size and density, as well as on the density and viscosity of the medium. The behavior can be described in terms of its *sedimentation coefficient* (*s*), defined as the velocity of the particle per unit of centrifugal field:

$$s = \frac{2r^2(p_p - p_m)}{9\eta}$$

where r is the radius of the particle and p_p its density; p_m is the density and η is the viscosity of the surrounding medium (all in egs units). The sedimentation can be expressed in seconds, or, more commonly, in Svedberg units, $S = s \times 10^{13}$ sec. The above equation applies to spherical particles; particles of other shapes sediment more slowly because of higher friction.

Centrifugal fractionation can be performed in three principal ways: as differential centrifugation, rate zonal centrifugation, and equilibrium centrifugation.

(1) *Differential centrifugation.* In differential centrifugation, the mixture is centrifuged at a certain speed for a certain period of time, the sediment is removed, and the supernatant centrifuged again at higher speed and/or for a longer time period; this pattern is repeated several times.

(2) *Rate zonal centrifugation.* In rate zonal centrifugation, the centrifugation tube is filled with a medium (e.g., sucrose, cesium chloride, or glycerol) that forms a gradient, with the most concentrated medium at the bottom of the tube and the most diluted at the top. (The gradient is prepared automatically by pumps that mix the medium with water in a decreasing ratio as the tube is filled.) The mixture of membrane particles dissolved in a light solvent is then layered on the gradient and centrifugal force is applied. Centrifugation causes each type of particle to sediment down at a specific rate determined by its sedimentation constant. If different classes of particles differ in their sedimentation constants, they segregate into separate bands or zones, which can be harvested individually.

(3) *Equilibrium (isopycnic) centrifugation.* In equilibrium (isopycnic) centrifugation, the particles are mixed with a medium, placed in a centrifugation tube,

and centrifuged for several hours or even days. During centrifugation, a stable density gradient of the medium is formed in the tube, and the particles segregate into bands according to their density. Each particle passing through the gradient stops its centrifugal motion (comes into buoyant equilibrium) at a position where its density exactly equals that of the surrounding medium (isopycnic density; $p_p = p_m$, and therefore, $s = 0$).

c. Column chromatography. Chromatography is a process of separating chemical compounds in a mixture by adsorption or extraction as the mixture flows over the adsorbend or extraction medium. Of the numerous chromatographic procedures, only two—exclusion chromatography and ion-exchange chromatography—will be described here.

(1) *Exclusion chromatography* (*gel filtration*). In exclusion chromatography (gel filtration), separation of molecular classes in a mixture is achieved on small polymer beads, usually composed of cross-linked sugar macromolecules. The polymer most widely used is Sephadex, a dextran that comes in different degrees of cross-linkage and hence fractionation range (G-10 through G-200). The beads are allowed to swell in water, buffer, or other solution, and the resulting gel is packed in a column. The mixture is applied to the top of the column, and a buffer solution is allowed to percolate through the gel at a constant rate. At the bottom of the column, the eluate is collected in small fractions, and the amount of protein in each fraction is determined by measuring the optical density of the solution at a 280μ wavelength. The hydrated beads have small pores, the size of which is determined by the degree of the sugar's polymerization. Small molecules in the mixture enter the pores (they are *included* in the gel), diffuse into the interior of the beads, and are thus retarded in their flow through the column. Large molecules, on the other hand, are unable to penetrate through the pores and hence pass rapidly through the gel (they are *excluded* from the gel). Each molecular class elutes from the column in a symmetrical peak of concentrations, the peaks of the largest molecules appearing first and the peaks of the smallest molecules last. Because elution of each class composed of molecules distinguished by a particular molecular weight requires a specific volume of eluting buffer, the elution time can be used for molecular-weight estimates. The position of the test peak is simply compared with that of a protein of known molecular weight.

(2) *Ion-exchange chromatography.* Ion-exchangers are materials consisting of an insoluble matrix (a synthetic resin, polysaccharide, or protein), fixed, electrically charged groups, and mobile ions of opposing charge. According to the charge, the exchangers can be distinguished into anionic (with positively charged fixed groups and negatively charged mobile anions), and cationic (with negatively charged groups and mobile cations). The anionic exchanger most frequently used in H-2 purification procedures is diethyl aminoethyl cellulose (abbreviated DEAE-cellulose), the matrix of which is cellulose, the charged group is DEAE, and the mobile ions are chloride anions. The swollen DEAE-cellulose is packed into a column, the sample dissolved in buffer and applied to the top of the bed, and the column is developed with an eluting buffer of

increasing ionic strength or pH. The electrostatically charged groups in the proteins of the sample displace some of the mobile Cl^- ions from the cellulose beads, the degree of displacement being dependent on three factors: the strength of the protein charge, and the pH and salt concentration of the eluting buffer. By changing the pH of the buffer and thus affecting the charge of the protein molecules, or by increasing the molarity of the buffer and thus introducing more ions to compete with the proteins for the charged groups, the proteins are released from the beads and move down the column. The various classes of proteins are released (eluted) at different rates and thus separate into different fractions (each in a characteristic peak) of the eluate.

d. Electrophoresis. When a protein mixture is placed in a buffer of a given pH and an electric current is applied, the proteins migrate to the positive or negative pole according to their charge at that pH. The migration of particles in an electric field is called *electrophoresis*. Of the numerous forms of electrophoresis that are currently available, only one will be described here, namely the polyacrylamide gel electrophoresis (PAGE). The advantage of this method is that it separates molecules according not only to their net charge but also to their size. Polyacrylamide is a cross-linked polymer that, under certain conditions, forms gels of a defined porosity, the size of the pores being determined by the concentration of the polymer. The porous gels act as a supporting medium for the protein mixture, as well as a filtering sieve separating the proteins into sharp bands which can be stained for better viewing. However, solubilized membrane proteins usually do not penetrate polyacrylamide gels at all, either because they are not completely dispersed, or because they reaggregate upon exposure to the low ionic-strength buffer used in electrophoresis. This obstacle is bypassed by carrying the electrophoresis at high ionic-strength and by saturating the protein mixtures with denaturants or detergents, most commonly with SDS (*SDS-PAGE system*). Proteins dispersed in SDS (in the presence of urea and SH reducers to split any possible —S—S— linkages) dissociate from each other and from membrane lipids as polypeptide-SDS complexes bearing the charge of the detergent; in addition, the polypeptide chains unwind and assume a uniform conformation and charge density. Because of their uniformity, the molecules separate primarily according to the logarithm of their molecular weights. The SDS-PAGE system can therefore be used not only for separation of proteins, but also for estimating their molecular weights (by comparison with the mobility of known-molecular-weight proteins).

e. Radioimmune precipitation. Among the most potent methods of H-2 antigen purification are those based on the use of isotopes to label the antigens, and the use of antisera to sort them out from solubilized preparations.

H-2 antigens can be labeled externally on the cell surface, or internally inside the cell. With external labeling methods, the cells are incubated with sodium iodide containing a radioactive iodine isotope ($Na^{125}I$), in the presence of the enzyme lactoperoxidase. The enzyme catalyzes the iodide incorporation into the exposed tyrosine (and, to some extent, histidine) groups on proteins. The lactoperoxidase molecules are too large to enter the cells, and consequently only proteins on the cell surface are iodinated. With internal labeling techniques, the cells are incubated in the presence of radioactive precursors of proteins (e.g., ^{14}C-leucine) or sugars (^{3}H-fucose), and the radioactive label is incorporated into the H-2 molecules during their biosynthesis.

The labeled H-2 antigens are then solubilized by one of the techniques described in the previous section, and separated from the rest of the labeled molecular species by immunoprecipitation, which consists of reacting the soluble preparation first with a specific H-2 alloantiserum and then with a xeno (e.g., rabbit) antimouse Ig serum. The reaction between the H-2 antigens and the alloantiserum produces soluble antigen-antibody complexes; the attachment of the xenoantibody to these complexes results in formation of insoluble precipitate, which can be removed from the mixture by centrifugation. The complexes can then be dissociated and the highly purified H-2 antigens released.

3. Characterization

Characterization of purified H-2 antigens rests upon determination of their physicochemical properties (such as molecular weight and subunit structure), chemical nature, and chemical composition. Many methods used in the characterization step are identical with the purification methods described in the preceding section; however, some special methods are also required, namely those used in protein biochemistry. The chemical characterization of proteins requires determination of their amino acid composition, peptide mapping, and amino acid sequencing.

a. Amino acid composition. The amino acid composition of a protein is determined by complete hydrolysis of its molecules, usually by boiling them with an excess of HCl (a process that cleaves the polypeptide chains into single amino acids). The types and number of amino acids in the hydrolyzate are then determined by ion-exchange chromatography. This analysis provides information about the proportional representation of individual amino acids in a given protein species.

b. Peptide mapping. In the second step of protein analysis, the polypeptide chains are fragmented into smaller peptides by partial hydrolysis and the peptides are then separated by ion-exchange chromatography, paper chromatography, or paper electrophoresis to form a two-dimensional map (*peptide map*), in which each peptide (revealed as a spot after proper staining) occupies a characteristic position. The arrangement of the spots in the peptide map is specific for each protein. Partial hydrolysis is usually performed in two stages. In the first stage, the proteins are incubated with trypsin, which cleaves the peptide bonds between lysine and arginine, and in the second stage the peptides are further fragmented by treatment with cyanogen bromide, which cleaves peptide bonds involving methionine residues.

c. Amino acid sequencing. The ultimate goal of chemical protein analysis is the determination of the protein's primary structure, that is, the sequence of amino acids in its polypeptide chains. Amino acid sequencing consists of splitting the polypeptide chains into small peptides, separating the peptides, and then determining (with special methods) the sequence of amino acids in each peptide.[3]

4. H-2 Antigen Assay Systems

During the entire procedure of chemical isolation, purification, and characterization, the presence of H-2 antigens must be monitored constantly through the use of a suitable assay system. The major systems of H-2 antigen detection are graft rejection, enhancement, elicitation of humoral antibodies, and inhibition of humoral antibodies in appropriate antisera.

In the graft rejection assay, mice are injected with the H-2 antigen preparation and the presensitized recipients are challenged with skin (or other tissue) grafts. Accelerated rejection of the grafts in comparison with control grafts transplanted to unsensitized mice is taken as an indication that the preparation contains H-2 activity. The test has many variables, such as the route of administration and the dose of the antigen, the interval between injection and grafting, the nature of the test graft, and the use of adjuvants (for a review, see Kahan 1972).

In the enhancement test, mice are challenged with the antigenic preparation, a graft (usually an allogeneic tumor) is subsequently placed on the same recipients, and prolonged survival of the graft is taken as an indication of the preparation's H-2 activity. The assumption is that the preparation induces humoral antibodies which then interact with the host's immune system in such a way as to prevent or delay the rejection of the graft (for a review, see Kandutsch 1972).

The humoral antibodies induced by the antigenic preparation can be detected directly by any of the available serological techniques.

In antibody inhibition assays, the solubilized antigens are incubated with a corresponding alloantiserum for a certain period of time, after which target cells are added to the system (D. Davies and Hutchinson 1961). If the preparation contains H-2 activity, the antibodies in the antisera bind to the soluble antigen and thus become unavailable for subsequent binding to the target cells (the reactivity of the antiserum with the target cells is inhibited by reaction with the soluble antigens). In this assay, therefore, absence of activity against the target cells (usually measured by the cytotoxic test) indicates presence of activity in the H-2 preparation. (The method as applied to the human HL-A system has been reviewed extensively by Pellegrino *et al.* 1972). Other histocompatibility antigen-detection systems include induction of tolerance (Medawar 1963; Graff and Kandutsch 1969; Law *et al.* 1972), preimmunization of parental strain spleen cells used as donors for induction of graft-versus-host reaction in F_1 hybrid recipients (D. Davies 1963), induction of delayed hypersensitivity

---

[3] For additional information regarding protein analysis the reader is referred to textbooks of biochemistry. A textbook that can be recommended highly is A. L. Lehninger: *Biochemistry. The Molecular Basis of Cell Structure and Function*, Worth, New York, 1970.

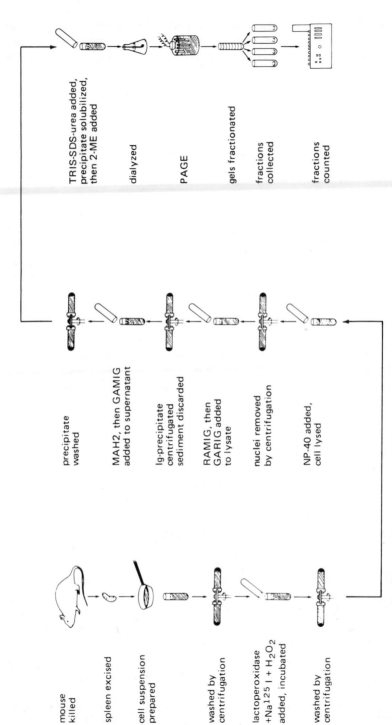

mouse
killed

spleen excised

cell suspension
prepared

washed by
centrifugation

lactoperoxidase
+Na^{125}I + H$_2$O$_2$
added, incubated

washed by
centrifugation

NP-40 added,
cell lysed

nuclei removed
by centrifugation

RAMIG, then
GARIG added
to lysate

Ig-precipitate
centrifugated
sediment discarded

MAH2, then GAMIG
added to supernatant

precipitate
washed

TRIS-SDS-urea added,
precipitate solubilized,
then 2-ME added

dialyzed

PAGE

gels fractionated

fractions
collected

fractions
counted

Fig. 15-5. An example of a procedure for solubilization and purification of H-2 antigens. RAMIG = rabbit antimouse Ig serum; GAMIG = goat antimouse Ig serum; GARIG = goat antirabbit Ig serum; MAH2 = mouse anti-H-2 serum; SDS = sodium dodecylsulfate; 2ME = 2-mercaptoethanol; PAGE = polyacrylamide gel electrophoresis.

(Ranney *et al.* 1973), suppression of the production of hemolytic plaques by spleen cells of mice injected with sheep erythrocytes (Kerman *et al.* 1972), and *in vitro* activation of lymphocytes (Manson and Simmons 1969, 1971).

The various methods of H-2 solubilization, purification, characterization, and detection have been used in many different combinations by numerous investigators. One specific combination, probably the best at present, is depicted diagrammatically in Fig. 15-5.

B. Properties of Purified H-2 Antigens

Antigenic preparations obtained through various solubilization methods differ considerably in their physicochemical and biological properties (Amos *et al.* 1963a), apparently because of the different mechanisms of antigen release. The properties will therefore be described briefly before an attempt is made to summarize and evaluate the current status of H-2 biochemistry. Some of the data have only historical value and are presented here merely to illustrate the long and difficult struggle the H-2 biochemistry has been going through in its quest of the nature of H-2 molecules.

1. Detergent- and Organic Solvent-Solubilized Antigens

a. **Triton- and cholate-solubilized antigens.** These treatments have been used by Kandutsch and Reinert-Wenck (1957), Kandutsch (1960, 1964), Kandutsch and Stimpfling (1963, 1965), Al-Askari *et al.* (1964), Kandutsch *et al.* (1965), Moreno (1966), Graff and Kandutsch (1966, 1969), Hilgert *et al.* (1969), Harris *et al.* (1971a, b), Kerman and Harris (1972), and Kerman *et al.* (1972).

According to Kandutsch and Stimpfling (1965), treatment of a particulate fraction obtained from Sarcoma I (an A strain tumor) with Triton X-100 produces a preparation that is insoluble in water at neutral pH, but soluble in 1 percent Triton solution. The preparation is essentially a lipoprotein containing less than 3 percent carbohydrate (hexose, hexosamine, and sialic acid), 15–30 percent lipid, the remainder being protein. Lipid extracted from this preparation shows no H-2 activity, indicating that the antigenicity resides either in the carbohydrate, in the protein, or in both. The protein contains all the common amino acids (including cysteine and methionine), with a predominance of glutamic acid, aspartic acid, and leucine. Incubation with snake venom, purified phospholipase A, or lysolecithin converts the lipoprotein, without any appreciable change in chemical composition, into a form soluble at neutral pH in the absence of detergent. Approximately 90 percent of the phospholipase-treated antigenic material is excluded from a Sephadex G-200 column (the high-molecular-weight fraction); the remainder (the low-molecular-weight fraction) is retained by the gel and is eluted with the enzyme, from which it can be separated by fractionation with ammonium sulfate. The lysolecithin-solubilized lipoprotein is excluded from the gel. The Triton-phospholipase A- and lyso-lecithin-solubilized materials are homogeneous by electrophoretic criteria but are highly heterogeneous when examined at pH 8.4 ultracentrifugation. Centrifugation at pH 12 produces a single broad peak with a sedimentation coefficient of 3.9; lowering of the pH back to 8.4 causes reversion to the original hetero-geneity. This behavior has been explained as being caused by the tendency of the lipoprotein toward formation of aggregates; partial dissociation of the aggregates is achieved by the addition of Triton, lysolecithin, or phospholipase A, but complete dissociation is achieved only when the action of phospholipase A is supplemented by elevation of the pH to 12. The high-molecular-weight fraction can be separated into two subfractions by chromatography on DEAE-cellulose, one subfraction (the larger) eluted at pH 7.4, and the other (the smaller) at pH 10.2. The presence of Triton and other complicating factors does not permit a molecular-weight estimate of the basic monomeric unit, but the retention of a part of the antigenic material by Sephadex G-200 suggests a molecular weight of less than 200,000 daltons. Antigenicity of the three fractions (large and small subfractions of the low-molecular-weight fraction and the high-molecular-weight fraction) has been demonstrated by at least one of the follow-ing assays: enhancement of tumor grafts, elicitation of hemagglutinins, and inhibition of hemagglutinins.

According to Kerman *et al.* (1972), digestion of Triton X-100-solubilized preparations with trypsin or papain yields two fractions of smaller molecular weights that retain H-2 activity. Trypsin digestion yields one fragment that is excluded by Sephadex G-50 but not by G-75, and another fragment that is ex-cluded by G-25 but not by G-50. Papain digestion yields one fragment that is excluded by G-25 but not by G-50, and another fragment that is excluded by G-10 but not by G-15, and, as determined by gel filtration, has a molecular weight slightly lower than vitamin B_{12} (1355).

The preparation obtained after treatment of Sarcoma I with Triton X-114 (Hilgert *et al.* 1969) is insoluble in the absence of the detergent at neutral pH. When dissolved in 1 percent Triton at pH 7.6, it is eluted as a single peak from agarose and Sephadex G-200 columns, indicating a molecular weight between 100,000 and 200,000 daltons. The preparation inhibits cytotoxic antibodies in the ^{51}Cr-release assay.

Of the material produced by treatment with potassium cholate in 4M NaCl, only a small fraction is retained by a Sephadex G-200 column (molecular weight less than 200,000 daltons), while the remainder is excluded (Hilgert *et al.* 1969). Digestion of the cholate extract with trypsin solubilizes approximately two-thirds of the protein.

b. NP-40-solubilized antigens. This treatment has been used by Schwartz and Nathenson (1971a), Schwartz *et al.* (1973a), Vitetta *et al.* (1972b), and DiPadua *et al.* (1973). According to Schwartz *et al.* (1973a), the NP-40-solubilized antigens are eluted from a Bio-Gel A 15-m column as a single peak at a position corresponding to a molecular weight of 380,000 daltons. Boiling of the solu-bilized, immunoprecipitated material in SDS produces two peaks by PAGE, one corresponding to a molecular weight of 88,000 and the other to a molecular weight of 43,000–47,000 daltons. Treatment with SDS and 2-mercaptoethanol produces only a single peak (molecular weight 43,000–47,000 daltons) on

PAGE. The NP-40-solubilized material is composed of protein and carbohydrate and is devoid of choline-containing lipids, although the presence of other lipids has not been ruled out.

c. SDS/SST-solubilized antigens. H-2 antigens solubilized from spleen cells by the combined action of SDS and SST, and detected by inhibition of humoral cytotoxicity, have a molecular weight in the range of several million, as indicated by Sephadex G-200 exclusion and Sepharose 4B inclusion (U. Hämmerling *et al.* 1971). The antigenic material is apparently composed of aggregates that dissociate spontaneously into smaller units, the molecular weight of the basic unit being about 50,000 daltons.

d. Organic solvent-solubilized antigens. This treatment has been used by Kandutsch and Reinert-Wenck (1957), Castermans (1961), Castermans *et al.* (1965), D. Davies (1966), Graff and Kandutsch (1966), Halle-Pannenko *et al.* (1968), Manson and Palm (1968), Harris *et al.* (1971a, b), and Kerman *et al.* (1972).

Extraction of normal lymphoid and tumor cells with 20 percent *n*-butanol (Castermans *et al.* 1965) produces water-soluble preparations containing approximately 50–65 percent proteins, 17 percent lipid, 2 percent hexosamine and about 1 percent saccharides (galactose, mannose, and ribose). The predominant amino acids in the protein portion are aspartic acid, glutamic acid, and leucin. The sedimentation coefficient of the solubilized fragments is between 0.5×10^{-13} and 1×10^{-13}, which indicates a relatively low molecular weight. The preparations sensitize mice to subsequent grafts, elicit hemagglutinin formation, and inhibit hemagglutinins in H-2 antisera.

Extraction of normal lymphoid and tumor cells with an ether-benzene (2:1, v/v) mixture (Halle-Pannenko *et al.* 1968) produces a fraction loosely retained on Sephadex G-200, and a single, H-2 activity-containing peak on DEAE-cellulose, separating into three bands on PAGE.

2. Proteolytically Solubilized Antigens

a. Autolytically solubilized antigens. This treatment has been utilized by Nathenson and D. Davies (1966a); Summerell and D. Davies (1969, 1970); O'Neill and D. Davies (1971); Halle-Pannenko *et al.* (1968, 1970); McPherson *et al.* (1971); and J. Young and Gyenes (1973).

Autolysis of spleen cells produces water-soluble fragments with molecular weights greater than 75,000 and lower than 200,000 (the fragments are excluded from Sephadex G-75 and partially included on Sephadex G-200; cf. Nathenson and D. Davies 1966a). The fragments, consisting of protein (60–65 percent) and carbohydrate (15 percent), inhibit cytotoxic reactions and elicit production of H-2 antibodies.

b. Papain-solubilized antigens. Work in this area has been done by Shimada and Nathenson (1967), Yamane and Nathenson (1970a, b), Cherry *et al.* (1970), Law *et al.* (1971, 1972), and Hess and D. Davies (1974).

According to Shimada and Nathenson (1967), optimal conditions for the release of H-2 antigens by papain digestion of homogenized spleen cells are incubation for 1 hr at 37°C and enzyme dilution 1:10 (one part of enzyme and ten parts crude particulate extract); longer incubation periods or higher enzyme concentrations destroy H-2 activity. The released H-2 antigens are soluble in water and are eluted in the included volume on Sephadex G-200. Chromatography on Sephadex G-150 separates the H-2 preparation into two peaks containing fragments with different H-2 specificities: Class I fragments in the first peak and Class II fragments in the second peak. Each class can be further purified by CM-Sephadex and DEAE-Sephadex chromatography and PAGE at pH 9.4. The purified material forms a single, protein-staining band on PAGE-SDS and can therefore be considered essentially homogeneous. Class I fragments have a molecular weight of about 58,000–65,000 daltons, and contain about 80–90 percent protein, 4 percent neutral carbohydrate, 3–4 percent glucosamine, and 1 percent sialic acid, but no detectable phosphate or lipid. Class II fragments have a molecular weight of about 33,000 to 37,000 daltons, and contain approximately 70–80 percent protein, 7 percent neutral carbohydrate, 1–5 percent glucosamine, 1–3 percent sialic acid. Fragments of both classes inhibit immune cytolysis and induce second-set rejection of skin grafts. An odd and unexplained observation is that in H-2^b preparations, K-series antigens (H-2.5 and 33) are present in Class I fragments and D-series antigens (H-2.2) in Class II fragments; in H-2^d preparations, on the other hand, K-series antigens (H-2.31) are present in Class II fragments and D-series antigens (H-2.3 and 4) in Class I fragments.

c. Trypsin-solubilized antigens.   Work with these antigens has been done by Edidin (1967), Hilgert *et al.* (1971) and Cherry *et al.* (1970).

Trypsin digestion of lymphoid and liver cell stroma, followed by treatment with a chelating agent (EDTA), releases H-2 antigens detectable by their capacity to inhibit cytotoxic alloantisera (Edidin 1967). The solubilized antigens are found in the included volumes of Sephadex G-25 and G-10, which indicates that they are extremely small in size.

Digestion of spleen and tumor cell fractions with trypsin in the presence of potassium cholate releases antigens that can then be fractionated by filtration through Diaflo membranes of defined porosity (Hilgert *et al.* 1971). The filtration separates three fractions with molecular-weight ranges 1,000–50,000, 50,000–100,000, and over 100,000. The first fraction exhibits a low but clearly detectable capacity to inhibit cytotoxic alloantisera, but it does not accelerate tumor graft rejection; the second fraction displays a strong antibody-inhibiting activity but only weak sensitizing activity, and the third fraction moderately inhibits cytotoxic alloantisera and sensitizes strongly against tumor grafts.

d. Antigens solubilized by other proteolytic enzymes.   Antigens solubilized by chymotrypsin, subtilisin, and thermolysin (Cherry *et al.* 1970) have not been sufficiently characterized; antigens solubilized by ficin (Nathenson and Davies 1966b) and bromelin (Summerell and Davies 1969) resemble those solubilized by papain.

3. Antigens Solubilized by Sonication

The sonication preparations have been explored by Billingham *et al.* (1956, 1958); Duplan *et al.* (1960); Manson *et al.* (1960a, 1962); Brent *et al.* (1962); Herzenberg (1962); Kahan (1965); Kahan *et al.* (1964); Zajtchuk *et al.* (1966); Al-Askari *et al.* (1966); Haenen-Severyns *et al.* (1968); Koene *et al.* (1971); McKenzie *et al.* (1971); and Svehag and Schilling (1973).

In the preparations obtained by Kahan (1965), a large portion of H-2 activity was excluded from Sephadex G-200, indicating a molecular weight greater than 200,000. The excluded fraction was soluble in water, was probably largely devoid of lipids, and had buoyant density (as measured by equilibrium centrifugation in 26 percent sodium bromide or in 1.5 M sucrose) of 1.23.

The preparation obtained by Haenen-Severyns *et al.* (1968) was soluble in water, was excluded from Sephadex G-200, contained 30 percent protein, and separated by ultracentrifugation or paper electrophoresis at pH 8.6 into two components, one predominantly proteinaceous and the other lipidic.

McKenzie *et al.* (1971) and Koene *et al.* (1971) obtained a preparation that precipitated in ammonium sulfate at 50 percent saturation, and was excluded from a Sephadex G-200 column. Fractionation of the excluded peak by starch gel electrophoresis produced a material that formed one major band on PAGE. The material was 8 percent carbohydrate, 92 percent protein, and contained no lipid. Lowering of the pH to 4.0 produced fragments that separated into the excluded fraction upon application to Sephadex G-25. The fragments had a molecular weight of 13,000 daltons (compared to 150,000 at pH 7.0). H-2 activity of the fractions was demonstrated by presensitization to skin and tumor grafts and by elicitation of humoral antibody formation.

4. Antigens Solubilized by Other Methods

a. KCl-solubilized antigens. This method has been used by Ahmed *et al.* (1973); Ranney *et al.* (1973) and Götze and Reisfeld (1974). Ahmed *et al.* (1973) obtained from spleen cells a 3 M KCl extract that separated, upon Sephadex G-200 gel filtration, into three peaks, the middle peak containing most of the cytotoxicity-inhibition capacity and corresponding to a molecular weight between 60,000 and 180,000 daltons. Electrophoresis of the crude extract in 7.5 percent polyacrylamide gels produced several not easily discernible bands. The capability of the KCl-extracted H-2 antigens to elicit formation of H-2 antibodies, to cause delayed hypersensitivity, and to accelerate graft rejection was demonstrated by Ranney *et al.* (1973).

b. EDTA-solubilized antigens. The treatment of 10-day-old embryos with EDTA released water-soluble material possessing H-2 activity, which was detected by inhibition of cytotoxic alloantisera (Edidin 1966). The material could be separated by chromatography on Sephadex G-25 into two H-2 active peaks, one slow-eluting peak corresponding to a molecular weight of approximately 2000 daltons, and another faster-eluting peak with a molecular weight of about 8000 daltons. Digestion of the 8000-molecular weight-material with trypsin reduced the molecular weight of the fragments to less than 2000 daltons, while still retaining the material's H-2 inhibiting activity. Since EDTA-extractable H-2 antigens appeared to be present only during early stages of embryo development, Edidin speculated that they might represent precursors of cell-bound antigens.

C. Current Status of H-2 Biochemistry

1. Chemical Nature of H-2 Antigens

All major components of living matter have, at one time or another, been implicated as carriers of H-2 antigenicity. First it was DNA, when Billingham and his co-workers (1956) found that the capacity of nuclear subcellular fractions to presensitize mice against skin grafts was destroyed by DNase but not by RNase or trypsin. The involvement of DNA was subsequently disproved by Hašková and Hrubešová (1958) and by Medawar (1958), who demonstrated that purified DNA fails to elicit accelerated graft rejection, and by Castermans and Oth (1956), who presented evidence that sodium chloride extracts from nuclear homogenates can be divided into two fractions, one containing DNA but having no H-2 activity, and another containing H-2 activity but no DNA.

The attention then focused on another component of the cell membrane, the lipids. Several investigators (Herzenberg and Herzenberg 1961; Lejeune *et al.* 1962; D. Davies 1962a, b; Manson *et al.* 1963) obtained H-2-active, water-insoluble material containing approximately equal amounts of lipids and proteins. D. Davies (1966) directly implicated the lipids as the active agent by demonstrating that organic solvent extraction produced an inactive fraction, consisting primarily of proteins, and an active fraction consisting predominantly of lipids, and that gradual purification of the H-2 material was accompanied by a parallel increase in lipid content. However, the lipid hypothesis had to be abandoned when Shimada and Nathenson (1969) obtained a soluble H-2 antigenic preparation that contained no detectable lipid, and when Graff and Kandutsch (1966) failed to find any H-2 activity in lipid fractions obtained by chloroform-methanol or methanol-ethanol extraction. It was then the carbohydrates' turn.

Carbohydrates were suspected of involvement in H-2 antigenicity as early as 1957 (Kandutsch and Reinert-Wenck 1957). The three main arguments suggesting that carbohydrates may participate in determining H-2 antigenicity are the following. First, H-2 antigenicity is destroyed by treatment with dilute solutions of sodium periodate (Kandutsch and Reinert-Wenck 1957; Brent *et al.* 1961; Kerman and Harris 1972), believed to be responsible for splitting carbon-carbon bonds in carbohydrates. Periodate is known to inactivate mucoprotein and mucopolysaccharide (human blood group) antigens. However, because periodate could also be inactivating proteins by reacting with their hydroxylysine or terminal amino acid residues, this evidence is ambiguous at best. Recent studies by Kerman and Harris (1972) suggest that the inactivation of H-2 antigens by periodate is due to deformation of the molecule in carbohydrate-containing areas outside the antigenic sites, with loss of structural support on which the configurational integrity of the antigenic determinant depends. Second, H-2 antigenicity is destroyed by incubation with a crude extract of *Trichomonas foetus* (Billingham *et al.* 1958), known to contain enzymes that inactivate human ABH polysaccharides. However, because the specificity of the extract was not rigorously tested to establish that it did not destroy protein activity as well, this evidence is also ambiguous. Third, the activity of H-2 alloantisera is inhibited by purified human blood group A mycopolysaccharides, by type XIV pneumococcal polysaccharide, and by a *Shigella shiga* polysaccharide (Brent *et al.* 1961). Similarly, D. Davies (1965) demonstrated a partial, nonspecific inhibition of H-2 antisera by D-galacto-pyranosyl-(1,4)-β-D-glucasomine residues and by N-glycolylneuraminic acid, and Stetson and Esko (1967) found that various antibacterial (presumably anticarbohydrate) sera were capable of discriminating among erythrocytes of various mouse strains. This third argument, however, can be criticized on the basis of nonspecific inhibition, which could involve both carbohydrate and noncarbohydrate structures of the H-2 glycoprotein.

Hence, at present there is no compelling and unambiguous evidence that carbohydrates are part of the H-2 antigenic sites. On the contrary, there is the following strong evidence indicating that carbohydrates are *not* involved in H-2 antigenicity. First, when the papain-solubilized H-2 glycoprotein is fragmented into peptides and the peptide bearing the carbohydrate chain is isolated, no H-2 antibody inhibitory or binding activity is found (Muramatsu and Nathenson 1970a, b). If the carbohydrate portion carried the antigenic sites, the isolated glycopeptide should have carried at least a small amount of hapten activity. Second, removal of all the sialic acid, over 70 percent of the galactose, and about 25 percent of the glucosamine from the purified H-2 glycoprotein does not alter its H-2 antibody binding activity (Shimada and Nathenson 1971). Third, a comparison of the composition and structure of carbohydrates from different *H-2* haplotypes reveals no major difference among them (Shimada and Nathenson 1971; Muramatsu and Nathenson 1971). It therefore appears highly unlikely that the H-2 antigenic sites reside in the carbohydrate portion of the H-2 glycoprotein.

And so one is left with the proteins. Although the presence of proteins in H-2 preparations has never been seriously questioned, their conjectured role as sites of H-2 antigenicity has been challenged on the basis of the fact that H-2 activity is not destroyed by proteolytic enzymes. But it is now known that proteolysis leaves a considerable portion of the H-2 protein intact, so the challenge is thwarted. Furthermore, it has been demonstrated that *prolonged exposure* of H-2 preparations to the proteolytic action of enzymes does destroy H-2 activity. The main arguments in favor of protein participation in H-2 antigenicity are the following.

First, H-2 activity, as measured by hemagglutinin inhibition and induction of immunological enhancement, is lost from preparations exposed to protein-denaturing agents (such as urea, 90 percent phenol, aqueous alcohol, acid, or alkali), low (below 4) or high (over 9) pH values, heat, and pronase (Kandutsch and Reinert-Wenck 1957; Brent *et al.* 1961, 1962; Kandutsch and Stimpfling 1965). Second, H-2 antigens are inactivated by reagents binding to amino acids in the polypeptide chain. Pancake and Nathenson (1973) demonstrated that modification of tyrosine residues using N-acetylimidazole or tetranitromethane was followed by inactivation of all H-2 antigens measured. Reagents thought to be specific for amino groups inactivated some antigens but not others. Similarly, DiPadua *et al.* (1973) observed that "blocking" of lysine residues with citraconic anhydride rendered the H-2 preparations antigenically inactive in both the ^{51}Cr-inhibition test and in *in vivo* tests; after deblocking, 13 percent of the H-2 activity found on whole cells was recovered in soluble form. Third, protein is a major component of all H-2 antigenic preparations. For instance, the papain-solubilized preparations are glycoproteins, in which proteins constitute 90 percent of the material (Shimada and Nathenson 1967). Fourth, glycoproteins isolated from different *H-2* haplotypes differ in their amino acid composition and in their peptide maps (see below).

Thus, the controversy that spanned almost three decades appears finally to be resolved in favor of the protein model of H-2 antigenicity. It could, of course, still be argued that the carbohydrate moiety at least *contributes* to the antigenic site residing in the protein, or that some H-2 antigens are protein-aceous whereas others are sugar based. However, the latter possibility is unlikely, because it would require the genes for the enzymes glycosylating the carbohydrate chain to reside in the *H-2* complex (otherwise, the sugar-based antigens would segregate independently of the *H-2* system).

In summary, it seems reasonable to conclude that the H-2 products are glycoproteins composed of 90 percent protein and 10 percent carbohydrate. H-2 antigenicity appears to reside in the protein portion of the H-2 molecules, and the antigenic variation seems to result from differences in amino acid sequences. According to this interpretation, the *H-2* loci code for polypeptide chains, whereas the enzymes responsible for glycosylation are determined by loci probably segregating independently of the *H-2* complex.

2. Molecular, Genetic, and Antigenic Relations

The finding that papain-solubilized H-2 fractions can be separated into two classes, one carrying the H-2D and the other the H-2K antigens, suggests that each *H-2* haplotype codes for at least two distinct polypeptide chains, D and K. This suggestion has recently been confirmed by Cullen *et al.* (1972a), using the NP-40 method of antigen solubilization and the radioimmunoprecipitation method of antigen separation. The authors labeled *H-2^b* antigens with ^{3}H-fucose, solubilized them with the NP-40 detergent, and reacted the soluble material with anti-H-2.2 antibodies in the indirect immunoprecipitation assay. After removal of the precipitate, they reacted the supernatant with anti-H-2.33 serum and found that the pretreatment removed all the H-2.2 activity but did not change the H-2.33 activity. Similarly, pretreatment with anti-H-2.33 serum removed all the H-2.33 activity but did not significantly alter the H.2.2 activity. Hence, the two private antigens of the *H-2^b* haplotype behaved as two independent units, presumably carried by two different polypeptide chains. The authors also demonstrated a similar independent behavior for private antigens H-2.4 and H-2.31, controlled by the *H-2^d* haplotype. Preparations isolated from *H-2^a/H-2^b* heterozygotes contained a mixture of four molecular classes carrying four private antigens controlled by the two *H-2* haplotypes: antigens 4 and 11 controlled by the *H-2^a* haplotype, and antigens 2 and 33 controlled by the *H-2^b* haplotype (Cullen *et al.* 1972b). There is thus little doubt that the *H-2* complex codes for at least two separate polypeptide chains, one carrying the private antigens of the K series and the other those of the D series.

An important question then arises with regard to the behavior of public H-2 antigens in this type of experiment. Cullen *et al.* (1972a) tested two such antigens, H-2.3 and H-2.5, and found that pretreatment with anti-H-2.4 (but not with anti-H-2.31) removed the H-2.3 activity, and pretreatment with anti-H-2.3 significantly lowered the H-2.4 (but not the H-2.31) activity. Similarly, pretreatment with anti-H-2.33 (but not with anti-H-2.2) removed all the H-2.5 activity. These results, which are in agreement with previous studies performed using papain-solubilized antigens (Cullen and Nathenson 1971), indicate that antigen H-2.3 is carried by the same polypeptide as antigen H-2.4 and antigen H-2.5 by the same polypeptide as antigen H-2.33, and hence that antigen H-2.3 is controlled by the same region controlling antigen H-2.4 (*D* region), and antigen H-2.5 by the same region controlling antigen H-2.33 (*K* region). These biochemical data thus disprove the existence of *C* and *E* regions, separate from regions *D* and *K*.

D. Davies and his co-workers (Davies 1969; Summerell and Davies 1969, 1970; O'Neill and Davies 1971) observed that most of the H-2 antigens they tested were present in separate peaks during chromatography on ion-exchange columns, suggesting that they might be present on different molecular fragments. These experiments were performed using autolytically- and/or papain-solubilized fractions, however, so they do not necessarily contradict the conclusions reached by Nathenson and his group. It is possible that the procedure used by Davies and his co-workers caused fragmentation of the native polypeptide chains and thus separation of some antigens.

A rather unorthodox view of the *H-2* gene-antigen relationship has recently been expressed by Hess and D. Davies (1974) on the basis of their experiments with papain-solubilized preparations. The authors solubilized *H-2^d* antigens, purified them by ion-exchange chromatography, gel filtration, and PAGE, and then subjected them to two-dimensional protein mapping using PAGE in one dimension and isotachophoresis in the second dimension. The final products showed a diffuse staining pattern and a broad serological profile when tested with monospecific anti-H-2.4 and 31 sera. (The anti-H-2.4 activity was present in at least two peaks after PAGE.) Because other proteins not related to H-2 produced sharp, well-defined bands, the authors concluded that the H-2 diffuse patterns were not artifacts of the methods but rather a reflection of the existence of true heterogeneity among the H-2 molecules. They postulate that H-2 polypeptides consist of two regions—one relatively constant and carrying the private antigen, and another variable and carrying the public H-2 antigens—and that the latter region is responsible for the observed heterogeneity.

An insight into the relationship among H-2 antigens presumably carried by the same polypeptide chain has been provided by the experiments of Pancake and Nathenson (1973). These authors observed that formaldehyde- or ethyl acetamidate-mediated reductive alkylation and acetamidation of amino groups in the polypeptide chain inactivated some H-2 antigens more easily than others. For example, in the *H-2*^{b} haplotype, antigen H-2.33 was almost totally lost and antigen H-2.5 almost totally retained. Because the two antigens are on the same polypeptide chain, the results suggest that the amino acids involved in the H-2.5 and H-2.33 sites are different and that the two antigens represent two separate sites on the single molecule.

3. Physical Properties

Because of the association of H-2 macromolecules with other components in the membrane, their native form is difficult to determine. The various isolation procedures have produced "molecules" that range in their molecular weight from 2000 to several million daltons. It is therefore most likely that some isolation procedures fragment the H-2 chains into smaller peptides, whereas others release H-2 molecules from the membrane with unrelated molecules bound to them. The matter is further complicated by the fact that the native H-2 macromolecules seem to be complexes, each consisting of several structural units. It appears that at present the closest approximation to free (noncovalently bound), native-state H-2 macromolecules is achieved through NP-40-mediated solubilization. On the basis of this method, the H-2 macromolecules can be viewed as having a molecular weight of approximately 400,000 daltons and consisting of two dimers held together by noncovalent bonds (Schwartz *et al.* 1973a). Each dimer has a molecular weight of 43,000–47,000 daltons and consists of a single polypeptide chain with two carbohydrate chains attached to it.

4. Chemical Composition

a. The carbohydrate moiety. Investigations in this area have been made by Muramatsu and Nathenson (1970a, b; 1971); Nathenson and Muramatsu (1971), and McPherson *et al.* (1971). According to Nathenson and Muramatsu (1971), carbohydrates are covalently linked to the protein portion of the H-2 glycoprotein and have a molecular weight of approximately 3300 daltons. Each polypeptide chain has two carbohydrate chains attached to it, and each carbohydrate chain consists of 12–15 monosaccharides. The monosaccharides include neutral sugars (mannose, galactose, and fucose), the amino sugar galactosamine, and sialic acid. Because all the sialic acid, most of the galactose (at least 70 percent), and part of the glucosamine (approximately 50 percent) can easily be released as monosaccharides using their corresponding enzymes, they apparently comprise the outer portion of the carbohydrate chain. Mannose and some glucosamine are released as oligosaccharides, leaving behind fucose and glucosamine (approximately 25 percent) attached to the peptide portion of the glycopeptide. From these results, Muramatsu and Nathenson (1971) proposed a hypothetical model of the carbohydrate chain, depicted in Fig. 15-6. The size and composition of the carbohydrate chains obtained from cells of different *H-2* haplotypes appear to be identical, lending strong support to the conclusion that the sugars are not involved in H-2 antigenic sites. The function of the carbohydrate moeity is not known, but Nathenson and Muramatsu (1971) speculate that the carbohydrate chains could be involved in either biosynthesis and turnover of the H-2 glycoprotein or positioning of the antigens in the membrane (for instance, by orienting the antigenic sites toward the outside of the membrane).

b. The protein moiety. Data on the chemical composition of the protein moiety (Shimada and Nathenson 1969; Shimada *et al.* 1970; Yamane and Nathenson 1970a, b; Yamane *et al.* 1972 and J. Brown *et al.* 1974) are available for the H-2 glycopeptides released by papain digestion and NP 40 solubilization. Because it is now known that papain fragments are smaller than native H-2 polypeptides (the molecular weight of papain-solubilized fragments is about 6000 daltons less than that of intact glyoproteins liberated by NP-40 solubilization, and this difference represents approximately 45 amino acid residues), the papain data must be interpreted with caution.

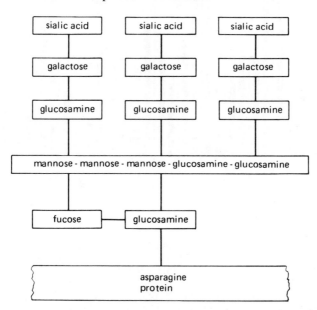

Fig. 15-6. Hypothetical structure of the H-2 carbohydrate chain. (Based on S. G. Nathensen and T. Muramatsu: "Properties of the carbohydrate portion of mouse H-2 alloantigen glycoproteins." In *Glycoproteins of Blood Cells and Plasma*, G. A. Jamieson and T. J. Greenwalt (eds.), pp. 245–262. Lippincott, Philadelphia, 1971.)

The amino acid analysis of papain-solubilized fragments reveals the presence of all common amino acids, and the predominance of glutamic acid and aspartic acid and a relatively low content of histidine, methionine, and tyrosine (Fig. 15–7). The Class I fragments obtained from H-2^b and H-2^d haplotypes differ to only a small extent, in that one (H-2^d) contains 1 mole percent more arginine and glutamic acid than the other. The Class II fragments of the H-2^b and H-2^d haplotypes are somewhat more diverse, with difference of 4 moles percent in serine, 2 moles percent in aspartic acid and about 1 mole percent in valine, isoleucine, leucine, and tyrosine. Taken together, amino acid analyses of Class I and II fragments seem to indicate that the K^b fragment is chemically more related to the D^d than to the K^d fragments, and the D^b fragment is more related to the K^d than to the D^d fragments. The possible implications of this highly unexpected finding will be discussed in Chapter Twenty.

Peptide mapping of Class I fragments reveals that approximately 90 percent of the peptides produced by cyanogen bromide and trypsin treatment are

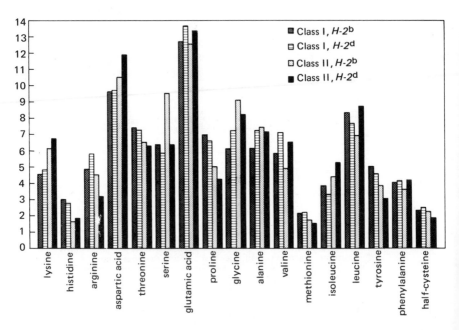

Fig. 15-7. Amino acid composition of papain-solubilized H-2 antigens. (Reproduced with permission from A. Shimada and S. G. Nathenson: "Murine histocompatibility-2 (H-2) alloantigens. Purification and some chemical properties of soluble products from H-2^b and H-2^d genotypes released by papain digestion of membrane fractions." *Biochemistry* **8**:4048–4062. Copyright © 1969 by American Chemical Society. All rights reserved. K. Yamane and S. G. Nathenson: "Murine histocompatibility-2 (H-2) alloantigens. Purification and some chemical properties of a second class of fragments (class II) solubilized by papain from cell membranes of H-2^b and H-2^d mice." *Biochemistry* **9**:1336–1341, Copyright © 1970a by American Chemical Society. All rights reserved.)

identical for both $H-2^b$ and $H-2^d$ preparations, and only 10 percent are different (Fig. 15–8). The $H-2^b$ preparations contain three unique peptides, and the $H-2^d$ preparations contain four unique peptides, whereas 38 peptides are shared by both preparations.

J. Brown *et al.* (1974) NP-40 solubilized H-2K and H-2D glycoproteins labeled with two different isotopes (e.g., H-2K glycoprotein labeled with ^{14}C-arginine and H-2D glycoprotein labeled with ^{3}H-arginine) and compared their peptide structure following trypsin digestion and chromotagraphy of the trypsin peptides on Spherix resin columns. The comparison of $H-2K^b$ and $H-2D^b$ products revealed similar chromatographic behavior of only 11 peptide peaks of a total of 21 and 24 peaks obtained respectively. Products of the $H-2K^d$ and $H-2D^d$ loci shared only 7 peptides of 20 and 25 visualized. The most striking finding, however, was that products of alleles at the same locus (e.g., $H-2K^b$ versus $H-2K^d$; $H-2D^b$ versus $H-2D^d$) contained only about 8 to 9 out of 20 to 26 peptide peaks at similar positions, suggesting again that the interallelic variability is almost as great as the intergenic variability.

5. Evaluation

After almost 20 years of intensive work and several hundred publications, the accomplishments of H-2 biochemistry are not very impressive. The facts established during those 20 years can be summarized in three sentences: (1) the H-2 molecules are membrane-bound glycoproteins; (2) the H-2 antigenicity most likely resides in the protein moiety of the molecule; and (3) one haplotype controls at least two H-2 molecules carrying the *K* and *D* region antigens,

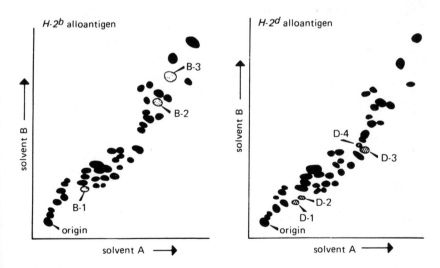

Fig. 15-8. Thin-layer peptide maps of $H-2^b$ Class I fragment (left) and $H-2^d$ Class I fragment (right) after cyanogen bromide and trypsin treatment. (Reproduced with permission from A. Shimada *et al.*: "Comparison of the peptide composition of two histocompatibility-2 alloantigens. *Proc. Nat. Acad. Sci. USA* **65**:691-696, 1970.)

respectively. The rest of the biochemical knowledge of the H-2 antigens is controversial, mainly because the data are based on heterogeneous mixtures rather than pure preparations. Homogeneous H-2 preparations still have not been obtained and a method for obtaining such preparations still is not available. The size of the basic structural unit of the H-2 product is not known. Almost nothing is known about the supramolecular structure of the H-2 products. The biochemical basis of H-2 antigenic variability has not been established, and amino acid sequencing of H-2 molecules is merely a biochemists' dream. Obviously, there are many more years of hard work ahead for H-2 biochemistry.

At present, the NP-40 solubilization method combined with radioimmunoprecipitation is clearly the most promising approach to the characterization of H-2 antigens. Among the questions that this method can answer, the most critical are those concerning H-2 antigen distribution among individual polypeptide chains controlled by different regions of the *H-2* complex, the chemical relationship between these polypeptides, and the relationship of the H-2 products to products of functionally related loci, such as *Ia* or *Lad*.

III. Biosynthesis of H-2 Antigens

A. Cellular Aspects

During a study designed to select *H-2* variants from heterozygous lymphomas by treatment of cells *in vitro* with alloantisera, E. Klein and G. Klein (1964) observed an odd phenomenon (see Chapter Twelve). When H-2 antibodies and complement were applied to the culture, a certain proportion of the cells was killed; however, when the survivors were allowed to multiply, the new population behaved in the same way as the original, in that most of the cells were again susceptible to the antibodies. The clue to this failure to select *H-2* variants was provided by Bjaring *et al.* (1969), who cultured mouse lymphoma cells *in vitro* for periods varying from 5 to 240 min, and tested the sensitivity of these cells to the cytotoxic action of H-2 antisera in the presence of complement at regular intervals. They found that the sensitivity was subject to cyclic variations with consecutive high and low values. The authors therefore concluded that the expression of H-2 antigens fluctuates during *in vitro* cultivation in a periodic fashion. On the basis of this observation, the "reappearance" of sensitive cells in the Kleins' experiment can be explained by assuming that the survivors were not true variants but merely cells that happened to be in the "low" period of cyclic variation.

The periodicity of the quantitative variation prompted Cikes (1970a, b; 1971a, b) to investigate its relationship to the life cycle of the cell.[4] The investiga-

---

[4] The life cycle of a dividing cell can be separated into four periods: M or mitotic period in which the cell divides; S or synthetic period in which DNA is synthesized, as determined by incorporation of radioactive thymidine; G_1 or gap period between the end of mitosis and the beginning of DNA synthesis, and G_2 or gap period between the end of DNA synthesis and the beginning of mitosis. The sequence of the periods is $M—G_1—S—G_2$. If a small number of

tion revealed that the percentage of cells killed by H-2 antiserum and complement was inversely proportional to the cell volume as well as to the growth rate. A seemingly logical explanation of this relationship was that the increase in cell surface area resulted in a sparser distribution of H-2 antigens, and hence in lower sensitivity of the cells to cytotoxic action of H-2 antibodies. This explanation was ruled out, however, by the demonstration that large immunoresistant cells have lower absorptive and fluorescent-antibody-binding capacities than small immunosensitive cells, implying a reduced number of H-2 sites on large cells. Analysis of the cells' life cycle suggested that the growth rate of the cultures was primarily determined by the duration of the G_1 period: the fast-growing cells had a relatively short G_1 period and as the growth rate declined, cells accumulated in G_1. The implication of this finding was that H-2 antigens are maximally expressed during the G_1 period. Direct proof of this implication was provided by experiments on synchronized cell cultures (Cikes and Friberg 1971) in which the highest proportion of antigen-positive cells was found during the G_1 period; during S and G_2 periods the antigen concentration was low, and increased again only when the majority of the cells divided and entered the G_1 period of the next cycle. Markedly decreased concentration of H-2 antigens during the S period was also observed by Pasternak *et al.* (1971). The variation of H-2 antigenicity in "asynchronous" cultures was explained by Cikes and G. Klein (1972a, b) and by Cikes *et al.* (1972) as being caused by synchronizing effects of dilution and resuspension of cells in fresh medium and the subsequent increase in cell density. The authors found the smallest amount of H-2 antigens during the early exponential phase, when the population-doubling time was shortest (apparently because most cells were dividing); as the growth rate slowed down, the relative antigen concentration increased until the stationary phase, when the maximum concentration of H-2 antigens was present on the cell surface. Exponentially growing cells (mostly cells in the S period) carried approximately one-third to one-half the number of H-2 antigens carried by stationary (mostly G_1) cells. Stationary cells were reversibly arrested in the G_1 period and could be released by dilution and incubation in a fresh medium. Reexpression of H-2 antigens after the first cell division following release from the G_1 block

---

cultured cells is transferred into a fresh medium, the cells continue to divide at a constant rate and their number increases in an *exponential* (logarithmic) fashion. The exponential growth continues until the conditions in the culture begin to deteriorate, at which point the growth slows and enters a *stationary phase*. The rate of growth in the exponential phase can be characterized mathematically by the formula

$$\log N = \log N_0 + kt \log 2$$

where N is the number of cells at time t, N_0 is the number of cells at time 0, and k is the growth-rate constant. The growth rate is determined primarily by the duration of the life cycle of the individual cells: the shorter the life cycle, the steeper the growth curve (i.e., the change in the number of cells as a function of time). In a standard tissue culture at any given moment, cells exist at various stages of their life cycles, so the culture is said to be *unsynchronized*. However, through the use of special treatments, the life cycles can be *synchronized* for several generations so that at any given moment most of the cells in the culture are at the same stage. A synchronized culture becomes unsynchronized when minor random variations in the duration of the life cycle of individual cells cause each cell to grow at its own pace.

depended on the final cell density of the culture. If the cells reached the final density after the first cell division following release from the G_1 block, H-2 antigens were fully reexpressed, but if the final cell density was higher than the density attained after the first division, the H-2 antigen concentration remained low.

The maximal expression of H-2 antigens during the G_1 period logically explains the inverse relation between the cell size and H-2 antigen content, because small cells are probably those in early interphase, primarily the G_1 period.

Cikes (1971b) postulated that the life cycle-dependent variation in H-2 antigen content was the result of derepression of H-2 genes occurring only during a limited time (the G_1 period). This conclusion was challenged by Lerner *et al.* (1971), who observed variations in sensitivity to immune cytolysis, but failed to confirm Cikes's data on life cycle-dependent changes using immuno-fluorescent staining. They suggested instead that the cytotoxic sensitivity variations were caused by differences in the mechanical properties of the membrane, by the ability of cells to repair membrane damage, or by the extent of the complement system's activation. However, Cikes and G. Klein (1972a) recently were able to demonstrate that extracts from cells arrested reversibly in the G_1 period (cells in the stationary phase) displayed approximately three times more H-2 activity (as measured by inhibition of ^{51}Cr cytolysis) than extracts from exponentially growing (S-phase) cells, implying a true variation in H-2 antigen expression.

The expression of H-2 antigens in logarithmically growing cultures is enhanced by the addition of actinomycin D (inhibitor of RNA synthesis), and this enhancement can be blocked by inhibitors of protein synthesis (mitomycin C, hydroxyurea, and cytosine arabinoside, cf. Cikes and G. Klein 1972b). On the other hand, cells cultured in medium with a low concentration of fetal calf serum ("starved" cells) show a decreased expression of H-2 antigens. When starved cells (i.e., cells presumably deprived of intracellular macromolecular pools) are transferred to fresh medium with 10 percent fetal calf serum, the antigens reappear within a few hours. The increase of H-2 antigens on refeeding can be blocked by protein and RNA inhibitors, but not by DNA inhibitors, suggesting that in "starved" cells the synthesis of RNA and protein is required for the reappearance of the antigens. Cikes and G. Klein (1972b) interpret these results as suggesting that H-2 antigen expression is regulated at the transcriptional[5] or the posttranscriptional level, depending on the cell's physiological state.

B. Molecular Aspects

The cyclic variation of H-2 antigen content of cultured cells suggests that the antigens are in a highly dynamic state and have a relatively rapid turnover

---

[5] Transcription is a process whereby the genetic information contained in DNA is transferred to a complementary sequence of RNA nucleotides.

rate. This suggestion is supported by the regeneration studies of Schwartz and Nathenson (1971b), in which the authors digested intact tumor cells with papain for 1 hr and then tested the H-2 antigen content using inhibition of ^{51}Cr cytolysis. The digestion removed approximately 70 percent of the H-2 activity present on untreated cells, and released about 15 percent of this activity into the solution (the rest was inactivated by the papain treatment). Approximately 90 percent of the cells remained viable during and after the papain treatment, and were able to regenerate the lost antigenicity. After a lag period of 1.5 hr, the H-2 activity of the papain-treated cells began to increase, rising from the initial 30 percent value to 100 percent after 6 hr. The 6-hr period necessary for complete restoration of H-2 activity is considerably shorter than the cell's 24-hr doubling time. However, the restoration may be due to "compensatory" synthesis of H-2 and may not reflect the turnover time.

The rate of H-2 antigen disappearance from whole cells and from cell surfaces was determined by Schwartz *et al.* (1973b). The authors incubated mastocytoma cells in the presence of ^{3}H-fucose or ^{14}C-leucine for 24 hr, then transferred the labeled cells into radiolabel-free medium, removed samples at various intervals, and determined the whole, as well as H-2-specific radioactivity in Triton X-100 extracts and in the material obtained by papain digestion of intact cells. The rate of radiolabel disappearance in cell extracts and in external cell surface fractions followed a typical exponential decay curve, with the time required for disappearance of half the H-2 radioactivity ($t_{1/2}$) equal to 10 hr in the former and 7 hr in the latter case. In comparison, the average turnover rate for the proteins in the crude detergent extract of whole cells had a $t_{1/2}$ of about 20–24 hr. Hence, the turnover rate of H-2 antigens is more than twice as rapid as that of an average protein. According to Wernet *et al.* (1973) and Vitetta *et al.* (1974b), the rapid disappearance of H-2 antigens from the cell surface is not due to a secretion in an antigenically active form, because only 1–2 percent of the H-2 glycoprotein is spontaneously released from spleen lymphocytes and recovered in the incubation medium over a period of 6 hr (compared to 40 percent release of cell surface Ig).

Wernet *et al.* (1973) studied the synthesis of H-2 antigens by labeling spleen cells *in vitro* with ^{3}H-amino acids, homogenizing the cells at various intervals after the incubation, separating microsomes from cell sap, and determining H-2 activity in the two fractions by immunoprecipitation. The experiments indicated that whereas most of the newly labeled non-H-2 proteins were found in the cell sap, the vast portion of H-2 activity was present in the microsomal fraction. These results suggest that contrary to most other proteins, which are released into the cell sap, H-2 antigens remain membrane bound from inception as nascent chains to their exteriorization. Apparently, the synthesis and intracellular transport of H-2 antigens in lymphocytes occur within membranes, presumably on polyribosomes attached to the endoplasmic reticulum.

Part Three

Central Regions of the *H-2* Complex

Section Five

I-Region Associated Traits

Chapter Sixteen

Genetic Control of Virus Susceptibility

I. Leukemia Viruses

The discovery that inbred strains differ in their susceptibility to tumor-inducing (oncogenic) viruses (for a review, see Gross, 1970) triggered a search for genes specifically involved in the control of viral oncongenesis. It was hoped that identification of such genes would provide clues to the mechanism of the neoplastic process itself, but the search was only partially successful. The several genes that were implicated in the viral induction of tumors failed to reveal the mechanism of their involvement. The discovery by Lilly and his co-workers (1964) that viral leukemogenesis could be influenced by the *H-2* system raised new hopes. Here the relationship between the gene and the neoplastic process seemed more apparent and more easily accessible to genetic analysis. Soon after this discovery, six other viruses were also demonstrated to be influenced by the *H-2* system: Tennant virus, radiation-induced leukemia virus, Bittner virus, Friend virus, lymphocytic choriomeningitis virus, and vaccinia virus. Of these, the first five are RNA-containing viruses and the last is a DNA-containing virus. As the mechanism of action is probably different in each of the six, each will be described separately. A brief description of the properties of each virus will also be provided.

A. Lymphatic Leukemia Viruses

1. Gross Virus

Although the incidence of spontaneous leukemia in mouse inbred strains is generally low, the existence of a few high-leukemic strains has been known for some time. Of these strains, two—AKR and C58—were studied in great detail by Gross (1970), who demonstrated that up to 90 percent of AKR and C58 mice develop leukemia spontaneously and that the disease can easily be transferred to other animals of the same strain by inoculating normal adult mice with cell suspensions prepared from spleen, lymph nodes, and liver of the leukemic individuals. He assumed that the disease was of viral etiology, and the virus presumably causing the disease became known as Gross virus (GV).

Gross virus is a spherical particle about 100 mμ in diameter, consisting of RNA surrounded by a protein coating. With an electron microscope, the mature particle (*C particle*) can be seen to have an electron-dense center (nucleoid) and two or three concentric membranes. In leukemic mice, virus particles can be found in almost any organ of the body, but great numbers of them are present in the thymus, bone marrow, lymph nodes, and spleen. Most of the virus particles are located in the cytoplasm of the infected cells, which they leave by budding through the cell membrane.

The fact that thymectomy inhibits development of spontaneous leukemia in AKR mice indicates that the disease begins in the thymus. According to Goodman and Block (1963), the earliest change noted in the thymus is cortical atrophy, that is, the disappearance of small lymphocytes from the circumference of the thymus with subsequent thinning or loss of the cortex. The atrophy begins between 70 and 130 days after inoculation of the virus. It is usually followed by proliferation of the medullary reticular cells and an increase in the number of medium and large lymphocytes. This regeneration phase occurs between 100 and 150 days after inoculation, and is followed by malignant transformation of the reticular cells and eventual development of thymic lymphosarcoma, that is, replacement of thymic architecture by large monomorphous cells packed into a syncytial arrangement. Invasion of lymphosarcoma cells into other organs— primarily spleen, lymph nodes, and liver—follows, and the enlargement of these organs is usually taken diagnostically as a sign of leukemia. The latent period of the disease, that between the inoculation of the virus and the earliest detection of leukemia, differs in different strains of mice; in the AKR strain the mean latent period for induced leukemia is 67 days and for spontaneous leukemia 8–11 months.

Attempts to transfer GV leukemia to adult animals of other inbred strains, such as C3Hf/Bi or C57BR, invariably failed. However, Gross demonstrated in 1951 that AKR leukemia could be transferred to C3Hf/Bi or C57BR mice by inoculation of *newborn* or suckling animals of these strains with extracts prepared from the leukemic organs of AKR animals. By comparison, mice of strains C57BL/6 or I/St were highly resistant to GV leukemia even when inoculated in early infancy (3–5 days after birth). The inbred strains thus fell into three categories with regard to susceptibility or resistance to GV leukemia: strains with a high incidence of both spontaneous and induced leukemia (AKR, C58), strains with a low incidence of spontaneous and a high incidence of induced leukemia (C3Hf/Bi, C57BR), and strains with a low incidence of both spontaneous and induced leukemia (C57BL/6, I/St).

Association between the disease and the *H-2* complex was first noted by Gorer and Boyse (quoted by Lilly 1971a), who were struck by the fact that all the strains showing a high incidence of spontaneous or induced leukemia had the same *H-2* haplotype (*H-2^k^*). Experimental evidence for the involvement of the *H-2* complex in GV leukemogenesis was provided by Lilly and his co-workers (Lilly *et al.* 1964; Lilly 1966a, b, 1970, 1971a, b) and can be summarized as follows. First, the distribution of susceptibility or resistance to GV among the inbred strains correlates with the distribution of *H-2* haplotypes. Thus, all strains carrying *H-2^k^* or *H-2^d^* haplotypes are susceptible to GV, and all strains carrying *H-2^b^* or *H-2^j^* haplotypes are resistant (Fig. 16–1). Second, in *H-2* congenic lines, the susceptibility or resistance to GV is determined primarily by the *H-2* haplotype, and not by the genetic background. For example, strain C57BL/6 (*H-2^b^*) is resistant to GV, but its congenic line, B6.AK (*H-2^k^*), which is identical with C57BL/6 except for the *H-2* complex, is susceptible, as is the strain from which the *H-2^k^* of B6.AK is derived (AKR). A similar situation also

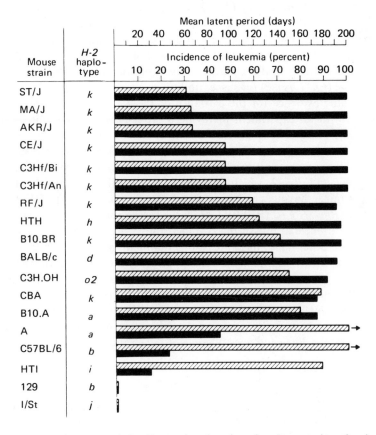

Fig. 16-1. Leukemogenesis by Gross virus in mice of various strains after inoculation at birth. Solid bar = percent of leukemic mice; hatched bar = mean latent period. (Based on Lilly 1966a, b, 1970, 1971a.)

occurs in congenic pairs C57BL/10 and B10.BR, C57BL/10 and B10.D2, C3H and C3H.SW, and C57BL/10 and B10.A. Third, analysis of segregating F_2 or backcross generations revealed a close genetic linkage between susceptibility to GV and the *H-2* complex. For instance, in cross (C3Hf/Bi × C57BL)F_1 × C3Hf/Bi, the proportion of GV-resistant animals was 28 percent. However, the incidence of GV-induced leukemia among mice of *H-2*^{k}/*H-2*^{k} homozygotes was more than 90 percent. In contrast, *H-2*^{k}/*H-2*^{b} heterozygotes had a much lower incidence (56 percent). Susceptibility of the *H-2*^{k}/*H-2*^{k} segregants clearly indicates the presence in the C3H genome of a GV susceptibility gene in close proximity to the *H-2* complex. Similar results were obtained from crosses (B10.BR × C57BL)F_1 × B10.BR, (BALB/c × C57BL)F_1 × BALB/c, (C3Hf/Bi × C57BL/6)F_2, (C3Hf/Bi × 129)F_1 × C3Hf/Bi, (C3Hf/Bi × I/St)F_1 × C3Hf/Bi, and (AKR × C57BL/6)F_1 × AKR. Statistical analysis of GV susceptibility in these crosses led to the conclusion that at least two genes were involved: *Resistance to Gross virus-1* (*Rgv-1*), which appears to be closely linked to the *H-2* complex, and *Resistance to Gross virus-2* (*Rgv-2*), which seems to segregate independently of *H-2*. Because the F_1 hybrids in all the crosses between susceptible and resistant strains are always resistant, it appears that resistance to GV is inherited as a dominant trait and susceptibility as a recessive trait, and that each of the two *Rgv* genes has two allelic forms: dominant (*Rgv-1*, *Rgv-2*) for resistance, and recessive (*rgv-1*, *rgv-2*) for susceptibility.

Compelling evidence for the existence of the *Rgv-2* gene was obtained by Lilly (1971b) in an experiment involving a cross between two inbred strains, B10.BR (*H-2*^{k}) and C3H.OH (*H-2*^{o2}). Both these strains are highly susceptible to GV leukemogenesis, but surprisingly, their F_1 hybrid is virus resistant. The simplest way to explain this result is to postulate two independently segregating genes, *Rgv-1* and *Rgv-2*, which complement each other genetically. The two parental strains, having genotypes *Rgv-1*/*Rgv-1*, *rgv-2*/*rgv-2* (C3H.OH) and *rgv-1*/*rgv-1*, *Rgv-2*/*Rgv-2* (B10.BR), are virus susceptible because of the absence of a dominant allele at one of the two loci; the F_1 hybrid (*Rgv-1*/*rgv-1*, *Rgv-2*/*rgv-2*), on the other hand, has at least one dominant allele at each locus and is therefore resistant. This explanation is supported by the testing of the (B10.BR × C3H.OH)F_2 generation. Assuming that the *Rgv-1* and *Rgv-2* genes are not linked, one would expect $(\frac{3}{4})^2$ of the F_2 progeny to be resistant, and the observed figure (56 percent) is in agreement with this prediction.

Taking into account the origin of the inbred strains and their response to GV infection, the *Rgv* genotypes of some of the strains can be listed as follows:

BALB/c(*H-2*^{d})		
DBA/2(*H-2*^{d})	*rgv-1*/*rgv-1*, *rgv-2*/*rgv-2*	
C3H(*H-2*^{k})		GV susceptible
C3H.OH(*H-2*^{o2})	*Rgv-1*/*Rgv-1*, *rgv-2*/*rgv-2*	
C57BR(*H-2*^{k})	*rgv-1*/*rgv-1*, *Rgv-2*/*Rgv-2*	
B10.BR(*H-2*^{k})		
C57BL/10(*H-2*^{b})	*Rgv-1*/*Rgv-1*, *Rgv-2*/*Rgv-2*	GV resistant

Hence, there are two categories of susceptible strains: those carrying recessive alleles at both *rgv* loci, and those carrying a recessive allele at one and a dominant allele at the other *Rgv* locus (resistant strains carry dominant alleles at both *Rgv* loci). This assignment of genotypes is based on the assumption that the recessive allele at the *rgv-1* locus is associated not only with the $H-2^k$ haplotype, where it was originally discovered, but with other *H-2* haplotypes as well, with $H-2^d$ of DBA/2 or BALB/c, for instance. An alternative explanation is that DBA/2 or BALB/c mice are susceptible because they carry only one recessive allele (at the *rgv-2* locus). However, this possibility was ruled out by Lilly (1970) in an experiment involving inoculation of (BALB/c × C57BL) × BALB/c segregants with GV. Were the susceptibility of the BALB/c strain due to a dominant allele at the *Rgv-1* locus, it would be expected to segregate independently of *H-2*. However, this is not the case, because in the backcross, the heterozygous $H-2^b/H-2^d$ mice have a much lower incidence of leukemia than their homozygous $H-2^d/H-2^d$ littermates. The association of the recessive *rgv-1* allele with the $H-2^d$ haplotype is also supported by the fact that mice of the B10.D2 strain, which received the *rgv-1* allele from DBA/2 and the *Rgv-2* allele from strain C57BL, are susceptible to GV (Lilly 1970).

The association between *rgv-1* and *H-2* is apparently very close, as indicated by the fact that inbred strains carrying the same *H-2* haplotype also display similar GV response. Some of these strains have been separated for many generations and some could even be of independent origin.

A clue to the location of the *rgv-1* gene with respect to the *H-2* complex has been provided by analysis of three *H-2* recombinant strains, HTH ($H-2^h$), HTI ($H-2^i$), and HTG ($H-2^g$) (Lilly 1970). The HTH and HTI recombinants are derived from a cross involving strains A ($H-2^a$ *rgv-1/rgv-1*, ?/?) and C57BL/10 ($H-2^b$ *Rgv-1/Rgv-1*, *Rgv-2/Rgv-2*). Haplotype $H-2^h$ carries the *K* end of $H-2^a$ and the *D* end of $H-2^b$ and is GV susceptible; haplotype $H-2^i$ carries the *K* end of $H-2^b$ and the *D* end of $H-2^a$ and is GV resistant. Similarly, the HTG recombinant, which is derived from a cross between BALB/c ($H-2^d$ *rgv-1/rgv-1*, *rgv-2/rgv-2*) and C57BL/10, and carries the *K* end of $H-2^d$ and the *D* end of $H-2^b$, is susceptible to GV infection, as is the donor of the *K* end. Thus, in all three recombinants, the GV response is determined by the origin of the *K* end; the *D* end of the *H-2* complex appears to be irrelevant. It can be concluded, therefore, that the *rgv-1* gene is located near the *K* end of the *H-2* complex, either outside *H-2* between the *H-2K* locus and the centromere, or within *H-2*, between the *K* and *S* regions.

2. Tennant Virus

In 1962, Tennant isolated a leukemogenic virus by the inoculation of cell-free extracts from spontaneous or transplanted C58 leukemias into newborn mice of strain BALB/c (Tennant 1962). The incidence of the disease in the BALB/c mice was relatively low at first (11–25 percent), but was later increased to 100 percent by serial passage of the virus through suckling mice. The virus, called *BALB/Tennant leukemia (B/T-L)* virus, induces lymphoid leukemia, similar to that induced by Gross virus. Mice of the BALB/c strain inoculated intraperitoneally with the virus before 3 days of age succumb to leukemia after a latent period of 3 months. The host range of the Tennant virus (Fig. 16–2) is different from that of the Gross virus (Tennant 1965): BALB/c and A are highly susceptible (93–100 percent inoculated mice develop leukemia), strains C57BL/10, C57BR, and C3HeB are highly resistant (0–25 percent incidence of leukemia), and strains B10.D2, A.BY, and B10.A are intermediate (68–80 percent incidence of leukemia).

The influence of the *H-2* system on B/T-L virus leukemogenesis was demonstrated in two ways: by inoculation with the virus of *H-2* congenic lines and by inactivation of the virus by H-2 antisera. Of the *H-2* haplotypes available in various B10 congenic lines, the most favorable for the development of leukemia is *H-2^d* (83 percent susceptibility), the haplotype of strain BALB/c in which the Tennant virus originated. Second to *H-2^d* is the *H-2^a* haplotype (73 percent susceptibility), which has the *D* end of the *H-2* complex derived from the *H-2^d* haplotype. Thus, the introduction of the *H-2* complex from a susceptible strain (DBA/2 or A) onto the background of a resistant strain (C57BL/10) resulted in increased susceptibility of the congenic lines (B10.D2 and B10.A). Similarly, introduction of the *H-2* complex from a resistant strain (C57BL/10) onto the genetic background of a susceptible strain (A) resulted in decreased susceptibility of the congenic line (A.BY). However, in none of these instances did the introduction of the *H-2* complex accomplish the complete alteration of a resistant strain to a susceptible one or vice versa, so it is clear that the *H-2* system is not the only genetic system involved in Tennant virus leukemogenesis. A number

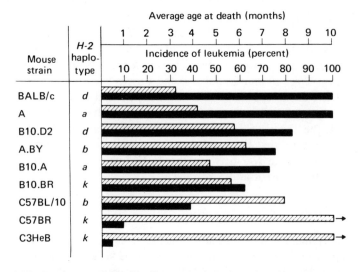

Fig. 16-2. Leukemogenesis by Tennant virus in mice of various strains after inoculation at birth. Solid bars = percent of leukemic mice; hatched bars = average age at death from leukemia. (Based on Tennant and Snell 1966, 1968.)

of other loci must also be important, some of which could be other *H* loci (i.e., *H-1* and *H-9*, cf. Tennant 1965).

In the inactivation experiments, Tennant (1968) incubated the virus preparations with monospecific H-2 alloantisera prior to inoculation into infant mice and observed partial neutralization of the viruses' leukemogenic potential as reflected in the prolongation of the latent period and in decreased leukemia incidence.

3. Radiation-Induced Leukemia Virus

M. Lieberman and Kaplan (1959) discovered that extracts from leukemias induced by X-irradiation of C57BL mice contained a virus capable of provoking leukemias in untreated mice of the same strain. This virus, called *radiation-induced leukemia virus* (*RadLV*; cf. Kaplan 1967), resembles GV in many respects, but the two differ in their host range. Mice of the C57BL strain are highly susceptible to RadLV but relatively resistant to GV, whereas mice of strain C3H/Bi are resistant to RadLV and susceptible to GV.

The RadLV was not studied with the intention of determining the *H-2* effect on its leukemogenesis, but there is some circumstantial evidence suggesting *H-2* complex involvement. The evidence rests on the observation by Kaplan (1967) that C3H (*H-2^k*) mice are more susceptible to RadLV than C3H.SW (*H-2^b*) mice, the latter sharing their *H-2* haplotype with the resistant C57BL strain.

B. Erythroid Leukemia (Friend) Virus

Friend virus (*FV*) was isolated by Friend in 1956 from a transplantable mouse carcinoma (Ehrlich ascites tumor), but had no apparent etiological relationship to the tumor (Friend 1957); it was probably picked up by the tumor cells during their serial passaging (passenger virus). FV induces a type of leukemia entirely different from that induced by GV or B/T-L. The earliest manifestation of the FV syndrome is the production of characteristic foci of rapidly proliferating cells in the spleen. The foci, which appear as early as 3 days after infection, are first microscopic, but grow so rapidly that they are visible to the naked eye 7–10 days after infection. The rapidly proliferating cells in the foci are of two main types—nucleated red cells (reticulum cells) and immature mononuclear cells (erythroblasts). The massive outgrowth of cells in the foci leads to enlargement of the spleen (splenomegaly), followed by widespread infiltration of the malignant cells into other organs of the body. Between the fifth and seventh week after infection, a sharp rise occurs in the white blood cell count—one of the symptoms for which this complex disease is classified as leukemia. Outwardly, the animals show almost no sign of illness until a few days before death, which usually occurs 2–3 months after infection. In sharp contrast to GV leukemia, the FV leukemia does not involve thymus or lymph nodes, and it affects adult as well as newborn animals.

The response to FV can be measured by two different assays: the spleen focus assay (Axelrad and Steeves 1964), which is based on the enumeration of macroscopic spleen foci in the infected animals, and the spleen weight assay (Rowe and Brodsky 1959), which measures the degree of splenomegaly.

The disease was first observed in mice of a random-bred Swiss albino strain, but was later shown to affect mice of other strains as well. FV is currently known in two variants (strains) with somewhat different host ranges: F-S (Swiss-origin) and F-B (BALB/c-adapted). The original F-S virus is propagated in the Swiss albino or in DBA/2 mice; the BALB/c mice are relatively resistant to it as adults and susceptible as infants. The F-B variant was obtained by Lilly (1967a), who forcibly passaged the FV through BALB/c mice and adapted it to the new environment. The F-B strain grows as well in the BALB/c as in the DBA/2 or Swiss mice; otherwise, the F-S and F-B variants are indistinguishable.

Recent evidence indicates that the FV is not a single virus but rather a virus *complex* consisting of at least two infectious agents: one that is the actual pathogenic agent (the *lymphatic leukemia virus* or LLV) and another that augments and accelerates the leukemogenic activity of the former (*spleen focus-forming virus* or SFFV).

The FV infection is a complicated process in which several genes of the host are involved. At least eight have been implicated so far: three histocompatibility loci (*H-2, H-4,* and *H-7*), three genes with an effect on erythropoiesis (W^v, Sl, and f) and two genes whose only known function is the effect on FV susceptibility (*Fv-1* and *Fv-2*). The influence of *H-2* on FV response was demonstrated by Lilly (1968) in low doses of the F-B virus variant. In his experiment, Lilly inoculated $(C57BL/6 \times DBA/2)F_1 \times C57BL/6$ backcross animals with the F-B virus at full strength, diluted 1:10, and diluted 1:100. The full-strength virus preparation induced splenomegaly in 47 percent of the animals, a proportion consistent with the interpretation that the response to FV under these conditions is determined by a single gene. Among the FV-susceptible animals, approximately half were H-2^b/H-2^d heterozygotes and half were H-2^b/H-2^b homozygotes. From these data Lilly concluded that at this high virus dosage, the *H-2* complex and the gene for the splenomegaly response (i.e., *Fv-2*) segregated independently. At a dilution of 1:10, the virus preparation induced splenomegaly in 45 percent of the backcross animals, and of these susceptible animals only 38 percent were H-2^b/H-2^b homozygotes. This latter figure is significantly different from the 50 percent expected on the basis of independent segregation of *H-2* and the gene for virus susceptibility. At the dilution 1:100, the virus preparation induced splenomegaly in only 17 percent of the segregants, and in none of the susceptible animals of the H-2^b/H-2^b type. In all three groups, some animals that developed splenomegaly recovered from it at later stages and regained usual spleen size. This recovery occurred more frequently among H-2^b/H-2^b homozygotes than among H-2^b/H-2^d heterozygotes. From these experiments, Lilly concluded that the *absolute* susceptibility to high doses of the F-B virus was controlled by a single gene segregating independently of *H-2*. However, *relative* susceptibility to moderate and low doses of the F-B virus was influenced by the *H-2* complex. This *H-2* influence was reflected in the incidence of the Friend disease among animals with different *H-2* haplotypes, and in the incidence of recovery from the early phase of the disease.

The influence of *H-4* and *H-7* loci was described by Axelrad and Van der Gaag (1969). Mice of congenic lines B10.129(21M) and B10.C(47N), which are known to differ from the background strain (C57BL/10Sn) at *H-4* and *H-7*, respectively, were shown to be susceptible to large doses of FV in terms of spleen focus formation. (Strain C57BL/10Sn is highly resistant to induction of spleen foci by FV.) However, the involvement of the *H-4* locus could not be confirmed by later experiments (F. Lilly, *personal communication*), and the effects ascribed to *H-7* were probably caused by *Fv-2*, which appears to be linked to *H-7* (Lilly

GENES $Fv\text{-}2$: alleles 2^s and 2^r
$Fv\text{-}1$: alleles 1^n and 1^b

DBA/2: $\dfrac{1^n\ 1^n}{2^s\ 2^s}$ (1)   C57BL: $\dfrac{1^b\ 1^b}{2^r\ 2^r}$ (3)

F_1: $\dfrac{1^n\ 1^b}{2^s\ 2^r}$ (2)

F_2:

Gametes	$1^n\ 2^s$	$1^b\ 2^s$	$1^n\ 2^r$	$1^b\ 2^r$
$1^n\ 2^s$	$\dfrac{1^n\ 1^n}{2^s\ 2^s}$ (1)	$\dfrac{1^n\ 1^b}{2^s\ 2^s}$ (2)	$\dfrac{1^n\ 1^n}{2^s\ 2^r}$ (1)	$\dfrac{1^n\ 1^b}{2^s\ 2^r}$ (2)
$1^b\ 2^s$	$\dfrac{1^n\ 1^b}{2^s\ 2^s}$ (2)	$\dfrac{1^b\ 1^b}{2^s\ 2^s}$ (2)	$\dfrac{1^n\ 1^b}{2^s\ 2^r}$ (2)	$\dfrac{1^b\ 1^b}{2^s\ 2^r}$ (2)
$1^n\ 2^r$	$\dfrac{1^n\ 1^n}{2^s\ 2^r}$ (1)	$\dfrac{1^n\ 1^b}{2^s\ 2^r}$ (2)	$\dfrac{1^n\ 1^n}{2^r\ 2^r}$ (3)	$\dfrac{1^n\ 1^b}{2^r\ 2^r}$ (3)
$1^b\ 2^r$	$\dfrac{1^n\ 1^b}{2^s\ 2^r}$ (2)	$\dfrac{1^b\ 1^b}{2^s\ 2^r}$ (2)	$\dfrac{1^n\ 1^b}{2^r\ 2^r}$ (3)	$\dfrac{1^b\ 1^b}{2^r\ 2^r}$ (3)

(1) $\dfrac{1^n\ 1^n}{2^s\ 2^-}$ highly susceptible $\left(\dfrac{3}{16}\right)$

(2) $\dfrac{1^b\ 1^-}{2^s\ 2^-}$ relatively resistant $\left(\dfrac{9}{16}\right)$

(3) $\dfrac{1^-\ 1^-}{2^r\ 2^r}$ absolutely resistant $\left(\dfrac{4}{16}\right)$

Fig. 16-3. The *Fv* genotype of strains DBA/2 and C57BL and their hybrids. (Reproduced with permission from F. Lilly and T. Pincus: "Genetic control of murine viral leukemogenesis." *Advances in Cancer Research* 17:231–277. Copyright © 1973 by Academic Press. All rights reserved.)

and Pincus 1973). [The B10.C(47N) strain carries not only the *H-7* allele, but also the *Fv-2* allele of the BALB/c strain.]

As it appears that the primary target cells for FV are the hematopoietic progenitor cells in spleen and bone marrow, it is not surprising that mutant genes that affect these cells also affect the response to FV. So far three genes

Table 16-1. Summary of susceptibility or resistance of inbred strains to different oncogenic viruses*

		Virus					
				Friend			
Strain	*H-2* haplotype	Gross	Tennant	F-S	F-B	Bittner	Vaccinia
A	a	rS	S	rR	rS	S(BR)	rS
B10.A	a	S	S	·	R	S	·
A.BY	b	·	S	·	rS	·	·
C57BL/6	b	R	·	R	R	·	·
C57BL/10	b	R	rR	R	R	R	·
C3H.SW	b	R	·	·	S	·	·
129	bc	R	·	S	S	·	·
BALB/c	d	S	S	rR	S	·	S
B10.D2	d	S	S	R	R	S	R
C57BL/Ks	d	·	·	R	R	·	·
DBA/2	d	rS	·	S	S	S	R
NZB	d	·	·	S	S	·	·
HTH	h	S	·	·	·	·	·
HTI	i	R	·	·	R	·	·
I/St	j	R	·	S	S	·	·
AKR	k	S	·	rS	rS	·	R
B10.BR	k	S	rS	·	R	·	·
CBA	k	rS	·	·	S	·	·
CE/J	k	S	·	·	·	·	·
C3H/Bi	k	S	·	S	S	S	S
C57BR	k	S	·	R	R	·	·
C58	k	S	·	R	R	·	R
MA/J	k	S	·	·	·	·	·
RF/J	k	S	·	·	S	·	·
C3H.OH	o2	S	·	·	S	·	·
DBA/1	q	·	·	S	S	·	R
RIII	r	·	·	·	·	S	·
SJL	s	·	·	S	S	·	·
GR	?	·	·	·	·	S	·

*   R = resistant
     rR = relatively resistant
      S = susceptible
     rS = relatively susceptible
   (BR) = breeders
      · = not tested

known to disturb erythropoietic differentiation—W^v, Sl, and f—have been shown also to influence susceptibility to FV. In all three cases, an FV-susceptible strain is made resistant by the presence of any of these three mutant alleles (M. Bennet *et al.* 1968; Steeves *et al.* 1968; Axelrad and Van der Gaag 1969). The W^v gene may adversely affect leukemogenesis by making hematopoietic progenitor cells unavailable, and the Sl gene may have a similar effect by creating an environment that is not conducive to spleen focus formation.

The two FV susceptibility loci, *Fv-1* and *Fv-2*, were discovered by testing segregating populations involving strains C57BL and DBA/2 (Lilly 1970; cf. Fig. 16–3). The *Fv-1* locus determines relative resistance to F–S virus but has no influence on susceptibility to F-B virus. It has two alleles, $Fv\text{-}1^n$ (originally called $Fv\text{-}1^s$), determining susceptibility, and $Fv\text{-}1^b$ (originally called $Fv\text{-}1^r$), determining relative resistance, with the $Fv\text{-}1^b$ allele dominant over the $Fv\text{-}1^n$ allele. The locus is in chromosome 4 (LG VIII, cf. W. Rowe *et al.* 1973; W. Rowe and Sato 1973), and it appears to act on LLV, but not on SFFV. The *Fv-2* locus, originally described by Odaka and Yamamoto (1962) as *Fv*, determines virtually absolute resistance to focus formation by both F-S and F-B viruses. It also has two alleles, $Fv\text{-}2^s$ for susceptibility and $Fv\text{-}2^r$ for resistance, with the susceptibility allele dominant over the resistance allele. The locus is in chromosome 9 (LG II) about 15 map units from *dilute* (*d*). It appears to act on SFFV but not on LLV.

The strain distribution of the alleles at the *Fv-1* and *Fv-2* loci is shown in Table 16–1.

C. In Vitro Studies of Leukemia Virus Genetics

Until recently, the only assay available for studying the genetics of host-virus interactions was the lengthy and time-consuming assay of leukemogenesis. This situation was changed a few years ago when it was discovered that susceptibility or resistance to leukemia viruses could also be studied *in vitro* by infecting cells in tissue culture. Using this approach, Hartley *et al.* (1970) found that naturally occurring leukemia viruses could be divided into three categories according to their capacity to propagate in a culture of mouse embryo cells: those that grow efficiently in BALB/c cells but poorly in NIH Swiss cells (*B-tropic*), those that grow efficiently in NIH Swiss cells but poorly in BALB/c cells (*N-tropic*), and those that grow equally well in BALB/c and NIH Swiss cells (*NB-tropic*). In the BALB/c strain, the most studied strain with regard to tropism, leukemia viruses isolated from young mice are predominantly N-tropic, whereas those isolated from older mice are predominantly B-tropic. (The NB-tropic category is represented by viruses with long laboratory passage histories.) When the studies were extended to include other inbred strains, it was discovered that all strains fall into one of two categories, the *B-type* category, resembling the BALB/c strain in their relative response to N- and B-tropic viruses, and the *N-type* category, resembling the NIH Swiss strain (Pincus *et al.* 1971a). Moreover, it was realized (Pincus *et al.* 1971b) that the classification into B- and N-types fully correlated with classification of strains for the *Fv-1* allele: all N-type strains (i.e., strains susceptible to N-tropic viruses) carried the *Fv-1ⁿ* allele, and all B-type strains (i.e., strains susceptible to B-tropic viruses) carried the *Fv-1ᵇ* allele. It thus became clear that the *Fv-1* locus, originally defined only as one of the loci determining the response of the host to the Friend virus, was probably identical with the locus determining the N- or B-tropism *in vitro*, and that, therefore, it represented a major genetic factor controlling the host's response to many other leukemia viruses (W. Rowe 1972; W. Rowe and Hartley 1972). The NB-tropism apparently represents an escape by the virus from the regulatory effects of the *Fv-1* locus. It now appears it is the helper component (LLV) that determines the N- or B-tropism of FV *in vitro*.

II. Mammary Tumor (Bittner) Virus

Bittner virus, also known as *mammary tumor virus* (*MTV*) or *mammary tumor agent* (*MTA*), causes mammary gland tumors originating in the epithelium (carcinomas or adencarcinomas; for reviews and references, see Bittner 1938, 1947; Law 1954; DeOme and Nandi 1966). The mature MTV particle (*B particle*) is spherical, about 105 mμ in diameter, with an eccentrically located electron-dense nucleoid surrounded by a thin membrane. The particles appear to be formed by budding from the cell membranes of mammary epithelium. After detachment from the cell, the particles accumulate in the intercellular spaces and then make their way into the lumen of the mammary duct. During lactation, the particles are excreted with the milk and infect the suckling progeny. Infection by way of mother's milk is the primary route of transmission of MTV, and for this reason the MTV has long been known as the "milk factor" or "milk agent." However, transmission via the ovum or sperm has also been described.

The MTV particles apparently pass unharmed through the gastrointestinal tract into circulating blood. It has been postulated (Nandi *et al.* 1971) that they are carried into the liver, picked up there by macrophages, and then incorporated into erythrocytes. Thus, there are two forms of MTV, *mammary tissue-borne MTV* (*M-MTV*) and *red blood cell-borne MTV* (*R-MTV*). M-MTV activity is associated with the presence of B particles; no such particles have been demonstrated as yet in erythrocytes with R-MTV activity. The R-MTV-containing erythrocytes are assumed to be engulfed eventually by macrophages and the virus transferred to the mammary gland epithelium. The infection of the mammary cells probably occurs only after the cells are suitably prepared by certain hormones. After the infection, the mammary epithelium is changed to nodular tissue, first visible at the age of 3–4 months. Histologically (and by other criteria), the nodules do not resemble neoplasms; however, it has been demonstrated that they can develop into neoplasms and must, therefore, be considered preneoplastic. The change of the preneoplastic nodules to typical mammary neoplasms takes several additional months, and the mammary carcinomas develop at the age of about 1 year or later. With the development of mammary tumors, the life cycle of the MTV is completed and more mature B particles are excreted into the milk.

The cycle described above is that of the classic Bittner virus. There are other viruses with slightly different properties, such as the degree of virulence, the types of lesions produced, and antigenicity, known to belong to the same family. But their life cycles are probably different from the classic mammary tumor virus. For example, C3H mice are known to harbor MTV, which is transmitted in milk from lactating females to suckling young. The mice have a high incidence of spontaneous mammary tumors, and most of the tumors begin to develop at about 8 months. From a litter of C3H mice born by Caesarean section and foster-nursed on C57BL/6 females (a strain virtually free of MTV), a new line of mice, designated C3Hf, was developed. The C3Hf mice carry virus particles that are indistinguishable from those seen in C3H mice, but the C3Hf virus differs from the C3H virus in at least two essential features. First, the C3Hf virus is not transmitted by way of milk; instead, it is probably transmitted at conception. Second, alveolar nodules induced by the C3Hf virus appear late in life and have low carcinogenic potentials. (For this reason, the virus has been designated NIV, nodule-inducing virus.)

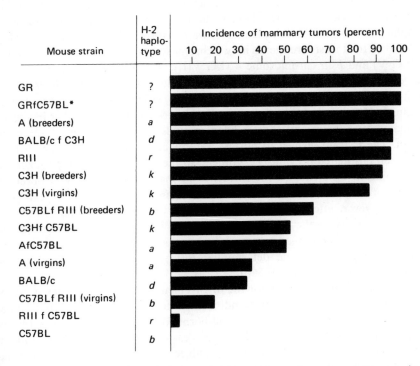

Fig. 16-4. Incidence of spontaneous mammary tumors in various mouse strains. *f = foster-nursed on mothers of indicated strain. (Based on D. H. Moore *J. Nat. Cancer Inst.* **48**:1017–1019, 1972.)

The development of mammary tumors in mice (Fig. 16–4) depends upon the interaction of three factors: the MTV, hormonal stimulation, and genetic susceptibility. The presence of MTV is, of course, the prime factor in mammary tumorigenesis. The virus is known to be present in some inbred strains of mice (C3H, BALB/c, A, and RIII) and absent in others (C57BL/10 and C57BL/6). Strains carrying the MTV can be freed of the virus by foster nursing; MTV-free strains can be artificially reinfected. However, mice carrying MTV do not develop mammary cancer unless a suitable hormonal environment, usually associated with pregnancy and lactation, is provided. For example, in A strain mice, known to harbor MTV, only breeding females develop spontaneous mammary carcinoma; the incidence of mammary cancer in virgin females is low. However, in some strains, such as C3H, the incidence of mammary cancer is high in both breeding and virgin females, indicating that the hormonal influence is overridden by genetic factors. The most striking example of the role of genetic factors in mammary tumorigenesis is the C57BL strain. In this strain, even after MTV is provided (by C57BL babies foster nursing from C3H females) and hormonal stimulation (using breeding C57BL females) is induced, the incidence of mammary carcinoma remains low.

Analysis of the genetic component of MTV tumorigenesis led first to the conclusion that the difference between high- and low-mammary cancer strains is due to a single gene. It was later realized that this conclusion was an over-simplification, and that multiple factors were involved. The MTV susceptibility was linked to at least three genes in two chromosomes: A^y and A in chromosome 2 (LG V) and b in chromosome 4 (LG VIII). An attempt to associate MTV susceptibility with the *H-2* system was first made by Lilly (1966b). He crossed a high-mammary cancer strain, C3H/An ($H-2^k$), with a low-mammary cancer strain, I ($H-2^j$), and observed that the F_1 females had an even higher incidence of mammary tumors and shorter latent periods than the susceptible parental strain. The I strain seemed to possess a dominant "accelerator factor," which had been postulated previously by others. In the $(C3H \times I)F_1 \female \times I \male$ backcross, no significant difference in the incidence of mammary tumors was observed between the $H-2^k/H-2^j$ and $H-2^j/H-2^j$ segregants during the first year after birth. However, after about 400 days, the curve representing the cumulative tumor incidence in the $H-2^j/H-2^j$ segregants leveled off, while that in the $H-2^k/H-2^j$ group continued to rise. Lilly concluded that "these results suggest inconclusively that a gene determining Bittner virus susceptibility may be associated with *H-2*" (Lilly 1966b).

More conclusive evidence for the involvement of the *H-2* complex in MTV tumorigenesis was obtained by Nandi and his co-workers (Nandi 1967; Nandi *et al.* 1971), who used the red blood cell-borne form of MTV. The susceptibility of different inbred strains to R-MTV was measured by the *noduligenic assay*, in which mice inoculated with R-MTV are subjected to intense hormonal stimulation and the MTV activity is measured by the incidence of hyperplastic alveolar nodules. The assay considerably shortens the length of the observation period (from the 2 years necessary with the classical mammary tumor assay to about 4 months). The results demonstrated that R-MTV from BALB/c ($H-2^d/H-2^d$) mice was capable of infecting 50 percent or more of mice that were either homozygous (DBA/2) or heterozygous [(BALB/c × C3Hf)F_1, (BALB/c × Af)F_1, (BALB/c × I)F_1, (BALB/c × C57BL)F_1] for the $H-2^d$ haplotype. In contrast, only 22 percent of mice with haplotypes other than $H-2^d$ [i.e., $H-2^a$ in strain Af, $H-2^k$ in C3Hf, and $H-2^b/H-2^j$ in (C57BL × I)F_1 hybrids] were susceptible to this form of the virus. Similarly, R-MTV obtained from C3H ($H-2^k/H-2^k$) mice was capable of infecting mice homozygous or heterozygous for the $H-2^k$ haplotype and virtually incapable of infecting strains carrying other $H-2$ haplotypes. In [(BALB/c × C3Hf)F_1 × C3Hf]BC and (BALB/c × C3Hf)F_2 mice inoculated with R-MTV from BALB/c donors, the nodule incidence was consistently higher in animals homozygous or heterozygous for the $H-2^d$ haplotype than in $H-2^k/H-2^k$ homozygotes. Similarly, in [(BALB/c × C3Hf)F_1 × BALB/c]BC and (BALB/c × C3Hf)F_2 mice inoculated with R-MTV from C3H donors, the incidence was higher in animals homozygous or heterozygous for the $H-2^k$ haplotype than in the $H-2^d/H-2^d$ homozygotes. The $H-2$ barrier could not be overcome by prolonging the hormone stimulation of the recipients or by treating the host with antithymocytic serum. Treatment of the R-MTV preparation with anti-H-2 antisera or spleen and lymph node cells from mice immunized against H-2 antigens did not decrease the noduligenic activity of the preparation. However, a considerable reduction in nodule incidence was observed in mice injected with a mixture of peritoneal macrophages from animals presensitized against H-2 antigens and R-MTV.

Hence, it appears that the RBC-borne MTV activity depends on $H-2$ compatibility of the R-MTV donor and the recipient. However, because the nodule incidence in $H-2$-compatible F_2 and backcross individuals never reached that of the parental strain from which the virus was derived, it is likely that in addition to $H-2$, other factors (genetic and/or epigenetic) are also involved in mammary noduligenesis. The mechanism leading to the resistance of the $H-2$ allogeneic recipients does not seem to operate at the level of the target (mammary) tissue, because BALB/c and C3Hf mammary tissues, transplanted into parenchyma-free mammary fat pads of (BALB/c × C3Hf)F_1 hybrids, are infectible by R-MTV from both C3H and BALB/c donors. Nandi and his co-workers suggested that the association of R-MTV resistance with $H-2$ incompatibility might be caused by incorporation of H-2 antigens from the host into the virus particles, and that this incorporation occurs during the budding of the virus through the cell membrane.

Evidence for the involvement of the $H-2$ complex in susceptibility to the M-MTV form was obtained by Mühlbock and Dux (1971a, b), who transmitted C3H-MTV into mice of congenic strains carrying different $H-2$ haplotypes (or other H loci) on a B10 background. The transmission was accomplished either by way of milk, that is, by foster nursing the young of the congenic strain on (C3H♀ × 020♂)F_1 females, or by intraperitoneal injection of purified tumor extract at the age of 2 months. To accelerate the appearance of mammary tumors, the infected females of the congenic strain were forced to have several pregnancies in rapid succession (by removal of each litter immediately after birth). These experiments demonstrated that congenic lines carrying haplotypes $H\text{-}2^a$, $H\text{-}2^d$, $H\text{-}2^f$, $H\text{-}2^k$, and $H\text{-}2^m$ had a significantly higher incidence of mammary tumors than the B10 strain. Congenic lines carrying different alleles at the minor histocompatibility loci ($H\text{-}1$, $H\text{-}3$, $H\text{-}4$, $H\text{-}7$, $H\text{-}8$, $H\text{-}9$, $H\text{-}12$, and $H\text{-}13$) had the same tumor incidence as the B10 strain. Similar experiments with the GR-MTV form (form transmitted in the GR strain equally well by mother's milk and by sperm and ovum at conception) did not show any significant difference in tumor incidence among the lines carrying various histocompatibility loci.

The results obtained by Mühlbock and Dux contradict those of Nandi and his co-workers. Not only were Mühlbock and Dux able to force the C3H-derived MTV to overcome the $H\text{-}2$ barrier, but in some cases, they achieved higher tumor incidence in incompatible strains than in compatible ones. For example, the C3H-MTV transmitted via milk induced 100 percent mammary tumors in strain B10.A, which carries a foreign $H\text{-}2$ haplotype ($H\text{-}2^a$), and only 50 percent in strain B10.BR, which has the same $H\text{-}2$ haplotype as C3H ($H\text{-}2^k$). A likely explanation of this discrepancy is that Nandi observed resistance not to the virus, but to the erythrocytes (his R-MTV was never free of erythrocytes), whereas Mühlbock and Dux observed a true $H\text{-}2$-associated virus resistance (F. Lilly, *personal communication*).

III. Vaccinia Virus

Vaccinia virus is a representative of the group of pox viruses, the largest animal viruses known. Vaccinia virus particles have dimensions of 2500–3000 Å, are rectangular in shape with rounded corners, and have a complex structure consisting of an inner DNA core (the nucleoid) surrounded by two membrane layers. The virus has a rather broad host range that includes many different species of animal, that is, man, rabbit, calf, sheep, and others. The targets of the vaccinia infection are usually epidermal cells, but the virus can multiply in other tissues as well. The virus multiplies inside the infected cells, and its life cycle from attachment and penetration to lysis of the cell and release of new particles lasts about 10–12 hr. Multiplication of the virus in epidermal cells of the skin causes the characteristic lesions or pocks.

The role of genetic factors in the vaccinia virus infection was studied by Duran-Reynals and Lilly. Duran-Reynals (1972), and Duran-Reynals and Lilly (1971) observed that vaccinia inoculated intradermally into the flank failed to elicit any detectable skin response in mice of eight inbred strains: BALB/c, C3HeB, A, C58, DBA/2, DBA/1, B10.D2, and AKR (Fig. 16–5). However, pretreatment with cortisone rendered some strains (i.e., BALB/c, C3HeB, A, and C58) susceptible, while others remained resistant. In the susceptible strain, vaccinia elicited a local skin response consisting of edema, superficial ulceration, and scabbing. The lesions healed in 10–15 days and no further response was observed. Of the four responding strains, BALB/c and C3H reacted strongly, A moderately, and C58 very weakly. The effect of the virus was further enhanced by paintings of the recipient's skin with 3-methylcholanthrene (MC) solution, prior to vaccinia inoculation. After this treatment, severe skin lesions were observed in strains BALB/c and less severe lesions in strains C3H, A, and C58. Mild skin reaction was also observed in strains DBA/2, DBA/1, and B10.D2, while almost no reaction was elicited in strain AKR. In the most susceptible strains (BALB/c, C3H, A, and C58), the skin lesions evolved on healing into papillomas, which were usually followed by the development of malignant tumors (fibrosarcomas and carcinomas) in the same site. Although skin tumors appeared in these strains even when the virus treatment was omitted (i.e., in mice treated with cortisone and MC or with MC alone), the virus significantly increased the incidence of tumors. No skin tumors appeared in the remaining four strains (DBA/2, DBA/1, B10.D2, and AKR) even after a combined treatment with cortisone, MC, and vaccinia. Thus, the skin response of the eight strains to both vaccinia and MC can be classified as severe in BALB/c and C3H, moderate in A, weak in C58, very weak in DBA/1, DBA/2, and B10.D2, and undetectable in AKR mice. Skin response to vaccinia inoculation and MC paintings was inversely correlated with the incidence of leukemia in mice of the eight strains; strains with low skin response had a high incidence of leukemia, either spontaneous (AKR and C58) or MC-induced (DBA/1 and DBA/2); strains with severe skin response (BALB/c, C3H, and A) did not develop leukemias at all.

For further analysis of the genetic factors involved in the combined effects of vaccinia virus and MC, two strains representing the extremes in the response to this treatment were selected: strain BALB/c, with a high susceptibility to the

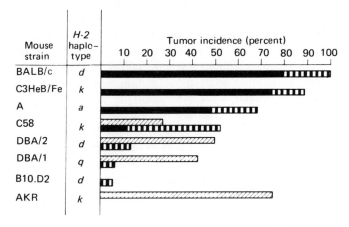

Fig. 16-5. Incidence of skin tumors and leukemia in mice of various strains treated with cortisone, inoculated with vaccinia virus and painted with 3-methylcholanthrene. Striped bar = incidence of early benign skin tumors; solid bar = incidence of late malignant skin tumors; hatched bar = incidence of leukemia. (Based on Duran-Reynals 1972.)

dermal effects of the virus and the carcinogen and with virtual absence of leukemia incidence, and strain AKR, virtually resistant to vaccinia and MC painting but demonstrating a high incidence of spontaneous leukemia (Lilly and Duran-Reynals 1972). The (BALB/c × AKR)F_1 hybrids were susceptible to vaccinia, although the degree of susceptibility was lower by comparison with BALB/c strain. The susceptibility of the F_1 hybrids to MC painting was also greatly reduced in comparison to BALB/c mice. In the (BALB/c × AKR)F_1 × AKR backcross generation, 78 percent of the mice treated with cortisone, vaccinia, and MC developed skin ulcers, suggesting that the response to vaccinia virus is controlled by two independently segregating genes, with the dominant alleles for susceptibility present in BALB/c mice and the recessive alleles for resistance present in AKR mice. Serological typing of the backcross animals demonstrated that the two genes also segregate independently of *H-2* and that *H-2* had no effect on the infection.

The overall incidence of skin tumors among the F_1 × AKR backcross mice treated with cortisone, vaccinia, and MC was 42 percent, and the tumors developed almost exclusively among mice that had previously exhibited skin ulcers, again indicating enhancement of MC tumorigenesis by active infection with vaccinia virus. However, not all the segregants susceptible to vaccinia infection developed skin tumors after MC painting; the tumor incidence among these segregants was only 52 percent (as compared to 86 percent incidence among the F_1 hybrids). These results suggested that MC tumorigenesis in the presence of vaccinia infection is probably controlled by one or more genes segregating independently of the two genes for vaccinia virus susceptibility. The incidence of malignant skin tumors after cortisone-MC-vaccinia treatment of the F_1 × AKR backcross mice was significantly higher in *H-2^k*/*H-2^d* heterozygotes (26 percent) than in *H-2^k*/*H-2^k* homozygotes (6 percent), indicating that the MC skin tumorigenesis is controlled by the *H-2* complex or by a gene closely linked with *H-2*. Spontaneous leukemia, which appeared in 41 percent of the treated backcross mice, occurred less frequently among mice with MC-induced tumors than among mice without the skin tumors, confirming the previously observed inverse correlation between MC tumors and leukemia. There was no correlation between leukemia incidence and the *H-2* haplotype among the backcross mice, which is not surprising because both *H-2^k* and *H-2^d* haplotypes are known to be favorable to Gross virus leukemogenesis.

The conclusion reached by the authors of these experiments is that *H-2* does not influence the early infectious response to vaccinia virus, but does influence the neoplastic consequences of this response—a situation strikingly similar to that observed with Friend leukemia virus.

IV. Lymphocytic Choriomeningitis Virus

Lymphocytic choriomeningitis (LCM) is a disease affecting meninges (i.e., the three membranes—pia mater, dura mater, and arachnoic—that envelop the brain and spinal cord), particularly the choroid plexus (i.e., the highly vascular portion of the pia mater thought to secrete the cerebrospinal fluid). The disease is marked by the presence of numerous lymphocytes in the leptomeninges (the pia mater and the arachnoid) and in the choroid plexus. It is caused by a virus (LCM virus) that, when injected into the brain (intracerebrally) of an adult susceptible mouse, kills the recipient, usually within 1 month after the injection.

The influence of the *H-2* complex on susceptibility to LCM virus has recently been demonstrated by Oldstone *et al.* (1973). In a cross of the resistant strain C3H (*H-2^k*) to the susceptible strain SWR/J (*H-2^q*), the F_1 hybrids were susceptible to the virus, and among the progeny from a backcross to the resistant parent, 75 percent of the *H-2^q/H-2^k* heterozygotes were susceptible, whereas only 30 percent of the *H-2^k/H-2^k* homozygotes succumbed to the disease. Congenic line C3H.Q, carrying the *H-2^q* haplotype of the susceptible strain, was susceptible. The lack of a strict 1:1 segregation ratio in the backcross generation suggests that several genes apparently are involved in the control of susceptibility to the LCM virus, and that the *H-2* complex is only one of them. The correlation of the susceptibility with the *H-2* haplotype is clear only at a low dose of the virus, whereas at higher doses all strains respond equally.

V. Interpretation

The *H-2* effect on viral infection can be demonstrated by two tests: one based on segregating populations (backcross and F_2 generation) and one involving congenic lines differing at the *H-2* complex. The disadvantage of the segregating population test is that large numbers of animals are required to obtain meaningful results; its advantage is that information can be obtained about the number of genes determining the susceptibility of the virus. Methods based on congenic lines usually provide answers more quickly and require fewer animals, but they are limited to testing a single (differential) locus. In both tests, it is difficult to distinguish between an effect caused by the *H-2* complex itself and one caused by loci closely linked to *H-2*. In the segregating population test, a rare recombinant between H-*2* and the linked gene would probably be missed, and in the congenic lines, even after 10 or 15 generations of backcrossing, a considerable amount of "foreign" chromatin (chromatin derived from the donor strain) can be expected to be present at both ends of the *H-2* complex. However, congenic lines carrying the different *H-2* recombinant haplotypes can potentially be of great help, because they can narrow down the position of the virus susceptibility locus in chromosome 17.

In all cases in which association of virus susceptibility with the *H-2* system has been demonstrated, the *H-2* is not the sole gene complex governing the response of the host to the virus; genes segregating independently of *H-2* have also been implicated in the infection process. Evidently, the host-virus interaction is a complex phenomenon in which the genetic component is always polygenic in nature and the *H-2*-associated factor is only one facet of the system.

Because the viruses for which association with the *H-2* system has been demonstrated differ from each other (vaccinia is a DNA virus, while the remaining six are RNA viruses; Gross and Tennant viruses induce lymphocytic leukemia, while Friend virus induces primarily erythrocytic leukemia, etc.), it is unlikely that the mechanism of the *H-2* effect is the same in each. It is, therefore, somewhat surprising that the strains of the C57BL family are uniformly resistant to all viruses so far tested (except RadLV, which is derived from C57BL mice). The explanation for this unusual resistance undoubtedly lies in the origin of the C57BL strains. Because the strains seem to be genetically unrelated to most, if not all other inbred strains, it has been speculated that the C57BL family was derived from a different subspecies of *Mus musculus* (Potter and R. Lieberman 1967). Because most oncogenic viruses have been isolated from strains other than C57BL, it is conceivable that the C57BL genome is too foreign to be overridden by recent host-range mutants of these viruses.

The actual mechanism of the interaction between the *H-2* complex and the viruses is not known; however, at least four hypotheses have been proposed (Snell 1968; Lilly 1971b): the receptor hypothesis, cross-tolerance hypothesis, steric interaction hypothesis, and immune response hypothesis.

The receptor hypothesis in its simplest form assumes that the H-2 molecules act as receptor sites for attachment of the virus to the cell surface. According to this hypothesis, there is a key-lock type of specificity between certain viruses and certain H-2 molecules, and an antigen that serves as a receptor for one type of virus is completely inert for another type. *H-2* polymorphism is then explained as being a result of a continuing attempt on the part of the animal to escape catastrophic viral epidemy. There is evidence (see Snell 1968, for discussion and references) that at least some animal viruses do, indeed, require special attachment sites on the cell surface. Although the receptor hypothesis is very attractive, mainly for its simplicity, it is contradicted by three experimental findings. First, because the *H-2* loci are codominant, an F_1 hybrid between susceptible and resistant strains should express half of the virus receptors and should, therefore, be susceptible; but in many situations this is not so. In the case of Gross virus, the F_1 hybrids are even more resistant than the resistant parent. Second, because the attachment of the virus to the cell is the very first step in virus infection, one would expect that *H-2* would exercise its influence on viral oncogenesis in an early stage of the infection; but again, this is not so. In the case of Friend and vaccinia viruses, it seems that loci other than *H-2* determine whether a mouse is infected with the virus; the *H-2* then determines whether the infection will lead to the development of a tumor. Third, incubation of Gross or Friend viruses with spleen, thymus, and bone marrow cells from susceptible strains does not significantly decrease the infectivity of these viruses (Lilly 1971b). Hence, the receptor hypothesis does not seem to be a plausible explanation of *H-2*-virus interaction.

The cross-tolerance hypothesis is based on the assumption that susceptibility to viruses represents a failure of the host to recognize antigens of the virus as foreign and to respond to them immunologically. The failure is presumably caused by a close resemblance between viral and H-2 antigens (*molecular mimicry*). According to this hypothesis, in the resistant strains, the viral antigens are dissimilar enough to be recognized immunologically and destroyed. The viral antigens mimicking H-2 antigens of the host could be either on the virus particle itself or, more likely, could represent cell surface antigens induced by the virus (tumor-specific antigens, or TSA). Both the Gross and Friend viruses are known to induce TSA in infected cells (Old and Boyse 1965). An argument in favor of the cross-tolerance hypothesis is that young animals (immunologically immature) are usually much more susceptible to viral infection than adult animals. An argument against it is the resistance of F_1 hybrids in the crosses between susceptible and resistant strains; according to the cross-tolerance hypothesis, all the F_1 hybrids should be tolerant to the TSA, and therefore susceptible.

A variant of the cross-tolerance hypothesis was proposed by Nandi and his co-workers (1967) for the Bittner virus case. According to Nandi, virus particles, in their process of maturation and release from the infected cells, incorporate fragments of the host's cell membrane into their outer coats. If the fragments carry H-2 antigens, the virus particles become histoincompatible for allogeneic hosts differing at the *H-2* complex. However, so far there is no evidence that particles of any virus carry H-2 antigens. On the contrary, Aoki *et al.* (1970) and Dorfman *et al.* (1972) have demonstrated that viruses bud through areas devoid of H-2 antigens in the membrane.

The steric interaction hypothesis assumes that a cell infected by a virus becomes malignant only after it acquires new antigens on the cell membrane (most likely TSA), and that the acquisition of the new antigen is somehow dependent on the presence of a particular H-2 molecule on the membrane. Lilly (1971b) has suggested three ways in which such an interaction between the TSA and H-2 molecules might occur. First, the TSA might need the H-2 molecule as an attachment site to the membrane; second, the space near the H-2 molecules on the membrane could be the most suitable for anchoring the TSA molecule; and third, the TSA molecule might be replacing the H-2 molecule. The first possibility seems to be ruled out by the observation that cells of *H-2* homozygotes have twice the number of H-2 sites as similar cells of *H-2* heterozygotes, while the Friend virus-infected *H-2* homozygotes and heterozygotes do not differ in their levels of TSA (Lilly 1971b). If the TSA molecules were attached to the H-2 molecules, one would expect that the dose effect observed with the H-2 antigens would also be seen in the case of TSA. The second possibility is also unlikely, because Friend virus-infected cells saturated with H-2 antibodies absorb about the same amount of TSA antibodies as untreated cells, and vice versa (Lilly 1971b). Apparently, there is no steric hindrance between the H-2 and the TSA sites on the cell membrane, suggesting that the sites are far apart. Evidence against the third possibility comes from measurements of the quantitative expression of H-2 antigens and TSA in Friend virus-infected cells (Lilly 1971b). In the course of the development of the Friend virus disease, the quantity of both H-2 and TSA in the spleen cells changes, the maximum quantity of both antigens being reached 6–10 days after infection.

If TSA were simply replacing H-2 molecules, one would expect an inverse relationship between the two.

Despite the fact that experimental data do not support any of the possibilities suggested by Lilly (1971b), some kind of interaction between H-2 and TSA in FV-infected cells does seem to exist, as indicated by the following observation. After the period of 6–10 days, when the concentration of both H-2 and TSA have reached peak values, the antigens begin to decrease until 18–21 days after infection, when they level off at about 60–70 percent of their maximum value. However, this is true only for the antigens determined by the *H-2D* locus; *H-2K* locus antigens (namely, antigen H-2.31 of the $H-2^d$ complex) decrease much more rapidly and to a much greater extent, so that by the twenty-first day the cells seem to be completely without them (Lilly 1971b). The disappearance of the $H-2K^d$ antigens in the FV-infected cells could be either phenotypic (antigenic modulation) or genotypic. In the second case, it would be tempting to speculate that the virus genome is actually integrated into the *H-2K* region of the *H-2* chromosome (Lilly 1971b).

According to the immune response hypothesis, a hypothetical immune response gene that is part of the *H-2* complex controls the ability of the host to respond either to the antigens of the virus particle or (more likely) to a viral-induced TSA. There are four arguments in favor of this hypothesis. First, as will be discussed in the next chapter, the *H-2* region, in which the factor controlling resistance to Gross virus is also located (Lilly 1970), carries a series of genes controlling immune response to a variety of antigens. Second, in the *H-2*-associated immune response genes, the responsiveness is a dominant trait, as is the resistance in the *H-2*-associated virus-susceptibility genes. Third, the immune response hypothesis predicts that the difference between virus-susceptible and resistant strains would disappear once the cells of the two strains were transferred into tissue cultures. An indication that this does, indeed, happen has been obtained recently by Pincus *et al.* (1971a, b). Mouse embryo fibroblasts, cultivated *in vitro* and obtained from GV-susceptible and resistant strains, show no correlation between *H-2* haplotype and susceptibility to GV infection. Fourth, it has been demonstrated that both the resistant strain and the F_1 hybrids obtained from a cross between susceptible and resistant animals have "natural" antibodies to the Gross virus TSA (Aoki *et al.* 1966), indicating that these mice respond immunologically to the virus. These four arguments strongly suggest that the immune response hypothesis is probably the most likely explanation of the mechanism of the *H-2* effect on viral oncogenesis. However, direct evidence for *H-2*-associated *Ir* genes' controlling immunological reactivity to viral antigens is still missing.

Chapter Seventeen

Genetic Control of Immune Response

I. The *Ir-1* System

In 1962 Humphrey and McDevitt (quoted by McDevitt and Sela 1965) made an important chance observation. While studying immunogenicity of certain synthetic polypeptides prepared and analyzed by Sela and his colleagues (see Sela 1969 for a review), they found a marked quantitative difference between two rabbit strains (Sandylops and Himalayans) in the ability to form antibodies against these antigens. The difference suggested that the antibody response to synthetic polypeptides was genetically controlled. Intrigued by this possibility and at the same time realizing the disadvantages of genetic studies on outbred rabbits, McDevitt began a genetic analysis of immune response, employing inbred strains and congenic mouse lines. McDevitt and his colleagues were soon able to demonstrate that the antibody response to synthetic polypeptides was, indeed, genetically controlled and, moreover, that it was determined primarily by a single, autosomal dominant gene (or gene cluster), *immune response-1* (*Ir-1*),[1] located within the *H-2* complex. This was not the first report in the mouse to indicate that immune responsiveness was genetically controlled, but it was the first report to imply a relatively simple basis for genetic control. In all previous studies, the correlation between the responses of parents and offspring had been complex and difficult to interpret. The two factors mainly responsible for the simplicity of the correlation in McDevitt's system are the use of antigens with a rather limited range of determinants, and the employment of highly inbred strains.

The discovery and subsequent analysis of the *Ir-1A* gene added a new dimension to knowledge of the *H-2* system, and, together with similar studies in guinea pigs by Benacerraf and his colleagues, it signalled a new era in cellular immunology (for reviews, see McDevitt and Benacerraf 1969; Benacerraf and McDevitt 1972). Soon after the discovery, by McDevitt and his co-workers, of simple genetic control of the immune response to synthetic polypeptides, similar discoveries were made by others, using various other antigens. However, the McDevitt system has remained the best defined and, for this reason, it will be described here in detail, while the other systems will be only briefly summarized.

A. The *Ir-1A* Locus

1. Antigens

The antigen originally used by McDevitt and Sela (1965) is a branched, multichain polypeptide—poly-L-(*Tyr*,*Glu*)-poly-D,L-*Ala*-poly-L-*Lys*, or (T,G)-A--L. It consists of a poly-L-lysine backbone with poly-D,L-alanine side chains attached to it, and peptides containing L-tyrosine and L-glutamic acid attached to the amino-terminal groups of the polyalanine (Fig. 17–1, top). The molecular weight of the polypeptide can vary considerably, but most of the studies have

---

[1] The designation of the locus was later changed from *Ir-1* to *Ir-1A* to comply with standardized nomenclature (J. Klein *et al.* 1974a). The rules for assigning *Ir* gene symbols are the following: "Whenever they are shown to be separable by recombination, the *H-2*-associated *Ir* loci should be given symbols consisting of *Ir-1* followed by a capital letter (i.e., *Ir-1A*, *Ir-1B*, *Ir-1C*, ... *Ir-1Z*, *Ir-1AA*, *Ir-1AB*, ... *Ir-1AZ*, ...). The letters should be assigned in the order of discovery of the *Ir-1* loci. ... The *H-2*-associated immune response determinants not yet separated by recombination ... should not be assigned standard gene symbols, but should instead be referred to by provisional symbols consisting of the prefix *Ir* and an abbreviation of the antigen to which a particular immune response is directed (*Ir-OA* stands for immune responsiveness to ovalbumin, *Ir-BGG* for responsiveness to bovine gammaglobulin, etc.). If the immune response to a given antigen later proves to be controlled by one of the already known *Ir-1* loci, the provisional symbol will be dropped; if, on the other hand, the responsiveness proves to be controlled by a separate locus, the provisional symbol will be replaced by a genetic symbol in the *Ir-1* series (*Ir-1C*, *Ir-1D*, etc.). The alternative forms (alleles) at the *Ir-1* loci or subregions are designated by small superscript letters indicating their genetic origin (*Ir-1A^b* and *Ir-1B^b* in the case of the *H-2^b* haplotype; *Ir-1A^k* and *Ir-1B^k* in the case of the *H-2^a* haplotype, etc.)." (J. Klein *et al.* 1974a).

been done using polymers with an average molecular weight of 232,000 daltons and molar ratios of the amino acids 1 Tyr:2 Glu:4 Ala:19 Lys. Preparations of (T,G)-A--L of different molecular weights give the same pattern of response at the optimal antigen dose (McDevitt and Sela 1967). Other synthetic polypeptides used by McDevitt and his co-workers are poly-L(*His*,*Glu*)-poly-D,L-*A*la-poly-L-*Lys* [(H,G)-A--L] (Fig. 17–1, middle), and poly-L(*Phe*,*Glu*)-poly-D,L-*A*la-poly-L-*Lys* [(Phe,G)-A--L] (Fig. 17–1, bottom), with histidine and glutamic acid, or phenylalanine and glutamic acid attached to the polyalanine sidechains. Simpler synthetic polypeptides, such as branched polymers poly-L-*Glu*-poly-D,L-*A*la-poly-L-*Lys* (G-A--L), poly-L-*Tyr*-poly-L-*Gly*-poly-D,L-*A*la-poly-L-*Lys* (T-G-A--L) and linear polymer poly-L(*Tyr*,*Glu*-*A*la) (T,G,A) have also been used by McDevitt and Sela (1967).

2. Immunization

The immunization schedule used by McDevitt and his co-workers consists of two injections: first, adult mice are given from 1 to 100 μg of antigen, for example, (T,G)-A--L, in complete Freund's adjuvant, followed 5 weeks later by a similar dose of the same antigen in saline. The mice are bled 10 days after

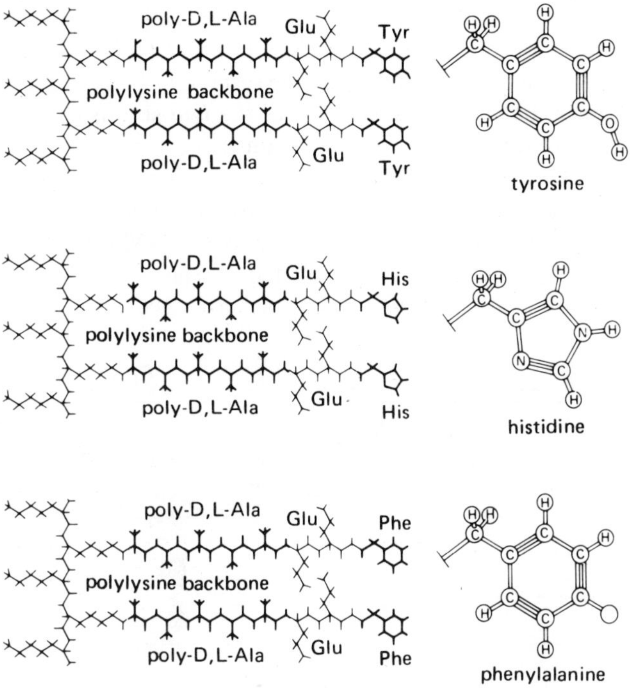

Fig. 17-1. Structure of three branched synthetic polypeptide antigens: (T,G)-A--L (top), (H,G)-A--L (middle), (Phe,G)-A--L (bottom). (Reproduced with permission from H. O. McDevitt: "Genetic control of the antibody response." *Hospital Practice* 8:61–74. Copyright © 1973 by Hospital Practice Co. All rights reserved.)

the second injection and individual sera are tested for the presence of (T,G)-A--L antibodies.

The titer of (T,G)-A--L antibodies is determined by their antigen-binding capacity (ABC). The antiserum is serially diluted and a constant amount of ^{125}I-labeled (T,G)-A--L is added to each dilution. After incubation, a constant amount of polyvalent rabbit antimouse gamma globulin antiserum is added to the mixture, and all the mouse antibodies present are precipitated. After another incubation period, the complexes composed of anti-(T,G)-A--L antibodies, ^{125}I-(T,G)-A--L antigen, and rabbit antimouse IgG antibodies are sedimented by centrifugation, and the amount of radioactivity left in the supernatant is counted. The results are expressed as the percentage of antigen bound in the complexes (see McDevitt and Sela 1965).

3. Genetic Analysis

Immunization of two inbred strains (C57 and CBA) with (T,G)-A--L demonstrated quite clearly that the antibody response to this antigen is genetically controlled (McDevitt and Sela 1965). C57 mice are good producers of (T,G)-A--L antibodies (high responders, HR), while CBA mice are poor producers (low responders, LR, Fig. 17–2), the difference in antibody production between the high and low responders being about tenfold. However, the response is dose dependent: at a low dose [1 μg of (T,G)-A--L], both strains respond poorly; at a high dose (100 μg), the response of CBA mice is lower than that of C57 mice, but the responsiveness of the two strains overlaps to a large extent. The difference between the two strains is most pronounced at a dose of 10 μg, at which the response ranges of CBA and C57 mice are widely separated.

An insight into the nature of genetic control of responsiveness to (T,G)-A--L was obtained by immunization of CBA and C57 hybrids (Fig. 17–2). The (CBA × C57)F$_1$ hybrids showed intermediate response compared to the two parental strains. The hybrids of the two backcross generations (F$_1$ × CBA and

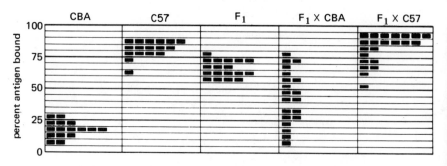

Fig. 17-2. Antibody response of CBA and C57BL mice and their hybrids to synthetic polypeptide (T,G)-A--L. Each rectangle represents one mouse. (The drawing is based on experiments of H. O. McDevitt and M. Sela.) (Reproduced with permission from H. O. McDevitt: "Genetic control of the antibody response." *Hospital Practice* 8:61–74. Copyright © 1973 by Hospital Practice Co. All rights reserved.)

$F_1 \times C57BL$) can be, with a certain degree of presumption, divided into two or possibly three classes. In the $F_1 \times CBA$ backcross, one class displays a range of responsiveness roughly coinciding with that of CBA mice (low responders); the responsiveness of the second class coincides with the range of F_1 hybrids (intermediate responders); a third, rather small group of animals could, perhaps, be interpreted as high responders (C57 type). In the $F_1 \times C57$ backcross, the two major classes of animal show intermediate (F_1) and high (C57) responsiveness, and the possible third minor class a low (CBA) responsiveness. If one ignores the minor third class, the simplest explanation of the bimodal distribution of the responsiveness in both backcross generations is that it is controlled by a single dominant gene, *immune response-1A* (*Ir-1A*). The gene has at least two alleles, one for high responsiveness (*Ir-1A^h*), and the other for low responsiveness (*Ir-1A^l*). For reasons that will later become apparent, the allelic symbols were subsequently changed (see J. Klein *et al.* 1974a) to reflect the origin of the *Ir-1A* gene, rather than the level of antibodies it controls. Thus, the designation of the *Ir-1A^h* allele carried by the *H-2^b* haplotype of strain C57 was changed to *Ir-1A^b*, and that of the *Ir-1A^l* allele carried by the *H-2^k* haplotype of strain CBA was changed to *Ir-1A^k*. According to the single-dominant-gene interpretation, the CBA strain is an *Ir-1A^k/Ir-1A^k* homozygote, the C57 strain an *Ir-1A^b/Ir-1A^b* homozygote, and the F_1 hybrid is an *Ir-1A^b/Ir-1A^k* heterozygote. The $F_1 \times CBA$ backcross produces two classes of animal: *Ir-1A^b/Ir-1A^k* (intermediate) and *Ir-1A^k/Ir-1A^k* (low); the $F_1 \times C57BL$ backcross also produces two classes of animal: *Ir-1A^b/Ir-1A^k* (intermediate) and *Ir-1A^b/Ir-1A^b* (high). If, on the other hand, the third minor class of animal in each backcross is taken into account, this simple interpretation must be modified by assuming that the *Ir-1A* gene is the major factor in the immune response, and that, in addition to it, an unknown number of modifying factors, which obscure the simple 1:1 segregation ratio, exist.

4. Nature of Antigenic Determinant

The *Ir-1A* gene has a remarkable capacity to discriminate among related antigens. After immunization with a closely related copolymer, (H,G)-A--L, the CBA mice respond well and the C57 mice poorly, a response diametrically opposite to the reactivity of these two strains to (T,G)-A--L (McDevitt and Sela 1967). After immunization with yet another related antigen (Phe,G)-A--L, both strains respond well, but a third strain, SJL, responds poorly (McDevitt and Sela 1967; McDevitt and Chinitz 1969). Because the only difference among (T,G)-A--L, (H,G)-A--L, and (Phe,G)-A--L is that the first carries tyrosine, the second histidine, and the third phenylalanine on the tips of the sidechains, the obvious conclusion is that responsiveness is directed against the (T,G), (H,G), and (Phe,G) portions of the polypeptides. This conclusion is supported by the finding that the G-A--L polymer, which represents the carrier portion of the three antigens without the tips, is nonantigenic (McDevitt and Sela 1967). A polymer called T-G-A--L, which has an amino acid composition similar to that of (T,G)-A--L except that it carries tyrosine and glutamic acid residues dispersed throughout the sidechain rather than on the tips, elicits the same pattern of response as (T,G)-A--L, but ten times lower, perhaps because of the low tyrosine content (McDevitt and Sela 1967). And finally, a random linear sequence of tyrosine, glutamic acid, and alanine (T,G,A) elicits the same response in both CBA and C57 mice. The difference in responsiveness to branched and linear polymers could be caused either by a difference in processing the two antigens, or by the fact that the linear polymer contains a much greater variety of antigenic determinants than the short terminal sequence in branched polymers and that this variety obscures the differences in responsiveness between CBA and C57 (McDevitt and Sela 1967).

5. Cross-reactivity and Cross-stimulation

The discriminating capacity of the *Ir-1A* gene is all the more remarkable in view of the fact that the three antigens cross-react extensively. For instance, anti-(T,G)-A--L serum binds not only (T,G)-A--L but also (H,G)-A--L and (Phe,G)-A--L, although the percentage of antigen bound is highest with (T,G)-A--L (McDevitt and Sela 1967). In spite of this cross-reactivity *in vitro*, cross-stimulation of the three antigens *in vivo* usually does not occur. For instance, (CBA × C57)F_1 hybrids immunized with (T,G)-A--L and then boosted with (H,G)-A--L make only low-titer (T,G)-A--L antibodies, which is typical of primary response to this antigen; no secondary response can be detected (McDevitt and Sela 1967).

6. Primary and Secondary Response

Analysis of the kinetics of antibody formation in mice immunized with (T,G)-A--L has revealed that the *Ir-1A* gene exerts its effect on the secondary, but not on the primary response. The effect was first demonstrated using the original immunization regimen, in which the first injection is given in Freund's adjuvant and the second in aqueous solution (McDevitt 1968). However, it is difficult to distinguish secondary response from primary response in this regimen, because the adjuvant retains the antigen for long periods of time, and only gradually releases it in small doses. Clearer results are obtained when both (T,G)-A--L injections are administered in aqueous solution. Grumet (Grumet *et al.* 1971a, b; Grumet 1972) demonstrated that the first injection of (T,G)-A--L administered in aqueous solution stimulates a prompt primary response in both HR (C3H.SW) and LR (C3H) strains. The response reaches its peak in the first week after immunization and then slowly declines over the next 3 weeks. The second injection elicits rapid secondary response only in the HR strain (Fig. 17-3). The difference in secondary response between the HR and LR strains can be obliterated if the antigen is complexed with methylated bovine serum albumin (MBSA), which causes both the C57 (HR) and CBA (LR) mice to respond to secondary stimulus with high titers of (T,G)-A--L antibodies (McDevitt 1968).

The low responders' inability to mount a secondary reaction seems to be linked in some way to the presence of (T,G)-A--L antibodies induced by the first immunization. Ordal and Grumet (1973) have demonstrated that non-immune LR cells transferred into irradiated syngeneic recipients containing (T,G)-A--L antibodies fail to respond to (T,G)-A--L immunization.

7. *Immunoglobulin Class*

Although McDevitt (1968) originally demonstrated that (T,G)-A--L antibodies are present in all four major immunoglobulin classes (IgG_1, IgG_2, IgA, and IgM), more recent studies indicate that the defect in the immune response to (T,G)-A--L primarily affects the IgG class (Grumet *et al.* 1971a, b; Grumet 1972). The first injection of the antigen in aqueous solution elicits an antibody production that is almost entirely of the 2-mercaptoethanol-sensitive (19S, IgM) type in both HR and LR strains. The titers of these antibodies reach their peak during the first week after immunization and then gradually decline. The second injection of (T,G)-A--L elicits 2-mercaptoethanol-resistant (7S, IgG) antibodies in the HR strain but not in the LR strain (Fig. 17-3), indicating that the LR strain is unable to produce the IgG class of (T,G)-A--L antibodies.

8. *Adoptive Transfer*

McDevitt and Tyan (1968) demonstrated that LR mice can be converted into high responders by replacing their lymphoid cells with cells derived from an HR strain. This replacement can be achieved by lethally irradiating the LR recipients and injecting them with spleen cells from HR animals. However, the difficulty with such an adoptive transfer experiment is that spleen cells from an *H-2*-incompatible donor display strong graft-versus-host reaction, which can kill the recipient. To avoid GVHR after the cell transfer, cells from an (HR × LR)F_1 hybrid must be used. Immunization in the cell transfer experiment can be carried out in two ways: by administering the first injection of (T,G)-A--L to the donor before the cell transfer, and the second injection to the recipient after the

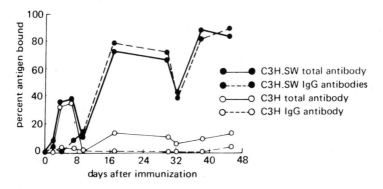

Fig. 17-3. Primary and secondary response of C3H and C3H.SW mice to aqueous solution of (T,G)-A--L. (Reproduced with permission from H. O. McDevitt: "Genetic control of the antibody response." *Hospital Practice* 8:61–74. Copyright © 1973 by Hospital Practice Co. All rights reserved.)

cell transfer (adoptive transfer of a secondary antibody response), or by administering both injections to the recipient after the cell transfer (adoptive transfer of a primary antibody response). Using this approach, McDevitt and Tyan (1968) demonstrated that the ability to elicit both primary and secondary response to (T,G)-A--L can be transferred to a low responder by injecting spleen cells from a moderate $(HR \times LR)F_1$ responder into the LR recipient. Their experiments can be summarized as follows:

Cell donor	Recipient	Response
HR	LR	H
HR	HR	H
LR	LR	L

(H = high response, L = low response). High responsiveness can be transferred with fetal liver cells (Tyan *et al.* 1969), bone marrow cells (G. Mitchell *et al.* 1972), or with partially purified peripheral blood leukocytes (Tyan and McDevitt, quoted by McDevitt and Benacerraf 1969), as well as with spleen cells. Thoracic duct lymphocytes can transfer secondary, but not primary response (Tyan *et al.* 1969).

9. Role of the Thymus

Experiments on thymectomized (Tx) mice (Table 17–1) led to the following observations (McDevitt and Tyan 1968; Tyan *et al.* 1969). First, adult Tx and lethally irradiated mice, whether of the HR or LR strain, behave as high responders do when protected with spleen cells derived from HR mice. Second,

Table 17-1. Responsiveness to (T,G)-A--L of adult thymectomized (Tx) and lethally irradiated mice protected with spleen or fetal liver cells from high (HR) and low (LR) responders*

Donor		Tx recipient	Response**
Responsiveness	Tissue		
HR	spleen	HR	H
HR	spleen	LR	H
HR	fetal liver	HR	L
LR	fetal liver	HR	L
HR	fetal liver	LR	L
LR	fetal liver and intact thymus	HR	L
HR	fetal liver and intact thymus	LR	H

* Based on experimental data of McDevitt and Tyan 1968, and Tyan *et al.* 1969.
** H = high response; L = low response.

adult Tx and lethally irradiated mice, whether of the HR or LR strain, behave as low responders do when protected with fetal liver cells derived from HR or LR mice. Third, adult Tx and lethally irradiated mice grafted with intact LR or HR thymuses and protected with fetal liver cells derived from HR mice behave as high responders do; the same mice protected with fetal liver cells derived from LR mice behave as low responders do.

These experiments allow the following conclusions to be drawn. First, the high or low responsiveness does not depend on the genotype of the thymus epithelium. Intact thymus is needed for the response, but whether the donor of the thymus is a high or low responder is irrelevant; thymus from an LR strain supports responsiveness as well as thymus from an HR strain. Second, high or low responsiveness does not depend on the genotype of the antibody-forming cells (or their precursors, B cells). B cells from LR strains can be stimulated to differentiate into HR antibody-producing cells. Third, high or low responsiveness does depend on the genotype of the thymus repopulating cells (e.g., fetal liver cells). Only thymocyte precursors derived from HR strains can provide conditions for high responsiveness; precursors from LR strains cannot. And finally, the experiments suggest, but do not prove, that the responsiveness is determined by the genotype of T cells.

10. Role of T Cells

McDevitt and his co-workers attempted to provide direct evidence for the involvement of T cells by proving that T cells from an HR strain can stimulate B cells from an LR strain to behave as if they were HR cells [i.e., to produce high titers of (T,G)-A--L antibodies]. The authors used two approaches in this attempt, one based on radiation chimeras (Chesebro *et al.* 1971, 1972), and the other on tetraparental mice (McDevitt *et al.* 1971, 1974a, b). Both chimeras and tetraparental mice can be produced in such a way as to create a situation in which HR T cells are mixed with LR B cells, and antibodies produced by the LR B cells can be identified by virtue of immunoglobulin allotype markers. Chesebro *et al.* (1972) obtained 39 chimeras by inoculation of B10 (HR) fetal liver cells into lethally irradiated adult CBA (LR) recipients, and by inoculation of CBA fetal liver cells into B10 recipients. Upon immunization with (T,G)-A--L, 19 of the chimeras (12 B10 → CBA and 7 CBA → B10) proved to be low responders, whereas the remaining 20 (15 B10 → CBA and 5 CBA → B10) proved to be high responders. Most LR chimeras had relatively low levels of B10 immunoglobulins, but there were several animals that had nearly normal levels. Using Simonsen's discrimination spleen assay (injecting lymphoid cells from the chimeras into newborn CBA and B10 mice and determining the degree of GVHR), the authors were able to demonstrate that most of the LR animals contained B10 lymphoid cells. The HR chimeras had very low levels of CBA immunoglobulins and nearly normal levels of B10 immunoglobulins. The discrimination spleen assay proved that most of the chimeras contained both B10 and CBA lymphoid cells. The allotype of (T,G)-A--L antibodies produced by the HR chimeras was determined by precipitating out from the anti-(T,G)-A--L serum the B10 (or CBA) immunoglobulins with antiallotype antisera, and then assaying the sera for remaining (T,G)-A--L activity. In all of the 11 HR chimeras that contained anti-(T,G)-A--L titers high enough for such determination, only (T,G)-A--L antibodies of the B10 (HR) allotype were detected. There was no evidence of production of (T,G)-A--L antibodies carrying the LR strain allotype. Thus, this experiment failed to prove that T cells of HR origin could stimulate B cells of LR origin to produce (T,G)-A--L antibodies. The failure to obtain such antibodies could mean either that the original assumption was incorrect, or that the interaction between the B10 T cells and CBA B cells was not possible because of the strong histocompatibility difference between these two strains, or it could mean that the methods used were not sensitive enough to detect low levels of (T,G)-A--L antibodies produced by the small fraction of CBA B cells.

In the experiment with tetraparental (allophenic) mice (McDevitt *et al.* 1971; Freed *et al.* 1973; Bechtol *et al.* 1974; McDevitt *et al.* 1974a, b), chimeras were obtained by fusion of cleavage-stage embryos from C3H (LR, Ig-1^a/Ig-1^a, H-2^k/H-2^k) and CWB (HR, Ig-1^b/Ig-1^b, H-2^b/H-2^b) or (CKB × CWB)F$_1$ (HR, Ig-1^b/Ig-1^b, H-2^b/H-2^b) and by development of the fused embryos in pseudopregnant "incubator mothers." Adult tetraparental animals were immunized with (T,G)-A--L (two injections, the first in Freund's adjuvant, the second in saline) and tested for the production of (T,G)-A--L antibodies (using the ABC assay) and immunoglobulin allotype (using antiallotype sera). In addition, individual lymphoid cells of the chimeras were also tested for (T,G)-A--L antibody production and *H-2* haplotype in a plaque-forming assay. The plaque-forming assay was performed with (T,G)-A--L conjugated to chromium chloride and then attached to sheep red blood cells. The *H-2* haplotype of the plaque-forming cells was determined indirectly by treatment of the cell suspension before plating in agar with anti-H-2^b (or anti-H-2^k) antibodies and complement. Of the 44 tetraparental mice obtained, eight produced 6–70 times more LR-type antibodies than standard C3H mice. This result proves that the progeny of LR B cells are capable of producing (T,G)-A--L antibodies, and suggests that the genetic defect is in T cells, rather than in B cells.

11. In Vitro System

Because of the difficulties in identifying the cells involved in the immune response to (T,G)-A--L and other synthetic polypeptides, attempts have been made to simplify the experimental system by duplicating it in tissue culture. To study genetically determined immune responses, an *in vitro* system based on measuring the proliferative response of lymphoid cells in the presence of the antigen has recently been described by Tyan (Tyan and Ness 1971; Tyan 1972). In this system, the prospective donor is given one injection of (T,G)-A--L in Freund's adjuvant and sacrificed 3 weeks later. Peripheral blood leukocytes from the immunized (and also unimmunized) donors are transferred into tissue cultures, (T,G)-A--L is added to the cells, and the cells are incubated for 5 to 7 days. Shortly before the termination of the cultures, ^{3}H-thymidine is added to the cells as a marker of the proliferative response. After harvesting the cultures, incorporation of the ^{3}H-thymidine into DNA of the cell nuclei is measured by scintillation counting. The experiments indicate that peripheral blood leukocytes from both HR and LR strains respond to stimulation with (T,G)-A--L by DNA synthesis, but at the peak of the response (5–6 days after transfer into tissue culture), leukocytes from HR mice synthesize from 10–100 times more DNA than do leukocytes from LR mice. Also, leukocytes from HR mice can be stimulated significantly at an antigen concentration of 3–6 μg/ml, while concentrations of 12–25 μg/ml are required to achieve the same response with cells from LR mice. There is no significant difference between cells from sensitized and normal mice in the response to (T,G)-A--L stimulation *in vitro*. Comparison of the response of different cell types from HR and LR to two antigens, (T,G)-A--L and DNP-BGG (2,4-dinitrophenyl conjugate of bovine gammaglobulin) demonstrated that peripheral blood leukocytes are the most responsive to *in vitro* antigenic stimulation, followed by spleen, bone marrow, and fetal liver cells, in that order. (Fetal tissues that do not contain precursors of antibody-producing cells, such as yolk sac, placenta, lung, brain, and skin, are not stimulated by the antigen *in vitro*.) At the peak of the response, HR mice seem to have from 10 to 100 times more leukocytes, 2 to 4 times more spleen cells, and 1.5 to 3 times more bone marrow cells proliferating as a result of *in vitro* stimulation with (T,G)-A--L, than the LR mice.

In vitro responsiveness is antigen-specific; cells responding poorly to one antigen [i.e., (T,G)-A--L] are capable of responding well to another antigen (i.e., DNP-BGG). Fetal liver tissues respond equally, regardless of the genotype (HR versus LR) and the antigen used [(T,G)-A--L versus DNP-BGG], suggesting that HR and LR embryos have the same number of lymphoid cells capable of response *in vitro* to either (T,G)-A--L or DNP-BGG. Addition of adult spleen or thymus cells to the culture of fetal liver cells does not cause a significant increase in the response to (T,G)-A--L. The *in vitro* response of HR and LR blood leukocytes and bone marrow cells to (T,G)-A--L can be greatly reduced by incubation of these cells (prior to culturing) with anti-Thy-1.2 serum. The antigen-induced proliferation of fetal liver cells is not influenced by anti-Thy-1.2 serum, but is completely ablated by antiserum produced in rabbits immunized with normal mouse serum.

These studies were extended by Lonai and McDevitt (McDevitt *et al.* 1974b) who demonstrated that the *in vitro* transformation of immune lymphocytes in the presence of (T,G)-A--L is clearly a T cell dependent function. The authors also demonstrated that cells carrying the *H-2^b* haplotype responded to (T,G)-A--L and (Phe,G)-A--L but not to (H,G)-A--L; cells carrying the *H-2^k* haplotype responded to (H,G)-A--L and (Phe,G)-A--L, but not to (T,G)-A--L; cells carrying the *H-2^q* haplotype responded only to (Phe,G)-A--L, while *H-2^s* cells did not respond to any of the three antigens. This pattern of *in vitro* responsiveness is identical to that observed *in vivo* and measured by antibody formation.

Lymphocytes from animals immunized with (T,G)-A--L responded *in vitro* only to (T,G)-A--L and did not respond to (H,G)-A--L or (Phe,G)-A--L, suggesting that the *in vitro* system is more specific than the *in vivo* system, in which antibodies produced against (T,G)-A--L cross-react with both (H,G)-A--L and (Phe,G)-A--L.

The *in vitro* stimulation of T cells by (T,G)-A--L is temperature dependent with low temperatures preventing the antigen binding by the T cells.

The stimulation is inhibited by preincubation of the cells with anti-H-2 sera directed against the antigens carried by the transforming lymphocytes. Addition of polyvalent antimouse Ig sera has no measurable effect.

12. Antigen Binding

The capability of lymphocytes to bind (T,G)-A--L has been studied by G. Hämmerling and McDevitt (1973, 1974a, b). In these experiments, lymphoid cells of different origins were incubated *in vitro* with ^{125}I-(T,G)-A--L for 15 min, and then washed, smeared thinly on gelatin-coated slides, and processed autoradiographically. Morphologically intact cells with more than nine grains over the cell surface were classified as antigen-binding cells (ABC's). Photographic exposure of the slides for 4 days detected only antigens binding to B cells, but when the exposure was increased to 11 days, the presence of antigens binding to T cells was revealed.

The T cell binding differed from B cell binding in four aspects. First, B cells bound much more antigen [between 500 and 15,000 (T,G)-A--L molecules/cell] than T cells (200–500 molecules/cell). Second, in contrast to B cells, the antigen-binding to T cells was temperature dependent, being three to four times higher at 37°C than at 4°C, and the dependence seemed to be related to metabolic activity (it was inhibited by sodium azide). Third, preincubation of cells with anti-H-2 sera did not affect B-ABC's, but completely inhibited T-ABC's. Similar inhibition of T-ABC's was observed after preincubation with anti-Thy-1 and with rabbit antimouse T cell sera, suggesting that it was caused by some topographical peculiarity of the T cell surface, rather than by cross-reaction between H-2 (Thy-1, T cell-specific antigen)- and (T,G)-A--L-recognizing receptors. Fourth, in contrast to T-ABC's, the ^{125}I-(T,G)-A--L binding to B cells can be inhibited by preincubation, not only with (T,G)-A--L but also (H,G)-A--L, suggesting a broader range of cross-reactivity for B cell receptors than for T cell receptors.

Preincubation of T cells from normal and immunized mice with anti-IgM (but not with anti-IgG) sera partially inhibited ^{125}I-(T,G)-A--L binding. The inhibition could mean either that the T cell receptor is an immunoglobulin, or that the B cells release cytophilic IgM molecules which then secondarily bind to T cell surfaces. In the latter case one has to assume further that binding of anti-immunoglobulin antibodies to the IgM on T cells sterically interferes with the actual T cell receptor. A third possibility is that T cells contain small amounts of IgM, which is not the T cell receptor, and that the inhibition is again through steric interference.

The B-ABC's have the following properties. Unimmunized HR and LR mice have about the same number of ABC's in their lymphoid organs, (approximately 10 $ABC/10^4$ cells in spleen and lymph nodes), and the (T,G)-A--L-binding receptors are almost exclusively of the IgM type. After primary immunization with (T,G)---AL in saline, the frequency of ABC's is much greater in the HR strain than in the LR strain, although both strains produce the same amount of IgM (T,G)-A--L antibody, suggesting that HR mice produce more memory cells after antigenic stimulation than do LR mice. After secondary immunization, the difference in the frequency of ABC's between HR and LR mice is even more striking. Surprisingly, however, the majority of ABC's (70–90 percent) in both HR and LR strains bind the antigen via IgG receptors, despite the fact that low responders are not able to produce detectable levels of IgG (T,G)-A--L antibodies.

The finding that LR mice give rise to a cell population with IgG receptors, although they fail to produce IgG antibodies, implies that the *Ir-1A* locus is not involved in the switch from IgM to IgG receptors, but rather affects the proliferation and differentiation of precursor B cells into IgG-producing plasma cells after the expression of IgG receptors.

13. Association with the H-2 Complex

The two strains in which the difference in (T,G)-A--L responsiveness was originally discovered differ not only in the *Ir-1A* locus, but also in a number of histocompatibility loci, in *H-2*, among others (CBA is $H-2^k$ and C57 is $H-2^b$). The strong histocompatibility barrier was the major obstacle in all attempts to study *Ir-1A* gene expression by transferring spleen cells from C57 donors to CBA recipients. The cell transfer experiments failed because of radiation death of the recipients or because of death caused by GVHR. McDevitt and his associates, therefore, began a systematic search for a combination of strains that would differ in (T,G)-A--L responsiveness but would share the same *H-2* haplotype. But they discovered that such a combination was not possible to find because of a strong correlation between (T,G)-A--L responsiveness and the *H-2* haplotype, suggesting that the two traits are genetically linked. The linkage was later proved by *Ir-1A* typing of various inbred strains and congenic lines and by linkage tests (McDevitt and Chinitz 1969; McDevitt *et al.* 1971, 1972).

As shown in Table 17–2, all inbred strains sharing the same *H-2* haplotype display the same pattern of responsiveness not only to (T,G)-A--L, but also to (H,G)-A--L and (Phe,G)-A--L. The only exceptions are strains carrying the $H-2^d$ haplotype, which, for some reason, are quite variable in their responsiveness to synthetic polypeptides. The data obtained by *Ir-1A* typing of congenic lines are even more compelling (McDevitt and Chinitz 1969; Grumet and McDevitt 1972), the pattern of responsiveness being determined almost exclusively by the *H-2* haplotype. For example, strains A ($H-2^a$) and C57BL/10

Table 17-2. H-2-associated immune responses to various antigens*, **

Strain	H-2 haplotype	(T,G)-A--L	(H,G)-A--L	(Phe,G)-A--L	OA	BPO-OA	BPO-BGG	BPO-OM	BPO-RNase	DNP-BGG	OM	TNP-MSA	GAT¹⁰	GAT⁺	GLA⁵ and GLA¹⁰	GLφ	TG	IgA(MOPC 467)	IgG(MOPC 173)	IgH(MOPC 195)	Thy-1.1 (θ-AKR)	Thy-1.2 (θ-C3H)	H-Y	H-2.2	Ea-1	Slp	Nase
A	a	l	h	h	l	l	h	h	h	h	h	l	h	h	h	l	m	h	l	h	l		m	h			h
B10.A	a	l	h	h	l							l	l	h	h	l	m	h	l	m	l		m	l			h
AL	a												h						h		m							
A.AL	al			l	l								h				h											
DKR	al	h	h	h									h	m														
C57BL/10	b	h	l	h	h		l	l	l	l	l	h	h	l	l	n	l		h		l		h	l	l	n	l
B10.T	b		m/h										l	m					h				h					
C57	b	h											h	h		n			h									
C57BL/6	b	m/h					l	l	l	l	l	h	h	h		n			h				h		l			l
C57L	b	h											h										h					
CWB	b	h																									n	
C3H.B10	b	h	l	h	h		l	l	l	l	l		l	l					h				m/h					
C3H.SW	b	h	l	h									h						h		m		h					
A.BY	b	h	l	h														l	n									l
D1.LP	b	h	l																h		h		m/h			n	
129	bc				h		l	l	l	l	l		h	h	l	n	l	l	n				h				
B10.129(6M)	bc	h																			h		l(m)				h
LP	bc	h			h								l	l		h			h		l		h			n	h
BALB/c	d	m	m	h	h		l	l	l	l	l		h	h	h			n	h	n			h				
DBA/2	d	m	m	h									h	h	h				n								
C57BL/Ks	d	m/h			m/h								h	h	h									h			

Strain	*H-2*
NBL	*a*
YBR	*d*
B10.D2	*d*
WH/Re	*d*
C.B6	*d*
C.AL	*d*
B6.C-*H-2²*	*d*
A.CA	*f*
B10.M	*f*
RFM	*f*
HTG	*g*
D2.GD	*g2*
HTH	*h*
B10.A(1R)	*h1*
B10.A(2R)	*h2*
B10.A(4R)	*h4*
HTI	*i*
B10.A(3R)	*i3*
B10.A(5R)	*i5*
I	*j*
C	*j*
C3H.JK	*ja*
WB/Re	*k*
C3H/He	*k*
C3H/Di	*k*
CBA	*k*
AKR	*k*
RF	*k*
C57BR	*k*
C58	*k*
CE	*k*
MA	*k*

Table 17-2. (Continued)

Strain	H-2 haplotype	(T,G)-A--L	(H,G)-A--L	(Phe,G)-A--L	OA	BPO-OA	BPO-BGG	BPO-OM	BPO-RNase	DNP-BGG	OM	TNP-MSA	GAT^{10}	GAT^4	GLA^5 and GLA^{10}	$GL\phi$	TG	IgA(MOPC 467)	IgG(MOPC 173)	IgH(MOPC 195)	Thy-1.1 (θ-AKR)	Thy-1.2 (θ-C3H)	H-Y	H-2.2	Ea-1	Slp	Nase
ST/b	k	·	·	·	·	·	h	·	·	·	·	·	·	·	·	·	h	n	·	·	·	·	·	·	·	·	·
B10.BR	k	l	h	h	l	·	·	·	·	·	h	·	h	h	h	l	h	h	l	m	m	·	m	l	·	h	·
B10.K	k	l	·	·	·	·	·	·	·	·	·	·	h	·	·	·	·	·	·	n	·	·	·	·	·	·	·
AKR.M	m	l	m/h	h	·	·	·	·	·	·	·	·	n	·	·	h	m	m	·	l	·	·	m	·	·	·	·
B10.AKM	m	l	h	h	·	·	·	·	·	·	·	·	h	·	·	n	·	m	h	·	·	·	·	·	·	·	·
B10.F	n	l	·	·	·	·	·	·	·	·	·	·	h	·	·	·	·	·	·	·	·	·	·	·	·	·	·
F	n	l	l	h	l	·	·	·	·	·	·	·	n	m	l	h	l	·	·	·	·	·	·	·	·	·	·
C3H.OH	o2	l	l	·	l	·	·	·	·	·	·	·	h	·	·	h	l	·	h	·	·	·	·	·	·	·	·
C3H.OL	o1	l	m	·	·	·	·	·	·	·	·	·	n	·	·	l	·	·	h	·	·	m	·	·	·	·	·
EDR	o1	l	·	h	·	·	·	·	·	·	·	·	n	n	l	·	·	m/h	h	·	l	·	·	·	·	·	l
P	p	l	m	·	·	·	l	·	·	·	·	·	n	·	·	·	m	·	n	·	·	·	·	·	·	·	·
BDP	p	l	l	h	·	·	l	·	·	·	·	·	n	n	l	h	·	·	·	·	·	·	·	·	·	·	·
B10.P	p	l	·	h	·	·	l	·	·	·	·	·	n	·	·	h	·	n	·	·	·	·	·	·	·	·	·
C3H.NB	p	l	l	·	·	·	·	·	·	·	·	·	n	n	h?	·	h	·	l	·	·	·	l(n)	·	·	·	·
B10.Y	pa	l	·	h	·	·	·	·	·	·	·	·	·	·	·	·	h	l	·	·	·	·	l(n)	·	·	h	·
DBA/1	q	l	·	h	h	·	·	·	·	m	l	·	n	·	·	h	h	·	·	·	·	m	·	·	·	·	·
BUB	q	l	·	·	h	·	·	·	m	m	·	·	·	·	·	h	·	·	·	h	l	·	·	·	·	·	·
SWR	q	l	·	h	h	·	·	m	m	m	l	·	·	·	·	·	·	·	·	·	·	m	·	·	·	·	·
T138	q	l	·	h	·	·	·	·	·	·	·	·	·	·	·	h	·	·	·	·	·	·	·	·	·	·	·
B10.G	q	l	·	·	·	·	·	·	·	·	·	·	n	·	h	·	·	·	h	h	l	·	·	·	·	h	·
RIII	r	l	·	·	·	·	·	·	·	·	·	·	·	·	h	·	·	h	h	h	l	·	·	·	·	h	·

Strain		(T,G)-A--L	(H,G)-A--L	(Phe,G)-A--L	OA	BPO-OA
LP.RIII	r			h	h	h
B10.RIII(71NS)	r	l		.	.	.
SJL	s	l	m	m	n	h
A.SW	s	l	m	h	n	h
TN	s	s	l	l	n	.
A.TH	t2				n	.
BSVS	t5				n	.
B10.S(7R)	t2	l			.	.
A.TL	t1	h	m	h	h	.
DSR	t1				.	.
PL	u				.	m
SM	v				l	.
AQR	y1	m/h h	l	h	.	.
B10.T(6R)	y2	l			l	l
NZW	z				l	l
CFW	?	h			.	.
SW-55	?	h h l			.	.
BRT	?	l			.	.
Swiss	?	l		n	.	.
BRSUNT	?			n	.	.
DD	?			n	.	.
STR	?			n	.	.
STR/1	?			n	.	.
DE	?			h	.	h
NH	?			h	l	.
RR	?			.	.	h

*Abbreviations:
(T,G)-A--L = synthetic branched multichain polypeptide poly-L(Tyr,Glu)-poly-D,L-Ala-Poly-L-Lys
(H,G)-A--L = synthetic branched multichain polypeptide poly-L(His,Glu)-poly-D,L-Ala-poly-L-Lys
(Phe,G)-A--L = synthetic branched multichain polypeptide poly-L-(Phe,Glu)-poly-D,L-Ala-poly-L-Lys
OA = ovalbumin
BPO-OA = benzylpenicilloyl$_6$(BPO) conjugate of ovalbumin (OA)

Table 17-2. (*Continued*)

BPO-BGG	= benzylpenicilloyl$_{125}$(BPO) conjugate of bovine gammaglobulin (BGG)
BPO-OM	= benzylpenicilloyl$_4$(BPO) conjugate of ovomucoid (OM)
BPO-RNAse	= benzylpenicilloyl$_4$(BPO) conjugate of bovine pancreatic ribonuclease (RNAse)
DNP-BGG	= dinitrophenyl$_{42}$(DNP) conjugate of bovine gammaglobulin
OM	= ovomucoid
TNP-MSA	= 2,4,6-trinitrophenyl (TNP) conjugate of mouse serum albumin (MSA)
GAT^{10}	= random linear copolymer (L-glu^{60}L-ala^{30}L-tyr^{10})$_n$
GAT^4	= random linear copolymer (L-glu^{58}L-ala^{38}L-tyr^4)$_n$
GLA^5 and GLA^{10}	= random linear copolymers (Glu^{57}Lys^{38}Ala^5) and (Glu^{56}Ly^{36}Ala^{10})
GLϕ	= random linear copolymer (L-Glu^{58}L-lys^{38}L-phe^4)$_n$ (the superscript is the molecular ratio of amino acids in the polymer)
TG	= thyroglobulin
IgA	= immunoglobulin A myeloma protein of BALB/c origin (MOPC 467)

IgG (G$_{2a}$)	= immunoglobulin G (γG$_{2a}$) myeloma protein of BALB/c origin (MOPC 173)
IgH (G$_{2b}$)	= immunoglobulin H (γG$_{2b}$) myeloma protein of BALB/c origin (MOPC 195)
Thy-1	= thymocyte alloantigen-1 (theta)
H-Y	= male histocompatibility antigen
H-2.2	= antigen 2 controlled by the *H-2* complex
Ea-1	= erythrocyte alloantigen 1
Slp	= sex-limited protein
Nase	= nuclease from *Staphylococcus aureus*
n	= no response
l	= low response
m	= moderate response
h	= high response
l/m	= borderline response between low and moderate
m/h	= borderline response between moderate and high
.	= not tested
l/(m)	= tested low by one laboratory and moderate by another
n	= recipient carries the same allotype as the immunogen

** References for antigens:

Columns 1–3:	McDevitt and Chinitz 1969; Grumet and McDevitt 1972
Columns 4–5:	Vaz *et al.* 1970, 1971; Dunham *et al.* 1973
Columns 6–9:	Vaz and Levine 1970
Column 10:	Vaz *et al.* 1971
Column 11:	Rathbun and Hildemann 1970
Column 12:	Martin *et al.* 1971; Merryman and Maurer 1972; Dunham *et al.* 1973
Column 13:	Merryman and Maurer 1972
Column 14:	Merryman *et al.* 1972
Column 15:	Maurer and Merryman 1974
Column 16:	Vladutiu and Rose 1971; Tomazic *et al.* 1974
Column 17:	R. Lieberman and Humphrey 1971
Column 18:	R. Lieberman and Humphrey 1972
Column 19:	R. Lieberman and Paul 1974
Column 20–21:	Fuji *et al.* 1971c, 1972; Zaleski *et al.* 1973; M. Zaleski 1974
Column 22:	Bailey and Hoste 1971; Bailey 1971c; Gasser and Silvers 1971a, b; Stimpfling and Reichert 1971
Column 23:	Lilly *et al.* 1971, 1973; Stimpfling and Durham 1972
Column 24:	Gasser and Shreffler 1972
Column 25:	H. C. Passmore, *personal communication*
Column 26:	Lozner *et al.* 1974b

(H-2^b) are LR and HR to (T,G)-A--L, respectively; congenic line B10.A, which has the background of strain C57BL/10 and the H-2 complex of strain A, is a low (T,G)-A--L responder, as is the donor of the H-2 complex. In contrast, congenic line A.BY, which has the A strain background but carries the H-2^b haplotype, is a high responder. Thus, the introduction of the H-2 complex from an HR strain onto a background of an LR strain leads to high responsiveness of the resulting congenic line.

Linkage with the H-2 complex was established using populations segregating for responsiveness to (T,G)-A--L (McDevitt and Tyan 1968), (H,G)-A--L (McDevitt and Tyan 1968), and (Phe,G)-A--L (McDevitt and Chinitz 1969). The linkage between the Ir-$1A$ locus and the H-2 complex is almost absolute; in the few cases in which crossing-over between H-2 and Ir-$1A$ was proved, the crossover event always took place *within* the H-2 complex, suggesting that the Ir-$1A$ locus actually lies between the K and D regions. The intra-H-2 location of the Ir-$1A$ locus was later confirmed by analysis of known H-2 recombinants (McDevitt *et al.* 1971, 1972; see Chapter Ten). The analysis established that the Ir-$1A$ locus occupies a chromosomal segment between the K and S regions. Because the Ir-$1A$ was the first locus identified in this segment, the segment was designated the Ir region and this designation was later changed to I region.

14. Other Ir Genes in the IA Subregion

Most recently three other Ir genes have been mapped into the same subregion (IA) as the Ir-$1A$ gene: Ir-l-OA, Ir-l-BGG, and Ir-l-OM, controlling the immune response to low doses of ovalbumin, bovine gammaglobulin, and hen ovomucoid, respectively (M. E. Dorf, F. Lilly and B. Benacerraf, quoted by Benacerraf and Katz 1974). These genes could be alleles at the Ir-$1A$ locus (see below). Genes controlling the immune response to antigens (T,G)-A--L (McDevitt *et al.* 1972), immunoglobulin A (R. Lieberman and W. Humphrey 1971), and ragweed extract (M. Dorf and B. Benacerraf, quoted by Benacerraf and Katz 1974), most likely are located in the IA subregion also, although genetically they have not yet been separated from genes in the K region.

B. The IB Subregion

The IB subregion controls the immune response to at least three antigens: myeloma protein MOPC 173 (R. Lieberman and Humphrey 1971, 1972; R. Lieberman *et al.* 1972), lactate dehydrogenase B (Melchers *et al.* 1974), and Staphylococcal nuclease.

1. The Ir-IgG Gene

Intraperitoneal injection of mineral (paraffin) oil into BALB/c mice leads to the development of plasma cell tumors, myelomas, which produce large amounts of structurally identical immunoglobulins (myeloma proteins). Each myeloma protein is unique, different from other myeloma proteins produced by other tumors in that each is of a particular immunoglobulin class (*IgG, IgA, IgM,* etc.), and has a particular allotype (*Ig-1ᵃ* if induced in a BALB/c mouse) and idiotype (a particular amino acid sequence in the Ig variable region). BALB/c mice are more susceptible to myeloma induction than most other inbred strains, and consequently a whole series of myelomas is available in this strain. The individual myelomas are most commonly designated by the symbol MOPC (mouse plasma cell tumor) and a serial number. The myeloma proteins can be readily isolated and used for immunization.

Immunization of various mouse strains with one such BALB/c myeloma protein, namely MOPC 173, previously shown to belong to the IgG_{2a} class, produces antibodies in some strains but not in others. If the responding recipient strain differs from BALB/c in its allotype, two types of antibody—antiallotypic (antibodies against antigenic determinants in the constant regions of Ig molecules) and antiidiotypic (antibodies against antigenic determinants in the variable regions of Ig molecules)—are formed. The antibodies can be detected, for example, by the passive hemagglutination assay, in which the myeloma protein is coupled to erythrocytes and the erythrocytes are then agglutinated by the antimyeloma protein antibodies.

R. Lieberman and her co-workers (R. Lieberman and Humphrey 1971, 1972; R. Lieberman *et al.* 1972) demonstrated that the production of anti-MOPC 1973 antibodies in various inbred strains is controlled by a single, autosomal, dominant gene that is closely linked to the *H-2* complex. Testing of *H-2* recombinants revealed that the gene resides within the *H-2* complex and is distinct from the *Ir-1A* gene. Lieberman originally designated the locus coding for response to the MOPC 173 protein *Ir-IgG*, but it has recently been recommended that the symbol be changed to *Ir-1B* to comply with standardized nomenclature (J. Klein *et al.* 1974a).

The separation of the *Ir-1B* locus from *Ir-1A* and *Slp* loci was discussed in Chapter Ten. Briefly, the separation is based on two *H-2* recombinants, B10.A(4R) or *H-2ʰ⁴*, and B10.A(5R) or *H-2ⁱ⁵*:

$$\frac{a}{b} = \begin{array}{|cc|c|cc}
\hline
K^k\ Ir\text{-}1A^k & LR & S^d\ D^d \\
\hline
K^b\ Ir\text{-}1A^b & HR & S^b\ D^b \\
\hline
\end{array}$$

with branches:

$$\rightarrow i5\ K^b\ Ir\text{-}1A^b\ HR\ S^d\ D^d$$
$$\rightarrow h4\ K^k\ Ir\text{-}1A^k\ HR\ S^b\ D^b$$

(In this diagram, HR and LR signify the alleles at the *Ir-1B* locus controlling high and low responsiveness to the allotypic determinants of MOPC 173 protein, respectively.)

2. The Ir-LDH_B Gene

Lactate dehydrogenase (LDH) is an enzyme found in various tissues of all vertebrates and many invertebrates. It catalyzes the conversion of pyruvic acid to lactic acid with the simultaneous oxidation of the reduced cofactor NADH:

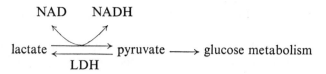

NAD   NADH

lactate ⇌ pyruvate ⟶ glucose metabolism

LDH

In the absence of oxygen, LDH generates a reservoir of hydrogen in the form of lactic acid and when oxygen becomes available again, the lactic acid is converted back into pyruvic acid, which then enters the metabolism pathway.

The structure of the enzyme is determined by two loci coding for two different polypeptide chains, A and B. Because the two chains can occur in any possible combination of four, there are five molecular forms (*isozymes*) of LDH present within the same species and often within the same individual: LDH-1 = B_4, LDH-2 = A_1B_3, LDH-3 = A_2B_2, LDH-4 = A_3B_1, and LDH-5 = A_4 (the subscript numerals indicate the number of A and B chains in each tetrameric molecule). Each of the molecular forms has a different electrophoretic mobility and is therefore identifiable, on starch gel electrophoresis, for example, as one of five separate bands.

Immunization of mice with pig LDH_B (= LDH-1 = B_4) in an adjuvant delineates high and low responders in the inbred strains. Crosses between the HR and LR strains indicate that the level of LDH_B antibodies is determined by a single, autosomal, dominant locus, $Ir\text{-}LDH_B$ (Melchers *et al.* 1974). Testing of *H-2* congenic lines, as well as linkage tests, suggests a close association between *H-2* and $Ir\text{-}LDH_B$ loci, and analysis of *H-2* recombinant strains places the $Ir\text{-}LDH_B$ gene within the *H-2* complex, in the *Ir-1B* subregion. The critical *H-2* recombinants in this respect are B10.A(4R) or *H-2^{h4}*, and B10.A(5R) or *H-2^{i5}*; the former places the $Ir\text{-}LDH_B$ locus to the right of *Ir-1B*, the latter places it to the left of the *Slp* locus (the two parental *H-2* haplotypes of 4R and 5R are *H-2^a*, a low responder to LDH_B, and *H-2^b*, a high responder to LDH_B):

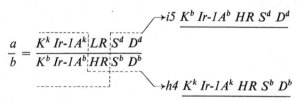

$$\frac{a}{b} = \frac{K^k\ Ir\text{-}1A^k \vert LR \vert S^d\ D^d}{K^b\ Ir\text{-}1A^b \vert HR \vert S^b\ D^b}$$

→i5 $K^b\ Ir\text{-}1A^b\ HR\ S^d\ D^d$

→h4 $K^k\ Ir\text{-}1A^k\ HR\ S^b\ D^b$

(In this diagram HR and LR signify the alleles at the $Ir\text{-}LDH_B$ locus controlling high and low responsiveness, respectively.) Whether the immune response to LDH_B is controlled by the same locus as the response to the IgG myeloma protein MOPC 173, or whether the two responses are controlled by closely linked but distinct loci remains to be resolved; so far, no recombinant that separates the two responses genetically is available. According to the agreement reached recently with regard to the nomenclature of loci in the *I* region (J. Klein *et al.* 1974a), the locus controlling immune response to LDH_B is only *tentatively* designated $Ir\text{-}LDH_B$. If it is ever demonstrated that $Ir\text{-}LDH_B$ is identical to *Ir-1B*, the former symbol will be dropped; if, on the other hand, the two loci are proved to be separate, the *Ir-LDH*$_B$ symbol will be changed to an *Ir-1*-series symbol.

Investigation of the mechanism of the LDH$_B$ response (Melchers *et al.* 1974) provides further evidence that the *Ir* loci in the *I* region primarily affect T cell functions. The evidence was obtained in a series of three experiments.

In the first experiment, Melchers and her co-workers transferred spleen cells from two donors, one donor primed with 4-hydroxy-5-iodo-3-nitrophenacetyl (NIP) conjugated to chicken gammaglobulin (CGG) and the other primed with LDH$_B$, into the same syngeneic irradiated recipients, immunized the recipients with NIP-LDH$_B$, and measured the level of anti-NIP antibodies formed. They observed that the levels of NIP antibodies depended on the recipients' responsiveness to LDH$_B$, LDH$_B$-HR, and LDH$_B$-LR strains producing high and low levels of NIP antibodies, respectively. In this experiment, the NIP functioned as a hapten and the CGG or LDH$_B$ as carriers, one donor cell population being primed against the hapten and the other against the carrier. The antihapten antibody production required collaboration between hapten-primed B cells and carrier-primed T cells (helper cells, cf. Chapter Eighteen). The experiment therefore indicates that the LR T cells are unable to perform the helper function in terms of the LDH$_B$ carrier. This conclusion is supported by the finding that the LR mice can be made to respond well to NIP if they are boosted with NIP-CGG, or if they receive a combination of NIP-CGG-primed B cells and NIP-BSA-primed T cells.

In the second experiment, the authors were able to convert LR mice into high responders by using LDH$_B$ as a hapten coupled to an immunogenic carrier. For this they took advantage of the fact that both LDH$_B$-HR and LDH$_B$-LR strains respond equally well to immunization with LDH$_A$. Therefore they immunized the LDH$_B$-HR and LDH$_B$-LR mice with the hybrid enzyme LDH$_{AB}$ and observed that both strains developed high titers of anti-LDH$_A$ as well as anti-LDH$_B$ antibodies. Apparently, upon immunization with the hybrid molecule, the A subunits function as carriers for the B subunits, and the purported carrier defect in the LDH$_B$-LR mice is thus circumvented.

In the third experiment, Melchers and her associates compared the LDH$_B$ antibodies of HR and LR strains for structural similarity. They subjected the LDH$_B$ antibodies to isoelectric focusing[2] in polyacrylamide gels, incubated the gels with LDH$_B$ and then with a stain reacting specifically with LDH$_B$. In this manner they were able to differentiate the LDH$_B$ antibodies from all other proteins in the sample. The method resolved several bands presumably reflecting the heterogeneity of the LDH$_B$ antibodies; however, the authors were unable to find any significant difference between HR and LR congenic lines in terms of antibody heterogeneity. They therefore interpreted the results as indicating that the HR and LR strains do not differ in genes coding for the structure of LDH$_B$

---

[2] Isoelectric focusing is a technique for separating proteins according to their isoelectric point (i.e., the pH at which a molecule carries no net charge and does not migrate in an electric field). The technique consists of developing a pH gradient from anode to cathode, with the proteins accumulating in the region of the gradient corresponding to their own isoelectric point.

antibodies and, hence, that the $Ir\text{-}LDH_B$ gene does not code for antibody specificity.

3. The Ir-Nase Gene

A third gene, *Ir-Nase*, has recently been mapped into the *IB* subregion by Lozner *et al.* (1974b). The gene controls the immune response to *Staphylococcal nuclease* (Nase), a well-characterized extracellular enzyme produced by *Staphylococcus aureus*. The mapping into the *IB* subregion is based on the observation that B10.A and B10.A(4R) are high responders to Nase, whereas B10, B10.A(2R) and B10.A(5R) are low responders.

C. The *IC* Subregion

A third subregion (*IC*) of the *I* region has recently been defined by Shreffler and David (1974). The *IC* subregion codes for antigens with restricted tissue distribution (Ia antigens) and for lymphocyte-activating determinants (Lad, see Chapter Eighteen). Preliminary data of Merryman and Maurer (1974) suggest that the *IC* subregion carries the gene controlling immune response to the random terpolymer GLT^5 (see Chapter Ten).

II. Other *Ir* Systems

In addition to *Ir-1A* and *Ir-1B*, a number of other immune-response genes have recently been described. They can be grouped into two classes: *H-2*-linked *Ir* genes and *Ig* allotype-linked *Ir* genes. A third group, genes that are neither *H-2*- nor allotype-linked, may also exist.

A. *H-2*-Linked *Ir* Genes

Currently, immune response genes to some 30 different antigens are known to be linked to the *H-2* complex (Tables 17–2, 17–3, and 17–4). The antigens are of a wide variety, although most of them seem to have one property in common: they are all of a restricted structural heterogeneity so that the animal is exposed to a limited number of antigenic determinants (Benacerraf and McDevitt 1972). The restriction of the antigens' heterogeneity is the result of the limited number of L-amino acids present in synthetic polypeptides, of the limited immunizing doses of complex protein antigens, or of small mutational differences among alloantigens.

The localization, with respect to the *H-2* complex, of the genes controlling the response to various antigens has been determined with differing degrees of accuracy. Some genes have been demonstrated simply to be linked to *H-2*, while others have been at least roughly positioned with respect to *H-2* regions (detailed mapping of many *Ir* genes is in progress in several laboratories). In general, there is, at present, no clear-cut evidence that any of the *Ir* genes map

Table 17-3. Essential features of the different systems used in studies of *H-2*-associated immune responses*

Antigen	Optimal dose	Immuni- zation schedule	Pattern of inheritance	Adjuvant	Assay system	Defect exerted during — Primary response	Defect exerted during — Secondary response	Nature of the difference	Association with *H-2* shown by tests with	Reference
(T,G)-A--L	2×10 g	A	AD	FCA	ABC	−	+	QT	SDP, CRL, LT	McDevitt and Sela 1965
(H,G)-A--L	2×10 g	A	AD	FCA	ABC	−	+	QT	SDP, CRL, LT	McDevitt and Sela 1967
(Phe,G)-A--L	2×10 g	A	AD	FCA	ABC	−	+	QT	SDP, CRL, LT	McDevitt and Sela 1967
OA	2×0.1 g	B	NT	$Al(OH)_3$	PCA or ABC	+	+	QT	SDP, CRL	Vaz *et al.* 1970, 1971
BPO_6OA	2×0.1 g	B	NT	$Al(OH)_3$	PCA or or ABC	−	+	QT	SDP	Vaz *et al.* 1970
$BPO_{25}BGG$	$n \times 0.1$ or 1.0 g	C	NT	$Al(OH)_3$	PCA or PH	−	+	QT	SDP	Vaz and Levine 1970
BPO_4OM	$n \times 0.1$ or 1.0 g	C	NT	$Al(OH)_3$	PCA or PH	−	+	QT	SDP	Vaz and Levine 1970
BPO_4RNAse	$n \times 0.1$ or 1.0 g	C	NT	$Al(OH)_3$	PCA or PH	−	+	QT	SDP	Vaz and Levine 1970
$DNP_{42}BGG$	$n \times 0.1$ or 1.0 g	C	NT	$Al(OH)_3$	PCA or PH	−	+	QT	SDP	Vaz and Levine 1970
OM	1 g	B	AD	$Al(OH)_3$	PCA or ABC	+	+	QT	SDP, CRL	Vaz *et al.* 1971
TNP-MSA	2×50 g	A	AR	FCA	ABC	NT	+	QT	CRL, LT	Rathbun and Hildemann 1970

GAT$_{10}$	2 × 1–10 g	A or B	AD	Al(OH)$_3$ or FCA	ABC	+	+	QL	SDP, CRL	Martin et al. 1971; Merryman and Maurer 1972
GAT$_4$	2 × 1–10 g	A or B	AD	FCA	ABC	+	+	QL	SDP, CRL	Merryman and Maurer 1972
GLφ	10 g	A	AD	FCA	ABC	+	+	QT	SDP, CRL, RIS	Merryman et al. 1972
TG	2 × 30–60 g	B	AD(?)	FCA	HA and HI	NT	+	QT	SDP, CRL	Vladutiu and Rose 1971
IgA	8 × 75 g	A	AD	FCA	DD and PH	NT	+	QT	SDP, CRL	Lieberman and Humphrey 1971; R. Lieberman and Humphrey 1972
IgG(γG$_{2a}$)	8 × 75 g	A	AD	FCA	DD and PH	NT	+	QT	SDP, CRL	R. Lieberman and Humphrey 1972
IgH(G$_{2b}$)	8 × 75 g	C	NT	FCA	DD and PH	NT	+	QT	SDP	R. Lieberman and Paul 1973
Thy-1	4 × 10^7 thymus cells	D	AD	–	PFC	+	±	QT	LT	Fujii et al. 1971c, 1972
H-Y	1 skin graft	D	AD	–	SGR	+	–	QT	SDP, CRL, RIS	Bailey and Hoste 1971; Bailey 1971c; Gasser and Silvers 1971a, b
H-2.2	n × 10^7 spleen or tumor cells	C	AD	–	HA	+	+	QT	CRL**	Lilly et al. 1971, 1973; Stimpfling and Durham 1972

Table 17-3. (*Continued*)

Antigen	Optimal dose	Immuni-zation schedule	Pattern of inheritance	Adjuvant	Assay system	Defect exerted during Primary response	Secondary response	Nature of the difference	Association with *H-2* shown by tests with	Reference
Ea-1	$n \times 0.2$ ml RBC+	C	AD†	FCA	HA	−	+	QT	LT	Gasser and Shreffler 1972
Slp	normal serum	C	AD	FCA	DD	NT	+	QL	SDP, CRL	H. C. Passmore, personal communication
Nase	100 μg	D	AD	FCA	EI	NT	NT	QT	LT, SDP, CRL	Lozner et al. 1974b

* Abbreviations:

Antigen
(T,G)-A--L = synthetic branched multichain polypeptide poly-L(Tyr,Glu)-poly-D,L-Ala-Poly-L-Lys
(H,G)-A--L = synthetic branched multichain polypeptide poly-L(His,Glu)-poly-D,L-Ala-poly-L-Lys
(Phe,G)-A--L = synthetic branched multichain polypeptide poly-L(Phe,Glu)-poly-D,L-Ala-poly-L-lys
OA = ovalbumin
BPO₆OA = benzylpenicilloyl (BPO) conjugate of ovaalbumin (OA)
BPO₂₅BGG = benzylpenicilloyl (BPO) conjugate of bovine gamma globulin (BGG)
BPO₄OM = benzylpenicilloyl (BPO) conjugate of ovomucoid (OM)

Adjuvant
FCA = Freund's complete adjuvant

Assay system
ABC = antigen-binding capacity
PCA = passive cutaneous anaphylaxis
PH = passive hemagglutination
HA = hemagglutination of allo- or autoantibodies
DD = double diffusion in agar gel
PFC = plaque-forming cell assay with thymocytes as target cells
SGR = skin-graft rejection
EI = enzyme inhibition

Nature of the difference

QL = qualitative difference between responder and nonresponder
QT = quantitative difference between responder and nonresponder

Association shown

CRL = congenic resistant lines
LT = linkage test
RIS = recombinant inbred strains
SDP = strain distribution pattern

Immunization schedule

A = first injection of antigen is adjuvant, booster injection in aqueous solution
B = two injections, both in adjuvant
C = multiple injections
D = single injection (or graft)

Pattern of inheritance

AD = autosomal dominant inheritance of the responsiveness
AR = autosomal recessive inheritance of the responsiveness

General

NT = not tested

BPO_4RNAse = benzylpenicilloyl (BPO) conjugate of bovine pancreatic ribonuclease (RNAse)
$DNP_{42}BCG$ = dinitrophenyl (DNP) conjugate of bovine gamma globulin
OM = ovomucoid
TNP-MSA = 2,4,6-trinitrophenyl (TNP) conjugate of mouse serum albumin (MSA)
GAT_{10} = random linear copolymer $(L\text{-}glu^{60}L\text{-}ala^{30}L\text{-}tyr^{10})_n$
GAT_4 = random linear copolymer $(L\text{-}glu^{58}L\text{-}ala^{38}L\text{-}tyr^{4})_n$
$GL\phi$ = random linear copolymer $(L\text{-}glu^{58}L\text{-}lys^{38}L\text{-}phe_4)_n$ (the superscript is the molecular ratio of amino acids in the polymer)
TG = thyroglobulin
IgA = immunoglobulin A myeloma protein of BALB/c origin (MOPC 467)
IgG (γG_{2a}) = immunoglobulin G (γG_{2a}) myeloma protein of BALB/c origin (MOPC 173)
IgH (γG_{2b}) = immunoglobulin G (γG_{2b}) myeloma protein of BALB/c origin (MOPC 195)
Thy-1 = thymocyte alloantigen-locus 1 (theta)
H-Y = male histocompatibility antigen
H-2.2 = antigen 2 controlled by the H-2 complex
Ea-1 = erythrocyte alloantigen locus 1

** Linkage test performed by Lilly *et al.* (1971) showed independent segregation of *H-2* and the *Ir*-gene for H-2.2.

† The immune response to Ea-1 is controlled, in addition to *H-2*, by the *Ir-2* gene, which segregates independently of *H-2*.

Table 17-4. Immune responses of independent *H-2* haplotypes. (Summary of Table 17-2)*

Region	Antigen	b	d	f	j	k	p	q	r	s
IA	(H,G)-A--L	–	–	–	·	+	–	–	·	–
	BGG	–	–	–	·	+	·	–	·	–
	OM	–	–	–	·	+	·	–	·	–
	OA	+	+	+	+	–	+	+	+	±
	(T,G)-A--L	+	±	–	–	–	–	–	–	–
	IgA	–	–	·	·	+	+	+	+	+
	RE	–	+	–	–	+	+	·	·	·
IB	IgG	+	–	·	·	+	–	+	+	+
	LDH_B	+	+	·	·	–	·	+	·	+
	Nase	–	+	·	·	+	·	–	·	–
	$GL\phi$	–	+	+	+	–	+	+	+	–
IC	GLT^5	–	+	–	+	–	–	–	+	–
	GAT^{10}	+	+	+	+	+	–	–	+	–
	$GLpro^5$	–	–	–	·	–	–	–	–	+
	(Phe,G)-A--L	+	+	+	+	+	+	+	+	–
	GLA^{10}	–	+	+	·	±	·	±	·	+
	GLA^{30}	+	+	+	·	+	–	–	+	+
	GA	+	+	+	+	+	–	–	+	+
Unassigned	$GL\phi^5$	–	+	–	+	–	+	+	+	–
	H-Y	+	±	–	·	–	–	±	±	·
	Thy-1.1	–	–	·	·	+	·	–	·	·
	Ea-1	–	(±)	·	·	·	·	·	·	·
	TG	–	–	–	·	+	±	+	·	+
	X.1	+	–	·	+	–	·	–	·	–
	BPO-OA	·	·	·	·	·	–	·	·	·
	BPO-BGG	–	–	·	·	+	·	–	·	±
	BPO-OM	–	·	·	·	+	·	±	·	±
	BPO-RNase	–	·	·	·	+	·	±	·	–
	DNP-BGG	–	·	·	·	+	·	±	·	±
	TNP-MSA	·	·	·	·	·	·	·	·	·
	IgH	–	–	+	·	+	+	+	+	+
	H-2.2	·	(±)	–	·	–	·	·	·	·
	Slp	–	·	·	·	+	·	+	·	·

+ = high responder;   – = low responder;   ± = intermediate responder;   · = not tested.

Antigens are divided into four groups: those that have been mapped into the *IA* (or *K+IA*) subregion; those that have been mapped to the *IB* subregion; those that have been tentatively mapped to the *IC* subregion; and those that have not yet been mapped. Antigens with indentical or antithetical distribution patterns of immune response are enclosed into rectangles of interrupted lines (See Text).

* For explanation of abbreviations and for references see Tables 17–2 and 17–3; for antigens not listed in Table 17–2 see Benacerraf and Katz (1974).

in the *D* end of the *H-2* complex; they all seem to be located in the *K* end, probably in the *I* region. The relationship of the individual genes among themselves and to the *Ir-1A* and *Ir-1B* loci is not known. Theoretically, the genes can represent alleles at the *Ir-1A* and *Ir-1B* loci, or each gene may represent a separate locus in the *I* region, although one can make an educated guess that the truth lies somewhere between the two extremes, and that a few genes will prove to be identical, while others will eventually be separated by genetic recombination.

Of the antigens listed in Table 17–4, the immune response to antigens (H,G)-G-A--L, BGG and OM shows the same strain distribution pattern which is antithetical to the distribution pattern of response to antigen OA; therefore, the response to these antigens could be controlled by two alleles at the same locus. Another antithetical relationship of response exists between antigens GLPro^5 and (Phe,G)-A--L; these responses, too, could be controlled by allelic genes. The response to closely related antigens GLA^{30} and GA is also identical.

Ir-genes that have been mapped with respect to the regions of the *H-2* complex are listed in Table 17–5.

The immune responsiveness to various antigens displays an uneven degree of genetic complexity. While with some antigens (e.g., LDH$_B$), the *H-2*-linked gene seems to be the sole controller of responsiveness, responsiveness to other antigens (e.g., Thy-1.1) is clearly controlled by a whole series of genes, some *H-2*-linked, others not.

The characteristics of the individual immune response systems are summarized in Table 17–2; the response patterns of different strains to individual antigens are given in Table 17–3. Almost all the immune response (IR) systems listed in Table 17–2 are dose dependent. In each system, the LR and HR strains respond equally well to a given antigen if the dose of that antigen is higher than the optimal dose. The dose dependence can be explained in two ways (Vaz and Levine 1970). First, it could be a property of the antigen receptor. Each receptor molecule has a certain affinity for a given antigen, high in the HR strain and low in the LR strain. At a very low antigen dose, even the receptors in HR mice are unable to bind the antigen in quantities sufficient for triggering of the receptor-bearing cells; at a very high antigen dose, on the other hand, even the receptors in LR mice can bind a sufficient quantity of the antigen to initiate the immune reaction. Second, at a high antigen dose, the animals respond to a large number of antigenic determinants, and this obscures the difference between the HR and LR strains. Lowering the antigen dose to optimum restricts the heterogeneity of the antigen by reducing the concentration of minor antigenic determinants to a subimmunogenic level.

There is no uniformity among the different IR systems with respect to their effect on the primary and secondary response. Some of them resemble the *Ir-1A* system in that they exert their influence only on the secondary response. However, because in almost all these systems the antigen is administered in adjuvant, it is questionable whether the reaction measured after the first injection is really a primary response.

Table 17-5. Mapping of *Ir* genes within the *H-2* complex

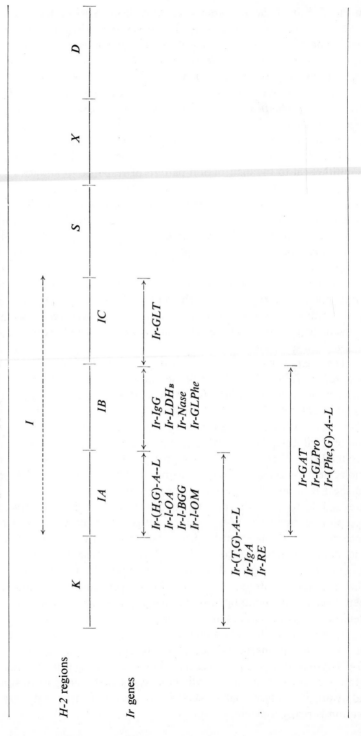

In only one IR system (*Ir-TNP-MSA*) are the (HR × LR)F$_1$ hybrids low responders, indicating a recessive pattern of inheritance (Rathbun and Hildemann 1970). In all the other systems, high responsiveness is inherited as a dominant trait.

In several IR systems, the only evidence for association with the *H-2* complex is the pattern of responsiveness of the different inbred strains and its correlation with the distribution of the different *H-2* haplotypes. Although such correlation certainly suggests an association between the two traits, it could not be considered a definitive proof of linkage. Ultimately, evidence based on congenic lines and linkage tests will be required in all systems. The correlation in various inbred strains between the pattern of responsiveness and *H-2* haplotypes is usually close but almost never absolute. The instance in which the strains all carry the *H-2^d* haplotype and yet respond variably to (T,G)-A--L has already been mentioned. Another example is the response to ovalbumin and ovomucoid in which, among *H-2^k* strains, the AKR strain responds much better than the others (Vaz *et al.* 1970, 1971). Still another example is the response of *H-2^b* strains to IgG allotypes: strain LP gives a very high response, strains C57BL/10 and C57BL/6 a moderate response, and strain C57BL/Ka a fairly low response (R. Lieberman and Humphrey 1972). These differences could be due either to the genetic background of the various inbred strains, which could modify the major effect of the *Ir* genes, or to diversity of the *H-2* haplotypes currently considered to be identical. It is conceivable that at least some haplotypes serologically typed as being identical differ in their *I* regions.

B. Allotype-Linked *Ir* Genes

Allotype-linked *Ir* genes control response to antigens such as streptococcal or pneumococcal polysaccharides, which induce antibodies of restricted heterogeneity. In contrast to the *H-2*-linked *Ir* genes, allotype-linked genes usually control qualitative rather than quantitative differences, such as those in antibody specificity, and are expressed in B cells rather than T cells. It is believed that allotype-linked *Ir* genes control the primary structure of the immunoglobulin's variable region.

C. Indeterminate *Ir* Genes

Indeterminate *Ir* genes are clearly not closely linked to the *H-2* complex, and apparently also segregate independently of Ig allotype markers. One of these genes, *Ir-2*, which controls the response to Ea-1 antigens, is located in chromosome 2 (LG V, cf. Gasser 1969). Because the same chromosome also carries at least two minor histocompatibility loci (*H-3* and *H-13*), it can be speculated that an association similar to that between *H-2* and *Ir-1* loci also exists between minor *H* and *Ir* loci. However, there is no experimental evidence to support such speculation, and the occurrence of the *Ir* and *H* loci in the same chromosome could be purely coincidental. If *Ir* loci are as numerous and as widespread throughout the mouse genome as *H* loci, then most, if not all *Ir* loci must be linked to *H* loci simply because the genome is not infinite. In any case, the linkage of the *Ir-2* locus to *H-3* or *H-13* is too loose to have any functional significance.

Another locus, segregating independently of *H-2* and allotype markers, is *Ir-3*, which controls the response to synthetic polypeptide (Phe,G)-Pro-L (Mozes *et al.* 1970; Shearer *et al.* 1971). The chromosomal location of the *Ir-3* locus has not been determined.

In the response to both Ea-1 (Gasser and Shreffler 1972) and (Phe,G)-Pro-L (McDevitt and Benacerraf 1969), *H-2* is also involved. Apparently, the response to each of these two antigens is controlled by at least two *Ir* loci, one *H-2*-linked and the other (*Ir-2* or *Ir-3*) segregating independently of *H-2*.

A rather complex genetic control of the immune response to antigens controlled by the *Thy-1* locus recently has been described by Fuji *et al.* (1972), Zaleski *et al.* (1973), Zaleski and Milgrom (1973), and Zaleski and Klein (1974). The control involves at least three different loci: *Ir-Thy-1A* and *Ir-Thy-1B*, which are closely linked to each other as well as to the *H-2* complex, and *Ir-5*, which is located on the noncentromeric arm of chromosome 17, about 17 map units to the right of the *H-2* complex (Zaleski and Klein 1974).[3]

III. *Ir* Systems in Other Species

Ir genes similar to those in the mouse have been described in several other mammalian species, including man. But one species, the guinea pig, has been analyzed in this respect to at least the same extent as the mouse. It is only because of lack of space that guinea pig experiments will not be fully covered here. (For a review and references, see Benacerraf 1973.) Instead, only those experiments that have not been (and, in some instances, could not be) done in the mouse will be mentioned briefly.

Benacerraf and his co-workers used a whole series of synthetic polypeptides, among them one called poly-L-lysine (PLL), because it is a polymer consisting of a single amino acid, L-lysine. PLL alone is usually only weakly immunogenic at best, but it can be coupled to a larger, more complex molecule such as BSA, and can then give rise to antibody formation. In the PLL-BSA complex, the BSA serves as a carrier and the PLL as a hapten. However, PLL can serve as a carrier itself when coupled to a smaller, simpler molecule such as 2,4-dinitrophenol (DNP). In the DNP-PLL complex, the DNP portion serves as a hapten and the PLL portion as a carrier.

When immunized with the DNP-PLL antigen dispersed in complete Freund's adjuvant, some guinea pigs (30 percent of animals of outbred Hartley strain and all animals of inbred strain 2) respond, whereas others (70 percent of

[3] Symbol *Ir-4* was used by Lilly *et al.* (1971) for the locus controlling the immune response to H-2 alloantigens. Because the locus is apparently a member of the *Ir-1* family of loci, the *Ir-4* designation should be dropped.

outbred Hartley animals and all inbred strain 13 animals) do not. The response can be measured by delayed hypersensitivity,[4] blast transformation *in vitro* upon exposure of lymph node cells to DNP-PLL, and synthesis of anti-DNP-PLL serum antibodies. The phenomena of delayed hypersensitivity and the *in vitro* blast transformation are usually classified as "cellular" immune responses, believed to be mediated by T cells and directed against the carrier portion of the carrier-hapten complex. The above observation suggests that the nonresponder guinea pigs do not respond to DNP-PLL because they fail to recognize the carrier (PLL). This conclusion is supported by the following four findings.

First, the same guinea pigs that respond to DNP-PLL also respond to other noncross-reacting haptens, such as benzylpenicilloyl, 5-dimethylamino-1-napthalene or *p*-toluenesulfonyl, conjugated to the PLL carrier. Guinea pigs that do not respond to DNP-PLL do not respond to any hapten coupled to the PLL carrier.

Second, responder (but not nonresponder) guinea pigs immunized with PLL in adjuvant develop delayed hypersensitivity to this polymer, but no detectable humoral antibodies.

Third, when DNP-PLL is complexed with BSA (DNP-PLL is a highly charged molecule that can form stable aggregates with negatively charged BSA molecules), the nonresponder animals produce high levels of anti-DNP antibodies, but still fail to produce delayed hypersensitivity or *in vitro* blast transformation. Apparently, in this experiment, the BSA acts as a carrier for the DNP hapten, indicating that the nonresponder animals are able to recognize DNP if it is presented on a proper carrier. In addition, the nonresponders can also produce humoral antibodies against the PLL portion of the complex if this portion is presented on an immunogenic carrier. However, they cannot develop cellular immunity against the PLL portion of the complex.

Fourth, nonresponder guinea pigs made tolerant to BSA and then immunized with DNP-PLL-BSA complexes fail to produce anti-DNP-PLL antibodies, indicating that it is, indeed, the carrier and not the hapten function that is defective in these animals.

All these data taken together strongly suggest that the defect in the nonresponder guinea pigs involves T cells, but not B cells.

In other respects, the immune response system of guinea pigs is amazingly similar to that of mice, suggesting that one is dealing not with a specialty of one species, but with a general biological phenomenon. In the guinea pig, as in the mouse, the immune response loci appear to be closely linked to the major histocompatibility complex, although the guinea pig MHC is still poorly defined.

---

[4] Delayed hypersensitivity is a form of immunological response characterized by a slowly evolving inflammatory reaction (reaching its maximum in 24–48 hr) at the site of antigen injection (usually skin) into a previously sensitized individual. The reaction is mediated by cells (lymphocytes) rather than antibodies, and its external expression is the appearance of a raised, erythematous, hardened lump. Delayed hypersensitivity is strongly pronounced in the guinea pig, but only weakly exhibited in the mouse. In contrast, immediate hypersensitivity is mediated by antibodies, and the reaction occurs immediately upon injection of the antigen.

IV. Mechanism of *Ir-1A* Gene Action

Despite the large body of experimental data, the mechanism of genetic control of the immune response to antigens exemplified by (T,G)-A--L and related synthetic polypeptides remains unknown. The possibilities have been narrowed down substantially, however, and several mechanisms have been ruled out. It is now clear that the low responsiveness of CBA mice to (T,G)-A--L is not caused by a nonspecific defect completely unrelated to antibody synthesis, such as enzymatic degradation of the antigen by the LR mice or production of a substance binding the antigen and making it unavailable for sensitization. Arguing against the existence of such a mechanism is the fact that CBA mice are capable of responding to closely related antigens such as (H,G)-A--L and (Phe,G)-A--L, and also to (T,G)-A--L coupled electrostatically to a highly charged immunogenic molecule (MBSA). Furthermore, the fact that LR mice can be converted into high responders by adoptive transfer of HR spleen, bone marrow, or fetal liver cells is also incompatible with the idea of a general nonspecific defect.

This leaves little doubt that the mechanism underlying low responsiveness has an immunological basis. One of the simplest immunological explanations of the *Ir-1A* defect is cross-tolerance, that is, the sharing of antigenic determinants between (T,G)-A--L and the LR animals's self-antigens. But experimental data once again rule out such a possibility. First, because most antigens are inherited codominantly, an F_1 hybrid of the HR and LR strains should possess all the self-antigens of the LR strain and should, therefore, be a low responder. In reality, however, the F_1 hybrids behave like high or moderate responders (McDevitt and Sela 1965). Second, alloantisera raised against spleen cells of LR strains do not bind (T,G)-A--L (McDevitt and Tyan 1968), although Ebringer and D. Davies (1973) claim that anti-CBA alloantisera have greater (T,G)-A--L-binding activity than other alloantisera and that this activity can be absorbed out to a greater extent by $H-2^k$ than by $H-2^b$ tissue homogenates. Third, fetal liver cells from an HR strain can transfer the ability to respond well to (T,G)-A--L when injected into irradiated LR recipients. Were cross-reaction with self-antigens a factor in the response of the LR strain to (T,G)-A--L, such a result would not be possible, because the transferred HR cells should become tolerant to LR antigens (McDevitt and Tyan 1968). Fourth, a survey of 33 strains carrying 20 different *H-2* haplotypes revealed no association, except one, among immune responses to (T,G)-A--L, (H,G)-A--L, and (Phe,G)-A--L and individual H-2 antigens. The one exception was antigen H-2.33, which seemed to be associated with high response to (T,G)-A--L, but this result was probably caused by the relatedness of the strains carrying the antigen (Grumet and McDevitt 1972).

The exclusion of cross-tolerance as a possible mechanism of low responsiveness of some strains leaves two possibilities: either the LR strains are defective in the genetic information coding for the (T,G)-A--L antibodies, or the LR strains have a defective antigen-recognition system. The first possibility would require the *Ir-1A* locus to be a structural locus coding for the constant or variable regions of the (T,G)-A--L antibody. However, such a possibility seems unlikely, because the *Ir-1A* locus is linked to the *H-2* complex, whereas the *Ig* loci coding for the constant regions of the immunoglobulin heavy chains segregate independently of *H-2* (Herzenberg *et al.* 1968). Because the genes for the constant and variable regions of the immunoglobulin molecules are believed to be carried by the same chromosome, the implication is that the *Ir-1A* locus is not linked to genes coding for the variable regions of the immunoglobulin molecules (V genes). The independent segregation of *Ig-1* and *Ir-1A* genes has been confirmed by a linkage test (McDevitt 1968). Because no allotype marker is available for the mouse immunoglobulin light chains, the linkage of *Ir-1A* with genes coding for the L-chains cannot be excluded. An argument against the *Ir-1A* locus's being the locus coding for the variable region of the antibody molecule is that the LR strains can mount a normal *primary* response to (T,G)-A--L, as well as primary and secondary response to (T,G)-A--L conjugated with MBSA, and to high doses of (T,G)-A--L. Therefore, they must have a nondefective structural gene coding for the (T,G)-A--L combining site of the antibody molecules. Direct evidence for the identity of the antibodies produced by HR and LR animals has recently been provided by Schlossman and Williamson (1972). Working with guinea pigs rather than mice, the author immunized PLL responder (HR) and PLL nonresponder (LR) animals with α-dinitrophenyl poly-L-lysine (DNP-PLL), isolated the antibodies, purified them on DNP-BSA immunoabsorbent, and investigated their specificities. They observed that the antibodies produced in responder and nonresponder guinea pigs had identical characteristics in isoelectrofocusing measurements, indicating that the B cell products from HR and LR animals were structurally identical. Taken together, these findings make possible the conclusion that the *Ir-1A* locus is probably not coding for immunoglobulin molecules.

According to the recognition hypothesis, the LR strains have all the information necessary for the synthesis of (T,G)-A--L antibodies, but are unable to recognize the antigen. The recognition defect could involve macrophages, bone marrow-derived lymphocytes (B cells) or thymus-derived lymphocytes (T cells). All three cell types have been shown to carry receptors capable of antigen binding on their cell membranes. Macrophages seem to bind the antigen indirectly; that is, the antigen must first be coupled to an antibody molecule, which is then linked to the cell membrane via the Fc portion of the molecule (for a review, see Nossal and Ada 1971). B cells bind the antigen directly via their immunoglobulin receptors (cf. Chapter Three). T cells are also presumed to be capable of direct antigen binding, but the nature of the antigen receptor is still a matter of controversy (cf. Chapter Eighteen). Of the three cell types, the macrophages seem to be the least likely candidates for the primary target of *Ir-1A* gene action, mainly because there is no evidence to implicate them in such a function. Also, they are not so much involved in recognition as in processing of the antigen. And finally, they do not display the degree of specificity that the *Ir-1A* gene product appears to possess.

B cells, which are directly involved in (T,G)-A--L antibody synthesis, might seem to be the most logical target of *Ir-1A* gene action. One could simply assume that the LR strains lack (or have a greatly reduced number of) B cells with receptors for the (T,G)-A--L antigen. However, because the B cell receptors are immunoglobulins, such an assumption would imply that there is something wrong with the synthesis of immunoglobulin in B cells of the LR strain. This implication, as discussed above, is contradictory to available experimental data.

Thus, one is left with the possibility that low responsiveness to (T,G)-A--L is a T cell defect. Almost all available experimental data agree with this conclusion, although direct proof that *Ir-1* genes are expressed exclusively in T cells is still lacking. Such proof can be obtained only by isolating the *Ir-1* gene product from T cells—a feat the achievement of which appears to be far away. The indirect experimental data that support expression of *Ir-1* genes in T cells are of two kinds. One is based on proving that there is nothing wrong with B cells of LR animals, the implication being that if HR and LR animals do not differ in their B cells, they must differ in their T cells. Such a line of reasoning is justifiable only under the assumption that the current theory of two (T and B cell-mediated) antigen-recognition systems is correct. The second kind of evidence is more direct, in that it purports to prove that there is something wrong with T cells of LR animals.

The nothing-wrong-with-B-cells evidence can be summarized as follows. First, lymphoid tissues of unimmunized HR and LR mice have the same frequency of B cells capable of binding (T,G)-A--L, suggesting that both HR and LR B cells have the same receptors for antigens (G. Hämmerling and McDevitt 1973). Second, B cells from LR mice, if properly stimulated, can differentiate into plasma cells producing antibodies in a high responder fashion, implying that B cells from HR and LR strains possess the same differentiation potential. The stimulation can be achieved by increased antigen dose (McDevitt and Sela 1965), complexation of the antigen to BSA (McDevitt 1968), by transferring HR T cells into T cell-deprived LR recipients (McDevitt and Tyan 1968), and, most important, by mixing HR T cells with LR B cells in tetraparental mice (Freed *et al.* 1973). Third, antibodies produced by HR and LR mice have the same specificity (Melchers *et al.* 1974; but see below) and therefore must be coded for by the same set of B cell-expressed genes. However, each of these three points can be criticized, and alternative explanations can be put forward. For example, the activation of LR B cells by HR T cells in tetraparental mice can also be explained as being a nonspecific, H-2-induced (allogeneic) effect (see Chapter Eighteen).

The something-wrong-with-T-cells evidence can also be summarized by three points. First, function usually attributed to T cells (i.e., cellular immunity, carrier effect, and helper effect, cf. Chapter Eighteen) are defective in LR animals. Thus, low-responder guinea pigs are unable to develop delayed hypersensitivity, and their cells are unable to undergo blast transformation *in vitro* upon stimulation with DNP-PLL (cf. Benacerraf 1973, for review and references); low-responder guinea pigs or mice fail to recognize the carrier in a hapten-carrier complex (Benacerraf 1973; Melchers *et al.* 1974), and finally, LR mice can mount normal primary IgM antibody response, but fail to initiate helper-dependent secondary IgG response (Grumet *et al.* 1971a, b). All these defects can be corrected by the addition of T cells from HR animals to the test system. Second, thymectomy abolishes reactivity of HR animals, and the reactivity can be restored with HR T cells but not with LR T cells (Tyan *et al.* 1969). Third, T and B cells differ in their antigen-binding specificity: binding of (T,G)-A--L to B cells, but not to T cells, can be blocked by (H,G)-A--L (G. Hämmerling and McDevitt 1974a); at the same time, B cell-derived anti-(T,G)-A--L antibodies cross-react with (H,G)-A--L, but (T,G)-A--L-immunized mice cannot be cross-stimulated with (H,G)-A--L (McDevitt and Sela 1967). In both situations, T cells appear to be more specific (less cross-reactive) than B cells.

Thus, the evidence for T cells' being affected by *Ir-1* loci is overwhelming, but the possibility that the same loci also affect B cells cannot be fully excluded. Side by side with the aforementioned evidence against B cell participation in the *Ir-1* defect, there is also evidence to the contrary.

Shearer and his co-workers (1971) injected irradiated HR and LR mice with a mixture of syngeneic bone marrow and thymus cells; 14 days later, at the peak of the response, they titrated individual antisera for (T,G)-A--L antibody activity, and expressed the results as the percentage of recipients giving positive response. In one experiment, the mixture consisted of an excess of thymocytes and limited graded doses of bone marrow cells; in another experiment, the bone marrow cells were in excess and the thymocytes were limited and graded (*limited dilution assay*). In both experiments, the HR recipients required a lower dose of cells (both bone marrow- and thymus-derived) to respond than did the LR recipients, suggesting that both T and B cells are defective in LR mice. However, one can argue that the events occurring in such a complex system are ill defined, and that the observed difference between HR and LR mice could have been caused by effects unrelated to *Ir-1* gene action.

B cell participation is also suggested by the observation that in some experimental systems MHC-linked *Ir* genes seem to affect not only the amount of antibodies produced but also their specificity. Thus, when strain 2 and 13 guinea pigs are immunized with a polymer of L-glutamic acid, L-alanine, and 10 percent L-tyrosine (GAT), they all respond equally well. However, the GAT antibodies produced in strain 2 animals also react with a linear polymer of glutamic acid and alanine (GA), whereas GAT antibodies produced in strain 13 animals do not cross-react with GA. Because, at the same time, strain 2 animals are responders and strain 13 animals are nonresponders to GA, the implication is that the presence of the GA response gene influences the specificity of the GAT antibodies (cf. Benacerraf *et al.* 1971).

And finally, an *Ir-1* gene effect on B cells must be postulated to explain the *H-2* influence on physiological T-B cell cooperation. (This phenomenon will be described in the next chapter.)

In summary, *H-2*-linked *Ir* loci seem to control the specificity of antigen recognition by thymus-derived, and possibly also by bone marrow-derived lymphocytes. The *Ir-1* gene product must, therefore, possess three important characteristics: it must be extremely variable (to recognize a wide variety of antigens), it must be specific [to distinguish between closely related antigens such as (T,G)-A--L and (H,G)-A--L], and it must be present on the surface of T cells (to act as a receptor for the antigen's carrier portion). Currently there is no known molecule possessing all three characteristics. Immunoglobulins come closest to filling the three requirements, because they are both variable and specific. However, the presence of immunoglobulins on T cell surfaces is still highly controversial, and in addition, as discussed earlier, *Ir-1* loci do not seem to code for any of the known Ig classes. Benacerraf and McDevitt (1972) therefore suggested that the *Ir-1* loci code for a new class of recognition molecules that are identical to the hypothetical T cell receptor, the existence of which was originally postulated for other reasons. The nature of the T cell receptor will be discussed in the next chapter.

On the basis of Benacerraf's and McDevitt's hypothesis, the mechanism of *Ir-1* gene action can be envisioned as follows. The *Ir-1* loci code for receptors on T cells, making them capable of recognizing carrier portions of antigenic molecules. T cells, with the antigen bound to them, then react (directly or via a third cell type, such as macrophage) with B cells and stimulate them to proliferate and differentiate into antibody-producing plasma cells. The B cells alone (in the absence of T cells) can also bind the antigen through their IgM receptors, but they recognize only the antigen's haptenic portion. The reaction of B cells with the hapten leads to production of antihaptenic IgM antibodies, and to the appearance of IgG receptors on some B cells. However, in the absence of T cells, the IgG-bearing precursor cells fail to differentiate further, and no IgG-secreting plasma cells appear. According to this hypothesis, the *Ir-1* gene provides the stimulus triggering proliferation and differentiation of B cells toward IgG-secreting cells.

Chapter Eighteen

Genetic Control of Cell Recognition and Interaction

I. *I* Region-Associated Antigens

A. Serology and Genetics

The *I* region of the *H-2* complex has been associated with several immunological functions that require the products of the region to behave as antigens.
Yet for a long time the entire central segment of the *H-2* complex was serologically undetectable. The situation changed recently when several laboratories
(Hauptfeld *et al.* 1973a, b; David *et al.* 1973a; Götze *et al.* 1973b; G. Hämmerling *et al.* 1974a; D. Sachs and Cone 1973) discovered simultaneously that
products of the *I* region can be detected by serological methods, provided the
methods are sensitive enough and that the right target cells are chosen. The
I-region-controlled, serologically detectable antigens were originally designated
Ir-1.1 and Ir-1.2 (to indicate that they were controlled by loci genetically
indistinguishable from *Ir-1*; cf. Hauptfeld *et al.* 1973a) and Lna (to indicate

Table 18-1. Antisera defining individual Ia antigens

Ia antigen	Antiserum	Target Cell
D1*	A.TH anti-A.TL	A.CA
D2	(A.TH × B10.D2)F$_1$ anti-A.TL (abs. with A.CA)	A.TL
D3	A.TH anti-A.TL	B10
D4	(A.TL × A.TFR3)F$_1$ anti-A.TH	A.TH
D5	A.TL anti-A.TH	A.CA
D6	B10.A(4R) anti-B10.A(2R)	B10.D2
D7	(B10 × HTI)F$_1$ anti-B10.A(5R)	A.TL
D8	B10.A anti-B10	B10.D2
D9	(A × B10.D2)F$_1$ anti-B10.A(5R)	B10.S
D10	AQR anti-B10.T(6R)	B10.T(6R)
H1**	B10.T(6R) anti-B10.AQR	B10.AQR
H2	B10.AQR anti-B10.T(6R)	B10.T(6R)
H3	(A.TL × B10)F$_1$ anti-B10.HTT	B10.S
H4	(A.TL × B10)F$_1$ anti-B10.HTT	B10.M

* Antigens defined by David *et al.* (1973a, 1974) and Shreffler and David (1974).
** Antigens defined by Hauptfeld *et al.* (1973a, b, 1974).

that they were originally detected on lymph node cells, cf. David *et al.* 1973a);
recently an agreement has been reached to refer to the antigens summarily as
Ia or *I* region-*a*ssociated antigens (Shreffler *et al.* 1974).

The first series of Ia antisera was produced by reciprocal immunization of
three pairs of congenic lines differing only in the central *H-2* regions: AQR
and 6R (Hauptfeld *et al.* 1973a, b), A.TL and A.TH (David *et al.* 1973a), and
2R and 4R (David *et al.* 1974); later the Ia antibodies were also found (along
with H-2 antibodies) in antisera produced in *H-2K* and/or *H-2D* disparate strain
combinations (Götze *et al.* 1973b; D. Sachs and Cone 1973; David and
Shreffler 1974).

From the data so far available, it appears that the antigens are numerous:
at least ten have already been described, and the number is likely to increase
rapidly, as production and typing of new *H-2* recombinants proceeds. Individual
antigens are designated by Arabic numerals (Ia.1, 2, 3, etc.), but the laboratories
involved have not yet agreed on a uniform sequence of numbering. The antisera
defining the eight known Ia antigens are listed in Table 18–1, and the strain
distribution of the antigens is given in Tables 18–2 and 18–3. The strain distribution pattern of the Ia antigens is that of a complex antigenic system, with some
antigens limited to one *I* allele and others shared by two, three, or more.
Although all the antigens so far detected are controlled by the *I* region, they do
not appear to be controlled by a single locus and may even be controlled by a
large number of loci.

If one chooses to follow the traditional serological approach and assign
antigens to individual loci on the basis of recombination, one can produce a
map of Ia antigens as shown in Fig. 18–1. However, because this approach
once before led H-2 serology into a blind alley, the interpretation presented in
Fig. 18–1 must be treated with caution. A more reliable genetic interpretation
of the *Ia* system will be possible only after the biochemistry of these antigens is
better defined.

Table 18-2. Distribution of Ia antigens in haplotypes of independent origin

H-2 Haplotype	Type Strain	Ia antigens described by David *et al.* (1973a, 1974) and Shreffler and David (1974)										Ia antigens described by Hauptfeld *et al.* (1973a, 1974)			
		1	2	3	4	5	6	7	8	9	10	1	2	3	4
b	C57BL/10	–	–	3	–	–	–	–	8	9	–	–	–	–	–
d	B10.D2	–	–	–	–	–	6	7	8	–	–	–	–	–	–
f	A.CA	1	–	–	–	5	–	–	–	–	–	–	–	–	4
k	B10.K	1	2	3	–	–	–	7	–	–	–	1	–	–	–
p	B10.P	–	–	–	–	5	6	7	–	–	–	–	–	–	–
q	B10.G	–	–	3	–	5	–	–	–	9	10	–	2	–	–
s	B10.S	–	–	–	4	5	–	–	–	9	–	–	–	3	4

Table 18-3. The Ia chart: Distribution of Ia antigens in recombinant *H-2* haplotypes.

H-2 haplotype	Type strain	Ia Specificities									
		1	2	3	4	5	6	7	8	9	10
a	A/Sn, B10.A	1	2	3	–	–	6	7	–	–	–
al	A.AL	1	2	3	–	–	–	7*	–	–	–
anl	A.TFR1	1	2	3	–	–	–	7	–	–	–
ap3	A.TFR3	1	–	–	–	5	–	–	–	–	–
ap5	A.TFR5	1	–	–	–	5	–	–	–	–	–
g	HTG	–	–	–	–	–	6	7	8	–	–
g2	D2.GD	–	–	3	–	–	–	–	8	–	–
h2	B10.A(2R)	1	2	3	–	–	6	7	–	–	–
h4	B10.A(4R)	1	2	3	–	–	–	–	–	–	–
i	HTI	–	–	3	–	–	–	–	8	9	–
i5	B10.A(5R)	–	–	3	–	–	6	7	8	9	–
m	AKR.M	1	2	3	–	–	–	7	–	–	–
ol	C3H.OL	–	–	–	–	–	6	7	8	–	–
o2	C3H.OH	–	–	–	–	–	6	7	8	–	–
sql	A.QSR1	–	–	–	4	5	–	–	–	9	–
tl	A.TL	1	2	3	–	–	–	7	–	–	–
t2	A.TH, B10.S(7R)	–	–	–	4	5	–	–	–	9	–
t3	B10.HTT	–	–	–	4	–	–	7	–	9	–
t4	B10.S(9R)	–	–	–	4	–	6	7	–	9	–
t5	BSVS	–	–	–	4	5	–	–	–	9	–
yl	AQR	1	2	3	–	–	6	7	–	–	–
y2	B10.T(6R)	–	–	3	–	5	–	–	–	9	10

* Adapted from Shreffler and David 1974.

As Fig. 18–1 shows, some of the *Ia* determinants map in the chromosomal segment between the *IB* and *S* regions. This fact, plus the observation that the same segment also is involved in mixed lymphocyte stimulation (see next section) led Shreffler and David (1974) to propose a separate designation, *IC*, for this subregion.

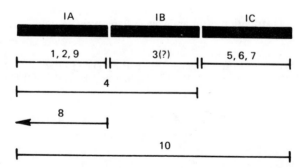

Fig. 18-1. Genetic map of the Ia antigens. *IA*, *IB* and *IC* are subregions of the *H-2* complex's *I* region. Arabic numerals indicate individual Ia antigens as defined by Shreffler's laboratory; horizontal bars designate position of determinants coding for indicated Ia antigens. Antigens that could not be positioned into one subregion are indicated by bars extending over two or three subregions.

B. Tissue Distribution

Anti-Ia sera react in direct cytotoxic and indirect immunofluorescence tests with lymphocytes from spleen and lymph nodes, but usually do not react with thymocytes and bone marrow cells (David *et al.* 1973a; Hauptfeld *et al.* 1973a; D. Sachs and Cone 1973; G. Hämmerling *et al.* 1974a). Although the sera may have relatively high titers, they never react with all cells in an unfractionated population of splenocytes and lymph node cells. The proportion of lymphocytes killed by anti-Ia antibodies in the dye-exclusion cytotoxic test varies, but usually does not exceed 70 percent in the case of spleen cells and 50 percent in the case of lymph node cells, suggesting that the antigens are expressed on a subpopulation of cells. After an initial confusion as to whether Ia antigens are expressed on T or B cells, their presence on B cells was definitely established by D. Sachs and Cone (1973), G. Hämmerling *et al.* (1974a) and by Hauptfeld *et al.* (1974). The presence of Ia antigens on T cells was a matter of controversy: G. Hämmerling and his co-workers (1974) and D. Sachs and Cone (1973) did not find any evidence of thymus-associated Ia activity; Hauptfeld and her co-workers (1974), on the other hand, were able to absorb anti-Ia sera with thymocytes, and obtained low but significant direct cytotoxicity of thymus cells after *in vivo* cortisone treatment of the donor.

Most recently Ia antisera have been produced with a clear-cut T cell activity measurable in the direct cytototoxic test (Götze 1974; Frelinger *et al.* 1974). Moreover, it appears that the T cell antibodies are produced more readily against antigens controlled by certain segments of the *I* region, particularly the *IC* subregion or the segment between *IB* and *S*. This finding might explain why some laboratories originally observed mainly T cell activity (Götze *et al.* 1973b) and others mainly B cell activity (D. Sachs and Cone 1973; G. Hämmerling *et al.* 1974a) in the Ia antisera. However, it is true that in most Ia antisera, the component reacting with mature B cells is predominant.

In addition to lymphocytes, the Ia antigens have recently been detected on spermatocytes, epidermal cells, and macrophages (G. Hämmerling *et al.* 1974b). The presence of Ia antigens on epidermal cells is also required to explain the formation of Ia antibodies following rejection of skin grafts transplanted across *I* region differences (J. Klein *et al.* 1974b). Anti-Ia sera do not react with, and are not absorbed by erythrocytes, and cells from brain, muscles, kidney, or lungs (Hauptfeld *et al.* 1974).

C. Chemistry

Preliminary biochemical analyses indicate that Ia antigens are associated with cell surface membranes, have a molecular weight of approximately 30,000 daltons, and are present on molecules that are distinct from molecules carrying classical H-2 antigens (Cullen *et al.* 1974; Vitetta *et al.* 1974a; Delovitch and McDevitt 1975). The demonstration of the distinctiveness of Ia and H-2 antigens was achieved by removing the H-2 antigens from a purified preparation with H-2-

specific antisera, and then demonstrating that Ia activity was unaffected by the treatment. Cullen and her co-workers (1974) obtained evidence that the native Ia molecule is a dimer with a molecular weight of approximately 61,000 daltons, and that different Ia antigens may be present on distinct molecular species. Vitetta and her colleagues (1974a) were able to detect Ia activity in the spleen cell incubation medium, suggesting that the antigens may either be actively secreted or shed from the membrane in relatively large quantities.

Chemical analysis of Ia antigens is complicated by the presence of autoimmune antibodies in many of the Ia antisera, by relatively low concentrations of the antigens on the cell surface, and by the fact that Ia activity forms relatively broad peaks upon immunoprecipitation and SDS polyacrylamide electrophoresis.

D. Relationship to H-2 Antigens

H-2 and Ia antigens differ in three important properties. First, H-2 antigens have been found on all thoroughly tested tissues, whereas Ia antigens have a more restricted tissue distribution. Second, H-2 antigens are carried by monomers having a molecular weight between 45,000 and 60,000 daltons, whereas Ia antigens are present on monomers with a molecular weight of between 28,000 and 32,000 daltons. And finally, the two classes of antigen are present on separate molecules. All this indicates that H-2 and Ia antigens are different; how much different they are remains to be seen.

According to the traditional model of the *H-2* complex, the two regions mapping in the vicinity of *I* regions are *A* and *E*, coding for H-2 antigens 1 and 5, respectively. One might therefore argue that some of the Ia antigens could be "rediscovered" antigens H-2.1 and H-2.5. However, such possibility is highly unlikely. Not only have Ia antigens different properties from H-2.1 and H-2.5, but also antigen H-2.5 is known to be present on the same molecule as *K* region antigen H-2.33 (Cullen *et al.* 1972a), whereas the *K* region products and the Ia antigens are known to be on separate molecules. Although the H-2.1 antigen has not been proved biochemically to belong to either the *K* or *D* region, the serological evidence for its presence in both regions is so strong that the existence of the *A* region cannot be easily warranted either.

For fuller discussion of the H-2-Ia relationship see Chapter Twenty.

II. Mixed Lymphocyte Reaction

A. Principle and Methods

For many years, immunologists attempted to establish *in vitro* cultures of normal lymphocytes, from either peripheral blood or lymphoid tissues, but they invariably failed. The lymphocytes remained viable for many days but did not divide, and so they could not be propagated in the way in which other cells in tissue culture are. A major breakthrough was achieved when Nowell (1960) discovered that the addition of a small amount of phytohemagglutinin (PHA), a mixture of glycoproteins extracted from the red kidney bean (*Phaseolus vulgaris*), to the culture medium induced changes in some of the cultured cells. The small lymphocytes began to enlarge, to synthesize DNA, RNA, and proteins, and on the third or fourth day of culture even began to divide. The large, active cells are variously referred to as *blast cells*, transformed cells, stimulated cells, or activated cells (Fig. 18–2), and the change from small lymphocytes to large blasts is known as *blast transformation*.

When it later became clear that lymphocyte activation could be induced by numerous other agents, many of which were strong antigens, the question naturally arose as to whether it could also be elicited by transplantation alloantigens. The first indication that this might be so was obtained accidentally by Schreck and Donelly (1961), who observed that in one of their lymphocyte cultures blast transformation occurred spontaneously, without the addition of PHA. The authors noted that the culture was a mixture derived from two different patients, but they failed to recognize the significance of this fact. The oversight was corrected three years later by Bain *et al.* (1964) and Bach and Hirschborn (1964), who demonstrated in a series of carefully controlled experiments that mixing of lymphocytes from unrelated persons in tissue culture leads to lymphocyte activation similar to that observed upon addition of PHA. The complex phenomena occurring when lymphocytes are cultured together later became known as the *mixed lymphocyte (leukocyte) reaction* (MLR), and the culture as the *mixed lymphocyte (leukocyte) culture* (MLC).

In the original technique described by Bain *et al.* (1964) and by Bach and Hirschborn (1964), cells from two donors, A and B, were mixed together; the

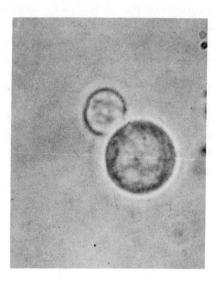

Fig. 18-2. Transformed lymphocyte (blast) and small lymphocyte from a mixed lymphocyte culture. Photograph taken using a phase contrast microscope. (Courtesy of Dr. J. Forman.)

A cells were then allowed to respond to antigens on B cells, and the B cells to respond to antigens on A cells (*two-way MLC*). This technique has many disadvantages, the major one being that because of the mutual stimulation it is not possible to assess separately the contribution of each of the two cell types to the reaction. For this reason, the two-way MLC has largely been replaced by its *one-way* modification, in which cells from one of the two donors are prevented from responding by being genetically tolerant (of F_1 hybrid origin), X-irradiated or pretreated with mitomycin C. (The latter two treatments inhibit cellular DNA synthesis and thus block blast transformation; other, less frequently used methods of producing unidirectional response include the use of macrophages, preparations of disrupted lymphocytes, and pretreatment with nitrogen mustard.) In the one-way MLC, the X-irradiated or mitomycin C-treated cells (*stimulating cells*) are used to stimulate the response of the untreated cells (*responding cells*) obtained from a different donor. The MLC can be set up with lymphocytes from spleen, lymph nodes, or peripheral blood, the last two being superior to the splenocyte culture because they display higher reactivity and lower background. MLC with thymocytes has also been reported, but bone marrow cells cannot be used, because they display high nonspecific stimulation.

The basic MLC technique exists in many modifications—probably as many as there are laboratories using it. However, in a typical test, 1 ml of irradiated or mitomycin C-treated stimulating cells is mixed with 1 ml of responding cells at concentrations 2×10^6 and 1×10^6 cells, respectively (however, for better results several concentrations of stimulating and responding cells should be used simultaneously). The mixture is placed in loosely capped, round-bottom test tubes and incubated at 37°C in a humidified atmosphere of 5 percent CO_2 in air. Eagle's minimal essential medium, supplemented with 5 percent fetal calf serum and antibiotics, is frequently used for the cell suspensions. The incubation period is usually 5–7 days. The response at the end of the incubation period is most commonly measured by pulse labeling with ^{3}H-thymidine. The radiolabel is added to each culture 16 hr before termination of the experiment, and the radioactive precursor is allowed to incorporate into the DNA of transforming cells. The cells are then harvested and trichloracetic acid (TCA) precipitable material is collected on filters. Each filter is dried, and its radioactivity is determined in a liquid scintillation spectrometer. The results are expressed either as counts per minute (CPM) per culture, or as a stimulation ratio (index), which is the ratio of ^{3}H-thymidine incorporated in allogeneic mixtures to ^{3}H-thymidine incorporated in syngeneic mixtures.

B. Responding Cells

1. Origin

Until recently, it has been generally accepted that the cells responding in MLC are predominantly, if not exclusively, thymus-derived lymphocytes (T cells). The evidence for this conclusion is provided by four categories of experimental data. First, cells from neonatally thymectomized animals fail to respond in MLC (Wilson *et al.* 1967), whereas cells from bursectomized chickens respond normally (Alm and Peterson 1970). Second, in experiments in which adult thymectomized, irradiated, chromosomally marked thymus/bone marrow chimeras were used as donors of responding cells, 77 percent (Festenstein *et al.* 1969) to more than 90 percent (Johnston and Wilson 1970) of the proliferating cells carried the karyotype of the thymus graft. Third, treatment of mouse spleen cells with anti-Thy-1.1 serum and complement abolishes the capacity of these cells to respond in MLC (Mosier and Cantor 1971; Tyan and Ness 1972), whereas treatment with MBLA antiserum has no effect on responsiveness (Häyry *et al.* 1972). Fourth, when mouse peripheral blood, spleen, or lymph node lymphocytes are separated into B and T cell fractions by free-flow cell electrophoresis, only the T cells respond in MLC (Häyry *et al.* 1972). However, in none of these experiments could participation of B cells be completely excluded. As a matter of fact, most recent data indicate that B cells can respond in MLC, provided that T cells are present in the stimulating population (Croy and Osoba 1973; v. Boehmer 1974). It appears that mitomycin C-blocked or X-irradiated T cells recognize allogeneic B cells, and as a consequence of this recognition release a factor that stimulates the proliferation of B cells (v. Boehmer 1974). Hence the proliferation of B cells in MLC is a secondary reaction requiring primary stimulation of T cells. The product of antigenic recognition released by T cells can stimulate not only B cells, but also T cells. This latter observation explains why mitomycin C-blocked or X-irradiated parental lymphocytes occasionally stimulate the proliferation of F_1 hybrid responding cells (e.g., Huemer *et al.* 1968). Apparently, the T cells in the stimulating population recognize the alloantigens of the second parent expressed in the F_1 hybrid cells and release a factor that triggers proliferation of the hybrid cells.

2. Frequency

In a typical MLC, only a minor fraction of cells respond. The exact frequency of responding cells is difficult to estimate, but for an MLC of cells differing in the major histocompatibility complex, the estimates are as low as 1 percent (Wilson *et al.* 1968; Jones 1973) and as high as 12 percent (Ford and Atkins 1973; the latter estimate was made for cells involved in graft-versus-host reaction rather than in MLR, but because the two phenomena parallel each other in their properties, the 12 percent figure probably applies to MLR as well). The frequency of lymphocytes responding to MHC antigens is thus much lower than that responding to such nonspecific stimuli as PHA or concanavalin A.

3. Effect of Preimmunization

Preimmunization of an animal prior to its use as a donor of responding cells enhances the MLC response against the immunizing MHC antigens (Virolainen *et al.* 1969). However, the nature of this enhancement remains controversial. Wilson and Nowell (1971), working with rat peripheral blood leukocytes, observed that preimmunization shortened the lag period before DNA synthesis can be detected, and that at the end of the second day of culture the majority of potentially responsive cells entered the mitotic cycle. However, the proportion of responding cells was unaltered. Because similar acceleration was not observed with thoracic duct lymphocytes (Wilson *et al.* 1972), the authors concluded that only T cells, which are the products of recent divisions, have the capacity to respond promptly in MLC. Adler *et al.* (1970), on the other hand, observed a marked increase in MLC activity in cell populations taken from preimmunized mice. Although the authors made no attempt to compare the frequency of responding cells in immunized and unimmunized cultures, the implication from the increase response was that there are more reacting cells in the former than in the latter culture. Obviously, additional experiments in better-defined systems are needed to resolve the question of the preimmunization effect.

C. Stimulating Cells

The identity of the cells providing the stimulus for MLR is far more controversial than that of the responding cells. Although there is general agreement that living lymphocytes provide a stimulus far superior to any other agent, the role of T- and B-stimulating cells is still a much-debated question. There are those who claim that it is the T cell that provides optimal stimulus and that MLR is basically a T cell-T cell interaction (MacLaurin 1972); there are others who maintain that optimal MLC stimulation is obtained by using T lymphocytes as responding cells and B lymphocytes as stimulating cells (Plate and McKenzie 1973); and there are some who believe that basically it makes no difference whether T or B lymphocytes are the stimulating cells (Cheers and Sprent 1973).

A sensible way out of this controversy has been suggested by recent experiments of Lonai and McDevitt (McDevitt *et al.* 1974b). The authors observed that in strain combinations differing in the *I* and *S* regions [A.TL anti-A.TH, B10.T(6R) anti-AQR)], T and B cells stimulated to an equal extent or in some cases (A.TL anti-A.TH) T cells stimulated slightly better than B cells; in combinations differing in the *IA* and *IB* subregions [(A.TL × B10)F$_1$ anti-B10.HTT] B cells gave a significantly weaker stimulation than T cells; and finally in combinations differing in the chromosomal segment between *IB* and *S* (subregion *IC*) [(B10.HTT × A)F$_1$ anti-A.TH] only T cells stimulated. Apparently, the factor determining whether T or B cells stimulate is the genetic difference between the responder and the stimulator.

Stimulation by nonlymphoid cells and by subcellular fractions is even more controversial. It has been reported both that epidermal cells, fibroblasts, and thrombocytes do stimulate and do not stimulate in MLC (for references, see Sørensen 1972). Similarly, some investigators have been able to achieve MLC stimulation with killed or even disrupted cells, and others have not. The only conclusion one can make from these conflicting reports is that if nonlymphoid and nonliving cells stimulate at all, the stimulation is of a far lower magnitude than that exerted by living lymphocytes.

D. Genetics

1. Xenogeneic MLC

A myth prevailing among immunologists for some time has been that MLR in xenogeneic combinations is either nonexistent or extremely weak (e.g., Lafferty and Jones 1969; Wilson and Nowell 1970), and if it does exist that it is the consequence of stimulation by environmental antigens. This latter conclusion was based on the observation that conventional but not germ-free rats respond in xenogeneic MLC (Wilson and Fox 1971). However, several authors recently demonstrated by using various culture conditions, that in some species combinations MLC reactivity to xenogeneic cells is of the same magnitude as that to allogeneic cells (e.g., Widmer and Bach 1972; Shons *et al.* 1973; Asantila *et al.* 1974), and that conventional and germ-free animals respond equally well to xenogeneic cells (e.g., Nielson 1972). The degree of responsiveness in xenogeneic MLC is determined by phylogenetic distance between the two species involved: it decreases as the phylogenetic distance increases. For instance, fetal human lymphocytes respond strongly to rat lymphocytes, moderately to chicken lymphocytes, and weakly to frog lymphocytes (Asantila *et al.* 1974).

2. Allogeneic MLC

a. Minor loci differences. (1) *Multiple non-H-2 differences.* Cultures derived from various inbred strains presumably identical in their *H-2* haplotypes but different in multiple minor *H* loci range in their reactivity from cultures that do not differ from syngeneic controls to those that stimulate as strongly as cultures involving complete *H-2* differences (Dutton 1965, 1966; Festenstein 1966a, b; Tridente *et al.* 1967; Shorter *et al.* 1968; Rychlíková and Iványi 1969; Häyry and Defendi 1970; Adler *et al.* 1970; Mangi and Mardiney 1970; Peck and Click 1973a). The stimulation of *H-2* identical lymphocytes could be the result of the cumulative effect of multiple minor *H* loci, of a difference at the *M* or *Thy-1* loci (see below), or of serologically undetected *H-2* differences. (As discussed in Chapter Fourteen, some *H-2* haplotypes, particularly those present in presumably unrelated strains, carry the same *K* and *D* region, but may differ in the central regions.) In addition, the responsiveness in various *H-2*-identical combinations appears to be influenced by the *MLR capacitating locus* residing in the *H-2* complex (Rychlíková *et al.* 1973): MLR directed against non-H-2 antigens is strong in the presence of the *H-2^a* haplotype and weak in the presence of most other *H-2* haplotypes. Peck and Click (1973a), using cultures incubated in the presence and absence of normal mouse serum, observed a difference in the kinetics of the response against *H-2* and non-*H-2* barriers. While the responses of *H-2* disparate mixtures were almost always higher in the presence of normal mouse serum and the peak of activity occurred at 98 hr of culture, the non-*H-2* mixtures gave identical responses in the presence and absence of serum and peaked at 72 hr of incubation.

(2) *Single H loci.* The data in MLC stimulation in combinations differing at single minor *H* loci are contradictory: Dutton (1966) and Rychlíková and Iványi (1969), using two-way MLC, failed to observe stimulation in combinations involving *H-1, H-7, H-8, H-Y,* and *H-9* differences, whereas Adler *et al.* (1970) and Mangi and Mardiney (1970), using one-way MLC, observed a low but significant stimulation in combinations differing in *H-1, H-3,* and *H-4.* The discrepancy was probably caused by the differences in sensitivity of the assays employed by the different laboratories. It is possible that further improvements in MLR sensitivity will eventually prove that practically all minor *H* loci give some degree of stimulation.

Of the serologically detectable minor loci, relatively strong stimulation has recently been reported for antigens controlled by the *Thy-1* locus (Peck and Click 1973b; Peck *et al.* 1973), but no stimulation was observed in cultures involving differences at *Ly-1* and *Ly-2* loci (Festenstein *et al.* 1972), or at the *Tla* locus (Widmer *et al.* 1973d).

(3) *M locus.* Mixed lymphocyte cultures of *H-2*-identical inbred strains BALB/c and DBA/2 give a reaction equivalent to that in *H-2*-disparate strain combinations (Festenstein 1966a, b). Genetic analysis of segregating backcross populations revealed that the strong MLC is controlled by a single locus, tentatively designated *M* (Festenstein *et al.* 1971). The locus segregates independently of *H-2* and has at least four alleles with the following strain distribution:

M^1: DBA/2, AKR, BRVR
M^2: BALB/c, CBA/H, CBA/HT6T6, C57L, C57BL/6, C57BL/10
M^3: A/J, C3H/HeJ
M^4: CBA/J

The *M* locus appears to have a weak to moderate effect on graft-versus-host reaction as measured by the popliteal lymph node assay (no effect could be detected using the splenomegaly assay: cf. Huber *et al.* 1973a), or as detected after parabiosis (Nisbet and Edwards 1973), no strong influence on skin (J. Sachs *et al.* 1973) or heart (Huber *et al.* 1973b) graft survival, no effect on cell-mediated lymphocytotoxicity (Abbasi *et al.* 1973), very weak effect on bone marrow allograft survival (Peña-Martinez *et al.* 1973), and so far has not been detected serologically (Festenstein *et al.* 1971, 1972).

b. The role of the H-2 complex. Ever since the MLC assay was first applied to the mouse (Dutton 1965), it has been clear that the *H-2* complex plays a major role in it (Dutton 1965, 1966; Humer *et al.* 1968; Rychlíková and Iványi 1969; and others). The tacit assumption was that the classical H-2 antigens defined by various serological methods were actually responsible for the stimulation. The first indication that the situation may be more complex came from two important discoveries made almost simultaneously. The first was made in man, the second in the mouse. In man, Yunis and Amos (1971) observed that MLC responsiveness can be separated genetically, by rare recombinational events, from the two *HL-A* loci (*LA* and *Four*) coding for serologically detectable antigens. On the basis of this observation, the authors postulated the existence of a distinct MLR locus closely linked to *HL-A* but outside the *LA-Four* complex. This observation was later confirmed by several other laboratories. At about the same time, Rychlíková and her co-workers (1970, 1971) reported that MLC stimulation in the mouse was associated almost exclusively with the *K* end of the *H-2* complex; the *D*-end difference did not seem to stimulate at all. This finding was later confirmed by J. Klein *et al.* (1972). Further analysis of the *K-D* asymmetry in MLR stimulation by Bach and his co-workers (Bach *et al.* 1971a, b) revealed a startling finding; it was not the *K* region itself that was responsible for the *K*-end stimulation, but a region next to *K*—the *I* region. This observation was confirmed by Meo and his co-workers (1973a), as well as by several other laboratories. Bach and his co-workers explained the original observation by Rychlíková *et al.* (1970, 1971) by the fact that all the *K*-end differences explored by these authors included not only the *K*, but also the *I* region.

The picture currently emerging from studies in several laboratories (Bach *et al.* 1972a, b, 1973b; Widmer *et al.* 1973a, b, c; Meo *et al.* 1973a, b, c; Abbasi *et al.* 1973; Plate 1973) is that of a whole series of *H-2*-associated loci determining MLC stimulation (Table (18-4). The loci have been summarily designated *Lad* (i.e., loci coding for lymphocyte activating determinants, cf. Festenstein and Démant 1973) and the individual loci distinguished by Arabic numerals (*Lad-1*, *Lad-2*, *Lad-3*, etc.). The precise number of *Lad* loci in the *H-2* complex is not known, but the existence of at least four loci has been postulated (Meo *et al.*

Table 18-4. Strength of MLR and GVHR across various regions of the *H-2* complex*

H-2 region difference	MLR		GVHR	
	Average ratio of stimulation	Range	Mean spleen index	Range
K	2.0	0.7–4.7	1.4	1.2–1.6
D	1.8	0.8–5.4	1.4	1.2–1.7
IA	6.4	3.7–9.2	1.8	1.8
IB + S	2.7	1.1–4.4	1.5	1.1–1.8
I + S	5.8	2.7–12.8	2.6	2.6
K + I	6.6	3.2–18.3	2.8	2.6–3.1
D + S	2.0	0.7–4.7	1.5	1.3–1.6
K + D	3.4	3.0–3.8	1.8	1.1–2.5
K + S + D	3.3	1.5–8.6	2.3	2.2–2.4
K + I + S + D	7.2	1.2–33.6	2.8	2.4–3.1

* Based on Bach *et al.* 1973a; Widmer *et al.* 1973b, c; J. Klein and Park 1973; Livnat *et al.* 1973; and J. Klein, *unpublished data.*

1973b; cf. Fig. 18-3). The strongest of them is the *Lad-1* locus associated with the *IA* subregion and defined by the strain combination $(A.TL \times B10.D2)F_1$ anti-B10.HTT (Meo *et al.* 1973b). A similar strong stimulation has been observed in several other strain combinations involving differences between the responding and stimulating cells in the entire central segment of the *H-2* complex (Bach *et al.* 1972a, b; Widner *et al.* 1973b; Meo *et al.* 1973a). It seems likely that much of this stimulation can be attributed to the *Lad-1* locus (or loci). The relationship of the *Lad-1* locus to *Ir-1A*, *Ia* and *H-2I* loci mapping in the same region is not clear. Genetically, the four types of loci have not been separated, but this could be because of the low frequency of recombination in that region.

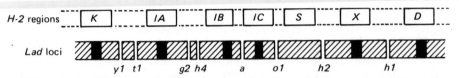

Fig. 18-3. Known *Lad* loci of the *H-2* complex. Positions of critical crossovers are indicated by recombinant symbols. (Based on experimental data of Bach, *et al.* 1972a, b, 1973a, b; Widmer *et al.* 1973a, b, c; and Meo *et al.* 1973a, b.)

The second *Lad* locus positioned in the central *H-2* segment has recently been identified by Widmer *et al.* (1973c), using strain combinations 1R and 2R. The MLR in this combination is relatively weak in a serum-free system, but much stronger in a serum-supplemented system, and has so far been observed in only one direction (1R responds to 2R but 2R does not respond to 1R). The possibility that the stimulation is due to residual background differences between the 1R and 2R lines has not been excluded, and the identification of this locus must therefore be considered tentative.

At least one more *Lad* locus probably exists in the central regions of the *H-2* complex, but its formal identification has not yet been achieved. The locus is involved in the unidirectional stimulation between the 2R and 4R strains (4R responds to 2R but 2R does not respond to 4R; cf. Bach *et al.* 1973b). The two strains differ in the *IB*, *S*, and *X* regions, and the postulated locus could therefore lie in any one of these. However, because of the association of the *Lad* and *Ir* loci in the *IA* subregion, one is tempted to speculate that a similar association exists in the *IB* subregion, and that the 2R-4R locus is actually located in this region. Alternatively, the 2R-4R locus could be identical to the 1R-2R locus in the *X* region.

The reason for the unidirectional MLC stimulation in the 1R-2R and 2R-4R combinations has not been determined. Because the stimulation is weak in both cases, it is possible that the reaction in the opposite direction is below the threshold of detection. It is also possible, however, that that stimulation is affected by *Ir* loci lying outside the *Ir-1B* or *X* subregions. A genetic model explaining the unidirectional MLC reaction in the 2R-4R strain combination has recently been proposed by Lozner *et al.* (1974a). The model is based on the author's observation that B10 anti-B10.A serum absorbed with 4R cells still reacts with 2R B cells; when absorbed with 2R cells, the same antiserum fails to react with 4R lymphocytes. Since the reciprocal antiserum (B10.A anti-B10) absorbed with 2R cells did not react with 4R cells, the authors postulated that the H-2^{h4} haplotype of the 4R strain arose by unequal crossing-over during which the *Lad* locus in the *IB* subregion was deleted. According to this hypothesis, the 2R strain carries in the *IB* subregion a locus coding for an antigen(s) expressed primarily on *B* cells, and this antigen acts as a lymphocyte-activating determinant in MLR. This locus was deleted in the 4R strain and, consequently, in MLC the 2R cells cannot respond to 4R stimulators. However, the hypothesis can be criticized on the basis that antibodies against the Ia^b antigens controlled by the *IB* subregion may be difficult to produce and that the immunization schedule used by the authors was inadequate. This criticism is strengthened by the data of David *et al.* (1974) who report that they were able to produce a weak 2R anti-4R serum.

The involvement of the *H-2K* and *H-2D* loci in the MLR was a much-debated question. Although both the *K* and *D* regions clearly stimulate in at least some strain combinations (J. Klein *et al.* 1972; Bach *et al.* 1972a, b; Meo *et al.* 1973a; Plate 1974), the stimulation could be due to *Lad* loci residing in the *K* and *D* regions but distinct from *H-2K* and *H-2D*. A strong argument against such an interpretation is the observation that the H-2da mutant causes significant stimulation in combination with the H-2^d haplotype (Rychlíková *et al.* 1972). Although the possibility that the H-2da mutation affects loci other than *H-2D* cannot be fully excluded, it seems rather unlikely (see Chapter Ten). Of the other *H-2* mutations tested, H-2^{ba} and H-2^{bb} are also known to stimulate their congenic partners in MLC (Bach *et al.* 1972a; J. Forman and J. Klein 1974), J. Klein *et al.* (1974e), and in these two cases, too, the mutations most likely affected the *H-2K* locus rather than loci in the *I* region (see Chapter Ten). The situation regarding the *H-2K* and *H-2D* loci can therefore be summarized by saying that there is no reason to believe that the two loci are not involved in MLC stimulation.

According to Plate (1974) the magnitude of the MLC response to the *D* region antigens (and presumably other antigens as well) is controlled by a minimum of two independently segregated loci. One of these loci is linked to the *H-2* complex, the other segregates independently of *H-2*. Certain alleles at these "response loci" promote a reaction against *D* region antigens that is comparable in strength to a typical *I* region response.

E. Mechanism

The basic postulate for any interpretation of MLR must be that the responding cells possess a determinant, generally R, that can interact with determinant S on stimulating cells, and that this interaction triggers DNA synthesis, blast transformation, and cell proliferation, This postulate is probably the only one on which all immunologists would agree; the rest are controversial. The nature of the interaction process, the nature of the R and S determinants, and the precise mechanism of triggering are not known. Shortly after MLR was discovered, its interpretation did not pose much of a problem. It was assumed that the reaction was immunological in nature and that it represented nothing more than recognition of H-2 (HL-A, RtH-1) antigens by cell-bound antibodies. However, in light of the advances in *H-2* genetics, this simplistic interpretation can be seriously questioned.

1. Nature of Interaction Between Responding and Stimulating Cells

Uncertainty begins with the question of the interaction between responding and stimulating cells. Is the interaction immunological in nature? Although there is no universally accepted definition of the term "immunological," most would probably agree that an immunological process is characterized by specificity of recognition and, in most cases, the capacity to develop memory. Can these two properties be proved unequivocally for the MLR?

a. Specificity. Although few would question that MLR possesses a certain degree of specificity, the exactness of the degree is not clear. Experimental evidence for specificity of MLR has been provided, for example, by Wilson and Nowell (1970), Zoschke and Bach (1971) and Salmon *et al.* (1971). The former two authors induced tolerance to rat Y cells in rat X and then used the tolerant X lymphocytes as responding cells in culture with Y stimulating cells in one experiment, and Z-stimulating cells (where Z is a third donor, unrelated to X or Y) in another experiment. They observed that the tolerant X cells were unable to respond to Y cells but responded normally to Z cells, indicating that they could distinguish between Y and Z stimulating determinants. Zoschke and Bach (1971), working with human peripheral blood leukocytes, mixed responding X and stimulating Y cells, killed all the dividing cells using a combination of 5-bromodeoxyuridine and light,[1] divided the surviving cells into halves and mixed one-half with fresh stimulating Y cells and the other half with stimulating Z cells. They observed that the culture responded to Z cells but did not respond to Y cells, indicating again a degree of MLR specificity. In a similar experiment, Salmon *et al.* (1971) observed that addition of lethal amounts of high specific activity ^{3}H-thymidine to MLC kills or inactivates the dividing cells. The cells surviving the exposure are incapable of responding to the original antigen, but still are able to respond to other, noncross-reacting antigens.

These experiments suggest that the MLR specificity has a clonal basis. The populations of responding cells apparently contains a clone of cells that recognizes stimulating determinant Y and another clone that recognizes stimulating determinant Z; the recognition is specific in that an activation or elimination of the Y clone leaves the Z clone intact.

The experimental data thus seem to support the immunological basis of

---

[1] Bromodeoxyuridine (BUdR) is a thymidine analogue that is incorporated into the DNA of DNA-synthesizing cells. When cells that have incorporated BUdR are exposed to visible light, they rapidly deteriorate and die.

MLR because they indicate a relatively high degree of specificity. However, difficulties arise when one attempts to tie together this specificity and the observation of a number of cells responding to any single stimulating cell type. If the estimates are correct and an average population of lymphocytes indeed contains 1–12 (an average of 6) percent of cells reacting to each stimulating cell type, one must assume that the responding cells are capable of distinguishing fewer than 60 S determinants. One is then faced with the dilemma that either the recognition repertoire ("dictionary") of the R determinants is very limited, or that the R determinants are broadly cross-reactive. The following explanations have been proposed to resolve the question. First, MLR represents secondary rather than primary reaction, with presensitization occurring unknowingly during the life span of the cell donor. Arguing against (but not ruling out) this possibility is the finding that cells from germ-free rats display the same degree of MLR to allogeneic antigens as cells from conventional animals (Wilson and Fox 1971). Second, because the frequency of responding cells is measured relatively late after the initation of response, the observed 6 percent value could be the result of clonal expansion and amplification, mediated, for example, by soluble substances, and the initial figure could be much lower. Because no assay is available for measuring the initiation of the response reliably, this possibility is difficult to rule out. As a matter of fact, the existence of soluble factors released into the medium and enhancing MLR has been reported by several laboratories (see Sørensen 1972, for references). Third, the response observed in an ordinary MLC may represent activation of a number of clones by a number of S determinants.

On the other hand, it is possible that the R determinants are broadly cross-reactive and that a single S determinant activates not one, but several cell clones.

b. Memory. As discussed earlier, preimmunization enhances MLR, but it is not clear whether the enhancement could be considered an expression of a second-set reaction. To test whether standard mixed cultures produce memory cells, Wilson *et al.* (1972) allowed cells to proliferate for 6–7 days in MLC and then injected them into T cell-deprived rats (i.e., rats that were thymectomized, lethally irradiated, and protected with syngeneic bone marrow from thymectomized donors subjected to thoracic duct drainage). The inoculum presumably contained only activated cells, because Mitomycin C-treated stimulating cells and most of the unstimulated cells did not survive the culture conditions. Following the transfer, peripheral blood lymphocytes and thoracic duct lymphocytes were obtained from the inoculated animals and were used in MLC against the same type of stimulating cells employed in the original culture. The experiments demonstrated that MLC reactivity can be restored with antigen-activated populations of lymphocytes to T cell-deprived animals. The secondary MLR was largely, but not completely specific for the stimulating cells used in the original MLC. Although the secondary MLC response was of the same order of magnitude as the primary MLR, a considerable clonal amplification must have occurred in the T cell-deprived animals, because the number of MLC-activated cells used to inoculate the animals was relatively small ($1.2–2 \times 10^7$ cells/rat).

These experiments, though not proving production of memory cells in MLC, nevertheless provide evidence that an effect resembling immunization may occur in the culture.

Hence, MLR seems to possess at least the potential for the two basic properties of an immunological phenomenon, specificity and memory, suggesting that the reaction is indeed immunological in nature. The immunological element in MLR, however, may not be so sophisticated as in other immunological systems. It may well be that the MLR represents a more primitive immunological interaction in terms of phylogeny.

2. Nature of R and S Determinants

At the time of this writing, the nature of the R and S determinants is an unresolved puzzle. Theoretically, there are the following possibilities:

1. Both the R and S determinants are coded for by the *H-2* complex.
   a. The R and S determinants belong to the same class of molecules controlled by the same type of loci.
   b. The R and S determinants are two different classes of molecules controlled by two types of loci (both types of loci residing in the *H-2* complex).
2. The S determinants are coded for by loci in the *H-2* complex, whereas loci for the R determinants reside somewhere else in the mouse genome. (The reverse possibility, namely that R determinants are controlled by the *H-2* complex and S determinants are controlled by loci outside chromosome 17, seems to be ruled out by the available data; see below.)

Experimental data on the nature of R and S determinants are so scarce that they do not allow, at present time, distinction between the above possibilities. Of the three possibilities, alternative (a) may seem heretical to a classical immunologist, since it requires interaction between like substances. Immunologists, drawing on three-quarters of a century of experience, are used to thinking in terms of clear-cut complementarity of determinants (antigens-antibodies, antigens-receptors). However, it may well be that in more primitive immunological systems strict complementarity does not always exist; one can visualize a system in which the same molecule functions as a receptor and as a stimulator.

The experimental data do establish one fact for certain, namely that the S determinants are controlled by the *H-2* complex (i.e., by the *Lad* loci). Another conclusion that can be drawn from the data, although with much lesser degree of certainty, is that the *Lad* and *Ia* loci are probably identical and that the S determinants are probably the Ia antigens. This conclusion is supported by three main findings: first, the *Lad* and *Ia* loci map in the same positions; second, the tissue distribution of the Ia antigens corresponds to that expected from S determinants (predominant presence on B lymphocytes); and third, the stimulating cells can be blocked with anti-Ia sera (M. Nabholz, *personal communica-*

tion V. Hauptfeld and J. Klein, *unpublished data*). However, an equally strong argument can be made in favor of *H-2K* and *H-2D* loci also coding for S determinants. The argument is based on two observations: first, *K* and *D* region differences cause weak but significant MLC; and second, congenic lines differing only at the *H-2D* (or *H-2K*) locus also display a significant MLR (see Chapter Ten). It must be concluded, therefore, that the H-2 antigens themselves can also function as S determinants. Nevertheless, it is clearly established that the *Lad*-associated MLR stimulation is usually much stronger than the *H-2K*- or *H-2D*-associated stimulation. This difference can be explained by one of the following three assumptions. First, the difference is quantitative rather than qualitative. One can interpret the superior MLR strength of the *IA* subregion over other regions and subregions of the *H-2* complex by assuming the existence of a great number of *Lad* loci and a different density of these loci over the *H-2* segment (Fig. 18–4). According to this hypothesis, the more *Lad* differences

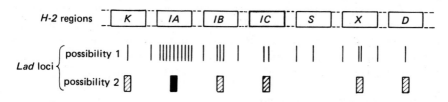

Fig. 18-4. Two possible interpretations of the unusual strength of the *IA* subregion in MLR. Each vertical line represents one *Lad* locus. Degree of shading indicates strength of *Lad* loci.

between two strains, the more cell clones are activated in MLC, and, consequently, the stronger the reaction. Since the *H-2K* or *H-2D* differences involve single loci, the MLR across this difference is relatively weak. Second, the carrier region of the H-2K and H-2D molecules (i.e., the region that is recognized in MLR) is less polymorphic than similar regions of the Ia molecules. Although the *H-2* loci are notorious for their polymorphism (see Chapter Twelve), the variability can be restricted to one region of the H-2 molecule, with other regions of the molecules being relatively constant. A low variability of the H-2 molecules' carrier portion would explain why some serologically distinct *H-2* haplotypes fail to stimulate in MLR. Third, the mechanism of MLR across *H-2K* or *H-2D* regions is different from that across the *I* region. It is not inconceivable, for instance, that in the former case MLR results from an interaction between H-2 antigens on both responding and stimulating cells, whereas the *I* region-associated MLR is the result of an interaction between receptors and antigens. It is even possible that MLR is a rather heterogeneous group of phenomena whose only common denominator is transformation of lymphocytes and that such transformation can be triggered by a number of different stimuli. In the case of *I* region-associated MLR it is generally believed that the R determinants are different from the S determinants.

This belief is largely based on the observation that antisera capable of blocking stimulating cells usually fail to block responding cells. However, since there is no antiserum whose responder-blocking activity is generally agreed on, the value of the above argument is dubious. It is possible, for instance, that the nature of the responding cells' reaction is such that the reaction could not be blocked with anti-S sera even if R and S determinants were the same.

Evidence supporting the identity of at least some R and S determinants has been recently obtained by Hirschberg *et al.* (1973) who observed that elimination of cells proliferating in response to a particular allogeneic cell population (A anti-B) significantly reduces the ability of the remaining A cells to stimulate cells from the donor that provided stimulating cells for the initial MLC (donor B).

If the R determinants are different from the S determinants, their identity is a complete mystery. It has been speculated that the R determinants are the *Ir* gene products, the latter being the hypothetical T cell receptor (see last section of this Chapter), however, so far, there is little evidence to support such hypothesis. There is almost no evidence that the R determinants are coded for by the *H-2* complex. The identity of the R determinants with the T cell receptor is a widely shared belief among immunologists, but because the nature of the T cell receptor is unknown, this hypothesis does not explain much.

3. Product of Antigen Recognition

According to Ramseier and his colleagues, the cell interaction in MLC is accompanied by the liberation of a substance that the authors designated *product of antigen recognition* (PAR; for review and references, see Ramseier and Lindenmann 1972; Ramseier 1973). The test system for PAR is as follows. Responding and stimulating lymphocytes (mouse, rat, or Syrian hamster) are mixed as in a standard MLC, and after 4–10 hr of incubation, the medium from the culture is concentrated by lyophilization and injected into the skin of normal Syrian hamsters. The presence of PAR in the concentrate is revealed by a cutaneous reaction characterized primarily by accumulation of poly-morphonuclear leukocytes (granulocytes) at the injection site. The intensity of the reaction is measured by excising and trypsinizing the skin lesions and count-ing the released granulocytes. According to Ramseier, PAR is released by nearly all allogeneic cell mixtures, including those differing at weak minor *H* loci, such as *H-Y*. The release of PAR can be inhibited either by incubating the stimulating cells with anti-H-2 sera or by incubating the responding cells with "antireceptor sera." The latter antisera are obtained by immunization of F_1 hybrids with parental cells. (Ramseier believes that the genes coding for the hypothetical receptors are recessive, and hence that the F_1 hybrid can produce antibodies against the parental recognition structures.) In both cases, the block-ing is highly specific. However, the same antisera were tested in a number of different laboratories and found to have no apparent effect on proliferation in MLC, survival of skin or heart allografts, cell-mediated lymphocytotoxicity *in vitro* or GVHR (Lindahl 1972).

III. Graft-Versus-Host Reaction

A. Principle and Methods

Inoculation of immunocompetent cells into immunoincompetent recipients (newborn or immunologically immature mice, F_1 hybrids injected with parental cells, or lethally irradiated mice) leads to a series of complex phenomena called the *graft-versus-host reaction* (GVHR; for reviews and references, see Simonsen 1962a; Billingham 1968; and Elkins 1971).[2] The source of immunocompetent cells may be any lymphoid organ, most commonly the spleen. There are numerous techniques for measuring GVHR, but the one most frequently used is the Simonsen or splenomegaly assay. In a typical test, newborn mice (less than 24 hr old) are injected intraperitoneally with several million spleen cells from an allogeneic adult donor. At 10 days after the injection, the recipients are sacrificed and their body and spleen weights are determined and compared with body and spleen weights of control mice (i.e., mice injected with syngeneic cells). The results are expressed as the spleen index, calculated from a formula

$$\text{spleen index} = \frac{\dfrac{\text{spleen weight}}{\text{body weight}} \text{ of experimental animals}}{\text{Mean } \dfrac{\text{spleen weight}}{\text{body weight}} \text{ of control animals}}$$

In theory, a spleen index larger than 1.0 indicates a positive GVHR, but in practice, many authors consider only indexes above 1.3 to be positive. Other GVHR assays are based on the death of the recipient, the presence of wasting syndrome (see below), increased phagocytosis, enumeration of microscopic foci of lymphocytic infiltrate in liver, skin, or kidney after local inoculation of cells, or incorporation of radioactive isotopes in the spleen or lymph node cells.

B. Mechanism

Following their inoculation into the immunoincompetent host, donor lymphocytes home to and settle in the spleen and lymph nodes. A small proportion of lymphocytes then begins to undergo blast transformation, which resembles transformation of lymphocytes in MLC in all respects. The blasts divide repeatedly for several days, expanding the initial small clone(s) of proliferating cells. Eventually, however, the blasts become smaller after each division and give rise to a population of small lymphocytes, which are then disseminated throughout the organs and tissues of the host. The new generation of small lymphocytes differs from those in the initial inoculum in that they have a killer capacity—they are committed to carrying out the destruction of the host tissue. However, the destruction of the host tissue begins even before the

---

[2] When immunocompetent cells are inoculated into immunocompetent hosts, they may be destroyed before they have a chance to react against the host, or the effects of the graft-versus-host reaction can be masked by concurrently occurring host-versus-graft reaction.

killer cells are generated, perhaps even before the donor cells begin to proliferate. In addition, the blast cells themselves also seem to have the capacity to
injure the tissues in which they proliferate. The proliferation of the donor cells
and the damage these cells inflict on the host tissue set into motion a complex
response from the host. The most prominent features of this response are
inflammation at the site of donor cell proliferation, increased phagocytic activity,
and increased proliferation of the reticulo-endothelial and lymphoid cells in the
spleen and liver. The proliferation of host cells enlarges the spleen (splenomegaly), liver (hepatomegaly), and often also the lymph nodes. In the meantime,
however, the donor-derived killer cells begin to attack the lymphoid tissue of the
host, destroying large populations of cells and causing atrophy of spleen and
lymph nodes, anemia, and lymphopenia. These effects weaken the host's resistance to pathogens, and as a result, secondary complications begin to appear
and the animal develops a typical runting (wasting) syndrome: loss of weight,
retarded growth, hunched appearance, ruffled fur, and diarrhea. In the most
severe cases of GVHR the animal eventually dies; in less severe cases the animal
may recover fully.

C. Relationship Between MLR and GVHR

The GVHR against antigens controlled by the major histocompatibility
complex closely resembles the MLR. Like MLR, the GVHR is mediated by
T lymphocytes, it involves an unusually high number of initially responding
cells, and it is not greatly enhanced by preimmunization of the donor. The initial
phase of the two reactions seems to be completely homologous, but the GVHR is
much more complex primarily because it also involves the nonspecific response
of the host to the graft.

D. Genetics of GVHR

1. Xenogeneic GVHR

It has been demonstrated repeatedly that donor cells from one species, when
inoculated into an immunologically unreactive host of another species, usually
induce a much milder GVHR than do cells of the same species. In many instances, xenogeneic cells induce no GVHR at all (for references, see Simonsen
1962a). The strength of the response depends on the phylogenetic relationship
between the donor and the host: the less related the two species, the lower the
GVHR. Simonsen (1962b) proposed two explanations for this unusual phenomenon. First, the lack of xenogeneic GVHR could be "a case of general
immunological depression from the encounter with too large a quantity of too
big an array of too strong antigens, leaving no grafted cells with much of their
immunological competence." Second, the lack of GVHR could be due to an
"inadequate physiological environment for the grafted cells to maintain suffi-

ciently normal function." However, both explanations seem to be ruled out by the observations that xenogeneic GVHR can be induced if the donor is pre-immunized against the host, and that donor cells can respond to allogeneic cells in the xenogeneic environment (Lafferty and Jones 1969). Assuming that the donor-host cell interaction in GVHR operates on the same principle as responder-stimulator interaction in MLR, one can propose two alternative explanations of the xenogeneic GVHR effect. If the interaction occurs between receptors of donor cells and antigens of host cells, one can postulate that each species has, for some reason, receptors for only allogeneic antigens or xenogeneic antigens of closely related species but not for xenogeneic antigens of an unrelated species (the receptor dictionary contains only slang words and no foreign words). If, on the other hand, one chooses to believe that the MLR and GVHR result from interaction of two antigens, one can postulate that the xenogeneic antigens are so dissimilar that they cannot interact.

2. Allogeneic GVHR

a. Minor H loci differences. GVHR across multiple or single minor *H* loci differences has been observed by some authors (Sankowski and Nouza 1968; Cantrell and Hildemann 1972), while others (Simonsen 1962a; Eichwald *et al.* 1969; Lengerová and Viklický 1969; Lengerová *et al.* 1971) have been unable to observe such a reaction. A recent systematic study by Cantrell and Hildemann (1972) seems to have resolved the controversy. The authors convincingly demonstrated that GVHR, as measured by the mortality assay, can be induced across almost any minor *H* locus difference, no matter how weak the difference is, if conditions conducive to the reaction are provided. Among the important variables determining the onset of the reaction are the dose of the donor cells, the route of injection, and preimmunization of the donor. The strength of the GVHR parallels the strength of the allograft reaction as measured by skin-graft rejection. Incompatibilities of decreasing strength require progressive increases in the doses of spleen cells to evoke GVHR, and correlate with a decreasing time of GVHR onset and a greater interval between onset and death. The weaker the *H* barrier, the stronger the potential efficacy of preimmunization's evoking GVHR.

b. H-2 differences. Since it was discovered that the *H-2* complex is involved in GVHR (Simonsen and Jensen 1959; Simonsen 1962a), its predominance in this reaction has never been questioned. The first indication that different regions of the *H-2* complex might not be equally important in GVHR was obtained by Eichwald and his co-workers (1969) and by Lengerová and Viklický (1969). These authors tested the severity of GVHR in combinations that were supposedly monoantigenic; that is, the graft was supposed to react against a single H-2 antigen. They noticed that some H-2 antigens caused a more severe GVHR than others. They failed to notice, however, that the strong antigens were those controlled by the *K* region and the weak antigens were those controlled by the *D* region. This oversight was corrected by Démant (1970), who demonstrated that *K*-end, but not *D*-end differences can cause GVHR. But in all the strain combinations used by Démant, the *K* differences always involved differences in the *I* region as well. The question thus arose as to whether the unusual strength of the *H-2K* antigens might not actually be due to their close association with the *I* region. This possibility was tested by J. Klein and Park (1973) and Oppltová and Démant (1973), who found that, as in the MLR, the *I* region plays a dominant role in GVHR, evoking a much stronger reaction than any other region of the *H-2* complex (Table 18-3). Mapping studies of GVHR-inducing loci are still in progress (J. Klein and Park 1973; J. Klein and Egorov 1973; Livnat *et al.* 1973; Oppltová and Démant 1973; J. Klein, *unpublished data*), but the results clearly indicate that there are at least four such loci coinciding with MLR-determining loci (Fig. 18-3). The coincidence of the genetic loci and the similarity of the reactions indicate that the GVHR- and MLR-determining loci are probably identical, and so a common designation, *Lad*, seems appropriate.

IV. Cell-Mediated Lymphocytotoxicity

A. Background

Because soon after its discovery it became apparent that the MLC represented only the early (recognitive) phase of the *in vitro* allograft reaction, an effort continued to define an *in vitro* analogue of the late (destructive) phase of the reaction. The first investigators to succeed in such an effort were Govaerts (1960), working with dogs, and Rosenau and Moon (1961), working with mice.

Govaerts transplanted a kidney from dog X to dog Y, and after its rejection obtained thoracic duct lymphocytes from the immunized animal and added them to cultured cells that he had established in the meantime from the second kidney of dog X. Within 48 hr of their addition to the culture, the immune lymphocytes produced specific lesions, which started with the retraction of processes and rounding and agglutination of the epithelial renal cells and ended with their complete destruction. Lymphocytes from unimmunized and unrelated dog Z displayed no such effect.

Rosenau and Moon (1961) immunized BALB/c mice with L cells (an established line of C3H origin) and then added spleen cells from the immune animal to the L cell culture. As in Govaerts' experiment, within 48 hr the lymphocytes had clustered around the individual L cells and destroyed them. In both experiments there was no evidence that antibodies or complement were needed for the cytotoxic effect, which appeared to result solely from cell-to-cell interaction.

The experiments were quickly confirmed by other laboratories and were followed by an avalanche of reports describing various modifications of the systems used by Govaerts and by Rosenau and Moon.

The various *in vitro* assays for lymphocyte-mediated cytotoxicity can be divided into two groups.[3] In the first group are assays based on the destruction of target cells by sensitized lymphocytes in the absence of antibodies and complement. Prototypes for this group are Govaerts' and Rosenau and Moon's assays, described above.

In the second group are assays based on a cell-to-cell interaction mediated by antibodies (*antibody-dependent cell-mediated lymphocytotoxicity*). This group's prototype assay was described by Perlmann and Holm (1968), who labeled chicken erythrocytes with ^{51}Cr and then attached (by means of tannic acid treatment) protein antigens such as PPD[4] to the erythrocytes. The labeled, antigen-coated erythrocytes were then incubated with a heat-inactivated antiserum obtained by immunization of guinea pigs with killed tuberculin bacilli and were mixed with normal guinea pig spleen cells. Lysis of the chicken erythrocytes followed and was measured by the release of radioactive ^{51}Cr.

Because all attempts to achieve H-2 antibody mediated cell lysis have failed (Nabholz *et al.* 1974a), of these two groups of assays, only the first group, summarily designated *cell-mediated lymphocytotoxicity* (CML) assays, will be given further consideration.

There is a large number of variants of the CML assays, which differ in the means of achieving sensitization of lymphocytes, the type of target cells, and the ways of measuring the cytotoxic effect. The sensitization can occur principally *in vivo* (by immunization of the prospective lymphocyte donor) or *in vitro* (in mixed lymphocyte culture). The latter is based on the finding, arrived at almost simultaneously by at least four laboratories (Häyry and Defendi 1970; Hodes and Svedmyr 1970; Hardy *et al.* 1970; Solliday and Bach 1970), that allogeneic lymphocytes undergoing blast transformation in one-way MLC are cytotoxic for proper target cells *in vitro*. A similar finding was made five years earlier by Ginsburg and Sachs (1965) in a xenogeneic system. These authors observed that rat lymphocytes exposed for 5 days to a monolayer of mouse embryo fibroblasts undergo blast transformation, followed by lysis of the target monolayer cells.

A wide variety of target cells, most of them derived from established cell lines on short-term cultures, have been employed by different laboratories. However, the three most popular target cell types are mouse mastocytoma P-815, PHA-stimulated blasts, and macrophages. The mastocytoma (mast cell tumor), originally obtained by Dunn and Potter (1957) from a DBA/2 mouse, was adapted to grow in suspension cultures and to serve as a CML target cell by

---

[3] A third group of *in vitro* assays based on destruction of target cells by sensitized macrophages has also been reported. A prototype assay for this group was described by Granger and Weiser (1964), who injected Sarcoma I cells (of A strain origin) intraperitoneally into C57BL/6K mice, harvested peritoneal macrophages from the immunized animals after 10 days, cultured the macrophages for 12 hr *in vitro*, and then added them in small drops to a culture of A strain embryonic cells. Destruction of the target cells followed within 60 hr. However, at present it is not clear whether the killing is really effected by specifically sensitized macrophages. The possibility of contamination by T lymphocytes or aquisition by macrophages of factors released by T cells has not been excluded.

[4] PPD, or purified protein derivative, is a mixture of proteins derived from *Mycobacterium tuberculosis* and employed in the tuberculin test.

Brunner *et al.* (1966). For reasons that are not understood, the cell line proved to be a superior CML target in that it produced high specific and low background lysis. PHA-stimulated blasts are used instead of normal lymphocytes, which are resistant to the cytotoxic action of sensitized cells (Miggiano *et al.* 1972) and usually display a high spontaneous release. The macrophages for the CML assays are usually obtained from peritoneal exudates, following nonspecific stimulation of the donor (Brondz 1968a, b).

The destruction of the growth inhibition of the target cells in CML assays can be determined visually (by counting cells prior to and after addition of sensitized lymphocytes, by counting clear plaques formed at the site of destruction in a confluent monolayer, or by counting colonies formed by target cells cultured with and without sensitized lymphocytes), or by measuring the release of isotope markers (e.g., ^{51}Cr from labeled target cells.

The two most frequently used CML assays are based on the use of mastocytoma and PHA-stimulated blasts as target cells. In the former assay (Brunner *et al.* 1966), allogeneic mice are inoculated with the DBA/2 mastocytoma and their spleen or lymph node lymphocytes are harvested 9–12 days later. A suspension of the sensitized lymphocytes (typically 2×10^7 cells/ml) is mixed in a test tube with an equal volume of mastocytoma cells (typically 2×10^5 cells/ml), grown in culture and labeled with ^{51}Cr. The mixture is incubated for 3–9 hr at 37°C, then centrifuged, and radioactivity of the supernatant is determined.

Typically, in the MLC-CML assay, lymphocytes are incubated for 70–90 hr in a standard one-way mixed culture, and at the end of the incubation period, the surviving activated cells are added to target cells, which are lymphocytes cultured for 3 days in the presence of PHA and labeled with ^{51}Cr. After 3 hr of incubation at 37°C, the cultures are centrifuged and the amount of radioactivity released in the supernatant is determined. The results are expressed in counts per minute (CPM) per culture, as a percentage of release, or as a percentage of specific ^{51}Cr release, calculated from a formula

$$\frac{\text{release with sensitized lymphocytes} - \text{spontaneous release}}{\text{maximum release} - \text{spontaneous release}}$$

where maximum release is obtained after nonspecific lysis of control cells, by Triton X-100 treatment, for example.

B. Mechanism[5]

The kinetics of CML are determined primarily by the ratio of *effector cells* (i.e., cells that actually carry out the killing) to target cells. Measurable cytotoxicity is usually obtained only with an excess of effector cells over target cells. Effector cells are derived from the thymus; B cells, in this particular system, are neither cytotoxic nor necessary for T cell-mediated lymphocytotoxicity. The

[5] For a review and references, see Brondz 1972; Feldman *et al.* 1972; Häyry *et al.* 1972, Cerottini and Brunner 1974.

killer T cells can act alone, in the absence of not only B cells but also macrophages (although macrophages are required for initiation of the sensitization in MLC and probably also *in vivo*). In populations of unsensitized lymphocytes, effector cells are either not present at all or are present in such low concentrations that they escape detection. (Although several investigators have obtained lympholysis with cells from unimmunized animals, their results could probably be explained by assuming that sensitization might have occurred *in vitro* in these tests.) The production of effector cells requires a cell proliferation such as that in MLC. In MLC the effector cells appear relatively late, but the potency to kill target cells increases beyond the peak of the proliferative response. Effector cells change their morphology during the course of sensitization: in the early phase they are large blast cells, but in the later stages medium- and small-sized lymphocytes with killer capacities begin to appear. It is assumed, but not proved, that the blasts themselves revert to the small effector cells.

Cytolysis requires direct cell-to-cell contact: target cells separated from effector cells by a Millipore membrane are not killed. The killing process, therefore, does not seem to be mediated by any diffuse, long-range, soluble substances such as lymphotoxins. Lysis starts immediately after contact between effector and target cells is established and is based on single-hit kinetics (a single contact between an effector and a target cell is sufficient to kill the latter). Most investigators agree that effector cells are not damaged extensively during the interaction with target cells, although claims to the contrary have been made. It appears that one effector cell is able to kill more than one target cell. The lytic process proceeds in two steps: in the first step, specific interaction between determinants on effector and target cells occurs; in the second, nonspecific step, the lytic reaction is activated. The first step is energy dependent.

C. Genetics

In most strain combinations tested in the past target and effector cells differed not only in the entire *H-2* complex but also in multiple non-*H-2* loci. In such combinations, strong CML reaction was observed (Abbasi and Festenstein 1973; Ax *et al.* 1971; Brondz 1964, 1965, 1966, 1968a, b; Brondz *et al.* 1971, 1972; Brondz and Goldberg 1970; Brondz and Snegiröva 1971; Brunner *et al.* 1968, 1970; Cerottini *et al.* 1970, 1971; Cohen *et al.* 1971; Ginsburg 1968; Howe *et al.* 1973; Mauel *et al.* 1970). An equally strong reaction was obtained in those relatively rare instances in which *H-2* congenic lines were employed (Brondz 1968a), suggesting that the CML was primarily directed against determinants controlled by the *H-2* complex. The role of minor *H* loci remains to be determined.

The first indication that various regions of the major histocompatibility complex may not be equally important in eliciting CML was the observation by Eijsvoogel *et al.* (1973a) that in man MLC activation by a locus distinct from the two *HL-A* loci (*LA* and *Four*) was a prerequisite for *in vitro* induction of lymphocytotoxicity. The specificity of this cytotoxicity, however, was found not to be directed toward the MLC-inducing determinants but toward the HL-A antigens (or antigens determined by loci closely linked to *HL-A*). This observation was confirmed by Alter *et al.* (1973) who demonstrated, using *H-2* recombinant strains of mice, that the CML occurred only when the cells in the culture differed simultaneously in the *K* (or *D*) and *I* regions; differences in the *I* (or *S*) region alone, or in the *K* (or *D*) region alone failed to elicit significant CML. Both groups of investigators explained these observations by postulating that CML was the result of an interaction between two distinct cell lineages. In the Bach's version of the two-cell model (Bach *et al.* 1973a), the responding cell population is visualized as consisting of two cell types, one recognizing the peripheral region differences and differentiating into cytotoxic lymphocytes (killer cells), and another recognizing the central region differences and differentiating into proliferating helper cells (PHCs). The stimulated PHC's collaborate with cytotoxic lymphocytes, and this collaboration leads to increased cytotoxicity.

In an attempt to provide experimental evidence supporting the two-cell model, Bach and his co-workers (1973a) took advantage of the observation that lymphocytes that mediate cytotoxicity adhere *in vitro* to target cell monolayers either prior to (Lonai *et al.* 1972) or following sensitization (Brondz and Goldberg 1970; Goldstein *et al.* 1971a, b). The authors demonstrated that adsorption of leukocytes from normal human donors on macrophage monolayers (prior to or following sensitization in MLC) specifically removed killer precursor cells but not, to any significant extent, the cells responding in MLC to leucocytes derived from the macrophage donor. According to the authors, the experiment can be interpreted as follows. The exposure to the monolayer removed from the responding culture clones of cells recognizing the serologically detectable antigens and predestined to produce killer cells, and thus abolished most of the CML activity. The proliferating helper cells recognizing the lymphocyte activating determinants were not affected and produced undiminished MLR. [An alternative explanation to that provided by Bach *et al.* (1973a) will be described below.]

However, the interpretation of CML genetics and physiology as originally put forward by Eijsvoogel and Bach and their respective co-workers is almost certainly an oversimplification. The main theses of this interpretation, namely the failure of peripheral region differences to elicit CML in the absence of central region differences, the failure of the central regions to serve as targets for CML, and the cooperation between central and peripheral *H-2* regions in the induction of CML, must now be qualified.

1. The Role of Peripheral H-2 Regions

It is now clear that the original claim by Alter *et al.* (1973) that central region differences are required for generation of lymphocytotoxicity against antigens controlled by peripheral regions is incorrect. The Alter data were first challenged by Nabholz and his colleagues (1974a) who pointed out that *K* and *D* region differences alone lead to significant CML in the absence of any known central region differences. Nabholz's data were then confirmed by several other investigators, including Bach and his colleagues (Schendel *et al.* 1973). Some of the combinations in which Nabholz *et al.* (1974a) observed significant CML were the following.

K region differences*			D region differences*		
Responder	Stimulator	Target	Responder	Stimulator	Target
A	A.SW	A.TL	A.TH	A.SW	A.SW
A	A.TH	A.TL	A.SW	A	A.TL
A	A.TL	A.TH	A.SW	A.TH	A
A	A.TL	A.SW	C3H.OH	B10.D2	B10.D2
			C3H.OH	B10.A	B10.D2
			HTG	B10.A(5R)	B10.D2
			B10.A(5R)	HTG	B10

* Region which the target shares with the stimulator and for which both are incompatible with the responder.

However, because all these combinations involve *H-2* recombinant strains, one can argue that unrecognized MLR differences remain closely linked to the serologically detectable difference and provide the necessary helper function in CML. This objection is largely (although not totally) eliminated in combinations involving *H-2* mutant strains. All the mutant strains that have been tested have been found to give significant CML in combination with their respective congenic partners carrying *H-2* haplotypes from which the mutant haplotypes were derived. Particularly illuminating in this respect is the B10.D2(M504) ($H\text{-}2^{da}$) strain, which gives significant CML with its congenic partner B10.D2 ($H\text{-}2^d$, cf. Brondz 1973; J. Klein *et al.* 1974e). If the $H\text{-}2^{da}$ haplotype were derived from $H\text{-}2^d$ by a single mutation, then by itself it invalidates the two-cell hypothesis, since there is ample evidence that the mutation occurred in the locus coding for serologically detectable antigens.

In contrast to reports that in man the Four antigens are considerably more important targets for the specific destruction *in vitro* than the LA antigens (Eijsvoogel *et al.* 1973b), in the mouse, there seems to be no difference between the *K* and *D* region antigens in their CML-eliciting capability (Freiesleben-Sørensen and Hawkes 1973; Nabholz *et al.* 1974). However, the two regions display a cumulative effect in that the combined *K*+*D* differences usually elicit stronger CML than *K* or *D* alone (Nabholz *et al.* 1974a).

A separate region (*ECS*) located between the *I* and *S* regions and controlling the generation of effector cell capacity was postulated by Festenstein *et al.* (1974). However, the currently available data do not support such a contention and even the authors were forced to concede that "a consistent assignment of *ECS* genotypes to individual *H-2* haplotypes is not possible . . ."

2. The Role of Central H-2 Regions

One of the most fascinating features of the CML is that the reaction (as measured by the release of radioactive chromium from PHA stimulated blasts), with a few exceptions, is either totally absent or extremely weak across central region differences. Even in strain combinations such as AQR-B10.T(6R) or A.TL-A.TH in which there is a strong MLR, there is almost no CML activity (Alter *et al.* 1973; Nabholz *et al.* 1974a). Various explanations have been offered for the lack of CML across central region differences (Howard 1973a, b; Nabholz *et al.* 1974a). One is that the *I* and *S* regions do not code for antigens serving as targets in CML. Although this is certainly the simplest and perhaps the most logical explanation, it is one that is hard to accept, particularly in view of the fact that graft rejection, of which the CML is supposed to be an *in vitro* analogue, does occur between *I* region disparate congenic lines (see discussion below).

Another possibility that has been considered is that the PHA-stimulated blasts are the wrong target cells for CML across the *I* region. Since PHA transforms mostly T cells, while the Ia antigens, a potential candidate for the CML target function, are predominantly on B cells, large magnitude killing of PHA blasts would not be expected.

Still another possibility is that the target antigens are inactivated, redistributed, or even lost during the transformation process. This possibility can be tested by replacing the blasts with normal lymphocytes as target cells. However, it is already known that at least the Ia antigens have not been inactivated by the transformation: mitogen stimulated blasts are as good targets for anti-Ia antisera in the presence of complement as normal lymphocytes (J. Forman, V. Hauptfeld, and J. Klein, *unpublished data*). Of course, one can argue that the transformation changed properties of the Ia antigens that are not important for antibody and complement mediated cytotoxicity but are important for cell-mediated cytotoxicity, or that Ia are the wrong antigens to look at.

Despite the fact that there is so far (i.e., at the time of this writing) no positive evidence one way or the other, one is still tempted to speculate that the lack of central region-associated CML is merely an artifact of the *in vitro* method.

It should be emphasized that weak to moderate CML across central *H-2* regions is occasionally observed. The two most notable examples are combinations B10 (responder)-HTG (stimulator)-B10.A(5R) (target; cf. Nabholz *et al.* 1974a), and B10.S(7R)-B10.S(9R) (V. Hauptfeld and J. Klein, *unpublished data*).

3. Collaboration Between Central and Peripheral H-2 Regions

Although *K* and *D* regions alone suffice for the induction of CML, the cytotoxicity against these regions is clearly considerably stronger if simultaneous stimulation across I region occurs. Bach and his associates (1973a) believe that the basis for this amplifying effect of the I region is a true collaboration between two cell lineages, one lineage leading to CML and the other to MLR. An alternative, and simpler, explanation of the effect is suggested by the recent findings on nonspecific MLR stimulation by soluble factors, as discussed in the previous section. One can postulate that the strong I region associated MLR is accompanied by the release of factors that nonspecifically enhance the K or D region-associated MLR and that the amplified K-D MLC activity leads to an increase in the number of cytotoxic lymphocytes. According to this hypothesis, there is only one cell lineage that starts from an antigen-sensitive lymphocyte, continues through typical MLC blasts, and ends in a cytotoxic lymphocyte. The hypothesis is supported by morphological observations suggesting a direct conversion of blasts into small lymphocytes presumed to be the killer cells (Häyry and Andersson 1973).

D. Nature of Target Antigens

The observation that the CML is primarily directed against the K and D regions suggests that the targets of the reaction are either the classical H-2 antigens or antigens controlled by loci closely linked to H-$2K$ and H-$2D$. The CML-target function of the H-2 antigens is supported by two types of observations. First, in the H-2da mutant the appearance of new serological character-istics is accompanied by a change in the CML-target characteristics. Second, the CML can be blocked by incubation of the target cells (but not of the effector cells) with anti-H-2 sera (Brunner *et al.* 1968; Mauel *et al.* 1970; Cerrotini *et al.* 1971; Nabholz *et al.* 1974a). The specificity of the blocking effect was demon-strated, for example, by Nabholz *et al.* (1974a) in a combination HTG (responder)-B10.A(5R) (stimulator)-B10 or B10.D2 (target), in which the sensitization occurs against the H-$2K^b$ allele of B10 and H-$2D^d$ allele of B10.D2. When an anti-H-$2K^b$ (anti-H-2.33) serum was added to the killer-target cell mixture, the lysis of B10 cells was completely blocked, whereas the activity of the killer cells against B10.D2 cells was not affected. Cerrotini and Brunner (1974) demon-strated that alloantiserum directed against one H-2 haplotype of an F_1 hybrid can block killer cells directed against antigens controlled by this haplotype without affecting killing against the antigens controlled by the other haplotype of the H-2 heterozygous cells.

Evidence against participation of H-2 antigens in CML has recently been obtained by Edidin and Henney (1973), who observed that stripping cells of their H-2 antigens by capping did not significantly affect their capability to function as targets for cytotoxic lymphocytes. However, it is possible that not all the H-2 antigens on the cell surface combine with antibodies and that those that do not are nevertheless capable of serving as CML-targets.

The assumption that H-2 antigens are the targets in CML, of course, does not exclude the possibility that other classes of antigens may also, under certain circumstances, assume this function. Also, the role of H-2 antigens as

CML targets does not imply that sites of the H-2 molecules recognized by H-2 antibodies and by cytotoxic lymphocytes are the same. On the contrary, there is every reason to believe that they are not the same. Because effector cells are thymus-derived, they probably recognize the "carrier" portion of the H-2 molecule, whereas the bone marrow–derived precursors of antibody forming cells recognize the "haptenic" portion. *A priori*, therefore, there is no reason to expect a strict correlation between H-2 serology summarized by the H-2 chart, and the results of CML typing—and, in fact, there is no such correlation. Brondz (1964, 1968) was the first to observe that effector cells sensitized against one *H-2* haplotype do not react with target cells of another haplotype, despite the fact that the haplotypes may share several public H-2 antigens. This observation was later confirmed by others (Ax *et al.* 1971; Berke *et al.* 1969; Hodes and Svedmyr 1970; Blomgren and Andersson 1974; Forman and Möller 1974). However, one can argue that the failure to detect lymphocyte cross-reactivity is due mostly to the insensitivity of the standard CML technique. Indeed, it has recently been demonstrated that in more sensitive CML techniques, lymphocytes sensitized against one *H-2* haplotype do react weakly with unrelated haplotypes (Phillips *et al.* 1973; Nabholz *et al.* 1974; M. Nabholz, *personal communication*). However, the cellular cross-reactivity patterns do not correlate with serological cross-reactions (M. Nabholz, *personal communication*) suggesting that the antigenic sites recognized by the CML effector lymphocytes and the B cell-precursors of antibody forming cells are indeed different.

E. Nature of CML Receptors

The CML reaction requires a specific recognition of the target antigens by receptors on the responding cells. Although the nature of the hypothetical receptors is not known, it is assumed that the receptors are expressed in clones of cells, each clone being capable of recognizing a specific group of antigens.

The clonal expression of the CML receptors is supported by adsorption experiments. Typically, lymphocytes derived from strain A and sensitized against cells from strain B can be adsorbed on B cell but not on A cell monolayer. The nonadherent cells from the B cell monolayer no longer react with B target cells but display undiminished reactivity against cells derived from an unrelated strain (Brondz 1968b, 1972; Brondz and Goldberg 1970; Brondz and Snegiröva 1971; Goldstein *et al.* 1971a, b; Lonai *et al.* 1972; Wekerle *et al.* 1972; Berke and Levey 1972; Altman *et al.* 1973). The experiments are explained by assuming that the original lymphocyte culture was a mixture of cells, each cell carrying specific receptors for a certain group of antigens. Removal of cells carrying anti-B receptors left behind cells with anti-C, D, E, etc. receptors. Brondz and Snegiröva (1971) also demonstrated that receptors recognizing the *K* and *D* region antigens are present in two different cell populations, by showing that B10(H-2^b) lymphocytes sensitized against A(H-2^a) strain stimulating cells can be adsorbed on C3H (H-2^k) monolayer and still exert cytotoxic effect on B10.D2(H-2^d) target cells; conversely, the sensitized lymphocytes can be adsorbed on B10.D2 monolayer without a loss of lymphocytotoxicity toward C3H target cells. Interestingly, the original cell mixture seemed to contain three times more lymphocytes sensitized against the *K* region than lymphocytes sensitized against the *D* region.

The clonal expression of CML receptors is also supported by recent experiments of Kimura (1974) who immunized rabbits with C3H lymphocytes sensitized *in vivo* against BALB/c antigens, adsorbed the antiserum thus obtained with C3H cells sensitized against C57BL/6 antigens (to remove species, strain, effector or blast specific antibodies), and purportedly demonstrated that the antiserum can specifically block the *in vitro* cytotoxicity of C3H anti-BALB/c effector cells without inhibiting C3H anti-C57BL/6 effector cells. If confirmed, these experiments may represent an important step toward characterization of the CML receptors.

The relationship between the CML receptors and the MLR receptors is not known. Bach and his colleagues (1973a) as well as some other investigators believe that the two receptor types are different, or at least that they are expressed in two different cell lineages. However, if one accepts the hypothesis that MLR is merely an intermediary step in the CML, there is no need for two classes of receptors in the original responding cells; of course, the nature of the site on the effector cell interacting with the target antigens is then still an open question.

F. Relationship Between CML and *in Vivo* Allograft Reaction

As mentioned earlier, the CML is generally considered an *in vitro* analogue of the allograft reaction's destructive phase. Accordingly, one would expect that those regions of the *H-2* complex that are involved in graft rejection also would be active in CML. However, this is true only for the two peripheral regions (*K* and *D*) and not for the *I* region: although skin grafts transplanted across *I* region differences are rejected as rapidly as grafts exchanged across *K* or *D* region differences (see Chapter Eight), the *I* region antigens are at best extremely poor targets for CML. One way to explain this discrepancy is to postulate, as discussed earlier, that the absence of CML across the *I* region is an *in vitro* artifact. Alternatively, one can speculate that the mechanism of graft rejection across the *I* region is different from that across the peripheral regions. It is conceivable, for instance, that humoral antibodies play a far greater role in *I* region-associated rejections than in *K* or *D* region-associated rejections.

G. MLR and CML *in Vivo*

In both the MLC and CML, the tests are carried out *in vitro*, that is, in a test tube. However, the test tube can be substituted by a living organism (lethally irradiated mouse) and tests analogous to MLC and CML can be carried out *in vivo*. The *in vivo* MLR has been studied by J. Sprent and J. R. A. P. Miller and their colleagues (for a review see Sprent 1973).

When parental-strain thymocytes or thoracic duct lymphocytes are injected into heavily irradiated F_1 hybrid mice, the cells home largely to the spleen and lymph nodes and there proliferate extensively in response to the alloantigens of the host (Sprent and Miller 1972b). The proliferating cells transform into blasts that accumulate in large masses around the central arterioles of the spleen and in paracortical regions of the lymph nodes. After 3–4 days, the spleens become enlarged, the enlargement being proportional to the number of parental cells injected. Up to this stage, the test does not differ from the various tests for GVHR.

When tritiated thymidine (^{3}H-TdR) is injected intravenously every 8 hr into the F_1 recipients, autoradiographs prepared from the spleen and lymph nodes show that virtually all the blasts in these organs are heavily labeled. The incorporation of ^{3}H-TdR can be quantitated by removing spleens 30 min after the radioisotope pulse, and level of radioactivity measured in a scintillation spectrophotometer. Within certain cell dose ranges, ^{3}H-TdR incorporation is directly proportional to the number of parental lymphocytes injected.

After 4 days of proliferation, the progeny of the responding cells enter circulation and appear in large numbers in thoracic duct lymph. More than 95 percent of the thoracic duct lymphocytes collected at this time is of the donor thymus origin (Sprent and Miller 1972c). These thymus-derived thoracic duct lymphocytes (T.TDL) are highly immunocompetent in that they can mediate skin graft rejection when transferred into appropriate host, lysis of target cells *in vitro*, and rejection of tumor cells *in vivo* (Sprent and Miller 1972a). The immunocompetency is specific in that it is directed toward the antigens that provoked the formation of the T.TDL. The T.TDL is incapable of eliciting splenomegaly when transferred to newborn mice (Sprent and Miller 1972a). In an *in vitro* MLC, approximately 25 percent of T.TDL synthesize DNA when exposed to the host antigens, but not when exposed to other antigens. However, in contrast to a standard MLC, the DNA synthesis of T.TDL is not accompanied by cell division, suggesting that the proliferative potential of the cells had been exhausted. Sprent and Miller consider T.TDL "a virtually pure population of specifically reactive lymphocytes" representing the effector cells generated against the host antigen (Sprent 1973). Most of the cells are short-lived, with only very few remaining in the recirculating pool for more than a few days. They apparently die soon after mediating their function.

V. T-B Cell Interaction[6]

A. Claman's Experiment

Since 1961, when thymectomy was first used in the study of immune response, it has been clear that thymus, although not directly involved, is nevertheless required for antibody production against at least some antigens. The first clue as to what the function of the thymus in antibody production might be was

[6] For references and review, see Katz and Benacerraf 1972; Katz 1972.

provided by the now classic experiment of Claman and his co-workers (1966). The experiment was beautifully simple. The authors injected lethally irradiated mice with varying numbers of either spleen, thymus, and bone marrow, or thymus and bone marrow cells from syngeneic donors that had previously been immunized (primed) against sheep erythrocytes. After the cell transfer, the recipients were challenged with sheep erythrocytes and tested at different time intervals for the production of sheep erythrocyte hemolysins. The results clearly demonstrated that bone marrow or thymus cells alone gave only a negligible response; but bone marrow and thymus cells combined together in the same recipient gave a strong response that was linearly related to the number of transferred cells. Claman and his colleagues concluded from these results that bone marrow contains cells capable of producing antibodies, but that the production of the antibodies by these cells requires the presence of thymus-derived cells. These experiments were confirmed and expanded by A. Davies *et al.* (1967), J. Miller and Mitchell (1967), and later by many other laboratories. Subsequent analysis of the synergy between bone marrow and thymus revealed that antibody production required interaction between two functionally distinct but morphologically indistinguishable cells. One cell (T cell), derived from the thymus but also present in the pool of recirculating lymphocytes, can bind and be stimulated by the antigen, but is incapable of secreting antibodies; the other cell (B cell), derived from bone marrow, gives rise to antibody-secreting cells but only after it has reacted with the T cell. Soon it also became evident that the two cell types, although reacting with the same antigens, recognized different portions of the antigenic molecule. Evidence supporting this conclusion was obtained from studies of the so-called carrier effect.

B. Carrier Effect

The most convincing demonstration of the carrier effect was provided by Mitchison (1971a, b), using hapten 4-hydroxy-5-iodo-3-nitrophenacetyl (NIP) conjugated to either ovalbumin (OVA) or bovine serum albumin (BSA). He injected lethally irradiated mice with spleen cells from syngeneic donors that had been immunized with NIP-OVA and observed that the recipients made a secondary anti-NIP response when challenged with NIP-OVA but not when challenged with NIP-BSA. However, when spleen cells from donors immunized with NIP-OVA were injected together with spleen cells from donors immunized with BSA, perfectly normal secondary anti-NIP response was observed. In these experiments, the addition of cells specific for the BSA carrier apparently permits the NIP-primed cells to develop a secondary anti-NIP response. The BSA-specific cells were later identified as T cells and the NIP-specific cells as B cells. It was also definitely established that the interaction of the NIP-specific B cells with the BSA-specific T cells operated on the same principle as the T-B cell cooperation in the hemolysin response to sheep erythrocytes. Because the carrier-specific T cells help to develop secondary response by cooperating with the hapten-specific B cells, they are often referred to as "helper" cells.

C. Allogeneic Effect

While studying the characteristics of the carrier-specific T cells, Katz and his co-workers (1970) made a surprising discovery that led to a description of a new phenomenon, the so-called allogeneic effect. They immunized strain 13 guinea pigs with 2,4-dinitrophenyl (DNP) ovalbumin (OVA), then injected them with lymphoid cells derived from bovine gammaglobulin (BGG)-sensitized syngeneic donor guinea pigs and observed a good secondary anti-DNP response after challenging the recipient with DNP-BGG. As a negative control, the authors injected allogeneic lymphoid cells from BGG-sensitized strain 2 guinea pigs. They expected the allogeneic cells to be rejected by the strain 13 recipients and that no secondary response would occur. However, to their surprise, they observed that the recipients of the allogeneic cells not only did develop secondary anti-DNP response when challenged with DNP-BGG, but also the response was 20–50 times greater than the secondary response of the recipients injected with syngeneic cells. Subsequent studies demonstrated that the *allogeneic effect* reflects the development of a specific GVHR in the lymphoid organs of the host. The effect can be explained by postulating that the T cells recognize foreign histocompatibility antigens on the allogeneic B cells and activate the B cells.

D. Physiological T-B Cell Cooperation

Hence, there are at least two types of T-B cell cooperation. In the one type, the antigen binds, through its carrier portion, to the T cell and this T cell then interacts with the B cell, which bound the same antigen through its haptenic portion. This *physiological cooperation* between syngeneic T and B cells is specific in that both the T and B cells bind the same antigen. In the second type, the T cell interacts with the B cells through the B cells' histocompatibility antigens, and if the B cell also happens to have another antigen bound to it, plasma cells are produced which secrete antibodies against the bound antigen (allogeneic effect). The question then arises: can physiological cooperation also occur between allogeneic cells?

Attempts to answer this question were made by Kindred and Shreffler (1972) and by Katz *et al.* (1973a, b, c). The former two authors injected BALB/c-*nu/nu* mice with *H-2*-compatible or *H-2*-incompatible thymus cells and then immunized the recipients with either sheep erythrocytes or bacteriophage T4. They observed that the mice formed antibodies only when injected with *H-2*-compatible thymocytes: disparity in the *H-2* complex prevented an effective cooperation between the B cells of the nude recipients and the T cells of the thymocyte donor.

Katz and his co-workers (1973a) used a more sophisticated experimental system. They injected spleen cells from A strain mice immunized against BGG into normal unimmunized (A × BALB/c)F$_1$ hybrids; 24 hr later, when the injected cells reached their destination in the lymphoid organs, they lethally irradiated the recipients. The irradiation killed all the lymphocytes in the recipients except those T cells that were immune to BGG (the authors had shown previously that carrier-primed T cells are relatively radioresistant, cf. Hamaoka *et al.* 1973). Shortly after the irradiation, they injected the recipients with B cells from mice immunized against 2,4-dinitrophenyl (DNP)-keyhole limpet hemocyanine (KLH), and boosted the recipients with DNP-BGG (the B cells were obtained by treatment of a spleen cell suspension with anti-Thy-1 in the presence of complement). The recipients produced relatively high titers of anti-DNP antibodies, indicating that the BGG-specific T cells cooperated with the DNP-specific B cells (KLH functions as a carrier for the DNP hapten). The authors then repeated the experiment, using instead A-derived T cells and BALB/c-derived B cells (or vice versa). This time they failed to detect a significant level of anti-DNP antibodies in the serum, indicating that the carrier-primed T cells did not cooperate with the histoincompatible hapten-primed B cells. One may ask why the B cells were not activated nonspecifically through the allogeneic effect. The authors explained the absence of the allogeneic effect in this experiment as being due to the restricted number of carrier-primed T cells (all the other T cells were presumably killed by the radiation), and to the fact that the hapten-primed B cells in the F_1 recipient constituted but a small proportion of the cells against which the carrier-primed T cells could react (the parental T cells could react against the cells of the F_1 host).

Experiments with congenic lines provided evidence that physiological T-B cell cooperation requires compatibility in the *H-2* complex: cells identical at all loci except *H-2* (e.g., A and A.BY) failed to cooperate, whereas cells identical in *H-2* but different at multiple non-*H-2* loci (e.g., A and B10.A) cooperate normally (Katz *et al.* 1973b). Furthermore, no physiological cell cooperation is observed when the T and B cells share the *D* end and differ in the *K* end of the *H-2* complex (for example, in strain combination A and BALB/c), suggesting that the locus controlling the cooperation resides in the *K* end (Katz *et al.* 1973a).

In an attempt to determine whether the *I* region of the *H-2* complex is involved in the control of T-B cell cooperation, Katz *et al.* (1973c) performed an experiment in which they utilized the fact that strain A is a nonresponder and strains BALB/c and $(A \times BALB/c)F_1$ hybrid are responders to synthetic terpolymer L-glutamic acid-L-lysine-L-tyrosine (GLT) and that this responsiveness is controlled by the *I* region. They immunized the F_1 hybrids with GLT, transferred the immune cells into a normal F_1 hybrid, and irradiated the recipient. Then they injected the recipient with DNP-KLH-primed B cells from either the responder (BALB/c) or nonresponder (A) strains and observed that after challenge with DNP-GLT, antibody response was obtained only with the responder and not with the nonresponder B cells. This result leads to two main conclusions. First, because the two parental strains differ with respect to GLT in the *I* region (controlling the responsiveness to this antigen), the responsiveness of the BALB/c-derived B cells and nonresponsiveness of A-derived B cells indicate that the *I* region is involved in the genetic control of T-B cell cooperation. Second, because the carrier-specific T cells in this experiment are derived from the responding strain (F_1 hybrid), the responsiveness of the BALB/c-derived B cells and nonresponsiveness of the A-derived B cells suggests that the *I* region genes are expressed on B cells (the responsiveness or nonresponsiveness in this system is determined by the GLT genotype of B, not of T cells).

Katz and his co-workers (1973b) postulate that *I* region loci code for acceptor molecules on the cell surface of B cells and some similar product in T cells (the T cell and B cell products are either controlled by the same loci or by different, but closely linked loci). The B cell binds the antigen and attracts, perhaps through the antigen, T cells. Upon contact with the antigen, the cells begin to secrete their *I*-controlled products, which bind to the acceptor molecule carried by the B cell and thus trigger in the B cell biochemical events that eventually lead to antibody synthesis (alternatively, the T cell product may be a cell surface component and the cooperation may be mediated through direct contact of T and B cell surfaces). In a histoincompatible situation, the T cell product is so different from the B cell acceptor that the B cell fails to bind it and so is not specifically stimulated. However, in this case, the T and B cells can be brought together into intimate contact by virtue of their histocompatibility differences, and can thus be activated nonspecifically (allogeneic effect). In this model, the question of how the T cell recognizes the antigen in the first place remains unanswered. Also, it is not clear whether the *I* region is the only one that matters in physiological T-B cell cooperation or whether the peripheral regions—particularly the *K* region—are also involved in some way.

The results of Katz and his co-workers on physiological cooperation are in sharp contrast to the data obtained using tetraparental mice (see Chapter Seventeen). In the tetraparental mice, *H-2* disparate lymphoid cells interact to produce high titered specific immune response. The basis for the discrepancy is not known.

VI. The T Cell Receptor

The fact that T cells display a high degree of specificity in immunological functions attributed to them (cell-mediated immunity, helper activity) suggests that they have the capacity to recognize the antigens specifically. As in the case of B cells, antigen recognition by T cells is believed to be mediated via cell surface receptors. However, in sharp contrast to the B cell receptors, which are clearly identified and well characterized, the nature and properties of the hypothetical T cell receptors are among the most controversial questions in modern immunology.

A. Methods

Most of the controversy surrounding the T cell receptor stems from the fact that no suitable methods are available for its study. The methods that are currently being used were developed for the study of B cell receptors and include the rosette formation test, binding of radiolabeled antigen, and antigen-mediated suicide test.

1. Rosette Formation

The rosette-formation technique, in its typical form, consists of mixing lymphoid cells with erythrocytes, incubating the mixture for 5 min at 40°C, followed by light centrifugation and inspection of the mixture under a light miscroscope. The lymphocytes bind the antigen on the surface of the red cells via their receptors and produce a *rosette*—a cluster consisting of one lymphocyte and several erythrocytes adhering to it. This *immunocytoadherence* is observed with both native erythrocytes (usually of chicken origin) and with erythrocytes artificially coated with foreign antigens or haptens. The number of erythrocytes fixed to one lymphocyte may vary, but an arbitrary definition of a rosette-forming cell (RFC) is a cell with at least five erythrocytes bound to its surface. RFC's are found in peripheral blood, lymph nodes, spleen, and thymus. Their number is small in unimmunized animals, but increases after immunization. Most RFC's are B cells: thymus-derived RFCs have been reported by some investigators, but others have failed to find them. The general concensus at present is that T cells are able to form rosettes but that the clusters readily dissociate and are therefore very difficult to detect. The dissociation is either the result of extremely weak binding between the lymphocytes and the antigen or the shedding of T cell receptors.

2. Binding of Radiolabeled Antigens

In binding of radiolabeled antigen tests, the antigen (e.g., BSA) is radiolabeled (e.g., iodinated to high-specific activity with ^{125}I), mixed with a suspension of spleen cells, and incubated for 1 hr at 4°C. The cells are then washed and smeared on slides, and the slides are processed autoradiographically. The antigen-binding cells appear as labeled spots on the slide. When normal spleen is processed in this fashion, a large proportion of the cells remains unlabeled, about 2 percent of the cells are lightly labeled, and about one cell in 1000 is heavily labeled. The proportion of labeled cells increases after immunization. Most of the labeled cells are B lymphocytes, but labeling of T lymphocytes has also been reported.

3. Antigen-Induced Suicide

In the antigen-induced suicide test, a suspension of spleen cells from normal unimmunized mice is mixed with ^{125}I-labeled antigen, and the mixture is incubated for 30 min. After the removal of the unbound antigen, the cells are incubated for an additional 24 hr at 4°C, and then transferred to lethally irradiated syngeneic recipients. One day later, the recipient is immunized with unlabeled antigen and the level of antibodies formed is determined 8 days after the immunization. If specific antigen-binding has occurred *in vitro*, the recipients fail to respond immunologically to the same antigen (although they respond normally to other antigens). The failure is explained as being the result of the elimination of lymphocyte clones capable of binding the particular antigen.

During its disintegration, the isotope carried by the antigen emits electrons of relatively low energy, and consequently, the cells to which the antigen is bound receive a high dose of irradiation and are inactivated (*antigen-mediated suicide*). Cells not carrying antigen remain largely intact.

B. Nature of the T Cell Receptor

The nature of the T cell receptor has been studied through two main approaches: chemical isolation and blocking of the receptor's function. However, neither of the two approaches provides any conclusive results.

The biochemical approach has been directed primarily toward answering the question of whether the T cell receptor, like the B cell receptor, is an immunoglobulin. Because the methods of immunoglobulin immunochemistry are well defined, one would expect that the results of the test would be unambiguous. And they are—except that they do not answer the question. Although in science there is no dearth of controversy, it can usually be blamed on differences in techniques and materials. With regard to the question of T cell-bound immunoglobulins, two laboratories used the same technique and the same material and yet arrived at diametrically opposite results: Marchalonis and his colleagues (1972) obtained clear evidence for the presence of large amounts of immunoglobulin in T cells; Vitetta and her colleagues (1972a) obtained clear evidence that no immunoglobulin was present on the surfaces of T cells. What is more, other laboratories, trying to resolve the controversy, increased it by neatly dividing between the two sides, confirming either Marchalonis's or Vitetta's results. There appears to be no room for compromise—one side must simply be wrong.

The results of the blocking studies are just as confusing. Typically, T cells are incubated with an antiserum directed against a certain specific antigen, and then are tested to determine whether the antibodies in the serum block T cell functions (antigen binding, helper activity, or cellular immunity). In a large number of studies performed to date, various laboratories have been able to block almost everything with almost anything, while other laboratories have been unable to confirm the results.

The message from this confusing situation appears to be that perhaps the methods currently employed are not suitable for the study of T cell receptors and that new techniques will have to be developed before a sensible attack on the receptor problem can be mounted.

Much has been speculated recently as to the nature of the T cell receptor. Although such speculations may be pleasurable, there seems to be little justification for them. First, the data are so scarce that there is not much on which to base the speculation, and second, the receptor problem will be resolved experimentally in a few years anyway. As of this writing, the available knowledge can be summarized in a simple statement: the T cell receptor does not appear to belong to any known immunoglobulin class (but could perhaps represent a new, thus far unrecognized immunoglobulin class), and the possibility exists that the receptor might be controlled by the *H-2* complex. According to Benacerraf and McDevitt (1972), the T cell receptor could be a new class of recognition molecule, controlled by *Ir-1* loci in the *I* region of the *H-2* complex. This hypothesis is based on the finding that the *Ir-1* loci appear to control the recognition of the carrier portion of an antigen via T cells. This is certainly an appealing speculation, but at present it is nothing more than one of several possibilities.

Section Six

S and *X* Region-Associated Traits

Chapter Nineteen

The *S* Region and Miscellaneous *H-2*-Associated Loci

I. The *S* Region

A. The *Ss* Locus

1. Genetics

The Ss substance was discovered by Shreffler and Owen (1963) during a search for serum protein variants in the mouse. The authors immunized several rabbits with globulin fraction obtained by ammonium sulfate precipitation of normal serum from Swiss mice and tested the antisera produced by Ouchterlony immunodiffusion in agar. The rabbits produced several antibodies that reacted with normal sera of the Swiss stock as well as with sera of inbred strains CBA and DBA/2. The number of precipitin bands formed with the three types of sera was the same, and the bands showed a reaction of identity (no spurring) when sera from different strains were placed in adjacent wells, indicating that all the detected antigens were present in all three strains and that there were no qualitative differences among the individual antigens. Moreover, with one exception, the position of corresponding bands obtained with the three sera was also the same, suggesting the absence of quantitative differences as well. The one exception was a precipitin band that, with the DBA/2 and Swiss sera, formed midway between the center (antiserum) and the peripheral (antigen) wells; with CBA sera it developed only as a faint line close to the peripheral well. The strong DBA/2 and weak CBA bands were continuous with each other when the two normal sera were placed in adjacent wells, the only difference between the two being their position and strength. Shreffler and Owen concluded from these results that the rabbit antibody responsible for the band was reacting with the same antigen in all three strains, but that the concentration of the antigen was higher in the Swiss and DBA/2 mice than in the CBA strain. Normal serum from (DBA/2 × CBA)F$_1$ hybrids formed a band intermediate in position and strength between the bands formed by DBA/2 and CBA sera and indistinguishable from a band formed by a mixture of equal quantities of DBA/2 and CBA sera. Absorption of the rabbit antiserum with normal serum removed all antibodies except the one detecting the quantitative difference of the antigen (Fig. 19-1a); absorption with DBA/2 normal serum removed all antibody activity. Analysis of segregating F$_2$ and backcross generations demonstrated that the quantitative difference in the level of the one component of the DBA/2 and CBA normal sera was under the genetic control of a single, autosomal, dominant gene. The component was designated *s*erologically detectable *s*erum variant, or serum substance Ss; the two alleles at the *Ss* locus were assigned symbols *Ss^h* and *Ss^l*, and the three phenotypes determined by these alleles were designated Ss-H (Ss-high; determined by the *Ss^h/Ss^h* homozygotes), Ss-L (Ss-low; determined by *Ss^l/Ss^l* homozygotes), and Ss-HL (Ss-intermediate; determined by *Ss^h/Ss^l* heterozygotes).

Testing of other inbred strains revealed that they too could be classified as either Ss-H or Ss-L and, in addition, that all the Ss-L strains carried the *H-2^k* haplotype or haplotypes derived from *H-2^k* by intra-*H-2* recombination. This peculiar distribution of the *Ss^l* allele among the inbred strains suggested a genetic linkage between the *Ss* locus and the *H-2* complex. The linkage was later proved by linkage tests involving several different strain combinations (Shreffler 1964, 1965). Screening of over 1000 segregants revealed that the linkage of *Ss* and *H-2* was extremely close, the only *Ss-H-2* recombinants being those in which the crossing-over took place within the *H-2* complex. This result suggested that the *Ss* locus was located within the *H-2* complex. Analysis of other available intra-*H-2* recombinants (Shreffler 1970, 1971; Shreffler and David 1972) fully confirmed this suggestion: of the ten *H-2* recombinants tested, five placed the *Ss* locus to the right of *H-2K* and the remaining five placed

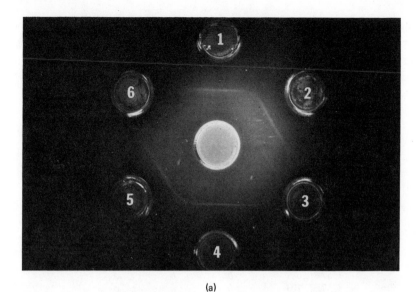

(a)

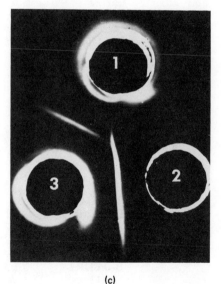

(b)   (c)

Fig. 19-1. Immunodiffusion patterns of anti-Ss and anti-Slp sera. (a) Rabbit anti-Ss serum is in the central well, DBA/2 normal serum in wells 1, 2, 4, and 5, C3H/He normal serum in wells 3 and 6. (Courtesy of Dr. D. C. Shreffler.) (b) Mouse anti-Slp serum is in the central well, peripheral wells contain normal sera from the following strains: well 1, A/J ♂; well 2, A/J ♀; well 3, C57BL/6 ♂; well 4, C57BL/6 ♀; well 5, DBA/2 ♀; well 6, DBA/2 ♂. (c) Mouse anti-Slp is in well 1, rabbit anti-Ss in well 2, and DBA/2 ♂ normal serum in well 3. [(b) and (c) reproduced with permission from H. C. Passmore and D. C. Shreffler: "A sex-limited serum protein variant in the mouse: Inheritance and association with the H-2 region." *Biochemical Genetics* 4:351–365. Copyright © 1970 by Plenum Press. All rights reserved.]

Table 19-1. Distribution of *Ss* and *Slp* alleles among inbred strains and congenic lines*

Strain	H-2	Ss	Slp
A/HeJ	a	h	a
A/J	a	h	a
A/Sn	a	h	a
B10.A	a	h	a
A.TFR1	an1	l	o
B10.M(11R)	ap1	h	o
A.TFR2	ap2	h	a
A.TFR3	ap3	h	a
A.TFR4	ap4	h	a
A.TFR5	ap5	l	o
B10.M(17R)	aq1	h	a
A.AL	al	l	o
A.BY	b	h	o
C3H.B10	b	h	o
C57BL/6	b	h	o
C57BL/10J	b	h	o
C57BL/10Sn	b	h	o
C57L/J	b	h	o
LP/J	b	h	·
129/J	bc	h	o
B6.M505	bd	h	o
D1.C	d	h	a
BALB/cJ	d	h	a
B10.D2	d	h	a
C3H.D	d	h	a
DBA/2J	d	h	a
YBR/H	d	h	a
SEC/J	d?	h	·
B10.D2(M504)	da	h	a
A.CA	f	h	o
B10.M	f	h	o
HTG	g	h	a
B10.HTG	g	h	a
B10.D2(R101)	g1	h	a
D2.GD	g2	h	a
B10.D2(R103)	g3	h	a
B10.BDR1	g4	h	a
B10.BDR2	g5	h	a
HTH	h	h	a
B10.A(1R)	h1	h	a
B10.A(2R)	h2	h	a
B10.AM	h3	l	o
B10.A(4R)	h4	h	o
B10.A(15R)	h15	h	o
HTI	i	h	o
B10.D2(R106)	ia1	h	o
B10.A(3R)	i3	h	a
B10.A(5R)	i5	h	a
B10.D2(R107)	i7	h	o

Table 19-1. (*Continued*)

Strain	*H-2*	*Ss*	*Slp*
JK/St	*j*	*h*	*a*
I/Ao	*j*	*h*	*a*
WB/Re	*ja*	*h*	*o*
B10.WB(69NS)	*ja*	*h*	*o*
AKR/J	*k*	*l*	*o*
B10.BR	*k*	*l*	*o*
B10.K	*k*	*l*	*o*
CBA/J	*k*	*l*	*o*
CE	*k*	*l*	·
CHI	*k*	*l*	·
C3H/J	*k*	*l*	*o*
C3H/St	*k*	*l*	·
C57BR/J	*k*	*l*	*o*
C58/J	*k*	*l*	*o*
C58/Wa	*k*	*l*	·
MA/J	*k*	*l*	*o*
RF/J	*k*	*l*	*o*
ST/bJ	*k*	*l*	·
C3H/FgLw	*k*?	*l*	·
CBA/Ca	*k*?	*l*	·
L/St	*k*?	*l*	·
FL/2	*k*	*l*	*o*
AKR.M	*m*	*l*	*o*
B10.AKM	*m*	*l*	*o*
F/St	*n*	*h*	*a*
C3H.OL	*o1*	*l*	*o*
C3H.OH	*o2*	*h*	*a*
BDP/J	*p*	*h*	*a*
B10.P	*p*	*h*	*a*
P/J	*p*	*h*	*a*
B10.Y	*pa*	*h*	?
C3H.Q	*q*	*h*	*o*
CBA/1J	*q*	*h*	*o*
B10.G	*q*	*h*	*o*
T138	*q*	*h*	*o*
STOLI/Lw	*q*	*h*	·
SWR/J	*q*	*h*	*o*
DA	*qp1*	*h*	*o*
C3H.R3	*r*	*h*	*o*
B10.RIII(71NS)	*r*	*h*	·
LP.RIII	*r*	*h*	·
A.SW	*s*	*h*	*a*
SJL/J	*s*	*h*	*a*
A.QSR1	*sq1*	*h*	*o*
B10.QSR2	*sq2*	*h*	*o*
A.TL	*t1*	*l*	*o*
B10.S(7R)	*t2*	*h*	*a*
A.TH	*t2*	*h*	*a*
B10.HTT	*t3*	*l*	*o*

Table 19-1. (*Continued*)

Strain	H-2	Ss	Slp
PL/J	u	h	a
SM/J	v	h	o
AQR	y1	h	a
B10.T(6R)	y2	h	o
DE/J	?	h	·
N/St	?	h	·
PBR/St	?	h	·
SEA/GnJ	?	h	·
WC/Re	?	h	·

* Based on Shreffler and Passmore 1971, and J. Klein, *unpublished data.*

it to the left of the *H-2D* locus. Several of these recombinants were obtained from crosses involving markers outside the *H-2* complex and were proved to be products of a single crossover event. Hence, the position of the *Ss* locus within the *H-2* complex is firmly established (see also Chapter Ten).

2. Strain Distribution

Over 100 strains, substrains, and CR lines have been tested for the Ss trait (Table 19-1), and all were shown to carry either the Ss^h or Ss^l allele; no other alleles have been discovered. In the inbred strains, the Ss^l allele is restricted to only the $H-2^k$ haplotype and its genetic derivatives; in wild mice from the Ann Arbor area, the Ss^l allele is found with a frequency of approximately one in 500 (J. Klein, *unpublished data*). In addition, the Ss^l allele was also found in one of the T/t balanced lethal stocks derived from wild mice (T/t^{w8}) (J. Petrů and J. Klein, *unpublished data*). The Ss^l allele found in wild and in the T/t^{w8} mice is associated with *H-2* haplotypes different from $H-2^k$. The Ss^h allele of different inbred strains may not be the same, because some inter-, as well as intrastrain variation in the quantity of Ss protein has been reported (Shreffler and Owen 1963; Hansen *et al.* 1974). For instance, the concentration of the Ss protein in males of Ss-H strains DBA/2, A, and C57BL/10 is about 24 times higher than that in Ss-L strains CBA or C3H, whereas males of Ss-H strains C57BL/6 and STOLI have only about 12 times as much Ss protein as Ss-L animals. Males of the Ss-H and Ss-L strains usually have higher concentrations of the Ss protein than do females. No significant change in the Ss level can be detected in females during pregnancy, but during disease or after X-irradiation, the level increases as much as twice (Shreffler 1962). The concentration of Ss protein in newborn males is only about 60 percent of that in adult males; in females the Ss concentration stays at a low level, in males it increases gradually, until it reaches the adult male level at approximately 6 weeks after birth. Castration of the newborn males keeps the Ss concentration at the level present in normal females. Females treated with testosterone develop the same level of Ss as normal males (Fig. 19-2; cf.

Shreffler and Passmore 1971). Thus, the secretion of the Ss protein seems to be, to a certain degree, under hormonal control.

The difference between the Ss-H and Ss-L phenotypes is strictly quantitative (Shreffler and Owen 1963). There is no indication of more than one band in Ss-HL sera or of a spur at the junction of precipitin bands produced by Ss-H and Ss-L antigens. Moreover, when an Ss-H serum is diluted to an appropriate degree, it forms a band of the same appearance and at the same position as the undiluted Ss-L serum. Finally, anti-Ss-L activity can be absorbed out by Ss-H antigen and vice versa. However, it usually is not possible to obtain anti-Ss serum by immunizing rabbits with Ss-L material; apparently, the concentration of Ss protein in Ss-L strains is so low that it fails to stimulate a detectable antibody response in rabbits.

3. Tissue Distribution

Examination of frozen tissue sections incubated first with rabbit anti-Ss serum and then with fluorescein conjugated goat antirabbit IgG serum reveals

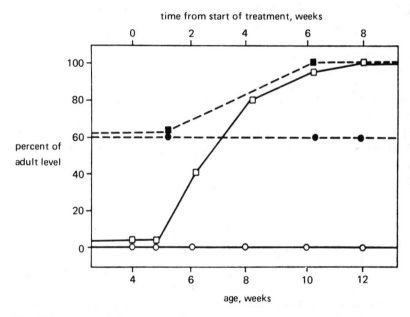

Fig. 19-2. Age and hormonal effects on Ss and Slp antigen levels in DBA/2 ($Ss^h/Ss^hSlp^a/Slp^a$) mice. ○ ——— ○ Slp levels in males castrated before 4 weeks of age and untreated females. ● — — — ● Ss levels in the same group (also applies to Slp^o/Slp^o animals). □ ——— □ Slp levels in normal males, castrated males given testosterone, and females given testosterone (bottom scale for females started at 1 or 3 weeks, top scale for females treated at 12 weeks). ■ — — — ■ Ss levels in the same group; also applies to Slp^o/Slp^o animals. (Reproduced with permission from D. C. Shreffler and H. C. Passmore: "Genetics of the H-2 associated Ss-Slp trait." In *Immunogenetics of the H-2 System.* A. Lengerová and M. Vojtíšková (eds.), pp. 58–68. Copyright © 1971 by S. Karger, Basel. All rights reserved.)

specific staining in the parenchymal cells of the liver (Saunders and Edidin 1974). However, the staining is always observed in the cytoplasm and never in the cell membrane. Adherent cells (macrophages) obtained from peritoneum, bone marrow, and peripheral blood also stain specifically for Ss in the cytoplasm. Cultured fibroblasts, on the other hand, stain almost exclusively in the cell membrane. Absorption of the anti-Ss serum by fibroblasts to a point at which it no longer stains the fibroblasts' membranes, reduces but does not eliminate the serum's staining of macrophage' cytoplasm. Immunodiffusion analysis of the absorbed serum shows spurring with the precipitine line formed by the un-absorbed anti-Ss serum reacting with normal mouse serum (Ss-H), suggesting "that the Ss-like material on the surface of . . . fibroblasts exposes some, but not all of the antigenic determinants of serum Ss" (Saunders and Edidin 1974). No Ss can be detected either in the cytoplasm or cell membrane of lymphocytes.

4. Physicochemical Properties

Relatively little is known about the physicochemical properties of the serum substance (Shreffler and Passmore 1971). The substance appears to be a protein with a molecular weight ranging from approximately 150,000 to 1,200,000 daltons. It can be dissociated into subunits, each having a molecular weight of approximately 75,000 daltons, by dialysis against 1 M NaCl or by treatment with 1 M 2-mercaptoethanol. The dissociated and undissociated antigens give a single continuous precipitin band when tested against anti-Ss serum by immunodiffusion. There is no indication of spurring or splitting of the band, indicating that the dissociated subunits represent relatively homogeneous material. The Ss antigen retains its activity at a high salt concentration (5.5 M KI), at a wide range of pH (3.2–11.0), and during heating up to 70°C for 20 min.

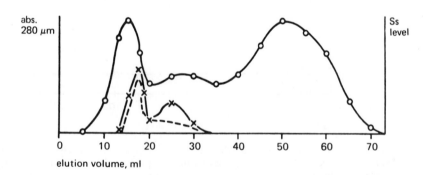

Fig. 19-3. Sephadex G-200 gel filtration pattern of Ss protein from Slp-a and Slp-o sera. ○ ────── ○ total protein (abs. at 280 μm); × ────── × Ss protein in Slp-a serum. ── ── ── Ss protein in Slp-o serum. Slp activity is detected only in the second peak of Slp-a sera. (Reproduced with permission from D. C. Shreffler and H. C. Passmore: "Genetics of the H-2 associated Ss-Slp trait." In *Immunogenetics of the H-2 System,* A. Lengerová and M. Vojtíšková (eds.), pp. 58–68. Copyright © 1971 by S. Karger, Basel. All rights reserved.)

When tested by immunoelectrophoresis, the Ss protein forms a band in the α_2-β globulin region. Upon gel filtration in Sephadex G-200 columns, Ss activity is found in two peaks, one large, the other considerably smaller (Fig. 19-3). So far, only partial purification of the Ss protein has been achieved with a combination of gel filtration, DEAE-Sephadex chromatography, and immuno-adsorption.

5. Biosynthesis

Peritoneal macrophages and liver parenchymal cells cultured for 10 days in a medium containing testosterone propionate and ^{14}C-labeled leucine produce radioactive material that can be specifically precipitated by anti-Ss serum (Saunders and Edidin 1974). At least one cultured liver cell line (ML-311) was found to produce Ss in quantities sufficient to be detected by immunodiffusion analysis of unlabeled medium.

6. Function

The Ss function is not known either. Although the *Ss* locus maps within the *H-2* complex, there is ample evidence that it is not coding for H-2 antigens or precursors of H-2 antigens. First, anti-Ss sera do not react with erythrocytes carrying different *H-2* haplotypes (Shreffler and Owen 1963). Second, erythrocytes or homogenates of spleen or liver do not absorb anti-Ss sera (Shreffler and Owen 1963). Third, there is no correlation between the distribution of the Ss trait among inbred strains with any H-2 antigens (Shreffler 1965). Fourth, congenic lines differing only at the *Ss* locus (e.g., C3H.OH and C3H.OL) permanently accept each other's skin grafts (J. Klein and Shreffler 1972a; D. C. Shreffler, *personal communication*). This is not to say, however, that the *Ss* locus is completely unrelated functionally to the *H-2* system. Relationship at a level other than that of biosynthesis of the products of the two systems has not yet been excluded.

7. Homologous Proteins in Other Species?

Only limited information concerning the existence of Ss-homologous proteins in other species is available. The rabbit anti-Ss serum reacts not only with different subspecies of *Mus musculus* (*M. poschiavinus*, *M. castaneus*, and *M. molossinus*), but also with different subspecies of the genus *Mus* (*M. cervicolor* and *M. caroli*; J. Klein 1971b, and *unpublished data*). The antigens of these species and subspecies show a reaction of complete identity with the antigen of *M. musculus*. Borovská *et al.* (1971) presented evidence that rabbit anti-Ss serum reacts with normal sera of different inbred strains of rats. The authors claim that the rat and mouse antigens show a reaction of complete identity, although the figure in their communication actually shows spurring of the corresponding precipitin bands. Similar spurring was also observed by C. S. David (*personal communication*). Borovská and her co-workers also observed that normal rat sera can absorb out antirat activity but not antimouse activity. Absorption of anti-Ss serum with normal sera from Ss-H (but not from Ss-L) mice removed the antirat and antimouse activity. The rat, therefore, appears to have a protein homologous to the mouse serum substance, but the rat and mouse antigens are probably slightly different. Borovská *et al.* (1971) observed no reactivity of rabbit anti-Ss serum with normal sera of cows, horses, pigs, guinea pigs, rabbits, and humans. An indication that even species unrelated to the mouse probably have an Ss homologue was obtained by C. S. David (*personal communication*). He used anti-Ss serum prepared by immunization of chickens with purified Ss fraction. The chicken antiserum reacted strongly with normal sera of rats and rabbits, and weakly with normal serum of rhesus monkey; it did not react with normal human sera. The rabbit, rat, and monkey antigens cross-reacted with the mouse Ss antigens. However, so far neither the rabbit nor the chicken anti-Ss sera can detect any genetic variants of the Ss homologues of the aforementioned species. Until such variation is found, the location of the homologous *Ss* loci in the genome of these species cannot be pinpointed.

B. The *Slp* Locus

1. Genetics

Because rabbit antiserum detected only quantitative variations of the Ss protein, the possibility existed that the *Ss* factor within the *H-2* complex was merely a regulatory locus, and that the structural locus for the Ss component was located elsewhere in the mouse genome. In an effort to rule out this possibility, Passmore and Shreffler (1970) attempted to find structural differences in the Ss protein by alloimmunization of different mouse strains with partially purified Ss preparations. The effort proved to be at least partially successful. Several alloantisera were obtained (i.e., RF/J ♂ anti-DBA/2J ♂, RF/J ♂ anti-A/J ♂, C3H ♂ anti-A/J ♂, and C3H ♀ anti-A/J ♂) that gave one well-defined precipitin band when tested by immunodiffusion against normal sera of the donor strain. All the antisera showed reaction of complete identity when compared with one another in adjacent wells (Fig. 19-1b). Apparently, all were directed against the same antigen, which was found to be present in some inbred strains and absent in others. However, in the positive strains, only normal sera of male mice reacted with the antisera; no reaction was observed with normal sera from females of any inbred strains tested. Several crosses made to determine the pattern of inheritance of the antigen showed it to be controlled by a single, dominant, autosomal locus; no indication of X or Y linkage was found. The females of the positive strains were shown to carry (but not express) the genetic information for the antigen. Because the protein appeared to be sex-limited, that is, its expression was confined to only one sex (males), it was denoted *sex-limited protein*, Slp. The two Slp phenotypes were designated Slp-a (the reactive or positive phenotype) and Slp-o (the nonreactive or negative phenotype); corresponding alleles at the *Slp* locus were designated *Slp^a* (coding for presence of the antigen) and *Slp^o* (coding for the absence of the antigen). Using linkage tests, the *Slp* locus was shown to be closely linked to the *H-2* complex (the only recombinants between *H-2* and *Slp* were those in which the crossing-over took place within the *H-2* complex) and by distribution pattern in inbred strains and congenic lines (strains with similar *H-2* haplotypes were shown to carry the same *Slp* allele). Analysis of intra-*H-2* recombinants placed the *Slp* locus within the *H-2* complex, at the same position as the *Ss* locus.

2. Strain Distribution

The strain distribution of the *Slp* alleles is shown in Table 19-1. All strains that carry the *Ss^l* allele are *Slp^o*; strains that carry the *Ss^h* allele are either *Slp^a* or *Slp^o*; combination *Ss^lSlp^a* has not been found. Although all the *Slp^a* strains give a precipitin band with the anti-Slp serum, it appears that at least some of them differ in quantitative levels of the Slp antigen, as indicated by the intensity and position of the band upon immunodiffusion. This quantitative variation appears to depend more on the genetic background than on the *Slp* locus itself. For instance, strains DBA/2 and B10.D2 carry the same *Slp^a* allele, yet the former gives a strong and the latter a weak reaction with anti-Slp serum. In inbred strains, the *Slp^a* allele is associated with *H-2* haplotypes *d, j, p, s,* and *u* and their genetic derivatives; the *Slp^o* allele is associated with *H-2* haplotypes *f, k, q, r,* and *v* and their derivatives. At least some of the *H-2* haplotypes carrying the *Slp^a* allele are probably of independent origin. Several hundred wild mice from the Ann Arbor area were tested, and all except one were found to carry the *Slp^o* allele (J. Klein 1970a, 1971a, 1972a, and *unpublished data*); the one exception will be discussed later. A few specimens of *Mus poschiavinus, M. castaneus, M. molossinus, M. cervicolor,* and *M. caroli* tested as *Slp^o* (J. Klein, *unpublished data*).

3. Genetic Control of Anti-Slp Response

Anti-Slp serum has been produced in several different strain combinations, all of which involve the immunization of animals from Slp-negative strains (both Ss-H and Ss-L) with an Ss preparation from a male of an Slp-positive strain. Extensive alloimmunization in other combinations has failed to produce antibodies against subtype antigens, antithetical antigens, or antigens defining other alleles (Passmore 1970). The immunization also demonstrated that females of *Slp^o* strains are capable of producing anti-Slp antibodies when immunized with *Slp^a* male serum. Similar immunization of *Slp^a* females produced no antibodies, indicating that the females are either tolerant to the Slp antigen or contain levels of Slp so low that they cannot be detected by presently available methods. The anti-Slp response appears to be controlled by an immune response gene located within the *H-2* complex (H. C. Passmore, *personal communication*; see Table 17-2).

4. Physicochemical Properties

The product of the *Slp* locus is a protein with a molecular weight of approximately 150,000 daltons and physicochemical characteristics similar to those of the Ss protein. Dialysis against 1 M NaCl or treatment with 1 M 2-mercapto-ethanol reduces the Slp molecules to subunits with the same molecular weight as the Ss subunits (75,000 daltons). On immunoelectrophoresis, the sex-limited protein, like the Ss protein, migrates to the α_2-β globulin region. Both antigens have the same pH stability (from 3.2 to 11.0) but differ in their heat stability (Slp is heat stable only to 52°C for 20 min) and salt stability (Slp is labile at 5.5 M KI). Upon gel filtration in Sephadex G-200, the Slp activity is found in a single peak that coincides generally with the second Ss peak (Fig. 19-3).

The Slp antigen has so far been found only in serum and ascitic fluid. It is absent in seminal fluid, testis homogenate, and urine. Its site of synthesis is not known.

5. Hormonal Control

The expression of the *Slp* locus is clearly under hormonal control (Fig. 19.2; cf. Passmore and Shreffler 1971). The Slp antigen is first detected in trace amounts in males at 5–6 weeks of age, a time that coincides approximately with the onset of sexual maturity. The concentration of the antigen then gradually increases until the adult level is reached at about 10 weeks of age. Males of the Slp-positive strains, if castrated at $3\frac{1}{2}$ weeks of age, fail to develop the antigen. Males castrated and then treated with testosterone propionate develop normal levels of Slp at a rate similar to that of untreated males. This rate cannot be accelerated by starting the hormone treatment at 1 week rather than $3\frac{1}{2}$ weeks: the Slp antigen never appears before 5 weeks of age. Young females of Slp-positive strains also develop normal male levels of Slp when treated with testosterone. Ovariectomy does not affect the appearance of the antigen. Males and females of Slp-negative strains fail to develop Slp even after testosterone treatment. Castration of mature males of Slp-positive strains leads to a sharp reduction in the level of the Slp in the 3 weeks following the operation and complete disappearance of the antigen by 200 days after the operation. Treatment of these males with testosterone can normalize the Slp level again. Testosterone treatment of mature females of Slp-positive strains also results in the development of normal male levels of Slp. Suspension of the treatment is followed by a decline in the antigen level. An increase in the testosterone dose does not seem to lead to an increase in either the rate of appearance or the final level of the Slp antigen. Incubation of Slp-negative serum with testosterone *in vitro*, or injection of *Slp^a* female serum into *Slp^o* males does not result in appearance of the Slp antigen. These results show that the presence of the Slp antigen is hormone dependent and that the hormone is required not only for the induction of Slp synthesis, but also for maintenance of the synthesis. However, it appears that the induction cannot take place until a differentiation step, independent of the hormone presence, has occurred during postnatal development. The male hormone does not seem to act directly on the Slp antigen, but rather on the locus that codes for the antigen.

One wild mouse in which the *Slp* locus seems to have escaped hormonal control has been found (J. Klein, *unpublished data*). The mouse, designated WOA 1, was a female captured at the WOA farm in the Ann Arbor vicinity. When tested with anti-Slp serum, it gave a strong positive reaction. This was not only the first female of any strain but also the first wild mouse to type as Slp-a; all other wild mice from the same farm, as well as mice from other farms, typed as Slp-o. Progeny tests with the WOA 1 female demonstrated that the trait was controlled by a single locus that was closely linked to *H-2* and apparently identical to the *Slp* locus. The genotype of the original WOA 1 female was demonstrated to be $Ss^hSs^hSlp^aSlp^o$. Reaction of complete identity was seen when WOA 1 and inbred Slp^a sera were placed in adjacent wells and tested against an anti-Slp reagent in the central well. Preliminary studies indicate that the Slp antigen in the WOA 1 strain is present at birth in males and females (T. H. Hansen, *personal communication*).

An attempt to correlate the presence or absence of the Slp antigen in different strains of mice with the level of testosterone and with testosterone-binding capacity of their plasma was made by Hampl *et al.* (1971). These authors observed that strains A and B10.A, which carry the Slp^a allele, have higher levels of endogenous testosterone than strains B10, B10.BR, and C3H, which are all Slp-negative (see Section IV of this chapter).

6. Function

The function of the Slp substance is an almost total mystery. An attractive possibility is that it represents one of the testosterone-binding proteins that have been shown to be present in the plasma of all mammalian species tested. Although testosterone is known to have an affinity for a number of different proteins in the plasma, a major portion of it is bound to a specific β-globulin that serves as its transportation vehicle. But there is no evidence so far that Slp can bind testosterone, or even that it has anything to do with this hormone. Although Hampl *et al.* (1971) claim that at least some of the Slp^o strains have lower testosterone-binding capacities than Slp^a strains, their own data do not support this claim. The data indicating hormonal control of the Slp antigen are clear-cut but they do not necessarily link Slp with testosterone. Both castration and testosterone treatment affect not only the level of testosterone itself but the levels of other hormones as well. The effect of testosterone on the Slp level could be only indirect, and direct interaction with Slp could be mediated by some other hormone.

7. Relationship Between Ss and Slp Loci

The Ss and Slp traits are similar in many respects. First, the *Ss* and *Slp* loci map in the same region of the *H-2* complex (the *S* region). Second, the *Ss* and *Slp* alleles have similar distribution patterns in inbred strains. Third, the Ss and

Slp products are both secreted into blood plasma, and they resemble each other in their physicochemical properties (Table 19-2). This close resemblance naturally raises the question of whether the Ss and Slp products are controlled by the same locus.

In mapping studies, several thousand segregants have been screened for intra-*H-2* recombination in different laboratories, but none of the crossovers obtained in these studies separated the *Ss* and *Slp* loci. This does not mean, however, that Ss and Slp are the products of a single locus. It is possible that the frequency of recombination between the *Ss* and *Slp* loci is far below the limits accessible through classical mating analysis.

The immunological relationship between Ss and Slp antigens (Passmore and Shreffler 1970) is illustrated in Fig. 19-1c, which shows an agar immuno-diffusion pattern in which normal serum from an *Slp^a* male is in one well, and the anti-Ss and anti-Slp in adjacent wells. A spur is visible at the juncture of the precipitin bands formed by the two antisera. The spur can be interpreted as indicating that some molecules in the normal serum contain both Ss and Slp sites, while others contain only Ss sites. Various manipulations with the antigen and antisera failed to reveal the additional band that would suggest that the two antigens are not identical.

The apparent cross-reactivity between Ss and Slp antigens has been confirmed by absorption studies (Passmore and Shreffler 1970), which demonstrated that mixing of *Slp^a* male serum with anti-Ss serum removes all Slp activity; mixing of the *Slp^a* male serum with anti-Slp substantially reduces, but probably does not completely remove Ss activity. (Because anti-Slp serum also contains the Ss antigen, it is not technically possible to decide whether the absorption of the Ss activity is complete in the latter case.) It appears, therefore, that anti-Ss serum can react with all the molecules carrying the Slp antigen, while anti-Slp serum can react with a substantial proportion but probably not all of the Ss molecules. The results obtained from attempts to purify the Ss and Slp products confirm this conclusion (Shreffler and Passmore 1971). As seen

Table 19-2. A comparison of properties of Ss and Slp antigens*

Property	Ss antigen	Slp antigen
Solubility	euglobulin	euglobulin
Electrophoretic mobility	α_2-β-globulin	α_2-β-globulin
Molecular weight	150,000–1,200,000	appr. 150,000
Subunit molecular weight	appr. 75,000	appr. 75,000
pH stability (in whole serum)	3.2–11.0	3.2–11.0
Heat stability (in whole serum)	70°C for 20 min	52°C for 20 min
Salt stability (5.5 M KI)	stable	labile

* Reproduced with permission from D. C. Shreffler and H. C. Passmore: "Genetics of the H-2 associated Ss-Slp Trait." *Immunogenetics of the H-2 system*, A. Lengerová and M. Vojtíšková (eds.), pp. 58–68. Copyright © 1971 by Karger, Basel. All rights reserved.

in Fig. 19-3, it is possible to separate partially the Ss and Slp antigens by Sephadex G-200 gel filtration. The Ss activity of *Slp^a* male serum is present in two peaks, whereas the Slp activity is found only in the second, lower-molecular-weight peak. Furthermore, in an immunodiffusion test, the first peak spurs over the second peak, indicating that the second is somewhat different antigenically from the first. However, when the eluate containing the material from the second peak is treated to destroy Slp activity, the spurring disappears and the first and second peaks show a reaction of complete identity. Gel filtration of *Slp^o* serum yields only the first Ss peak. These results indicate that all molecules that carry Slp sites also carry Ss sites, but not all Ss molecules carry Slp sites. In other words, *Slp^a* male serum seems to contain two types of Ss molecule, one type with and the other without Slp sites. This conclusion is in agreement with the hormonal studies (Passmore and Shreffler 1971), which demonstrated that Slp is completely under hormonal control while Ss is only partially so.

It can be speculated, therefore, that Ss and Slp are two separate loci coding for very similar products, and that the Slp locus is fully inducible by hormones and the Ss locus is partially so. However, other interpretations are also possible (cf. Shreffler and Passmore 1971).

II. Complement-Controlling Locus?

Complement (C′) is a system of at least 11 serum proteins which is activated by antigen-antibody reactions. The individual complement components (designated C1, C2, C3, etc.) act in concert with one another in a specific sequence. Complement is present in normal sera of all mammals that have been tested, but the quantitative representation of its individual components may vary considerably among species. It participates in most antigen-antibody reactions (except those involving IgA and IgE), but its effect is most pronounced in cytolytic and cytotoxic reactions. (The latter differ from the former in that the cell membranes are damaged by the action of complement, but the cells usually do not lyse.) It is relatively nonspecific in that complement from one species (e.g., rabbit) can be activated by antigen-antibody reactions in another species (e.g., mouse). Complement activity is destroyed by heating the serum at 56°C for 30 min.

Démant and his co-workers (Hinzová *et al.* 1972; Démant *et al.* 1973) determined the level of complement in normal sera of various inbred strains and *H-2* congenic lines. For this determination they obtained washed sheep erythrocytes, mixed them with rabbit antisheep hemolysins plus normal mouse serum, incubated the mixture for 60 min at 37°C and, after centrifugation, measured the degree of red blood cell lysis by determining either the amount of hemoglobin in the supernatant or the amount of radioactivity released from ^{51}Cr-labeled sheep erythrocytes. Theoretically, the normal mouse serum should be the only source of complement in the mixture, and so the degree of hemolysis should be proportional to the level of complement in the serum.

Examination of a large number of serum samples revealed small but significant interstrain variation in the activity of complement. Similar variation was also observed among congenic lines carrying the same genetic background but differing in the *H-2* complex, suggesting that complement activity could be influenced by loci residing in or linked to this complex. The association with the *H-2* complex was confirmed by segregation analysis. In addition, Démant and his co-workers observed that complement activity seemed to correlate with the genetic composition of the *S* region: the highest complement activity was associated with the $Ss^h Slp^a$ genotype, lower activity with the $Ss^h Slp^o$ genotype, and the lowest activity with the $Ss^l Slp^o$ genotype. Association with the *S* region was also suggested from typing of nine *H-2* recombinants. In each instance, complement activity of the recombinant strain resembled that of the strain from which the recombinant received its *S* region. Particularly informative was the pair of 2R and 4R strains, which differ only in the *IB* and *S* regions. The 2R strain is $Ss^h Slp^a$ and displays a high level of complement activity, whereas the 4R strain is $Ss^h Slp^o$ and has a low level of activity.

Démant and his co-workers (1973) also obtained some evidence directly implicating the Ss protein in complement activity by demonstrating that the addition of anti-Ss serum to normal mouse serum inhibits hemolytic activity of the latter. However, rigorous proof of this reaction's specificity has not been provided by the authors.

With the interstrain differences as minute as they are, one might feel more comfortable about the data if they were confirmed by another laboratory. If confirmed, the data would, for the first time, provide at least indirect evidence that the *S* region is functionally related to the rest of the *H-2* complex. The relationship between the Ss or Slp proteins and the various complement components is not clear. Although one can find a superficial resemblance in physicochemical properties of some C' components to the *S* region products, it may not be of any significance.

III. Complement Receptor Lymphocyte Locus

Many B lymphocytes bear a surface receptor for the activated complement component C3 and are capable of binding antigen-antibody-complement complexes through this receptor (*complement receptor lymphocytes*, CRL). Studies in inbred mice demonstrated that in some strains (e.g., AKR), CRL can be detected at the age of 1 week and represent a substantial fraction (27 percent) of splenic lymphocyte population at the age of 2 weeks (high CRL strains); in other strains (e.g., BALB/c, C57BL/6, and DBA/2), CRL occur in low frequency (7 percent) at 2 weeks of age (low CRL strains). Adult animals of both groups have the same frequency of CRL (25–30 percent). Analysis of CRL frequency at 2 weeks of age in the progeny of $(AKR \times DBA/2)F_1 \times DBA/2$ backcross suggests that the rate of CRL appearance is controlled by two independently segregating loci; presence of the "high" allele at either locus leads to an intermediate or high CRL frequency at two weeks of age (Gelfand *et al.* 1974). Analysis of congenic lines indicates that one of the two loci (the *CRL-1* locus) is closely linked to the *H-2* complex and most likely located in the chromosomal segment to the right of *Ss* and to the left of *Tla* loci. This latter conclusion is based on the observation that B10, B10.A(2R), B10.A(4R), B6-*Tla*^a and *B6-Tla*^b strains carry the "low" allele at the *CRL-1* locus, whereas strains B10.A, B10.A(5R), *A-Tla*^a and *A-Tla*^b carry the "high" allele (Gelfand *et al.* 1974).

The function of the complement receptors is not known but the two most likely possibilities are the following. First, the binding of antigen-antibody-complement complexes by the complement receptor serves as an antigen concentrating device that increases the likelihood of antigen interaction with the Ig receptors on B cells. Second, the binding of activated C3 could provide the hypothetical "second signal" believed to be necessary for B cell stimulation (the "first signal" being binding of an antigen to the Ig receptor).

IV. Locus Controlling Hormone Metabolism ?

Iványi and his colleagues studied the level of testosterone and testosterone-binding protein (Hampl *et al.* 1971; Iványi *et al.* 1972a, b, 1973), and the relative weight of hormone-influenced organs such as testes, the vesicular gland, thymus, and lymph nodes (Iványi *et al.* 1972b). Initially they concentrated on three strains, A, B10, and B10.A, and their hybrids, but more recently (Iványi *et al.* 1973; Gregorová and Iványi 1973), they extended the studies to other inbred strains and congenic lines as well. Their results are summarized in Table 19-3. The authors conclude that testosterone (and, more generally, androgen) metabolism in mice is controlled by a series of genes, with the major role played by a locus that they designated *Hormone metabolism-1* or *Hom-1*. They believe that the presumed *Hom-1* locus is linked to *H-2* and perhaps resides in the *K* end of the *H-2* complex. This conclusion is based on the observation that the level of testosterone and testosterone-binding protein in *H-2* recombinant strain 5R is close to that in B10, while the level in 2R is more similar to that in B10.A (Iványi and Micková 1971; Iványi *et al.* 1973; Gregorová and Iványi 1973). The *Hom-1* locus is believed to have two alleles: *Hom-1*^a, present in strain A and determining the high relative weight of testes, thymus, and lymph nodes, high relative weight of the vesicular gland, and low level of testosterone and testosterone-binding protein, and *Hom-1*^b, present in strain B10 and determining low relative weight of testes, thymus, and lymph nodes, high relative weight of vesicular gland, and low level of testosterone and testosterone-binding protein. This interpretation can be criticized, however, on several grounds. First, the segregation data show only very poor association, if any, with the *H-2* complex, while the strain distribution data are limited to only a few congenic lines. Second, as the authors admit, the traits are quantitative in nature, their genetic control is complex (multiple loci, influence of hybrid vigor, etc.), and they are strongly influenced by environmental factors. Third, when testosterone is in-

Table 19-3. Testosterone level, testosterone-binding capacity, and relative weights of hormone-influenced organs of inbred mice and their hybrids*

Strain	Level of		Relative weight of			
	Testosterone	TeBP**	Testis	Vesicular gland	Thymus	Lymph nodes
A	3.06 ± 0.31 (H)†	6.55 ± 0.29 (H)	0.67 ± 0.08 (H)	0.73 ± 0.13 (L)	1.18 ± 0.19 (L)	0.65 ± 0.25 (L)
B10.A	2.81 ± 0.19 (H)	6.70 ± 0.19 (H)	0.60 ± 0.09 (I)	0.87 ± 0.18 (L)	1.74 ± 0.35 (H)	1.28 ± 0.38 (H)
B10	2.10 ± 0.04 (L)	5.65 ± 0.29 (L)	0.53 ± 0.08 (L)	1.08 ± 0.16 (H)	1.29 ± 0.28 (L)	0.88 ± 0.30 (L)
(A × B10)F$_1$	2.22 ± 0.09 (L)	6.91 ± 0.49 (H)	0.75 ± 0.12 (H)	0.90 ± 0.14 (I)	1.14 ± 0.24 (L)	0.61 ± 0.16 (L)
F$_2$aa‡	2.93 ± 0.09 (H)	6.16 ± 0.22 (I)	0.69 ± 0.11 (H)	0.74 ± 0.16 (L)	1.26 ± 0.24 (L)	0.77 ± 0.33 (L)
F$_2$ab	2.51 ± 0.13 (I)	6.59 ± 0.16 (H)	0.66 ± 0.12 (H)	0.74 ± 0.16 (L)	1.10 ± 0.27 (L)	0.82 ± 0.26 (L)
F$_2$bb	2.06 ± 0.06 (L)	5.71 ± 0.34 (L)	0.65 ± 0.11 (H)	0.85 ± 0.23 (L)	1.10 ± 0.23 (L)	0.97 ± 0.38 (I)

* From Iványi et al., 1972a, b.
** Testosterone-binding protein.
† Mean value ± standard deviation (high, low, or intermediate).
‡ (A × B10)F$_2$ hybrid $H\text{-}2^a/H\text{-}2^a$, $H\text{-}2^a/H\text{-}2^b$ or $H\text{-}2^b/H\text{-}2^b$.

jected into males, the organ weight is influenced independently of the *H-2* haplotype (Gregorová and Iványi 1973). Fourth, even if the difference in androgen metabolism were controlled genetically by the *H-2* complex, there is still no need to postulate a separate locus for such control. The *I* region of the *H-2* complex is known to be involved in the genetic control of susceptibility to diseases, particularly viral diseases (see Chapters Seventeen and Eighteen), and the observed differences in organ weight and hormone levels may well be a secondary effect of such a control.

V. Loci Controlling the Outcome of Bone Marrow Transplantation

A. High-Dose Transplants

Irradiation of a mouse with a lethal dose of X-rays or gamma rays causes destruction of its bone marrow cells and death of the recipient, usually within 10 days of the exposure. However, if the irradiated animal is injected intravenously with as few as 10^5 syngeneic bone marrow cells, it often recovers from the ill effects of irradiation and becomes a *radiation chimera*, that is, an individual that has been successfully repopulated by cells transferred from another donor. If allogeneic bone marrow cells are used for the transfusion, the chimeras behave like those protected with syngeneic cells in the first 3–4 weeks after exposure, but signs of *secondary* or *allogeneic disease* begin to appear later. The animal may or may not recover from the secondary disease, depending on the strength of the histocompatibility differences between the host and the donor. The disease is characterized by lymphoid hypoplasia (amounting sometimes to complete aplasia), loss of weight, diarrhea, adoption of a hunched posture, and ruffling of the fur. It was originally believed to represent a secondary phase of radiation injury (hence the name), but later was proved to be primarily the result of GVHR, accompanied by lymphoid aplasia and secondary infections. Because all the immunocompetent cells of the host are destroyed by irradiation, the host cannot reject the graft, but the graft contains precursor cells that develop into immunocompetent cells and attack the recipient's tissue. Using congenic lines, Morgado *et al.* (1965) demonstrated that the secondary disease (as measured by mortality of the recipients) is strongest when the donor and recipient differ in the *H-2* complex, and is weak when differences occur at the minor *H-1* and *H-3* loci. In this respect, the genetics of the secondary disease appear to be governed by the same laws that apply to GVHR.

B. Low-Dose Transplants

The behavior of the allogeneic bone marrow transplants just described applies to situations in which the host has been injected with a relatively large dose of cells (more than 10×10^6). When the number of cells in the inoculum is reduced to about 1 million per mouse, a new set of laws governing the fate of the transplant becomes apparent. The laws appear to be different for semi-allogeneic (parent to F_1 hybrid) and allogeneic transplants.

1. Hybrid Resistance

a. Method.   The method for testing low dosages of bone marrow transplants (Cudkowicz and Stimpfling 1964a, b) consists of lethally irradiating adult recipients and injecting them 2 hr later with from 0.5 to 1×10^6 cells administered intravenously. Five days after irradiation, the recipients are injected with 5-fluoro-2'-deoxy-uridine (FUdR) and 1 hr later with 5-iodo-2'-deoxyuridine (IUdR) labeled with ^{125}I. The FUdR blocks the incorporation of thymidine into the DNA of DNA synthesizing cells, and thus assures the incorporation of the labeled IUdR. Seventeen hours after the injection of the isotope, at the time when most of the unincorporated isotope is excluded from circulation, the recipient is killed, its spleen is removed, and the radioactivity of the whole organ is counted. The results are expressed as the percentage of injected isotope retained in the spleen. The assay is based on the assumption that some transfused bone marrow cells migrate into the spleen, settle there, and begin to proliferate. The proliferating cells actively synthesize DNA, and this synthesis is measured by incorporation of the radioactive precursor. Cells that fail to proliferate do not incorporate the isotope. Irradiated mice that have not been inoculated with bone marrow cells or mice that have been inoculated with incompatible bone marrow cells show less than 0.1 percent incorporation; irradiated mice that have been inoculated with syngeneic bone marrow cells show between 0.3 and 1 percent incorporation.

An alternative method of measuring the outcome of low-dose bone marrow transplantation consists of counting grossly visible foci in the spleen. Owing to the low dose of injected cells, the initial settlement of the spleen by the donor cells is very sparse, each cell being separated from its neighbor by a wide area of "empty" space (the reticular scaffolding of the spleen). Therefore, when the cells divide and give rise to clones, they form distinct foci (nodules), which can be visualized after fixation in Bouin's fluid. Mice injected with compatible cells usually contain more than ten foci per spleen and sometimes so many foci that they cannot be counted; mice injected with incompatible cells usually have only one or two foci per spleen and often no foci at all.

b. Description of the Hybrid Resistance Phenomenon.   The initial study of low-dose bone marrow transplants was made in strains B10, C3H, and A and their F_1 hybrids (Cudkowicz and Stimpfling 1964a, b, 1965). Using the technique described above, Cudkowicz and Stimpfling (1964a) discovered that B10 bone marrow cells grew poorly in irradiated $(A \times B10)F_1$ or $(B10 \times C3H)F_1$ hybrids, as compared to their growth in syngeneic B10 or allogeneic A or C3H recipients. The hybrids were therefore designated resistant to grafted parental cells, to indicate that they were not capable of supporting optimal growth of these cells, and the phenomenon was designated *hybrid resistance*. Segregation analysis and tests involving various congenic lines revealed that the hybrid resistance trait was controlled by a single autosomal locus, which the authors designated *Hybrid histocompatibility-1* or *Hh-1*. Linkage studies indicated that the *Hh-1* locus was closely linked to *H-2*. The authors explained the hybrids' resistance by postulating that either the *Hh-1* locus coded for a recessive "parental antigen" (an antigen expressed in the *Hh-1* homozygous parent but not in the heterozygous F_1 hybrid), or that the two parental *Hh-1* alleles interacted in the F_1 hybrid in such a way as to produce a "hybrid antigen" (an antigen limited to the *Hh-1* heterozygote). The original study also indicated that the hybrid resistance phenomenon was restricted to certain strain combinations, because the C3H and A parental cells grew normally in the $(C3H \times B10)F_1$ and $(A \times B10)F_1$ hybrids, respectively.

c. Characteristics of the Hybrid Resistance Phenomenon. Subsequent studies, carried out primarily by Cudkowicz and his associates, revealed a number of interesting and often unorthodox characteristics of the hybrid resistance phenomenon. These are enumerated briefly below.

First, the grafted bone marrow cells are destroyed within a few days after infusion of the irradiated mice, and the destruction is caused by a reaction from the host (Cudkowicz and M. Bennett 1971a, b).

The conclusion that the failure of parental bone marrow grafts to grow in an irradiated F_1 hybrid recipient is due to host antigraft reaction is based on the following observations:

1. graft failure does not occur in infant mice until 3 weeks of age;
2. the failure can be prevented by several pretreatments of the prospective recipient (e.g., split-dose irradiation, cyclophosphamide, antilymphocyte serum, antibrain serum, antimacrophage agents);
3. hybrid resistance can be transferred adoptively to irradiated mice by F_1 bone marrow or spleen cells.

The conclusion that the transplanted cells are destroyed by the host within a few days is based on retransplantation experiments in which spleen cells of each primary recipient were transferred into a secondary recipient, syngeneic with the original bone marrow donor. The secondary recipients had previously been "immunized" against the second parental strain of the primary F_1 recipient. The results of this experiment indicated that only during the first few hours after transplantation could the parental cells be recovered from the secondary host, and that no cells could be recovered beyond 24–48 hr after transplantation.

Second, the host reaction is directed against products of homozygous *Hh-1* alleles (see below).

Third, rejection is accomplished without proliferation of host lymphoid cells. This conclusion is based on the observation that "rejection" of the parental cells could be detected as early as 9–48 hr after the lethal irradiation of the host, presumably when proliferation of the host's lymphoid cells has been arrested.

Fourth, the effector cells responsible for the "rejection" are derived from bone marrow (Cudkowicz 1965), have radiosensitive precursors (hybrid resistance is abrogated or weakened if the hybrids are exposed to a sublethal dose of irradiation before the lethal dose and the bone marrow transplants are administered, suggesting that the sublethal dose inhibits proliferation of effector cells' precursors; cf. Cudkowicz 1965), differentiate independently of thymus influences (resistance is not weakened by neonatal or adult thymectomy; cf. Cudkowicz and M. Bennet 1971a, b), and function after exposure to lethal irradiation.

Fifth, the rejection does not involve a sensitized state in the host, and the host is usually unable to mount a secondary response (Cudkowicz and Stimpfling 1964b; Cudkowicz 1968).

Sixth, the capability to reject bone marrow grafts develops only at 3 weeks after birth (Cudkowicz and M. Bennett 1971a, b).

Seventh, bone marrow rejection is prevented by administration to the prospective host of antimacrophage agents, such as silicate particles or carrageenens (Lotzová and Cudkowicz 1974), macrophage activators (Cudkowicz and M. Bennett 1971b; Lotzová and Cudkowicz 1972), or antilymphocyte agents such as antilymphocyte serum (Lotzová and Cudkowicz 1972), cyclophosphamide (Cudkowicz and M. Bennett 1971a, b; Lotzová and Cudkowicz 1972, 1973).

Eighth, although the rejection is directed against *Hh-1* products, it is influenced by genetic factors resembling *Ir* genes (strains with the same *H-2* haplotype but different backgrounds could be either susceptible or resistant, indicating the influence of background genes; cf. Cudkowicz 1971a, b).

d. Genetics. Lotzová and Cudkowicz (1973) believe that there are at least four distinct loci, all carried by chromosome 17, determining the resistance of irradiated F_1 hybrids to parental bone marrow grafts (Fig. 19-4).

The original *Hh-1* locus, which controls, for example, the resistance of $(B10 \times C3H)F_1$ hybrids to B10 bone marrow grafts, is located either in the *D* region of the *H-2* complex or in its vicinity. This conclusion is based on the observation that $(5R \times B10)F_1$ hybrids, but not $(2R \times B10)F_1$ hybrids are resistant to B10 bone marrow grafts (Cudkowicz and Stimpfling 1964c, 1965). According to Cudkowicz (1968), there are at least two alleles at the *Hh-1* locus:

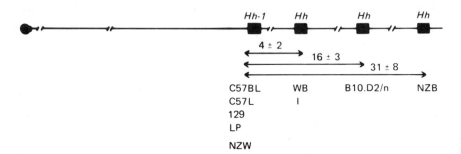

Fig. 19-4. Hypothetical loci controlling hybrid resistance. (Courtesy of Dr. G. Cudkowicz.)

Hh-1ᵃ, carried by strains C57BL/10, C57BL/6, C57L, LP, 129, A.BY, C3H.SW, D1.LP, HTH, HTG, and B10.A(2R), and *Hh-1ᵒ*, carried by strains C3H, A, AKR, BALB/c, C57BR, DBA/1, RFM, 101, A.SW, AKR.M, B10.A, B10.BR, B10.AKM, B10.M, C3H.K, HTI, and B10.A(5R). The *Hh-1ᵒ* allele is presumably silent, in that it does not express the *Hh-1* product. This conclusion is based on the observation that (C3H × B10)F₁ hybrids are susceptible to C3H bone marrow grafts. The genetic effect of the *Hh-1* locus is explained by the assumption that interallelic interaction in the *Hh-1ᵒ/Hh-1ᵃ* heterozygote leads to the suppression of the *Hh-1ᵃ* allele; consequently, no *Hh-1ᵃ* product is expressed in the heterozygote. Because no such interaction occurs in the *Hh-1ᵃ/Hh-1ᵃ* homozygote, the homozygote expresses the *Hh-1ᵃ* product, and this product is then recognized as foreign by the heterozygote.

The second *Hh* locus was postulated by Lotzová and Cudkowicz (1971) to explain the results obtained in studies involving strains NZB (*H-2ᵈ*) and NZW (*H-2ᶻ*). These two strains were selected because they were assumed to be unrelated to most other inbred strains and were therefore suitable for testing whether hybrid resistance was a widespread phenomenon or a specialty of the B10 family of strains. The authors were able to demonstrate that (NZW × NZB)F₁ hybrids were resistant to both NZB and NZW bone marrow transplants, and thus to prove that the capacity of hybrid resistance was shared by a wide variety of strains. They then proceeded to test the genetics of hybrid resistance in the NZW and NZB strains by producing backcross segregants and typing them for *H-2* and for resistance to parental grafts. They discovered that in the (NZW × NZB)F₁ × NZW backcross generation, approximately half the segregants were resistant and the other half were susceptible to NZW bone marrow grafts, and that in the majority of cases, the resistant animals were of the *H-2ᶻ/H-2ᵈ* genotype and the susceptible animals of the *H-2ᶻ/H-2ᶻ* genotype. There were some animals (2/80 = 2.5 percent) that appeared to be recombinants between *H-2* and *Hh* loci. However, because the number of segregants tested was relatively small, the authors could not determine whether the *Hh-NZW* locus was identical to or distinct from the *Hh-1* locus.

When the (NZW × NZB)F₁ × NZB backcross mice were inoculated with NZB bone marrow, they segregated in a ratio of three susceptible to one resistant, indicating that in this cross, two *Hh* loci were segregating (Lotzová and Cudkowicz 1973). Linkage tests involving *H-2* and *T* markers suggested that one of the two loci segregated independently of *H-2*, whereas the other was linked to *H-2* and was located in the noncentromeric end of chromosome 17, approximately 31 map units from *H-2D*. According to Lotzová and Cudkowicz (1973), the NZW and NZB strains share the same *Hh-1* alleles but differ at the *Hh-NZB* locus.

A third *H-2*-linked *Hh* locus was postulated by Lotzová and Cudkowicz (1972) to explain the results obtained by testing (B10.T × WB) × WB backcross animals. When inoculated with WB bone marrow, these animals segregated into susceptible and resistant individuals, with approximately 3.8 percent recombination between the hypothetical *Hh-WB* locus and the *H-2* complex.

A postulate of a fourth *H-2*-linked *Hh* locus is based on the observation that (B10.D2/n × B10.T) × B10.D2/n backcross mice show approximately 16 percent recombination between the *H-2* complex and resistance to B10.D2/n bone marrow grafts (E. Lotzová, *personal communication*).

A serious objection to the postulate of four distinct, *H-2*-linked *Hh* loci segregating in four different crosses is that none of the presumed recombinants was progeny tested. The recombinants thus could have represented phenotypic, rather than genotypic variations. Indeed, the possibility that the *H-2* complex itself is responsible for the hybrid resistance phenomenon cannot be ruled out. Furthermore, different recombination frequency values cannot be taken as evidence for distinctiveness of genetic loci. The results of the different crosses can be explained alternatively by postulating that there is only one *Hh* locus (*Hh-1*) and that the recombination frequency between *H-2* and *Hh-1* is influenced by genetic background.

2. Allogeneic Resistance

It was originally believed that the resistance to low-dose bone marrow transplants was limited to lethally irradiated hybrid recipients, but later it was discovered that at least some allogeneic donor-host combinations seemed to display a similar phenomenon. Subsequent detailed analysis revealed that allogeneic and hybrid resistance share the same characteristics: practically all the hybrid resistance properties described under Section 19.B.I.C. also apply to allogeneic resistance (Cudkowicz and Lotzová 1973). The only difference between the two phenomena appears to be in their genetics: hybrid resistance is a reaction of a heterozygote to homozygous cells, whereas allogeneic resistance is a reaction of a homozygote to homozygous cells. However, it is conceivable that even this difference is illusory, and that both reactions are elicited by products of the same loci. Recent data of M. Bennett (1972) might be interpreted as indicating that it is the homozygosity of the donor that is a prerequisite for the resistance to develop, and that the zygosity of the recipient is irrelevant. Bennett obtained (C57BL × DBA/2)F_1 × DBA/2 backcross animals, typed them for *H-2*, and then injected their bone marrow into lethally irradiated (C3H × C57BL)F_1 recipients. He found that the F_1 mice were susceptible to *H-2^b/H-2^d* grafts but resistant to *H-2^d/H-2^d* grafts. In other crosses he found no correlation between the presence of any particular H-2 antigen and the occurrence of the resistance phenomenon, so he interpreted the result as indicating that perhaps homozygosity at the *Hh* loci is all that matters for the induction of both hybrid and allogeneic resistance. However, he also found strain combinations in which it was the *H-2* heterozygous graft that was resisted and the *H-2* homozygous graft that was accepted by allogeneic F_1 hybrids. To explain this exception, Bennett introduced a complicated genetic interpretation that is difficult to validate.

In summary, there appears to be little doubt that the unorthodox behavior of low-dose bone marrow transplants is genuine and that it is determined by genetic laws different from those applicable to skin transplants, for instance. However, the nature of these laws remains a mystery.

C. F_1 Hybrid Effect

Snell (1958b) was the first to observe that B10 lymphomas grow better in syngeneic mice than in F_1 hybrids between B10 and allogeneic strains. His observation was later confirmed and extended to many other tumors and mouse strains by several investigators (for a review and references, see K. Hellström and I. Hellström 1967). The phenomenon of the F_1 *hybrid effect* can be observed only when low doses of tumor transplants are used (usually fewer than 10^5 cells/mouse). The poor growth in F_1 hybrids is manifested by a low tumor incidence and long latent periods (i.e., periods between inoculation of the tumor cells and the appearance of the tumor). The effect cannot be abrogated by prior irradiation of the F_1 hybrid host, nor is it influenced by "preimmunization" of the recipient with homozygous cells.

A host of other phenomena resembling the F_1 hybrid effect have also been reported. Gorer and Boyse (1959) demonstrated that B10 (but not A) spleen cells were eliminated by $(A \times B10)F_1$ hybrids within 2 weeks after transplantation. Cudkowicz (1961) observed a deficient growth of homozygous bone marrow cells transplanted into "preimmunized," lethally irradiated F_1 hybrids. Celada and Welshons (1962) observed a deficient growth of B10 spleen cells using an experimental system similar to that employed by Cudkowicz. K. Hellström and I. Hellström (1965) obtained evidence that the outgrowth of lymphoma cells in a syngeneic host was inhibited by preincubation of the tumor cells *in vitro* with F_1 hybrid lymphoid cells in the presence of PHA. K. Hellström *et al.* (1964) reported that homozygous tumor cells of A or B10 origin were killed in tissue culture when exposed to $(A \times B10)F_1$ hybrid lymphoid cells or homogenates prepared from the F_1 cells. And finally, G. Möller and E. Möller (1965) showed that monolayers of homozygous embryonic cells are killed by the addition of normal F_1 hybrid lymphocytes in a medium containing PHA.

Both the Hellströms and the Möllers interpret these phenomena as being caused by *allogeneic inhibition* (or *syngeneic preference*), that is, a nonimmunological interaction between H-2 antigens of a homozygous target and heterozygous lymphoid cells. Although the idea of allogeneic inhibition quickly became popular among immunologists, its principal postulate—the nonimmunological nature of the cytotoxic killing—is still unconfirmed. Furthermore, all the *in vitro* experiments require reexamination in light of the new facts concerning cell-mediated lymphocytotoxicity and the PHA effect on cultured cells.

Part Four

Conclusion

Chapter Twenty

Terra Incognita: Function and Evolution of the *H-2* Complex

I. Function

For years, the *H-2* complex has been viewed as merely a source of potent antigenic stimulation leading either to secretion of humoral antibodies by plasma cells or to various forms of lymphocyte-mediated (cellular) immunity. More recently, another dimension has been added to the H-2 studies by the speculation that the *H-2* complex may also code for molecules that specifically recognize antigens and serve as their receptor. According to this view, the *H-2* complex has two principal functions: one is to stimulate immunity and the other is to generate immunological specificity. Of these two functions, the stimulating function is clearly established, whereas the receptor function is so far purely hypothetical.

A. Stimulatory Function

The fact that the H-2 products (and by these we mean not only the classical H-2 antigens but also any other antigens with a clear cut stimulatory effect) stimulate immune reactions could mean one of two things. The antigenicity could be functionally irrelevant characteristics of the H-2 products and the true function of the products could be totally unrelated to any form of immunity. Alternatively, immune stimulation could be either the true H-2 function or could be somehow related to this function. Both views had been expressed in the history of the H-2 system and specific hypotheses had been advanced based on either the former or the latter alternative. Here, one example of the first and two examples of the second category of hypotheses will be given.

1. H-2 Molecules As Enzymes?

Probably the simplest way to interpret the *H-2* system is to assume that it consists of a series of loci coding for enzymes involved in some membrane-associated function. The antigenicity of the H-2 molecules would then be merely coincidental and primarily the result of the molecules' being located on the cell surface. However, the enzyme hypothesis of the *H-2* function is actually the least likely. Although association of H-2 activity with certain enzymes such as phosphatases (Basch and Stetson 1963) and triphosphatases (Sanderson and D. Davies 1963) has been reported, it could not be confirmed and was almost certainly due to contamination of the H-2 preparation. No enzymatic activity has been found in H-2 preparations produced by papain or NP-40 solubilization procedures. Furthermore, it is difficult to imagine that any enzymatic system would tolerate the degree of polymorphism known to be associated with at least the peripheral regions of the *H-2* complex.

2. Immune Surveillance Hypothesis

Because H-2 antigens are so strongly involved in tissue transplantation, one can speculate that the function of these antigens is to induce cellular immunity in histoincompatible situations. However, if such a postulate is correct, then one can ask: and what is the function of cellular immunity? The question was first raised by L. Thomas in a discussion following Medawar's presentation at a symposium, *Cellular and Humoral Aspects of the Hypersensitive States*. Thomas made the following observation:

> Dr. Medawar has shown us the operation of a precise, fastidious mechanism by which animals are enabled to destroy whole areas of living, vascularized tissue that they had previously incorporated into themselves. It is, moreover, a mechanism dependent upon an exquisite degree of immunologic specificity. For what purpose was such a mechanism designed? Not, certainly (or I cannot imagine it), as a means of defending one animal against surgically implanted homografts from another animal. Nature may have provided checks and balances for all conceivable kinds of untoward events, but I seriously doubt that she deliberately planned for this

one. It is an artificial situation, created by meddlesome human beings and, in itself, not a regular circumstance in biology.

On the other hand, it is equally doubtful that homograft rejection represents a meaningless phenomenon, or an artefact-response resulting from an artefact. I prefer to think that the events constitute a basic biological process, useful for something, and symbolizing something. What?...

... There are two possible functions that leap to the mind, both worth considering. One has to do with the universal requirement of multicellular organisms to preserve uniformity of cell type and to prevent mutant cells from colonizing and flourishing. This may be a real hazard, if we can judge from the readiness of bacterial cells to undergo mutation, or the weird cell forms of malignant appearance that develop and multiply, and outgrow and replace, normal epithelial cells in tissue cultures. Perhaps, in short, the phenomenon of homograft rejection will turn out to represent a primary mechanism for natural defense against neoplasia. The numerous analogies between this reaction and the immunologically induced destruction of experimental tumors (or their prolonged preservation after flooding an animal with tumor antigen) are consistent with this line of speculation (Thomas 1959, pp. 529–530).

The hypothesis that cellular immunity is the vehicle of immune surveillance was then expanded and made popular by Burnet; it became fashionable following the *Immune Surveillance* symposium organized by Smith and Landy (1970). Burnet's (1970a, b; 1973) version of the immune surveillance hypothesis can be described briefly as follows. Each individual possesses a specific array of histocompatibility antigens and a collection of lymphocytes carrying immunoglobulin receptors capable of binding the H antigens. The diversity of the H antigens determines the uniqueness of the individual and is responsible for the fact that no two outbred individuals are antigenically identical. The diversity of the Ig receptors enables the individual to recognize any invading cells carrying nonself-antigens. In other words, the antigenic uniqueness of a given individual ensures that invading cells from another individual of the same species are distinct from the host, are recognized as foreign by the Ig receptors, and are destroyed. According to Burnet (1973), "if there were no diversity of histocompatibility antigens and no corresponding arrays of immunoglobulin receptors to react with them, cancer of one animal would be contagious for others of its species, especially for the young."

The immune surveillance hypothesis can be criticized on several counts (cf. Smith and Landy 1970). First, it is too vague. Burnet (1973) states, for example, that "antigen diversity has evolved in relation to the immune system," but he explains neither how this evolution came about nor what the precise relationship between the histocompatibility antigens and the immunoglobulin receptors is. What is so special about an individual's having Ig receptors for H antigens? Since the individual is capable of producing antibodies against them, it *must* have the corresponding receptor. This does not prove, however, that there is a functional relationship between H antigens and receptors. Second, it is doubtful that histocompatibility antigens have anything to do with contagiousness of tumors (see Chapter Twelve). Third, animals in which the cellular immunity system is nonoperative (such as the congenitally athymic mice) do not display an increase in incidence of spontaneous (Rygaard and Povlsen 1974) or induced tumors (Stutman 1974).

3. H-2 Antigens As GOD?

A bold, intellectually pleasing, but unrealistic hypothesis of *H-2* function was formulated by Jerne (1971), who postulated that H-2 antigens act as *generators of diversity* (GOD) for immunoglobulin receptors on the surface of lymphocytes. According to Jerne, each mouse carries in its genome a series of genes coding for antibodies directed against H-2 and other histocompatibility antigens of the species *Mus musculus*. In each individual mouse, the genes can be divided into two groups: genes coding for antibodies against antigens present in a given individual (subset I genes), and genes coding for antibodies against antigens absent in a given individual but present in other individuals of the same species (subset II genes). In the precursor lymphocytes, the antibodies constitute the cell surface receptors, each lymphocyte expressing only one receptor type. When the precursor lymphocytes enter primarily lymphoid organs (thymus and mammalian equivalent of the bursa of Fabricius), subset I lymphocytes react with the antigens against which they are directed and are stimulated to intensive proliferation. Most cells produced by multiple divisions carry receptors identical to their progenitor cells; these cells react with the H antigen and die. However, during the many generations of cell divisions, somatic mutations occur that modify the antibody receptors so that they no longer fit the antigens against which they were originally directed. Mutant cells that are unable to react with the individual's antigens escape the elimination process and develop into mature lymphocytes. Subset II lymphocytes that do not find their corresponding *H* antigens in the particular individual also escape elimination, and they too— perhaps after limited proliferation—develop into mature cells. Consequently, the population of mature lymphocytes consists of cells carrying receptors against allogeneic H antigens diversified by mutations, but it lacks cells with receptors against self-antigens. The postulate that the population of cells having receptors against allogeneic H antigens is unselected, and is, perhaps, even amplified through limited proliferation could explain why the frequency of these cells in MLC and GVHR is so high (see Chapter Eighteen). According to Jerne, the elimination of cells having receptors against self-antigens explains the linkage of the *Ir* gene to the MHC, because it can be postulated that the nonresponders are individuals in which the particular cell clone reacting with a given H antigen and cross-reacting with an unrelated antigen has been eliminated.

Jerne's hypothesis has been criticized with regard to both its concept and its details (see Smith and Landy 1970; Bodmer 1972). Furthermore, its predictions could not be confirmed experimentally (see, for instance, Grant and Hood 1971). And finally, recent data (e.g., Premkumar *et al.* 1974) obviate any somatic generators of diversity by suggesting that the germ line contains enough genetic information to account for the extent of antibody variability.

In conclusion, there is no satisfactory explanation as to what the function of the H-2 antigens might be. When considered independently of the putative recognitive function, the stimulatory role of the *H-2* complex simply does not make sense.

B. Recognitive Function

The evidence that the *H-2* complex may also code for a class of molecules with a recognitive function is indirect and circumstantial. It is based mainly on two observations. First, a set of loci controlling the immune response to synthetic polypeptides, proteins, and alloantigens (the *Ir* loci) is located within the *H-2* complex. The control is highly specific and the specificity of the *Ir* loci is explained by the assumption that the *Ir* gene products function as antigen receptors. Second, the *H-2* complex controls the cooperation between syngeneic T and B cells: both cells interact with an antigen and the interaction results in production of antibodies by the B cell's progeny. The cooperation between the two classes of lymphocytes is specific and the specificity is attributed, as in the case of the *Ir* loci, to a recognitive capability of the H-2 products.

Three hypotheses based on the assumption of H-2 recognitive function are briefly described below.

1. The Differentiation Antigen Hypothesis

It is generally believed that differentiation of tissues in ontogeny involves an element of cell-to-cell recognition, mediated by cell surface structures. Bodmer (1972) speculated that the recognition process requires two classes of molecule: differentiation antigens and recognizers. Differentiation antigens are cell surface structures specific to a given cell type and/or to a given time during ontogeny, and detectable by serological methods. Recognizers are cell surface molecules "whose function is to recognize the differentiation antigens and so to mediate the interaction between appropriate types of cells during development" (Bodmer 1972). According to Bodmer, both the differentiation antigens and the recognizers are controlled by the *H-2* complex, by loci distinct from *H-2K* and *H-2D*. The function of the *H-2K* and *H-2D* antigens, which are present in practically all tissues, is envisioned by Bodmer as being similar to that of the constant regions of the immunoglobulin molecule. Bodmer also speculates that the differentiation antigen-recognizer system might have been the primordium from which the set of immunoglobulin genes [such as those postulated by Jerne (1971)] has evolved by duplication and transposition to other locations in the genome so as to "allow the evolution of the immune system to proceed without disturbing the control of multicellular development and differentiation" (Bodmer 1972).

2. The T Cell Receptor Hypothesis

The T cell receptor hypothesis postulates that the main function of the *H-2* complex, in particular of the *Ir* loci, is to code for structures expressed on the surfaces of T cells, and that these T cell receptors are distinct from known immunoglobulins (Benacerraf and McDevitt 1972). The T cell receptors are capable of specifically recognizing and binding antigen in a way similar to the antigen-binding of B cell receptors. The antigen-activated T cells then either differentiate into cells capable of destroying the antigen or cooperate with B cells to help them mount an efficient attack against the antigen.

The T cell receptor hypothesis suffers from three main drawbacks. First, the evidence that *Ir* loci are expressed in T cells is only indirect and there is even some evidence that the loci are expressed in B cells. Second, none of the H-2 products identified so far fulfills the requirement for a T cell receptor (specific antigen binding, clonal distribution, etc.). Third, despite an enormous effort aimed at its identification, the H-2 controlled T cell receptor remains elusive.

Several alternative interpretations of the *Ir* gene function (i.e., interpretations that do not require coding by the *Ir* loci for the T cell receptor) have been proposed by Feldman (1973).

3. The Second Immune System Hypothesis

To this author, the most appealing is the possibility that the *H-2* complex represents a second immune system, the first being that of classical immuno-globulins. The complex can be envisioned as coding for determinants, some of which are expressed predominantly on T cells, others predominantly on B cells, and still others on both T and B cells, as well as other cell types. The recognition of foreign bodies by the H-2 determinants is accomplished on the principle of structural dissimilarity, rather than strict complementarity between the two interacting cells. Whenever a cell carrying a particular determinant establishes contact with another cell carrying a different determinant, the foreignness of the determinants becomes the catalyst triggering a primitive immune response. The triggered T cells respond by blast transformation and production of effector cells that destroy the target cell. The target of this T cell-mediated immunity are primarily microorganisms, parasites, somatic cell variants, and so on, and secondarily, all allotransplants. As originally suggested by Kreth and Williamson (1971), a B cell that has bound one antigen through its Ig receptors is also recognized as foreign by the T cells; but instead of being killed, it is triggered, perhaps through special acceptor structures postulated by Katz and his co-workers (1973a, b, c; cf. Chapter Nineteen), to transform into antibody-producing cells.

C. Functional Interrelationships of *H-2* Loci

When considering the H-2 function, one of the major questions is whether the individual *H-2* loci are related in their origin (and thus in their function) or whether the complex is an accidental assembly of loci with different functions. This question can be definitely answered only after biochemical information on the nature of the H-2 products is available; in the absence of such information, the answers are speculative at best. The various classes of *H-2* loci will first be considered in groups, and later the complex will be considered as a whole.

1. H-2 (i.e., H-2K and H-2D) and Ia Loci

The main differences between the classical H-2 and Ia antigens are in their tissue distribution, molecular weights, and functions.

The tissue distribution of the Ia antigens appears to be more restricted than the tissue distribution of the ubiquous H-2 antigens. Nevertheless, it is clear that the Ia antigens are present in tissues other than lymphocytes (e.g., epithelial cells and spermatozoa). Moreover, it cannot presently be ruled out by the available methods that small quantities of Ia antigens are present in many other tissues as well.

The molecular weight data too are not a very convincing argument for the distinctiveness of the H-2 and Ia antigens. The Ia molecules appear to be smaller than the H-2 molecules but this difference means very little, considering the enormous difficulties the biochemists are having in characterizing any membrane components. Most of the biochemical information about the H-2 products, including molecular weight estimates, is highly unreliable. However, even if the molecular weight difference is not an artifact, one can still devise models accounting for the discrepancy. For example, in analogy with the immuno-globulin polypeptides, one can visualize the H-2 polypeptide chains as consisting of domains with each domain coded for by a single cistron. The *H-2* chromosomal segment would then be a series of duplicated cistrons with different number of cistrons participating in the synthesis of the H-2 and Ia polypeptide chains (e.g., four cistrons coding for one H-2 polypeptide chain and 2 cistrons coding for one Ia chain).

The functional difference between the *H-2* and *Ia* loci is also not absolute.[1] Although clearly the region harboring the *Ia* loci is more strongly involved in MLR than the *K* or *D* regions, there is little doubt that the H-2 antigens themselves have an MLR-stimulating capability. The difference between the two classes of antigens could be quantitative rather than qualitative. The difference in the capability of the Ia and H-2 antigens to serve as targets in CML is a more serious problem, but here again one cannot exclude the possibility of the difference being artifactual. Supporting this possibility is the fact that the *IA* region is strongly involved in graft rejection.

The *H-2I* locus itself is a good example of the *H-2-Ia* distinction's artificiality. On the one hand, the locus does not seem to code for classical H-2 antigens, is

---

[1] Most recently evidence has been obtained by Dickler and Sachs (1974) suggesting identity or close association of Ia antigens with Fc receptors, i.e. sites in the membrane of lymphocytes capable of binding antigen-complexed or heat-aggregated immunoglobulin. The authors demonstrated that when mouse spleen lymphocytes are pretreated with deaggregated antisera specific for Ia antigens, binding of Ig complexes to the Fc receptor is markedly inhibited. Other antisera that bind to lymphocytes, including antisera specific for antigens controlled by the *K* and *D* regions of the *H-2* complex, produced no inhibition. This report, if confirmed, would be the first evidence suggesting functional differentiation of Ia and classical H-2 antigens.

located in the *I* region and can well pose for an *Ia* locus since the *H-2I* incompatibility leads to production of Ia antibodies. On the other hand, the locus is strongly involved in graft rejection, a function usually attributed to the *H-2K* and *H-2D* loci. Should the locus be considered homologous to *H-2* or to *Ia* loci? Perhaps the answer is that one should not view the *H-2* and the *Ia* as two totally different classes of loci, but rather as members of the same family of loci. One can speculate that all loci in this family originated from the same primordial locus by gene duplication, and later differentiated by specializing to slightly different but similar functions.

2. Ia and Lad Loci

The relationship between the *Ia* and *Lad* loci was discussed earlier (see Chapter Eighteen), the conclusion from the discussion being that in all respects the loci appear to be identical. This being the case, it follows that all that was said about the *H-2-Ia* relationship also applies to the *H-2-Lad* relationship. If one accepts the relatedness of the *H-2* and *Lad* loci, then the MLR-stimulating capability of the H-2 antigens does not come as a surprise. The implication from the relatedness would be that, as far as the stimulating function is concerned, there is no qualitative difference between the peripheral and central regions of the *H-2* complex.[2]

3. Ir and Ia Loci

The question of the relationship between the *Ir* and other loci in the *H-2* complex is the most difficult to answer. Since virtually nothing is known about the nature of the Ir gene product, one can only speculate what the relationship might be. There are two basic possibilities: The Ir gene product could be distinct from all products of the *H-2* complex identified so far, or it could be related to the products of other *H-2* loci, most probably the *Ia* loci. So far there has been a good genetic correlation between the *Ir* and the *Ia* loci, but this could be simply because so few crossovers are known that occurred in the critical region of the *H-2* complex (the *I* region). In fact, Meo and Shreffler (quoted by McDevitt *et al.* 1974b) have recently found at least one strain combination in which the correlation breaks down. In this particular combination the two strains differ in an *Ir* gene but show no difference with respect to Ia antigens or MLR. The opposite situation is also known to occur. In the combination (B10.HTT × A) anti-A.TH, significant MLR stimulation is obtained in the absence of any known *Ir* difference between the responder and the stimulator (McDevitt *et al.* 1974b). The argument against both observations is that in these combinations *Ia*, *Lad*, or *Ir* differences might be found later after the improvement of the available techniques or after expansion of the spectrum

---

[2] Regardless of the relatedness or nonrelatedness of *H-2* and *Lad* loci, there is no justification for distinguishing the *H-2* complex into *lymphocyte-defined* (*LD*) and *serologically defined* (*SD*) regions, as advocated by Bach *et al.* (1972b) since the *LD* regions are also serologically defined and similarly the *SD* regions are "lymphocyte-defined."

of antigens tested. However, even if the particular combinations continue behaving the way they do now, it still will not necessarily mean that the *Ir* and *Ia* (*Lad*) loci cannot belong to the same class. Conceivably, the pleiotropism of the *Ia* (*Ir*) loci does not always have to be expressed to the same degree. One can argue that the product of one *Ia* (*Ir*) locus can function both as lymphocyte activating determinants and immune response controller, whereas the product of another locus fulfills only one or the other of the two functions.

If the *Ir* and *Ia* loci do belong to the same category of loci, then the hypothesis of the *Ir* gene coding for T cell receptor becomes untenable and an alternative explanation for the *Ir* gene's specificity must be found. One possibility is cross-tolerance between the Ia and the immunizing antigens in the low responder strains (see Chapter Seventeen).

4. Functional Relationships in the H-2 Complex as a Whole

Table 20-1 summarizes the functions attributed to the individual regions of the *H-2* complex. Based on the preceding discussion and ignoring loci whose functional relationships to the *H-2* loci is dubious, the table can be interpreted in three principal ways.

First, the *H-2* complex can consist of three types of loci, *H-2*, *Ia* (*Lad*) and *Ir*, which may be only distantly (if at all) related among themselves. The *H-2* loci would code for cellular immunity's target antigens, the *Ia* loci for cellular immunity's stimulating determinants, and the *Ir* loci for the T cell receptors or other types of recognizers.

Second, the *H-2* complex consists of two types of loci, *H-2* (*Ia*, *Lad*) and *Ir*. According to this interpretation, the *H-2* and *Ia* (*Lad*) loci would be members of the same family with some minor differences characterizing each of them.

Table 20-1. Function of *H-2* regions in immunity

Function	H-2 region						
	K	*IA*	*IB*	*IC*	*S*	*X*	*D*
Control of serologically detectable H-2 antigens	⧺	—	—	—	—	+	⧺
Control of transplantation antigens	⧺	⧺	—	—	—	+	⧺
Control of antigens with restricted tissue distribution (Ia)	—	⧺	⊹	⊹	—	—	—
Activation of lymphocytes in MLR and GVHR	+	⧺	+	+	+	+	+
Target cell function in CML	⧺	+	—	—	—	?	⧺
Production of killer cells in CML	+	⧺	?	?	—	?	+
Control of immune response	—	⧺	⊹	+	—	—	—
Physiological T-B cell cooperation	?	⧺	?	?	—	—	—

An alternative to this interpretation would be that the *H-2* loci are distinct from the *Ia*, but the *Ia* loci belong to the same category as the *Ir* loci.

Third, the *H-2* complex consists of only one category of loci and the differences between *H-2* and *Ia*, *H-2* and *Ir* and *Ir* and *Ia* are the result of relatively recent functional specialization during the evolution of the complex. At the time of this writing, the choice among the three possibilities is difficult to make; however, from the evolutionary point of view, the third possibility would make most sense.

II. Comparative Aspects

A. Homologous Systems in Other Species

In the more than 30 years since its discovery, *H-2* has remained the only system known to have the properties of a major histocompatibility complex. At one time it seemed possible that the *H-2* complex was a curiosity of the mouse, without any true counterparts in other mammalian species. But subsequent studies have clearly demonstrated that many other mammals possess a system closely resembling *H-2*. The best known homologue of *H-2* is the *HL-A* system in man, followed by similar systems in chimpanzee, rhesus monkey, pig, dog, guinea pig, rabbit, rat, and even chicken (Table 20-2; for a review, see Iványi 1970). Whenever sufficient effort is made, an MHC is discovered in every species studied. So it seems justified to conclude that the existence of MHC's is a general biological phenomenon characterizing not only all mammals, but perhaps other vertebrate classes as well. However, with the exception of *HL-A*, none of the homologous MHC's has been studied to a degree comparable to the analysis of the *H-2* system. Consequently, the knowledge of MHC's in other species is only fragmentary.

In general, the investigation of homologous MHC's has not produced a single feature not known in the *H-2* system. Comparative studies in different

Table 20-2. Major histocompatibility complexes of various species

Species	MHC symbol	Synonyms	Key reference
Man	*HL-A*	*Hu-1*	Kissmeyer-Nielsen and Thorsby 1970
Chimpanzee	*ChL-A*		Balner *et al.* 1971a
Rhesus monkey	*RhL-A*		Balner *et al.* 1971b
Dog	*DL-A*		Vriesendorp *et al.* 1971
Pig	*SL-A*		Vaiman *et al.* 1970
Guinea pig	?		Ellman *et al.* 1970
Rabbit	*RbH-1*	*RL-A*	Chai 1974; Tissot and Cohen 1972
Rat	*RtH-1*	*AgB*	Palm 1964; Štark *et al.* 1967
Mouse	*H-2*		This monograph
Chicken	*B*		Schierman and Nordskog 1961

species indicate that each species possesses only one MHC; that the one MHC consists of two regions coding for serologically detectable, highly polymorphic, and extremely complex antigens; that the antigens controlled by MHC's cause rapid rejection of skin and other tissue grafts, and that the MHC is always associated with *Ir* genes and genes coding for lymphocyte-activating determinants. These results strongly reinforce the notion that MHC's of various species are true homologues from the evolutionary point of view. This notion is further supported by data indicating the existence of biochemical similarities between MHC's of different species. Such data have been provided for the mouse *H-2* and human *HL-A* systems.

B. The *H-2-HL-A* Homology

The *human leukocyte system A* (*HL-A*) consists of a large number of antigens (Table 20-3) that can be separated into two series, each of which behaves as if its members were controlled by alleles at the same locus (for a review, see Kissmeyer-Nielsen and Thorsby 1970). It is therefore believed that the *HL-A* complex is composed of two loci, *LA* and *Four*, determining antigens that can be detected by serological methods (most commonly cytotoxic and leuko-agglutination tests) on the surface of lymphocytes. The two loci are closely linked, with a recombination frequency between them of about 0.8 percent.

Table 20-3. HL-A antigens of the *LA* and *Four* series and their corresponding frequencies in Caucasians*· **

LA		Four	
HL-A1	0.16	HL-A5	0.06
HL-A2	0.31	HL-A7	0.12
HL-A3	0.15	HL-A8	0.09
HL-A9	0.13	HL-A12	0.13
HL-A10	0.06	HL-A13	0.02
HL-A11	0.07	HL-A14	0.04
HL-A28	0.05	HL-A17	0.04
W19	0.06	HL-A27	0.04
Blank	0.01	W5	0.09
		W10	0.03
		W15	0.06
		W18	0.06
		W22	0.03
		Blank	0.17

* Reproduced with permission from W. F. Bodmer: "Evolutionary significance of the HL-A system." *Nature 237*:139–145. Copyright © 1972 by The Macmillan Company. All rights reserved.

** The HL-A numbers are the officially recognized antigens; the W numbers refer to antigens provisionally identified during the Fourth International Histocompatibility Testing Workshop.

The *LA* and *Four* loci are believed to be homologous to the *H-2K* and *H-2D* loci. The antigens controlled by one *HL-A* locus are mutually exclusive, in that the presence of one antigen precludes the presence of another controlled by that locus in an *HL-A* homozygote. Hence, HL-A antigens seem to correspond to private H-2 antigens. Although the existence of HL-A public antigens has never been officially acknowledged, there is little doubt that they exist. For example, HL-A investigators have been aware, practically from the beginning of HL-A studies, of the existence of a family of related antigens (the so-called 4a4b system) that did not fall into any easily recognizable serological or genetic pattern. In many respects, these antigens resemble the 1-family or the 3-family of the mouse *H-2* system. However, most of the public HL-A antigens are probably never analyzed, because the antisera detecting them are too complex. HL-A serology is based on the population approach described in Chapter Three, which requires a considerable degree of simplification for the serological pattern to become apparent. HL-A investigators have continually selected the strongest and simplest antisera and have tended to discard antisera that are more complex. It is probably the latter antisera that contain the anti-HL-A public antibodies. It is also possible that at least some of the officially recognized HL-A antigens are actually complexes of one private and one or more public antigens. The high phenotypic frequencies of some of the HL-A antigens (cf. Table 20-3) suggest indirectly that this might be so. (For further discussion of the relationship between H-2 and HL-A serology, see J. Klein and Shreffler 1971.)

The *HL-A*-linked *Ir* genes have not been mapped with respect to the loci coding for serologically detectable antigens, but the homologue of the mouse's strong *Lad* locus appears to be outside the *LA* and *Four* regions.

Evidence for serological homology of H-2 and HL-A antigens was obtained by Götze *et al.* (1972, 1973c) and David *et al.* (1973b). The former group obtained rabbit antisera against human lymphocytes and demonstrated human-mouse (most likely, *HL-A-H-2*) cross-reactivity by testing the antisera against lymphocytes from various *H-2* congenic lines. David and his co-workers (1973b) immunized chickens with soluble H-2 and HL-A substances and produced precipitating and cytotoxic antibodies that displayed cross-species reactivity.

However, testing of H-2 alloantisera against human lymphocytes failed to demonstrate a clear correlation with any of the known HL-A antigens (Ivašková *et al.* 1972).

Cross-reactivity between H-2 antigens and rabbit histocompatibility antigens has been reported by Abeyounis *et al.* (1968), and by Abeyounis and Milgrom (1969). Biochemical evidence for *H-2-HL-A* homology was described by D. Mann and Nathenson (1969), who compared papain-solubilized preparations obtained from mouse and human lymphoid cells. They found that the kinetics of papain solubilization from cell membranes, gel filtration, and electrophoretic behavior of H-2 and HL-A antigens were nearly identical. When the amino acid composition and carbohydrate content of the *H*-2 and HL-A preparations were compared, striking similarities between the two became apparent. From this compositional relatedness of the antigens, the authors concluded that "the genes determining these major transplantation antigen systems may have evolved from a common precursor" (D. Mann and Nathenson 1969).

C. Homologous Proteins

Theoretically, the possibility exists that the MHC's might have evolved from genes that had originally had a different function, or from genes that also served as precursors of loci coding for other proteins. In both cases, structural homology between the MHC antigens and the evolutionarily related proteins could be expected. Relatedness of MHC antigens to β_2-microglobulins, β-lipoproteins, and immunoglobulins has been considered recently by several investigators.

1. β₂-microglobulin

The serum of various mammals contains a group of proteins, summarily designated *microglobulins*, which have relatively low molecular weights (less than 40,000 daltons) and which, upon electrophoresis, migrate to the globulin region. The human β_2-microglobulin is present in low amounts in the serum, urine, and cerebrospinal fluid (and also on the surface of lymphocytes) of normal individuals; it is present in elevated amounts in the urine of patients with malfunctions of the renal tubules. In addition, the protein is also produced by a variety of mesenchymal and epithelial cell lines. The function of the protein is not known. Biochemical analysis of the β_2-microglobulin revealed that the protein consists of a single polypeptide chain having a molecular weight of 11,600 daltons corresponding to about 100 amino acid residues. The amino acid sequence of the smaller protein has recently been determined (Peterson *et al.* 1972) and shown to be strikingly similar to a portion of the IgG constant region of both the H and L chains. The similarity prompted Peterson and his co-workers (1972) to speculate that the gene for β_2-microglobulin and the gene for the basic unit (domain) of the IgG molecule have a common ancestry.

More recently, a homology between the β_2-microglobulin gene and the *HL-A* genes has also been suggested. Cresswell *et al.* (1973) and Tanigaki *et al.* (1973) observed that solubilization of HL-A antigens with papain yielded two polypeptide fragments, one larger and the other smaller. The larger polypeptide (molecular weight of about 33,000 daltons) carried the serological activity and appeared to be homologous to papain-solubilized H-2 fragments of the mouse. The smaller polypeptide had a molecular weight of 10,000–12,000 daltons, carried no serological activity, and was also present in serum and urine. The similarity in properties between the small HL-A fragment and β_2-microglobulin led Peterson *et al.* (1974) and Nakamuro *et al.* (1973) to investigate the relationship between the two proteins. Both groups came to the conclusion that the low-molecular-weight fragment found in papain-solubilized and purified HL-A antigens was very similar, if not identical to the β_2-microglobulin. It has therefore been speculated that the β_2-microglobulin is a basic unit from which the evolution of both immunoglobulins and HL-A antigens started and to which, in both cases, variable regions are added.

However, such far-reaching speculations are a bit premature, because it has not yet been proved that the β_2-microglobulin has anything to do with HL-A molecules in their native state. It is quite possible that the association between β_2-microglobulin and HL-A in purified preparations is an artifact caused either by the papain treatment or by the purification procedure. It must also be emphasized that no homology (serological or biochemical) has been found between the small and large fragment in the HL-A preparations.

Most recently, Neauport-Sautes *et al.* (1974) reported that when all β_2-microglobulin is redistributed (capped) on the lymphocyte membrane by specific rabbit antibodies and goat antirabbit Ig conjugates, the HL-A antigens are no more detectable with anti-HL-A conjugates outside the caps. However, when the HL-A antigens are capped first, the lymphocytes can still be stained on the whole surface with conjugated anti-β_2-microglobulin serum, indicating that HL-A antigens may be associated with β_2-microglobulin at the cell surface, but that all β_2-microglobulin molecules are not bound to HL-A antigens (Neauport-Sautes *et al.* 1974).

The mouse β_2-microglobulin has not yet been identified, although many H-2 preparations contain a small molecular weight fraction that some biochemists believe is homologous to the human β_2-microglobulin.

2. β-lipoproteins

Mammalian blood plasma contains several classes of β-lipoprotein distinguished by density and electrophoretic mobility. The β-lipoproteins contain about 80–90 percent lipid and have an average molecular weight of 10,000,000 daltons. Using antisera produced in rabbits or other animals, the human β-lipoprotein can be delineated into several antigenic types, presumably belonging to the same system, which is designated *Lp*.

A connection between Lp and HL-A antigens is suggested by several observations. Berg *et al.* (1968) reported that skin grafts exchanged between *Lp*-identical individuals survived significantly longer than those transplanted between *Lp*-disparate persons. Charlton and Zmijewski (1970) reported that the β-lipoprotein fraction inhibited anti-HL-A activity. And Berg (1971) compared the amino acid composition of Lp lipoproteins, papain-solubilized HL-A antigens, and H-2 antigens and found significant similarities among the three preparations; the resemblance between the Lp(a) lipoprotein of human serum and H-2 antigens appeared to be even greater than that between the H-2 and HL-A antigens. According to Berg, "the results of the analyses support the concept that a relationship exists between lipoprotein in the serum and histocompatibility antigens on cell membranes" (Berg 1971). However, all the data on the relationship between β-lipoproteins and histocompatibility antigens can also be explained as resulting from cross-contamination of the preparations, particularly because at least some of the data could not be confirmed by others (cf. Schultz and Shreffler 1972). *A priori*, it is difficult to see why such a relationship would exist.

3. Immunoglobulins

The most logical candidates for structural homology to H-2 antigens are the Ig molecules. An evolutionary relationship between the *Ig* and *H-2* genes has been postulated by several investigators (e.g., Bodmer 1972; Peterson *et al.* 1974). However, there is so far no experimental evidence to support the existence of such a relationship.

III. Evolution

In the orthodox multiple gene model, the *H-2* complex was interpreted as consisting of a series of more or less equivalent regions, with the *Ss* and *Slp* loci in the middle. The functional similarity of the regions (all were believed to code for classical H-2 antigens) led Shreffler and his co-workers (1971) to postulate that the regions evolved by gene duplication. The original duplication model (Fig. 20-1a) envisioned the evolution of the *H-2* complex as proceeding in two major steps: in the first step a primoridal *H-2* locus, adjacent to an unrelated *Ss* locus, duplicated to give two (or more) *H-2* loci; in the second step, the entire *Ss–H-2* segment underwent an inverted duplication centered around the *Ss* locus.

The new developments in the genetics of the *H-2* complex make the duplication model in its original form untenable. All the available evidence indicates that the *H-2* regions are not symmetrically distributed on both sides of the *S* region. On the contrary, the *K* end appears to be functionally distinct from the *D* end in that it contains *Ir*, *Ia*, and strong *Lad* loci. The functional *K-D* asymmetry was first discovered by Rychlíková *et al.* (1970) and was then con-

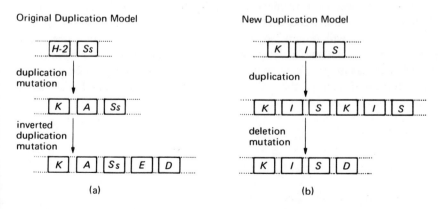

Fig. 20-1. Evolution of the *H-2* complex. Each rectangle represents one *H-2* region. (The original duplication model was proposed by Shreffler *et al.* 1971.)

firmed by many other laboratories. Although one can argue theoretically that there is an *I* region between the *S* and *D* regions, such an argument is not supported by experimental data; in several functional tests the *K* end always behaves differently from the *D* end (see Chapter Eight) and all the *Ir* and *Ia* loci map in the *K* end. As far as the lymphocyte-activating determinants are concerned, there appears to be at least one *Lad* locus in the *X* region, but it is much weaker than the *Lad* loci in the *I* region.

To account for the *K-D* asymmetry, and at the same time to preserve the duplication model, one has to postulate that the original *H-2* chromosome consisted of *K*, *I*, and *S* regions and that the *K-I-S* segment was duplicated without an inversion (Fig. 20-1b). This hypothesis raises the possibility of the *I* and *S* regions' existing outside *H-2* at the *D* end of the chromosome. Although there is no evidence to support such a possibility, it cannot be totally discounted. Most mapping studies of *Ir* genes have been carried out using congenic lines that were developed by selecting for *K* and *D* serologically detectable antigens. Theoretically, such lines should have lost the donor's regions outside the *H-2* complex during the repeated backcrossing. Admittedly, however, the chance that another *I* (and/or *S*) region outside *H-2* has been missed is rather slim. It seems more likely that the *I* and *S* homologues outside the *D* region were lost during subsequent evolution, as shown in Fig. 20-1b. It is conceivable, however, that they were preserved in other mammals; for example, the existence of a strong *I* region outside the *LA* and *Four* complex has been reported in man.

A disturbing observation is that the *K*-region antigens isolated by papain digestion from $H-2^b$ cells show more homology to D^d antigens than to K^d antigens (see Chapter Fifteen). Barring the possibility that the observation is an artifact of the isolation procedure, one would have to explain the observation by postulating either that the *H-2* complex is evolutionarily unstable and constantly subjected to gross structural rearrangements, or that products of other loci are joined to the H-2D and H-2K products to form a single H-2 monomer. These secondary points would have to be highly variable so as to mask the true homologies between the primary *D* and *K* products.

It must be emphasized that all consideration of H-2 evolution is highly speculative and will remain so until data on the primary structure of H-2 products become available. Judging from the pace at which H-2 biochemistry has been progressing, it can be expected that for some time to come, on the map of the H-2 studies the area of the function and evolution will bear an inscription: *Hic sunt leones!*

Appendix

Chronology of Major Events in the History of the *H-2* System

Year	Event	Author
1902–1908	Transplantable tumors in mice are discovered.	Jensen, Loeb
1909	Genetics of susceptibility to tumor transplants is studied.	Tyzzer
1914	Genetic theory of tumor transplantation is formulated.	Little
1915–1920	Development of several inbred strains of mice is initiated.	Little and others
1916	The genetic theory of tumor transplantation is confirmed experimentally.	Little and Tyzzer
1920–1935	Immunological mechanisms of tumor regression are sought.	Lumsden, Shinoi, and others
1933	Alloantigen hypothesis of tumor regression is formulated.	Haldane
1936	Four blood group antigens, among them antigen II, are discovered in the mouse.	Gorer
1937	Identity of the gene for antigen II with one gene for tumor resistance is established.	Gorer
1938	Immunological theory of tumor transplantation is formulated and confirmed experimentally.	Gorer
1943–1944	Immunological basis of rejection of normal tissue transplants is established.	Medawar and others
1946	First congenic resistant lines are initiated.	Snell
1948	Theory of congenic lines is formulated, and the term *histocompatibility* is introduced.	Snell
1948	Linkage of the gene for antigen II with the gene for *Fused tail* is established, and the gene for antigen II is designated *H-2*.	Gorer, Snell, and others
1951	Histogenetic methods are developed for analysis of *H* genes.	Snell
1951–1953	A number of alleles at the *H-2* locus are identified by histogenetic methods.	Snell
1953	*dk* effect is discovered and complexity of the *H-2* locus is hinted.	Snell
1953	Leukoagglutination method is introduced.	Amos
1954	Human serum-dextran hemagglutination test is developed.	Gorer and Mikulska
1954	Distinction between private and public H-2 antigens is made.	Hoecker and others

Year	Event	Author
1954–1955	Serological complexity of the *H-2* system begins to emerge.	Gorer, Amos, Hoecker, and others
1955	First two intra-*H-2* recombinants are discovered.	Allen, Gorer, and others
1956	Dye-exclusion cytotoxic test is developed.	Gorer and O'Gorman
1956	*H* genes are divided into strong or major (*H-2*) and weak or minor (non-*H-2*).	Counce *et al.*
1956	First attempt is made to isolate H-2 antigens.	Billingham *et al.*
1957	First H-2 variants from heterozygous tumors are isolated.	E. Klein *et al.*
1958	*H-2* congenic lines are described.	Snell
1959	First genetic map of the *H-2* complex is proposed.	Gorer and Mikulska
1961	PVP-hemagglutination technique is developed.	Stimpfling
1961	Fluorescent antibody technique is developed.	G. Möller
1961	Tissue distribution of H-2 antigens is determined.	Basch and Stetson, Pizzaro *et al.*
1961	Association of H-2 antigens with cell membrane fraction is demonstrated.	Herzenberg and Herzenberg
1963	The *Ss* locus is discovered.	Shreffler and Owen
1963	*Tla* locus is described.	Old *et al.*
1964	Close linkage of *Tla* locus with the *H-2* complex is established.	Boyse *et al.*
1964	Intra-*H-2* localization of the *Ss* locus is suggested.	Shreffler
1964	Nomenclature of the *H-2* system is revised.	Snell and others.
1964	Susceptibility to Gross virus is shown to be controlled by the *H-2* complex.	Lilly *et al.*
1964	Deficient growth of parental bone marrow cells in F_1 hybrids is associated with the *H-2* complex.	Cudkowicz and Stimpfling
1965	Congenic lines carrying recombinant *H-2* haplotypes are described.	Stimpfling and Richardson
1965	The *Ir-1A* locus is discovered.	McDevitt and Sela
1965	^{51}Cr-release cytotoxic test is introduced.	Wigzell and Sanderson
1967	First mutation in the *H-2* complex is described.	Egorov
1969	Two classes of glycoprotein fragments carrying H-2 antigens are isolated.	Shimada and Nathenson
1969–1970	Serological H-2 typing of wild mice is begun.	Iványi and J. Klein
1970	*Rgv-1* locus is positioned within the *H-2* complex.	Lilly
1970	*Slp* locus is discovered and positioned within the *H-2* complex.	Passmore and Shreffler
1970	Predominant role of the *K* end in MLR is demonstrated.	Rychlíková *et al.*
1970	Free movement of H-2 molecules in the cell membrane is demonstrated.	Frye and Edidin

Year	Event	Author
1971	Postulate of duplicate antigens in different regions of the *H-2* complex is made.	Shreffler *et al.*
1971	Two series of mutually exclusive private H-2 antigens are recognized.	Snell and others
1971	Families of H-2 antigens are described.	Snell *et al.*
1971	Two-locus model of the *H-2* complex is formulated.	J. Klein, Shreffler, Stimpfling, Snell and others
1971	Chromosome carrying the *H-2* complex is identified cytologically.	J. Klein
1971	Recombinant inbred strains are introduced.	Bailey
1972	The *Ir-1A* locus is positioned within the *H-2* complex.	McDevitt *et al.*
1972	*I* region is associated with MLC stimulation.	Bach *et al.*, Meo *et al.*
1972	*Ir-1B* locus is described.	Lieberman and Humphrey
1973	*I* region is associated with GHV reaction.	J. Klein, Park, Oppltová, Démant
1973	Ia antigens are discovered.	David, Götze, Hauptfeld, Hämmerling, Sachs, and others
1973	T-B cell cooperation is shown to be *I* region dependent.	Katz *et al.*
1973	Independent movement of H-2K and H-2D molecules in the cell membrane is demonstrated.	Neauport-Sautes *et al.*
1974	*H-2I* locus is described.	J. Klein *et al.*

References

Abbasi, K., and Festenstein, H.: Antigenic strength investigated by cell-mediated lympholysis in mice. *Eur. J. Immunol. 3*:430–435, 1973.

Abbasi, K., Démant, P., Festenstein, H., Holmes, J., Huber, B., and Rychlíková, M.: Mouse mixed lymphocyte reactions and cell-mediated lympholysis: Genetic control and relevance to antigenic strength. *Transplant. Proc. 5*:1329–1337, 1973.

Abeyounis, C. J., and Milgrom, F.: Tissue isoantigens shared by rabbits and mice. *Transplant. Proc. 1*:556–559, 1969.

Abeyounis, C. J., Edebo, L., and Milgrom, F.: Localization and characterization of mouse and rat tissue isoantigens. In *Advance in Transplantation*, J. Dausset, J. Hamburger, and G. Mathé (eds.), pp. 305–309, Williams & Wilkins, Baltimore, 1968.

Adamczyk, K., and Ryszkowski, L.: Settling of mice (*Mus musculus L.*) released in an uninhabited and an inhabited place. *Bull. Acad. Pol. Sci. 13*:631–637, 1965.

Adler, W. H., Takiguchi, T., Marsh, B., and Smith, R. T.: Cellular recognition by mouse lymphocytes *in vitro*. II. Specific stimulation by histocompatibility antigens in mixed cell culture. *J. Immunol. 105*:984–1000, 1970.

Ahmed, A., Thurman, G. B., Vannier, W. E., Sell, K. W., and Strong, D. M.: Cytotoxicity inhibition studies using 3M KCl solubilized murine histocompatibility antigens and a new multiple automated sample harvester. *J. Immunol. Methods 3*:1–16, 1973.

Al-Askari, S., Dumonde, D. C., Lawrence, H. S., and Thomas, L.: Subcellular fractions as transplantation antigens. *Ann. N.Y. Acad. Sci. 120*:261–269, 1964.

Al-Askari, S., Lawrence, H. S., and Thomas, L.: Transplantation antigens in normal mouse organs. *Proc. Soc. Exp. Biol. Med. 122*:1270–1273, 1966.

Albert, W. H. W., and Davies, D. A. L.: H-2 antigens on nuclear membranes. *Immunology 24*:841–850, 1973.

Allen, S. L.: Linkage relations of the genes histocompatibility-2 and fused tail, brachyury and kinky tail in the mouse, as determined by tumor transplantation. *Genetics 40*:627–650, 1955a.

Allen, S. L.: *H-2^f*, a tenth allele at the histocompatibility-2 locus in the mouse as determined by tumor transplantation. *Cancer Res. 15*:315–319, 1955b.

Alm, G. V., and Peterson, R. D. A.: Effect of thymectomy and bursectomy on the *in vitro* response of chick spleen cells to PHA, sheep erythrocytes (SRBC) and allogeneic cells. *Fed. Proc. 29*:430, 1970 (Abstract).

Alter, B. J., Schendel, D. J., Bach, M. L., Bach, F. H., Klein, J., and Stimpfling, J. H.: Cell-mediated lympholysis. Importance of serologically defined H-2 regions. *J. Exp. Med. 137*:1303–1309, 1973.

Altman, A., Cohen, I. R., and Feldman, M.: Normal T-cell receptors for alloantigens. *Cell. Immunol., 7*:134–172, 1973.

Amos, D. B.: The agglutination of mouse leucocytes by iso-immune sera. *Brit. J. Exp. Pathol. 34*:464–470, 1953.

Amos, D. B.: Serological differences between comparable diploid and tetraploid lines of three mouse ascites tumors. *Ann. N.Y. Acad. Sci. 63*:706–710, 1956.

Amos, D. B.: Genetic studies on tumor immunity: An analysis of C3H sublines and their tumors. *Ann. N.Y. Acad. Sci. 71*:1009–1021, 1958.

Amos, D. B.: Some iso-antigenic systems of the mouse. *Proc. 3rd Canad. Cancer Res. Conf. 3*:241–258, 1959.

Amos, D. B.: Isoantigens of mouse red cells. *Ann. N.Y. Acad. Sci. 97*:69–82, 1962.

Amos, D. B., Gorer, P. A., Mikulska, B. M., Billingham, R. E., and Sparrow, E. M.: An antibody response to skin homografts in mice. *Brit. J. Exp. Pathol. 35*:203–208, 1954.

Amos, D. B., Gorer, P. A., and Mikulska, Z. B.: An analysis of an antigenic system in the mouse (the H-2 system). *Proc. Roy. Soc. (London) B 144*:369–380, 1955.

Amos, D. B., Haughton, G., and Spencer, R. A.: A serological analysis and comparison of various preparations of mouse H-2 histocompatibility antigen. *Immunology 6*:370–381, 1963a.

Amos, D. B., Zumpft, M., and Armstrong, P.: H-5.A and H-6.A, two mouse iso-antigens on red cells and tissues detected serologically. *Transplantation 1*:270–283, 1963b.

Amos, D. B., Cohen, I., and Klein, W. J., Jr.: Mechanisms of immunologic enhancement. *Transplant. Proc. 2*:68–69, 1970.

Anderson, P. K.: Lethal alleles in *Mus musculus*: Local distribution and evidence for isolation of demes. *Science 145*:177–178, 1964.

Anderson, P. K.: The role of breeding structure in evolutionary processes of *Mus musculus* populations. In *Mutation in Population*. Proc. Symp. on the Mutational Process, R. Hončariv (ed.), pp. 17–21, Academia, Praha, 1966.

Anderson, P. K.: Ecological structure and gene flow in small mammals. In *Variation in Mammalian Populations*. Symp. Zool. Soc. London No. 26, R. J. Berry and H. N. Southern (eds.), pp. 299–325, Academic Press, New York, 1970.

Anderson, P. K., Dunn, L. C., and Beasley, A. B.: Introduction of a lethal allele into a feral house mouse population. *Amer. Nat. 98*:57–64, 1964.

Andersson, B., Wigzell, H., and Klein, G.: Some characteristics of 19S and 7S mouse isoantibodies *in vivo* and *in vitro*. *Transplantation 5*:11–20, 1967.

Andrzejewski, R., Petrusewicz, K., and Walkowa, W.: Preliminary report on results obtained with a living trap in a confined population of mice. *Bul. Acad. Pol. Sci. 7*:367–370, 1959.

Aoki, T., Boyse, E. A., and Old, L. J.: Occurrence of natural antibody to the G (Gross) leukemia antigen in mice. *Cancer Res. 26*:1415–1419, 1966.

Aoki, T., Izard, J., Hämmerling, U., deHarven, E., and Old, L. J.: Ferritin-conjugated antibody for the demonstration of isoantigens on the surface of murine cells. In *Proc. 26th Ann. Meeting Electron Micros. Soc. America*, C. J. Arceneaux (ed.), pp. 48–49, Claitor's Publ. Div., Baton Rouge, La., 1968.

Aoki, T., Hämmerling, U., deHarven, E., Boyse, E. A., and Old, L. J.: Antigenic structure of cell surfaces. An immunoferritin study of the occurrence and topography of H-2, θ and TL alloantigens on mouse cells. *J. Exp. Med. 130*:979–1001, 1969.

Aoki, T., Boyse, E. A., Old, L. J., deHarven, E., Hämmerling, U., and Wood, H. A.: G(Gross) and H-2 cell-surface antigens: Location on Gross leukemia cells by electron microscopy with visually labeled antibody. *Proc. Nat. Acad. Sci. USA 65*:569–576, 1970.

Aoki, T., McKenzie, I. F. C., Sturm, M. M., and Liu, M.: Distribution of the allo-antigen Ly-4.2 on murine B-cells. *Immunogenetics 1*:291–296, 1974.

Apt, A. S., Blandova, Z., Dishkant, I., Shumova, T., Vedernikov, A. A., and Egorov, I. K.: Study of *H-2* mutations in mice. IV. A comparison of the mutants M505 and Hzl by skin grafting and serological techniques. *Immunogenetics*, 1974 (*in press*).

Asantila, T., Vahala, J., and Toivanen, P.: Response of human fetal lymphocytes in xenogeneic mixed leukocyte culture: Phylogenetic and ontogenetic aspects. *Immunogenetics 1*:272–290, 1974.

Ax, A., Koren, H. S., and Fischer, H.: Cytotoxicity of allogeneic lymphocytes sensitized against H-2 antigens *in vitro*. *Exp. Cell Res. 64*:439–449, 1971.

Axelrad, A., and Steeves, R. A.: Assay for Friend leukemia virus: Rapid quantitative method based on enumeration of macroscopic spleen foci in mice. *Virology 24*:513–518, 1964.

Axelrad, A., and Van der Gaag, H. C.: Genetic and cellular basis of susceptibility or resistance to Friend leukemia virus infection in mice. *Proc. 8th Canad. Cancer Res. Conf. 8*:313–343, 1969.

Bach, F., and Hirschhorn, K.: Lymphocyte interaction: A potential histocompatibility test *in vitro*. *Science 143*:813–814, 1964.

Bach, F. H., Widmer, M. B., Segall, M., Bach, M. L., and Klein, J.: Genetic and immunological complexity of major histocompatibility regions. *Science 176*:1024–1037, 1972a.

Bach, F. H., Widmer, M. B., Bach, M. L., and Klein, J.: Serologically defined and lymphocyte-defined components of the major histocompatibility complex in the mouse. *J. Exp. Med. 136*:1420–1444, 1972b.

Bach, F. H., Segall, M., Zier, K. S., Sondel, P. M., and Alter, B. J.: Cell mediated immunity: Separation of cells involved in recognitive and destructive phases. *Science 180*:403–406, 1973a.

Bach, M. L., Widmer, M. B., Bach, F. H., and Klein, J.: Mixed leukocyte cultures and immune response region disparity. *Transplant. Proc. 5*:369–375, 1973b.

Bachman, K.: Genome size in mammals. *Chromosoma 37*:85–93, 1972.

Bailey, D. W.: Histoincompatibility associated with the X chromosome in mice. *Transplantation 1*: 70–74, 1963.

Bailey, D. W.: Heritable histocompatibility changes: Lysogeny in mice? *Transplantation 4*:482–487, 1966.

Bailey, D. W.: The vastness and organization of the murine histocompatibility-gene system as inferred from mutational data. In *Advances in Transplantation*, J. Dausset, J. Hamburger, and G. Mathé (eds.), pp. 317–323, Munksgaard, Copenhagen, 1968.

Bailey, D. W.: Private communication. *Mouse News Letter 41*:30, 1969.

Bailey, D. W.: Four approaches to estimating number of histocompatibility loci. *Transplant. Proc. 2*:32–38, 1970.

Bailey, D. W.: Recombinant-inbred strains, an aid to finding identity, linkage, and function of histocompatibility and other genes. *Transplantation 11*:325–327, 1971a.

Bailey, D. W.: Cumulative effect or independent effect? *Transplantation 11*:419–422, 1971b.

Bailey, D. W.: Allelic forms of a gene controlling the female immune response to the male antigen in mice. *Transplantation 11*:426–428, 1971c.

Bailey, D. W., and Hoste, J.: A gene governing the female immune response to the male antigen in mice. *Transplantation 11*:404–407, 1971.

Bailey, D. W., and Kohn, H. I.: Inherited histocompatibility changes in progeny of irradiated and unirradiated inbred mice. *Genet. Res. (Camb.)* 6:330–340, 1965.

Bailey, D. W., and Mobraaten, L. E.: Estimates of the number of loci contributing to the histoincompatibility between C57BL/6 and BALB/c strains of mice. *Transplantation 7*:394–400, 1969.

Bailey, D. W., and Usama, B.: A rapid method of grafting skin on tails of mice. *Transplant. Bull. 7*:424–425, 1960.

Bailey, D. W., Snell, G. D., and Cherry, M.: Complementation and serological analysis of an H-2 mutant. In *Immunogenetics of the H-2 System*, A. Lengerová and M. Vojtíšková (eds.), pp. 155–162, Karger, Basel, 1971.

Bain, B., Vaz, M. R., and Lowenstein, L.: The development of large immature mononuclear cells in mixed lymphocyte cultures. *Blood 23*:108–116, 1964.

Baldwin, W. M., III, and Cohen, N.: "Weak" histocompatibility antigens generate functionally "strong" humoral immunity. *Immunogenetics 1*:33–44, 1974.

Balner, H., Dersjant, H., van Vreeswijk, W., van Leeuwen, A., and van Rood, J. J.: Identification of chimpanzee leukocyte antigens (ChL-A) and their relation to HL-A. *Transplantation 11*:309–317, 1971a.

Balner, H., Gabb, B. W., Dersjant, H., van Vreeswijk, W., and van Rood, J. J.: Major histocompatibility locus of rhesus monkeys (RhL-A). *Nature New Biol. 230*:177–180, 1971b.

Barnes, A. D.: A quantitative comparison study of immunizing ability of different tissues. *Ann. N.Y. Acad. Sci. 120*:237–250, 1964.

Barnes, A. D., and Krohn, P. L.: The estimation of the number of histocompatibility genes controlling the successful transplantation of normal skin in mice. *Proc. Roy. Soc. (London) B 146*:505–526, 1957.

Barth, R. F., and Russell, P. S.: The antigenic specificity of spermatozoa. I. An immunofluorescent study of the histocompatibility antigens of mouse sperm. *J. Immunol. 93*:13–19, 1964.

Barth, R. F., Espmark, J. A., and Fagraeus, A.: Histocompatibility and tumor virus antigens identified on cells grown in tissue culture by means of the mixed hemadsorption reaction. *J. Immunol. 98*:888–892, 1967.

Basch, R. S., and Stetson, C. A.: The relationship between hemagglutinogens and histocompatibility antigens in the mouse. *Ann. N.Y. Acad. Sci. 97*:83–94, 1962.

Basch, R. S., and Stetson, C. A.: Quantitative studies on histocompatibility antigens of the mouse. *Transplantation 1*:469–480, 1963.

Batchelor, J. R.: Complement-fixing isoantibodies in mice. *Immunology 3*:174–178, 1960.

Batchelor, J. R., and Brent, L.: Histocompatibility in transplantation immunity. In *Immunogenicity*, F. Borek (ed.), pp. 409–451, North-Holland, Amsterdam, 1972.

Bateman, N.: High frequency of a lethal gene (t^e) in a laboratory stock of mice. *Genet. Res. (Camb.) 1*:214–225, 1960a.

Bateman, N.: Selective fertilization at the T-locus of the mouse. *Genet. Res. (Camb.) 1*:226–238, 1960b.

Bayreuther, K., and Klein, E.: Cytogenetic, serologic, and transplantation studies on a heterozygous tumor and its derived variant sublines. *J. Nat. Cancer Inst. 21*:885–923, 1958.

Bechtol, K. B., Wegmann, T. G., Freed, J. H., Grumet, F. C., Chesebro, B. W.,

Herzenberg, L. A., and McDevitt, H. O.: Genetic control of the immune response to (T,G)-A--L in C3H ↔ C57 tetraparental mice. *Cell. Immunol. 13*:264–277, 1974.

Benacerraf, B.: The genetic control of specific immune responses. *Harvey Lectures 67*:109–141, 1973.

Benacerraf, B., and Katz, D. H.: The histocompatibility linked immune response genes. *Adv. Cancer Res.*, 1974 (*in press*).

Benacerraf, B., and McDevitt, H. O.: Histocompatibility-linked immune response genes. *Science 175*:273–279, 1972.

Bennett, D.: Embryological effects of lethal alleles in the t-region. *Science 144*:263–267, 1964.

Bennett, D.: The karyotype of the mouse, with identification of the translocation. *Proc. Nat. Acad. Sci. USA 53*:730–737, 1965.

Bennett, D., and Dunn, L. C.: Effects on embryonic development of a group of genetically similar lethal alleles derived from different populations of wild house mice. *J. Morphol. 103*:135–157, 1958.

Bennett, D., and Dunn, L. C.: A lethal mutant (t^{w18}) in the house mouse showing partial duplications. *J. Exp. Zool. 143*:203–219, 1960.

Bennett, D., and Dunn, L. C.: Studies of effects of t-alleles in the house mouse on spermatozoa. I. Male sterility effects. *J. Reprod. Fert. 13*:421–428, 1967.

Bennett, D., and Dunn, L. C.: Genetical and embryological comparisons of semilethal t-alleles from wild mouse populations. *Genetics 61*:411–422, 1969.

Bennett, D., and Dunn, L. C.: Transmission ratio distorting genes on chromosome IX and their interactions. In *Immunogenetics of the H-2 System*, A. Lengerová and M. Vojtíšková (eds.), pp. 90–103, Karger, Basel, 1971.

Bennett, D., Dunn, L. C., and Badenhausen, S.: A second group of similar lethals in populations of wild house mice. *Genetics 44*:795–802, 1959.

Bennett, D., Boyse, E. A., and Old, L. J.: Cell surface immunogenetics in the study of morphogenesis. In *Cell Interactions*, Third Lepetit Colloquium, L. G. Silvestri (ed.), pp. 247–263, North-Holland, Amsterdam, 1972a.

Bennett, D., Goldberg, E., Dunn, L. C., and Boyse, E. A.: Serological detection of a cell-surface antigen specified by the T (brachyury) mutant gene in the house mouse. *Proc. Nat. Acad. Sci. USA 69*:2076–2080, 1972b.

Bennett, M.: Rejection of marrow allografts. Importance of H-2 homozygosity of donor cells. *Transplantation 14*:289–298, 1972.

Bennett, M., Steeves, R. A., Cudkowicz, G., Mirand, E. A., and Russell, L. B.: Mutant Sl alleles of mice affect susceptibility to Friend spleen focus-forming virus. *Science 162*:564–565, 1968.

Bennett, W. I., Gall, A. M., Southard, J. L., and Sidman, R. L.: Abnormal spermiogenesis in quaking, a myelin-deficient mutant mouse. *Biol. Reprod. 5*:30–58, 1971.

Berg, K.: Compositional relatedness between histocompatibility antigens and human serum lipoproteins. *Science 172*:1136–1138, 1971.

Berg, K., Ceppellini, R., Curtoni, E. S., Mattiuz, P. L., and Bearn, A. G.: The genetic antigenic polymorphism of human serum β-lipoprotein and survival of skin grafts. In *Advance in Transplantation*, J. Dausset, J. Hamburger, and G. Mathé (eds.), pp. 253–255, Williams & Wilkins, Baltimore, 1968.

Berke, G., and Amos, D. B.: Cytotoxic lymphocytes in the absence of detectable antibody. *Nature New Biol. 242*:237–239, 1973.

Berke, G., and Levey, R. H.: Cellular immunoabsorbents in transplantation immunity:

Specific *in vitro* deletion and recovery of mouse lymphoid cells sensitized against allogeneic tumors. *J. Exp. Med. 135*:972–984, 1972.

Berke, G., Ax, W., Ginsburg, H., and Feldman, M.: Graft reaction in tissue culture II. Quantification of the lytic action on mouse fibroblasts by rat lymphocytes sensitized on mouse embryo monolayers. *Immunology 16*:643–657, 1969.

Berrian, J. H., and Jacobs, R. L.: Diversity of transplantation antigens in the mouse. In *Biological Problems of Grafting*, F. Albert and P. B. Medawar (eds.), pp. 131–143, Blackwell, Oxford, 1959.

Berrian, J. H., and McKhann, C. F.: Transplantation immunity involving the *H-3* locus: Graft survival times. *J. Nat. Cancer Inst. 25*:111–123, 1960.

Billingham, R. E.: The biology of graft-versus-host reactions. *Harvey Lectures 62*: 21–78, 1968.

Billingham, R. E., and Medawar, P. B.: The technique of free skin grafting in mammals. *J. Exp. Biol. 28*:385–402, 1951.

Billingham, R. E., and Silvers, W. K. (eds.): *Transplantation of Tissues and Cells.* Wistar Institute Press, Philadelphia, 1961.

Billingham, R. E., Brent, L., Medawar, P. B., and Sparrow, E. M.: Quantitative studies on tissue transplantation immunity. I. The survival times of skin homografts exchanged between members of different inbred strains of mice. *Proc. Roy. Soc. (London) B 143*:43–58, 1954.

Billingham, R. E., Brent, L., and Medawar, P. B.: The antigenic stimulus in transplantation immunity. *Nature 178*:514–519, 1956.

Billingham, R. E., Brent, L., and Medawar, P. B.: Extraction of antigens causing transplantation immunity. *Transplant. Bull. 5*:377–381, 1958.

Billington, W. D.: Influence of immunological dissimilarity of mother and foetus on size of placenta in mice. *Nature 202*:317–318, 1964.

Bittner, J. J.: The transplantation of splenic tissue in mice. *Publ. Hlth. Rep. Wash. 51*:244–247, 1936.

Bittner, J. J.: The genetics of cancer in mice. *Quart. Rev. Biol. 13*:51–64, 1938.

Bittner, J. J.: The causes and control of mammary cancer in mice. *Harvey Lectures 42*:221–246, 1947.

Bjaring, B., and Klein, G.: Antigenic characterization of heterozygous mouse lymphomas after immunoselection *in vivo. J. Nat. Cancer Inst. 41*:1411–1429, 1968.

Bjaring, B., Klein, G., and Popp, I.: Cyclic variations in the H-2 isoantigenic expression of mouse lymphoma cells *in vitro. Transplantation 8*:38–43, 1969.

Bjaring, B., Bregula, U., Klein, G., and Levan, A.: Antigenic studies on mouse lymphomas bearing the T190 translocation chromosome. *J. Nat. Cancer Inst. 45*:921–935, 1970.

Blandova, Z. K., Shumova, T. E., Kryshkina, V. P., and Egorov, I. K.: Complementation study of three mutant alleles at the H-2 locus. In *Biology of the Laboratory Animals*, V. A. Dushkin (ed.), pp. 53–55, Acad. Med. Sci. USSR, Moscow, 1972. (In Russian).

Blankenhorn, E. P., and Douglas, T. C.: Location of the gene for theta antigen in the mouse. *J. Hered. 63*:259–263, 1972.

Blomgren, H., and Andersson, B.: Cross-reactivity patterns of mouse lymphocytes sensitized against the major histocompatibility complex using a graft-versus-host assay. *Cell. Immunol. 11*:122–129, 1974.

Bodmer, W. F.: Evolutionary significance of the HL-A system. *Nature 237*:139–145, 1972.

Bonmassar, E., Goldin, A., and Cudkowicz, G.: Differential reactivity of mice to alloantigens associated with the D and K end of H-2. Preliminary studies with bone marrow and lymphoma grafts. *Transplantation 12*:314–318, 1971.

Borges, P. R. F., and Kvedar, B. J.: A mutation producing resistance to several transplantable neoplasms in the C57 black strain of mice. *Cancer Res. 12*:19–24, 1952.

Borges, P. R. F., Kvedar, B. J., and Forester, G. E.: The development of an isogenic subline of mice (C57BL/6-H-2^d) resistant to transplantable neoplasms indigenous to strain C57BL. *J. Nat. Cancer Inst. 15*:341–346, 1954.

Borovská, M., Kořínek, J., Václavíková, I., and Démant, P.: Ss protein: Search for cross-reacting substances in different species. *Folia Biol. (Praha) 17*:283–285, 1971.

Boubelík, M., and Lengerová, A.: Genetic control of developmental expression of H-2 antigens. In *Proc. Symp. Immunogenetics of the H-2 System*, A. Lengerová and M. Vojtíšková (eds.), pp. 85–89, Karger, Basel, 1971.

Boyle, W.: An extension of the ^{51}Cr-release assay for the estimation of mouse cytotoxins. *Transplantation 6*:761–764, 1968.

Boyse, E. A., and Old, L. J.: Some aspects of normal and abnormal cell surface genetics. *Ann. Rev. Genetics 3*:269–290, 1969.

Boyse, E. A., Old, L. J., and Thomas, G.: A report on some observations with a simplified cytotoxic test. *Transplant. Bull. 29*:436–439, 1962.

Boyse, E. A., Old, L. J., and Luell, S.: Antigenic properties of experimental leukemias. II. Immunological studies *in vivo* with C57BL/6 radiation-induced leukemias. *J. Nat. Cancer Inst. 3*:987–995, 1963.

Boyse, E. A., Old, L. J., and Chouroulinkov, I.: Cytotoxic test for demonstration of mouse antibody. *Meth. Med. Res. 10*:39–47, 1964a.

Boyse, E. A., Old, L. J., and Luell, S.: Genetic determination of the TL (Thymus-leukemia) antigen in the mouse. *Nature 201*:779, 1964b.

Boyse, E. A., Old, L. J., and Stockert, E.: The TL (thymus leukemia) antigen: A review. In *Immunopathology*, 4th Internat. Symposium, P. Grabar and P. A. Miescher (eds.), pp. 23–40, Schwabe, Basel, 1966.

Boyse, E. A., Stockert, E., and Old, L. J.: Modification of the antigenic structure of the cell membrane by thymus-leukemia (TL) antibody. *Proc. Nat. Acad. Sci. USA 58*:954–957, 1967.

Boyse, E. A., Old, L. J., and Stockert, E.: An approach to the mapping of antigens on the cell surface. *Proc. Nat. Acad. Sci. USA 60*:886–893, 1968a.

Boyse, E. A., Stockert, E., and Old, L. J.: Isoantigens of the H-2 and Tla loci of the mouse. Interactions affecting their representation on thymocytes. *J. Exp. Med. 128*:85–95, 1968b.

Boyse, E. A., Stockert, E., and Old, L. J.: Properties of four antigens specified by the *Tla* locus. Similarities and differences. In *International Convocation on Immunology*, N. R. Rose and F. Milgrom (eds.), pp. 353–357, Basel, S. Karger, 1968c.

Boyse, E. A., Miyazawa, M., Aoki, T., and Old, L. J.: Ly-A and Ly-B: Two systems of lymphocyte isoantigens in the mouse. *Proc. Roy. Soc. (London) B 170*:175–193, 1968d.

Boyse, E. A., Stockert, E., Iritani, C. A., and Old, L. J.: Implications of TL phenotype changes in an H-2 loss variant of a transplanted H-2^b/H-2^a leukemia. *Proc. Nat. Acad. Sci. USA 65*:933–938, 1970.

Boyse, E. A., Itakura, K., Stockert, E., Iritani, C., and Miura, M.: Ly-C: A third locus specifying alloantigens expressed only on thymocytes and lymphocytes. *Transplantation* *11*:351–352, 1971.

Boyse, E. A., Flaherty, L., Stockert, E., and Old, L. J.: Histoincompatibility attributable to genes near H-2 that are not revealed by hemagglutination or cytotoxic tests. *Transplantation* *13*:431–432, 1972.

Braden, A. W. H.: Influence of time of mating on the segregation ratio of alleles at the T locus in the house mouse. *Nature* *181*:786–787, 1958.

Braden, A. W. H.: Genetic influences on the morphology and function of the gametes. *J. Cell. Comp. Physiol.* *56*:17–29, 1960.

Braden, A. W. H.: T-locus in mice, segregation distortion and sterility in the male. In *The Genetics of the Spermatozoon*, R. A. Beatty and S. Gluecksohn-Waelsch (eds.), pp. 289–305, Edinburgh, 1972.

Braden, A. W. H., and Gluecksohn-Waelsch, S.: Further studies of the effect of the T locus in the house mouse on male sterility. *J. Exp. Zool.* *138*:431–452, 1958.

Braden, A. W. H., and Weiler, H.: Transmission ratios at the T-locus in the mouse: Inter- and intra-male heterogeneity. *Austral. J. Biol. Sci.* *17*:921–934, 1964.

Braden, A. W. H., Erickson, R. P., Gluecksohn-Waelsch, S., Hartl, D. L., Peacock, W. J., and Sandler, L.: A comparison of effects and properties of segregation distorting alleles in the mouse (t) and in *Drosophila* (*SD*). In *The Genetics of the Spermatozoon*, R. A. Beatty and S. Gluecksohn-Waelsch (eds.), pp. 310–312, Edinburgh, 1972.

Brambilla, G., Cavanna, M., Parodi, S., and Baldini, L.: Time dependence of the number of histocompatibility loci in skin graft rejection of mice. *Experientia* *26*:1140–1141, 1970.

Brent, L., Medawar, P. B., and Ruszkiewicz, M.: Serological methods in the study of transplantation antigens. *Brit. J. Exp. Path.* *42*:464–477, 1961.

Brent, L., Medawar, P. B., and Ruszkiewicz, M.: Studies on transplantation antigens. In *Ciba Foundation Symposium on Transplantation*, G. E. W. Wolstenholme and M. P. Cameron (eds.), pp. 6–20, Churchill, London, 1962.

Brondz, B. D.: Interaction of immune lymphocytes with normal and neoplastic tissue cells. *Folia Biol.* (*Praha*) *10*:164–176, 1964.

Brondz, B. D.: Relationship between humoral and cellular isoantibodies. I. Inability of humoral isoantibodies to prevent the cytotoxic effect of immune lymphocytes. *Transplantation* *3*:356–367, 1965.

Brondz, B. D.: On the mechanism of the cytotoxic effect of immune lymphocytes on homologous tissue cells *in vivo*. *J. Gen. Biol.* *27*:80–88, 1966. (In Russian).

Brondz, B. D.: Complex specificity of immune lymphocytes in allogeneic cell cultures. *Folia Biol.* (*Praha*) *14*:115–125, 1968a.

Brondz, B. D.: Immunological specificity of cell-bound antibodies in the cultures of allogeneic target cells. In *Advance in Transplantation*, J. Dausset, J. Hamburger, and G. Mathé (eds.), pp. 47–53, Williams & Wilkins, Baltimore, 1968b.

Brondz, B. D.: Lymphocyte receptors and mechanisms of *in vitro* cell-mediated immune reactions. *Transplant. Rev.* *10*:112–151, 1972.

Brondz, B. D., and Golberg, N. E.: Further *in vitro* evidence for polyvalent specificity of immune lymphocytes. *Folia Biol.* (*Praha*) *16*:20–28, 1970.

Brondz, B. D., and Snegiröva, A. E.: Interaction of immune lymphocytes with the mixtures of target cells possessing selected specificities of the H-2 immunizing allele. *Immunology* *20*:457–468, 1971.

Brondz, B. D., Snegiröva, A. E., Rasulin, Y. A., and Shamborant, O. G.: Effect of some enzymes, polysaccharides and lysosome-active drugs on interaction of immune lymphocytes with allogeneic target cells. In *Progress in Immunology*, D. B. Amos (ed.), pp. 447–460, Academic Press, New York, 1971.

Brown, J. L., Kato, K., Silver, J., and Nathenson, S. G.: Notable diversity in peptide composition of murine H-2K and H-2D alloantigens. *Biochemistry 13*:3174–3178, 1974.

Brown, R. Z.: Social behaviour, reproduction and population changes in the house mouse (*Mus musculus L.*). *Ecol. Monogr. 36*:627–634, 1953.

Bruck, D.: Male segregation ratio advantage as a factor in maintaining lethal alleles in wild populations of house mice. *Proc. Nat. Acad. Sci. USA 43*:152–158, 1957.

Bruell, J. H.: Behavioral population genetics and wild *Mus musculus*. In *Contributions to Behavior-Genetic Analysis. The Mouse as a Prototype*, G. Lindzey and D. D. Thiessen (eds.), pp. 261–291, Appleton-Century-Crofts, New York, 1970.

Brunner, K. T., Mauel, J., and Schindler, R.: *In vitro* studies of cell-bound immunity; cloning assay of the cytotoxic action of sensitized lymphoid cells on allogeneic target cells. *Immunology 11*:499–506, 1966.

Brunner, K. T., Mauel, J., Cerottini, J. C., and Chapius, B.: Quantitative assay of the lytic action of immune lymphoid cells on ^{51}Cr-labelled allogeneic target cells *in vitro*; inhibition by isoantibody and by drugs. *Immunology 14*:181–196, 1968.

Brunner, K. T., Mauel, J., Rudolf, H., and Chapius, B.: Studies of allograft immunity in mice. I. Induction, development and *in vitro* assay of cellular immunity. *Immunology 18*:501–515, 1970.

Bryson, V.: Spermatogenesis and fertility in *Mus musculus* as affected by factors at the T locus. *J. Morph. 74*:131–187, 1944.

Buckland, R. A., Evans, H. J., and Sumner, A. T.: Identifying mouse chromosomes with the ASG technique. *Exp. Cell. Res. 69*:231–236, 1971.

Burnet, F. M.: *Immunological Surveillance*. Pergamon Press, Oxford, 1970a.

Burnet, F. M.: A certain symmetry: Histocompatibility antigens compared with immunocyte receptors. *Nature 226*:123–126, 1970b.

Burnet, F. M.: Multiple polymorphism in relation to histocompatibility antigens. *Nature 245*:359–361, 1973.

Calarco, P. G., and Brown, E. H.: Cytological and ultrastructural comparisons of t^{12}/t^{12} and normal mouse morulae. *J. Exp. Zool. 168*:196–186, 1968.

Cann, H. M., and Herzenberg, L. A.: *In vitro* studies of mammalian somatic cell variation. I. Detection of H-2 phenotype in cultured mouse cell lines. *J. Exp. Med. 117*:259–265, 1963a.

Cann, H. M., and Herzenberg, L. A.: *In vitro* studies of mammalian somatic cell variation. II. Isoimmune cytotoxicity with a cultured mouse lymphoma and selection of resistant variants. *J. Exp. Med. 117*:267–283, 1963b.

Cantrell, J. L., and Hildemann, W. H.: Characteristics of disparate histocompatibility barriers in congenic strains of mice I. Graft-versus-host reactions. *Transplantation 14*:761–770, 1972.

Capaldi, R. A., and Green, D. E.: Membrane proteins and membrane structure. *FEBS Letters 25*:205–209, 1972.

Čapková, J., and Démant, P.: Two new H-2 specificities: H-2.44 and H-2.45. *Folia Biol. (Praha) 18*:231–236, 1972.

Carter, T. C., and Phillips, R. S.: Three recurrences of mutants in the house mouse. *J. Hered. 41*:252, 1950.

Carter, T. C., Lyon, M. F., and Phillips, R. J. S.: Gene-tagged chromosome translocations in eleven stocks of mice. *J. Genetics 53*:154–166, 1955.

Carter, T. C., Lyon, M. F., and Phillips, R. J. S.: Further genetic studies of eleven
translocations in the mouse. *J. Genetics 54*:462–473, 1956.

Caspari, E., and David, P. R.: The inheritance of a tail abnormality in the house
mouse. *J. Hered. 31*:427–431, 1940.

Castermans, A.: *Étude des Antigènes de Transplantation Présénts Dans Les Cellules
Spléniques et Thymiques.* Éditions Arscia, Brussels, 1961.

Castermans, A., and Oth, A.: Transplantation immunity: Separation of antigenic
components from isolated nuclei. *Nature 184*:1224–1225, 1959.

Castermans, A., Philippart, F., Haenen, A. M., Lejeune, G., and Dieu, H.: Transplantation antigens extracted from normal mouse tissue. In *Immunopathology*,
4th Int. Symp., P. Grabar and P. Miescher (eds.), pp. 119–133, Schwabe, Basel,
1965.

Cavalli-Sforza, L. L., and Bodmer, W. F.: *The Genetics of Human Populations*,
Freeman, San Francisco, 1971.

Celada, F., and Rotman, B.: A fluorochromatic test for immunocytotoxicity against
tumor cells and leucocytes in agarose plates. *Proc. Nat. Acad. Sci. USA 57*:630–
636, 1967.

Celada, F., and Welshons, W. J.: Demonstration of F_1 hybrid antiparent immunological reaction. *Proc. Nat. Acad. Sci. USA 48*:326–331, 1962.

Cerottini, J-C., and Brunner, K. T.: Localization of mouse isoantigens on the cell
surface as revealed by immunofluorescence. *Immunology 13*:395–403, 1967.

Cerottini, J-C., and Brunner, K. T.: Cell-mediated cytotoxicity, allograft rejection,
and tumor immunity. *Adv. Immunol. 18*:67–132, 1974.

Cerottini, J-C., Nordin, A. A., and Brunner, K. T.: Competence of various cell populations for humoral and cell-mediated transplantation immunity. In *Immunopathology VIth International Symposium*, P. A. Miescher (ed.), pp. 97–107, Grune
& Stratton, New York, 1970.

Cerottini, J-C., Nordin, A. A., and Brunner, K. T.: Cellular and humoral response
to transplantation antigens. *J. Exp. Med. 134*:553–564, 1971.

Chai, C. K.: Genetic studies of histocompatibility in rabbits: Identification of major
and minor genes. *Immunogenetics 1*:126–132, 1974.

Chai, C. K., and Chiang, M. S. M.: A method of estimating the number of histocompatibility loci in a sib-mating mouse population. *Genetics 48*:1153–1161, 1963.

Chard, R.: Immunological enhancement by mouse isoantibodies: The importance of
complement fixation. *Immunology 14*:583–589, 1968.

Charlton, R. K., and Zmijewski, C. M.: Soluble HL-A7 antigen: Localization in the
β-lipoprotein fraction of human serum. *Science 170*:636–637, 1970.

Cheers, C., and Sprent, J.: B lymphocytes as stimulators of a mixed lymphocyte
reaction. *Transplantation 15*:336–337, 1973.

Cherry, M., and Snell, G. D.: A description of mu: a non-H-2 alloantigen in C3H/Sn
mice. *Transplantation 8*:319–327, 1969.

Cherry, M., Hilgert, I., Kandutsch, A. A., and Snell, G. D.: Effects of proteolytic
enzymes on murine H-2 antigens. *Transplant. Proc. 2*:48–58, 1970.

Chesebro, B. W., Mitchell, G. F., Grumet, F. C., Herzenberg, L. A., and McDevitt,
H. O.: Analysis of cell transfer studies in a genetic control of the immune response
in mice. In *Cellular Interactions in the Immune Response*, S. Cohen, G. Cudkowicz,
and R. T. McCluskey (eds.), pp. 83–92, Karger, Basel, 1971.

Chesebro, B. W., Mitchell, G. F., Grumet, F. C., Herzenberg, L. A., McDevitt, H. O., and Wegmann, T. G.: Cell transfer in a genetically controlled immune response. *Eur. J. Immunol. 2*:243–248, 1972.

Chesley, P.: Development of the short-tailed mutant in the house mouse. *J. Exp. Zool. 70*:429–455, 1935.

Chesley, P., and Dunn, L. C.: The inheritance of taillessness (anury) in the house mouse. *Genetics 21*:525–536, 1936.

Chutná, J., and Hašková, V.: Antigenicity of embryonic tissues in homotransplantation. *Folia Biol. (Praha) 5*:85–88, 1959.

Cikes, M.: Antigenic expression of a murine lymphoma during growth *in vitro*. *Nature 225*:645–647, 1970a.

Cikes, M.: Relationship between growth rate, cell volume, cell cycle kinetics and antigenic properties of cultured murine lymphoma cells. *J. Nat. Cancer Inst. 45*:979–988, 1970b.

Cikes, M.: Variations in expression of surface antigens on cultured cells. *Ann. N.Y. Acad. Sci. 177*:190–200, 1971a.

Cikes, M.: Expression of surface antigens on cultured tumor cells in relation to cell cycle. *Transplant. Proc. 3*:1161–1166, 1971b.

Cikes, M., and Friberg, S., Jr.: Expression of H-2 and Moloney leukemia virus-determined cell-surface antigens in synchronized cultures of a mouse cell line. *Proc. Nat. Acad. Sci. USA 68*:566–569, 1971.

Cikes, M., and Klein, G.: Quantitative studies of antigen expression in cultured murine lymphoma cells. I. Cell-surface antigens in "asynchronous" cultures. *J. Nat. Cancer Inst. 49*:1599–1606, 1972a.

Cikes, M., and Klein, G.: Effects of inhibitors of protein and nucleic acid synthesis on the expression of H-2 and Moloney leukemia virus-determined cell-surface antigens on cultured murine lymphoma cells. *J. Nat. Cancer Inst. 48*:509–515, 1972b.

Cikes, M., Friberg, S., Jr., and Klein, G.: Quantitative studies of antigen expression in cultured murine lymphoma cells. II. Cell-surface antigens in synchronized cultures. *J. Nat. Cancer Inst. 49*:1607–1611, 1972.

Claman, H. N., Chaperon, E. A., and Triplett, R. F.: Thymus-marrow cell combinations. Synergism in antibody production. *Proc. Soc. Exp. Biol. Med. 122*:1167–1171, 1966.

Clarke, B., and Kirby, D. R. S.: Maintenance of histocompatibility polymorphisms. *Nature 211*:999–1000, 1966.

Cohen, I. R., Globerson, A., and Feldman, M.: Autosensitization *in vitro*. *J. Exp. Med. 133*:834–845, 1971.

Cooper, S., and Lance, E. M.: A serological method for detecting the surface antigens of epidermal cells. *Transplantation 11*:108–109, 1971.

Corry, R. J., Winn, H. J., and Russell, P. S.: Heart transplantation in congenic strains of mice. *Transplant. Proc. 5*:733–735, 1973.

Counce, S., Smith, P., Barth, R., and Snell, G. D.: Strong and weak histocompatibility gene differences in mice and their role in the rejection of homografts of tumors and skin. *Ann. Surg. 144*:198–204, 1956.

Cresswell, P., and Sanderson, A. R.: Spatial arrangement of H-2 specificities: Evidence from antibody adsorption and kinetic studies. *Transplantation 6*:996–1004, 1968.

Cresswell, P., Turner, M. J., and Strominger, J. L.: Papain-solubilized HL-A antigens from cultured human lymphocytes contain two peptide fragments. *Proc. Nat. Acad. Sci. USA 70*:1603–1607, 1973.

Crippa, M.: The mouse karyotype in somatic cells cultured *in vitro. Chromosoma 15*:301–311, 1964.

Crowcroft, P.: Territoriality in wild house mice, *Mus musculus L. J. Mammal. 36*:299–301, 1955.

Crowcroft, P.: *Mice All Over.* Dufour Editions, Chester Springs, Pa., 1966.

Crowcroft, P., and Jeffers, J. N. R.: Variability in the behaviour of wild house mice (*Mus musculus L.*) towards live traps. *Proc. Zool. Soc. London 137*:573–582, 1961.

Crowcroft, P., and Rowe, F. P.: The growth of confined colonies of the wild house mouse (*Mus musculus L.*). *Proc. Zool. Soc. London 129*:359–370, 1957.

Crowcroft, P., and Rowe, F. P.: The growth of confined colonies of the wild house mouse (*Mus musculus L.*): The effect of dispersal on female fecundity. *Proc. Zool. Soc. London 131*:357–365, 1958.

Crowcroft, P., and Rowe, F. P.: Social organization and territorial behaviour in the wild house mouse (*Mus musculus L.*). *Proc. Zool. Soc. London 140*:517–531, 1963.

Croy, B. A., and Osoba, D.: Nude mice and the mixed leukocyte reaction. *Transplant. Proc. 5*:1721–1723, 1973.

Cudkowicz, G.: Evidence for immunization of F_1 hybrid mice against parental transplantation antigens. *Proc. Soc. Exp. Biol. Med. 107*:968–972, 1961.

Cudkowicz, G.: The immunogenetic basis of hybrid resistance to parental bone marrow grafts. In *Isoantigens and Cell Interactions*, Joy Palm (ed.), pp. 37–56, Wistar Institute Press, Philadelphia, 1965.

Cudkowicz, G.: Hybrid resistance to parental grafts of hematopoietic and lymphoma cells. In *The Proliferation and Spread of Neoplastic Cells. XXI Ann. M.D. Anderson Symp. on Fundamental Cancer Research*, pp. 661–691, Williams & Wilkins, Baltimore, 1968.

Cudkowicz, G.: Genetic control of bone marrow graft rejection I. Determinant-specific difference of reactivity in two pairs of inbred mouse strains. *J. Exp. Med. 134*:281–293, 1971a.

Cudkowicz, G.: Genetic regulation of bone marrow allograft rejection in mice. In *Cellular Interactions in the Immune Response*, S. Cohen, G. Cudkowicz, and R. T. McCluskey (eds.), pp. 93–102, Karger, Basel, 1971b.

Cudkowicz, G., and Bennett, M.: Peculiar immunobiology of bone marrow allografts. I. Graft rejection by irradiated responder mice. *J. Exp. Med. 134*:83–102, 1971a.

Cudkowicz, G., and Bennett, M.: Peculiar immunobiology of bone marrow allografts. II. Rejection of parental grafts by resistant F_1 hybrid mice. *J. Exp. Med. 134*:1513–1528, 1971b.

Cudkowicz, G., and Lotzová, E.: Hemopoietic cell-defined components of the major histocompatibility complex of mice. Identification of responsive and unresponsive recipients for bone marrow transplants. *Transplant. Proc. 5*:1399–1405, 1973.

Cudkowicz, G., and Stimpfling, J. H.: Deficient growth of C57BL marrow cells transplanted in F_1 hybrid mice. *Immunology 7*:291–306, 1964a.

Cudkowicz, G., and Stimpfling, J. H.: Induction of immunity and of unresponsiveness to parental marrow grafts in adult F_1 hybrid mice. *Nature 204*:450–452, 1964b.

Cudkowicz, G., and Stimpfling, J. H.: Hybrid resistance to parental bone marrow grafts: Association with the *K* region of *H-2. Science 144*:1339–1340, 1964c.

Cudkowicz, G., and Stimpfling, J. H.: Hybrid resistance controlled by *H-2* region: Correction of data. *Science 147*:1056, 1965.

Cullen, S. E., and Nathenson, S. G.: Distribution of H-2 alloantigenic specificities on radiolabeled papain-solubilized antigen fragments. *J. Immunol. 107*:563–570, 1971.

Cullen, S. E., Schwartz, B. D., and Nathenson, S. G.: The distribution of alloantigenic specificities of native H-2 products. *J. Immunol. 108*:596–600, 1972a.

Cullen, S. E., Schwartz, B. D., Nathenson, S. G., and Cherry, M.: The molecular basis of codominant expression of the histocompatibility-2 genetic region. *Proc. Nat. Acad. Sci. USA 69*:1394–1397, 1972b.

Cullen, S. E., David, C. S., Shreffler, D. C., and Nathenson, S. G.: Membrane molecules determined by the *H-2*-associated immune response region: Isolation and some properties. *Proc. Nat. Acad. Sci. USA 71*:648–652, 1974.

Darbishire, A. D.: On the result of crossing Japanese waltzing with albino mice. *Biometrika 2*:282–285, 1904.

David, C. S., and Shreffler, D. C.: Studies on recombination within the H-2 complex. II. Serological analyses of four, recombinants, H-2^{al}, H-2^{ol}, H-2^{tl}, and H-2th. *Tissue Antigens 2*:241–249, 1972a.

David, C. S., and Shreffler, D. C.: Adaptation of the ^{51}Cr cytotoxic assay for rapid H-2 classifications on peripheral blood cells. *Transplantation 13*:414–420, 1972b.

David, C. S., and Shreffler, D. C.: Lymphocyte antigens controlled by the *Ir* region of the mouse *H-2* complex. Detection of new specificities with anti-H-2 reagents. *Transplantation 17*:462–469, 1974.

David, C. S., Shreffler, D. C., and Frelinger, J. A.: New lymphocyte antigen system (Lna) controlled by the *Ir* region of the mouse *H-2* complex. *Proc. Nat. Acad. Sci. USA 70*:2509–2514, 1973a.

David, C. S., Shreffler, D. C., Murphy, D. B., and Klein, J.: Serological cross-reaction between H-2D and H-2K region antigens. *Transplant. Proc. 5*:287–293, 1973b.

David, C. S., Klein, J., and Shreffler, D. C.: Serologic homology between H-2 and HL-A systems. *Transplant. Proc. 5*:461–466, 1973c.

David, C. S., Frelinger, J. A., and Shreffler, D. C.: New lymphocyte antigens controlled by the *Ir-IgG* region of the *H-2* gene complex. *Transplantation 17*:122–125, 1974.

Davies, A. J. S., Leuchars, E., Wallis, V., Marchant, R., and Elliott, E. V.: The failure of thymus-derived cells to produce antibody. *Transplantation 5*:222–231, 1967.

Davies, D. A. L.: Chemical nature of mouse histocompatibility antigens. *Nature 193*: 34–36, 1962a.

Davies, D. A. L.: The isolation of mouse antigens carrying H-2-histocompatibility specificity: Some preliminary studies. *Biochem. J. 84*:307–216, 1962b.

Davies, D. A. L.: The presence of non-H-2 histocompatibility specificities in preparations of mouse H-2 antigens. *Transplantation 1*:562–568, 1963.

Davies, D. A. L.: Histocompatibility antigens of the mouse. In *Immunopathology*, P. Grabar and P. Miescher (eds.), pp. 111–118, Schwabe, Basel, 1965.

Davies, D. A. L.: Mouse histocompatibility isoantigens derived from normal and from tumour cells. *Immunology 11*:115–125, 1966.

Davies, D. A. L.: Soluble mouse H-2 isoantigens. *Transplantation 5*:31–42, 1967.

Davies, D. A. L.: The molecular individuality of different mouse H-2 histocompatibility specificities determined by single genotypes. *Transplantation 8*:51–70, 1969.

Davies, D. A. L.: Characterization of the *H-2^z* allele and some new H-2 specificities

(46 and 47). In *Immunogenetics of the H-2 System*, A. Lengerová and M. Vojtíšková (eds.), pp. 18–19, Karger, Basel, 1971.

Davies, D. A. L., and Hutchison, A. M.: The serological determination of histocompatibility activity. *Brit. J. Exp. Pathol. 42*:587–591, 1961.

Davies, D. A. L., Boyse, E. A., Old, L. J., and Stockert, E.: Mouse isoantigens: Separation of soluble TL (thymus-leukemia) antigen from soluble H-2 histocompatibility antigen by column chromatography. *J. Exp. Med. 125*:549–558, 1967.

Davies, D. A. L., Alkins, B. J., Boyse, E. A., Old, L. J., and Stockert, E.: Soluble TL and H-2 antigens prepared from a TL positive leukemia of a TL negative mouse strain. *Immunology 16*:669–676, 1969.

Davis, W. C.: H-2 antigen on cell membranes: An explanation for the alteration of distribution by indirect labeling techniques. *Science 175*:1006–1008, 1972.

Davis, W. C.: The relation of the enhancement phenomenon to the physical association of H-2 alloantigens. *Transplant. Proc. 5*:625–230, 1973.

Davis, W. C., and Silverman, L.: Localization of mouse H-2 histocompatibility antigen with ferritin-labelled antibody. *Transplantation 6*:535–543, 1968.

Davis, W. C., Alspaugh, W. M., Stimpfling, J. H., and Walford, R. L.: Cellular surface distribution of transplantation antigens: Discrepancy between direct and indirect labeling techniques. *Tissue Antigens 1*:89–93, 1971.

Delovitch, T. L., and McDevitt, H. O.: Isolation and characterization of Ia antigens. *Immunogenetics*, 1975 (*in press*).

Démant, P.: Genetic requirements for graft-versus-host reaction in the mouse. Different efficacy of incompatibility at *D*- and *K*- ends of the *H-2* locus. *Folia Biol. (Praha) 16*:273–275, 1970.

Démant, P., and Graff, R. J.: Transplantation analysis of the *H-2* system. *Transplant. Proc. 5*:267–270, 1973.

Démant, P., and Nouza, K.: Different sensitivity of H-2K and H-2D incompatibility to ALS immunosuppression. *Folia Biol. (Praha) 17*:410–413, 1971.

Démant, P., Cherry, M., and Snell, G. D.: Hemagglutination and cytotoxic studies of H-2. II. Some new cytotoxic specificities. *Transplantation 11*:238–241, 1971a.

Démant, P., Snell, G. D., and Cherry, M.: Hemagglutination and cytotoxic studies of H-2. III. A family of 3-like specificities not in the C crossover region. *Transplantation 11*:242–259, 1971b.

Démant, P., Graff, R. J., Benešová, J., and Borovská, M.: Transplantation analysis of H-2 recombinants. In *Immunogenetics of the H-2 System*, A. Lengerová and M. Vojtíšková (eds.), pp. 148–154, Karger, Basel, 1971c.

Démant, P., Benešová, J., Martínková, J., and Oppltová, L.: Serological and transplantation analysis of recombinant alleles at the histocompatibility-2 locus of the mouse. *XIIth Europ. Conf. Animal Blood Groups Biochem. Polymorph.*, pp. 615–620, Akedemiai Kiado, Budapest, 1972.

Démant, P., Čapková, J., Hinzová, E., and Voráčová, B.: The role of the histocompatibility-2-linked *Ss-Slp* region in the control of mouse complement. *Proc. Nat. Acad. Sci. USA 70*:863–864, 1973.

Deol, M. S.: Genetical studies on the skeleton of the mouse. XXIV. Further data on skeletal variation in wild populations. *J. Embryol. Exp. Morphol. 6*:569–674, 1958.

DeOme, K. B., and Nandi, S.: The mammary-tumor system in mice: A brief review. In *Viruses Inducing Cancer. Implications for Therapy*, W. J. Burdette (ed.), pp. 127–137, University of Utah Press, Salt Lake City, 1966.

DePetris, S., and Raff, C.: Normal distribution, patching and capping of lymphocyte surface immunoglobulin studied by electron microscopy. *Nature New Biol.* 241:257–259, 1973.

Dev, V. G., Grewal, M. S., Miller, D. A., Kouri, R. E., Hutton, J. J., and Miller, O. J.: The quinacrine fluorescence karyotype of *Mus musculus* and demonstration of strain differences in secondary constrictions. *Cytogenetics 10*:436–451, 1971.

Dhaliwal, S. S.: Studies on histocompatibility mutations in mouse tumor cells using isogenic strains of mice. *Genet. Res. (Camb.) 2*:309–332, 1961.

Dhaliwal, S. S.: Histocompatibility variations in mouse tumor cells and embryonic tissue with the use of C57BL/10Sn strain and its isogenic resistant strains. *J. Nat. Cancer Inst. 32*:1001–1022, 1964a.

Dhaliwal, S. S.: Use of "immunological enhancement" in the study of histocompatibility mutations. *J. Nat. Cancer Inst. 32*:1245–1258, 1964b.

Dhaliwal, S. S.: Histocompatibility variants in mouse tumor cells: Distribution of isoantigenic components in variants of a hybrid lymphoma. In *Genetic Variations in Somatic Cells*, J. Klein, M. Vojtíšková, and V. Zelený (eds.), pp. 373–384, Academia, Prague, 1966.

Dickie, M. M., Griffen, A. B., and Frazier, J. E.: Private communication. *Mouse News Letter 32*:43–44, 1965.

Dickler, H. B., and Sachs, D. H.: Evidence for identity or close association of the Fc receptor of B lymphocytes and alloantigens determined by the *Ir* region of the *H-2* complex. *J. Exp. Med. 140*:779–796, 1974.

DiPadua, D., McKenzie, I. F. C., and Russell, P. S.: The isolation and characterization of soluble murine H-2 alloantigens. *Transplant. Proc. 5*:435–438, 1973.

Dishkant, I. P., Vedernikov, A. A., and Egorov, I. K.: Study of H-2 mutations in mice. III. Serological analysis of the mutation 504 and its derived recombinant H-2 haplotypes. *Genetika (Moscow) 9*:83–90, 1973 (In Russian).

Dobrovolskaia-Zavadskaia, N.: Sur la mortification spontanée de la queue chez la souris nouveau-née et sur l'existence d'un caractère (facteur) héréditaire "non viable." *C.R. Soc. Biol. 97*:114–116, 1927.

Dobrovolskaia-Zavadskaia, N., and Kobozieff, N.: Les souris anoures et la queue filiforme qui se reproduisent entre elles sans disjunction. *C. R. Soc. Biol. 110*: 782–784, 1932.

Dorfman, N. A., Stepina, V. N., and Ievleva, E. A.: H-2 antigens on murine leukemia cells and viruses. *Int. J. Cancer 9*:693–701, 1972.

Doria, G.: Development of homotransplantation antigens in mouse hemopoietic tissues. *Transplantation 1*:311–317, 1963.

Dray, S.: Effect of maternal isoantibodies on the quantitative expression of two allelic genes controlling γ-globulin allotypic specificities. *Nature 195*:677–680, 1962.

Drysdale, R., Merchant, D. J., Shreffler, D. C., and Parker, F. R.: Distribution of H-2 specificities within the LM mouse cell line and derived lines. *Proc. Soc. Exp. Biol. Med. 124*:413–418, 1967.

Dumonde, D. C., Al-Askari, S., Lawrence, H. S., and Thomas, L.: Microsomal fractions as transplantation antigens. *Nature 198*:598, 1963.

Dunham, E. K., Dorf, M. E., Shreffler, D. C., and Benacerraf, B.: Mapping the H-2 linked genes governing, respectively, the immune responses to a glutamic acid-alanine-tyrosine copolymer and to limiting doses of ovalbumin. *J. Immunol. 111*:1621–1625, 1973.

Dunn, L. C.: The inheritance of taillessness (anury) in the house mouse. III. Taillessness in the balanced lethal line 19. *Genetics 24*:728–731, 1939.

Dunn, L. C.: A test for genetic factors influencing abnormal segregation ratios in the house mouse. *Genetics 28*:187–192, 1943.

Dunn, L. C.: Widespread distribution of mutant alleles (t-alleles) in populations of wild house mice. *Nature 176*:1275–1276, 1955.

Dunn, L. C.: Analysis of a complex gene in the house mouse. *Cold Spring Harbor Symp. Quant. Biol. 21*:187–194, 1956.

Dunn, L. C.: Variations in the transmission ratios of alleles through egg and sperm in *Mus musculus. Amer. Nat. 94*:385–393, 1960.

Dunn, L. C.: Abnormalities associated with a chromosome region in the mouse. *Science 144*:260–263, 1964.

Dunn, L. C.: Private communication. *Mouse News Letter 37*:20, 1967.

Dunn, L. C., and Bennett, D.: Sex differences in recombination of linked genes in animals. *Genet. Res. (Camb.) 9*:221–231, 1967.

Dunn, L. C., and Bennett, D.: A new case of transmission ratio distortion in the house mouse. *Proc. Nat. Acad. Sci. USA 61*:570–573, 1968.

Dunn, L. C., and Bennett, D.: Studies of effects of t-alleles in the house mouse on spermatozoa. II. Quasi-sterility caused by different combinations of alleles. *J. Reprod. Fert. 20*:239–246, 1969.

Dunn, L. C., and Bennett, D.: Further studies of a mutation (Low) which distorts transmission ratios in the house mouse. *Genetics 67*:543–558, 1971a.

Dunn, L. C., and Bennett, D.: Lethal alleles near locus *T* in house mouse populations on the Jutland peninsula, Denmark. *Evolution 25*:451–453, 1971b.

Dunn, L. C., and Caspari, E.: Close linkage between mutations with similar effects. *Proc. Nat. Acad. Sci. USA 28*:205–210, 1942.

Dunn, L. C., and Caspari, E.: A case of neighboring loci with similar effects. *Genetics 30*:543–568, 1945.

Dunn, L. C., and Gluecksohn-Schoenheimer, S.: The inheritance of taillessness (anury) in the house mouse. II. Taillessness in a second balanced lethal line. *Genetics 24*:587–609, 1939.

Dunn, L. C., and Gluecksohn-Schoenheimer, S.: Repeated mutations in one area of a mouse chromosome. *Proc. Nat. Acad. Sci. USA 36*:233–237, 1950.

Dunn, L. C., and Gluecksohn-Waelsch, S.: Genetic analysis of seven newly discovered mutant alleles at locus T in the house mouse. *Genetics 38*:261–271, 1953.

Dunn, L. C., and Gluecksohn-Waelsch, S.: A genetical study of the mutation "fused" in the house mouse, with evidence concerning its allelism with a similar mutation, "kink." *J. Genetics 52*:383–391, 1954.

Dunn, L. C., and Levene, H.: Population dynamics of a variant *t*-allele in a confined population of wild house mice. *Evolution 15*:285–292, 1961.

Dunn, L. C., and Morgan, W. C., Jr.: Alleles at a mutable locus found in populations of wild house mice (*Mus musculus*). *Proc. Nat. Acad. Sci. USA 39*:391–402, 1953.

Dunn, L. C., Beasley, A. B., and Tinker, H.: Polymorphism in populations of wild house mice. *J. Mammal. 41*:220–229, 1960.

Dunn, L. C., Bennett, D., and Beasley, A. B.: Mutation and recombination in the vicinity of a complex gene. *Genetics 47*:285–303, 1962.

Dunn, T. B., and Potter, M.: A transplantable mast-cell neoplasm in the mouse. *J. Nat. Cancer Inst. 18*:587–601, 1957.

Duplan, J. F., Foschi, G. V., and Manson, L. A.: Isolation and characterization of transplantation antigens. I. Methods of assay. *Transplant. Bull. 27*:143–145, 1960.

Duran-Reynals, M. L.: Combined neoplastic effects of vaccinia virus and 3-methylcholanthrene. I. Studies with mice of different inbred strains. *J. Nat. Cancer Inst. 48*:95–104, 1972.

Duran-Reynals, M. L., and Lilly, F.: The role of genetic factors in the combined neoplastic effects of vaccinia virus and methylcholanthrene. *Transplant. Proc. 3*:1243–1246, 1971.

Dutton, R. W.: Further studies of the stimulation of DNA synthesis in cultures of spleen cell suspensions by homologous cells in inbred strains of mice and rats. *J. Exp. Med. 122*:759–770, 1965.

Dutton, R. W.: Spleen cell proliferation in response to homologous antigens studied in congenic resistant strains of mice. *J. Exp. Med. 123*:665–671, 1966.

Dux, A., and Corduwener, D.: Private communication. *Mouse News Letter 47*:18, 1972.

Dux, A., Corduwener, D., and Mühlbock, O.: Analysis of the difference at the *H-2* locus between the C57BL/LiA and the C57BL/10ScSn strains. In *Immunogenetics of the H-2 System*, A. Lengerová and M. Vojtíšková (eds.), pp. 163–165, Karger, Basel, 1971.

Ebringer, A., and Davies, D. A. L.: Cross reactivity between synthetic (T,G)-A--L and transplantation antigens in CBA mice. *Nature New Biol. 241*:144–147, 1973.

Edelman, G. M.: The structure and function of antibodies. *Sci. Amer. 223*:34–42, 1970.

Edidin, M.: Transplantation antigen levels in the early mouse embryo. *Transplantation 2*:627–637, 1964.

Edidin, M.: The release of soluble H-2 alloantigens during disaggregation of mouse embryo tissue by a chelating agent. *J. Embryol. Exp. Morphol. 16*:519–539, 1966.

Edidin, M.: Preparation of single, soluble antigens of the mouse histocompatibility-2 complex. *Proc. Nat. Acad. Sci. USA 57*:1226–1231, 1967.

Edidin, M.: Histocompatibility genes, transplantation antigens, and pregnancy. In *Transplantation Antigens*, B. D. Kahan and R. A. Reisfeld (eds.), pp. 75–114, Academic Press, New York, 1972a.

Edidin, M.: The tissue distribution and cellular location of transplantation antigens. In *Transplantation Antigens*, B. D. Kahan and R. A. Reisfeld (eds.), pp. 125–140 Academic Press, New York, 1972b.

Edidin, M., and Church, J. A.: A quantitative fluorochromatic assay for alloantibodies. *Transplantation 9*:1010–1014, 1968.

Edidin, M., and Henney, C. S.: The effect of capping H-2 antigens on the susceptibility of target cells to humoral and T cell-mediated lysis. *Nature New Biol. 246*:47–49, 1973.

Edidin, M., and Weiss, A.: Antigen cap formation in cultured fibroblasts: A reflection of membrane fluidity and of cell motility. *Proc. Nat. Acad. Sci. USA 69*:2456–2459, 1972.

Egorov, I. K.: A new isoantigen of mouse erythrocytes. *Genetika (Moskva) 6*:80–85, 1965. (In Russian).

Egorov, I. K.: A mutation of the histocompatibility-2 locus in the mouse. *Genetika (Moskva) 9*:136–144, 1967a. (In Russian).

Egorov, I. K.: Interpretation of the genetic structure of the H-2 locus of mice, based on a statistical analysis of its alleles. *Folia Biol. (Praha) 13*:169–180, 1967b.

Egorov, I. K.: Genetic control of H-2 alloantigens as inferred from analysis of mutation. *Immunogenetics 1*:97–107, 1974.

Egorov, I. K., and Blandova, Z. K.: The genetic homogeneity of the inbred mice bred at the Stolbovaya farm. II. Skin grafting tests. *Genetika (Moskva) 12*:63–69, 1968. (In Russian).

Egorov, I. K., and Blandova, Z. K.: Private communication. *Mouse News Letter 45*:36, 1971.

Egorov, I. K., and Blandova, Z. K.: Histocompatibility mutations in mice: Chemical induction and linkage with the H-2 locus. *Genet. Res. (Camb.) 19*:133–143, 1972.

Egorov, I. K., and Zvereva, N. M.: A method of production of congenic resistant strains of mice involving the use of skin grafting. *Genetika (Moskva) 1*:114–121, 1967. (In Russian).

Egorov, I. K., Vedernikov, A. A., and Dishkant, I. P.: Private communication. *Mouse News Letter 48*:17–18, 1973.

Eichwald, E. J., and Silmser, C. R.: Note without title. *Transplant. Bull. 2*:148–149, 1955.

Eichwald, E. J., Wetzel, B., and Lustgraaf, E. C.: Genetic aspects of second-set skin grafts in mice. *Transplantation 4*:260–273, 1966.

Eichwald, E. J., Hart, E. A., and Eichwald, B.: Genetic aspects of the graft-versus-host reaction of mice. *Folia Biol. (Praha) 15*:254–258, 1969.

Eijsvoogel, V. P., duBois, M. C. J. C., Melief, C. J. M., deGroot-Kooy, M. L., Koning, C., van Rood, J. J., van Leeuwen, A., du Toit, E., and Schellekens, P. T. A.: Position of a locus determining mixed lymphocyte reaction (MLR), distinct from the known HL-A loci, and its relation to cell-mediated lympholysis (CML). In *Histocompatibility Testing 1972*, J. Dausset and J. Colombani (eds.), Munksgaard, Copenhagen, pp. 501–508, 1973a.

Eijsvoogel, V. P., DuBois, M. J. G. J., Meinesz, A., Bierhorst-Eijlander, J., Zeylemaker, W. P., and Schellenkens, P. Th. A.: The specificity and the activation mechanism of cell-mediated lympholysis (CML) in man. *Transplant. Proc. 5*:1675–1678, 1973b.

Elandt-Johnson, C.: Estimation of the number of histocompatibility loci in laboratory animals. *Transplantation 7*:12–40, 1969.

Elkins, W. L.: Cellular immunology and the pathogenesis of graft-versus-host reactions. *Progr. Allergy 15*:78–187, 1971.

Ellerman, J. E.: *The Families and Genera of Living Rodents.* Vol. I, II. The British Museum, London, 1940, 1941.

Ellman, L., Green, I., Martin, W. J., and Benacerraf, B.: Linkage between the poly-L-Lysine gene and the locus controlling the major histocompatibility antigens in strain 2 guinea pigs. *Proc. Nat. Acad. Sci. USA 66*:322–328, 1970.

Erickson, R. P.: Alternative modes of detection of H-2 antigens on mouse spermatozoa. In *The Genetics of the Spermatozoon*, R. A. Beatty and S. Gluecksohn-Waelsch (eds.), pp. 191–202, Edinburgh, New York, 1972.

Erickson, R. P.: Haploid gene expression versus meiotic drive: The relevance of intercellular bridges during spermatogenesis. *Nature New Biol. 243*:210–212, 1973.

Falconer, D. S.: *Introduction to Quantitative Genetics.* Ronald Press, New York, 1960.

Fass, L., and Herberman, R. B.: A cytotoxic antiglobulin technique for assay of antibodies to histocompatibility antigens. *J. Immunol. 102*:140–144, 1969.

Feldmann, M.: Histocompatibility-linked immune-response genes. What do they do? *Transplant. Proc. 5*:1803–1809, 1973.

Feldmann, M., Cohen, I. R., and Wekerle, H.: T cell-mediated immunity *in vitro*: An analysis of antigen recognition and target cell lysis. *Transplant. Rev. 12*:57–90, 1972.

Fellous, M., and Dausset, J.: Probable haploid expression of HL-A antigens on human spermatozoon. *Nature 225*:191–193, 1970.

Festenstein, H.: Antigenic strength investigated by mixed cultures of allogeneic mouse spleen cells. *Ann. N.Y. Acad. Sci. 129*:567–572, 1966a.

Festenstein, H.: Further investigations of antigenic strength by the mixed spleen cell reaction. *Exc. Med. Int. Congr. Series 131*:214–217, 1966b.

Festenstein, H., and Démant, P.: Workshop summary on genetic determinants of cell-mediated immune reactions in the mouse. *Transplant. Proc. 5*:1321–1327, 1973.

Festenstein, H., Davies, A., Leuchars, E., Wallis, V. J., and Doenhoff, M. J.: Mouse blood lymphocyte origins investigated by a simple cell culture technique. In *Lymphatic Tissue and Germinal Centers in Immune Response*, L. Fiore-Donati and M. G. Hanna, Jr. (eds.), pp. 121–124, Plenum Press, New York, 1969.

Festenstein, H., Sachs, J. A., and Oliver, R. T. D.: Genetic studies of the mixed lymphocyte reaction in H-2 identical mice. In *Immunogenetics of the H-2 System*, A. Lengerová and M. Vojtíšková (eds.), pp. 170–177, Karger, Basel, 1971.

Festenstein, H., Abbasi, K., Sachs, J. A., and Oliver, R. T. D.: Serologically undetectable immune responses in transplantation. *Transplant. Proc. 4*:219–222, 1972.

Festenstein, H., Abbasi, K., and Démant, P.: The genetic basis of the generation of effector capacity for cell mediated lympholysis in mice. *J. Immunogenetics 1*:47–50, 1974.

Finkel, S. I., and Lilly, F.: Influence of histoincompatibility between mother and foetus on placental size in mice. *Nature 234*:102–103, 1971.

Flaherty, L., and Bennett, D.: Histoincompatibilies found between congenic strains which differ at loci determining differentiation antigens. *Transplantation 16*:505–514, 1973.

Flanagan, S. P.: Nude, a new hairless gene with pleiotropic effects in the mouse. *Genet. Res. (Camb.) 8*:295–309, 1966.

Ford, W. L., and Atkins, R. C.: The proportion of lymphocytes capable of recognizing strong transplantation antigens *in vivo*. *Adv. Exper. Biol. Med. 29*:255–262, 1973.

Forman, J., and Ketchel, M. M.: Resistance to non-strain-specific variant tumor cells by H-2 allogeneic mice receiving strain-specific cells. *J. Nat. Cancer Inst. 48*:933–939, 1972.

Forman, J., and Klein, J.: Analysis of *H-2* mutants: Evidence for multiple CML target specificities controlled by the *H-2K^b* gene. *Immunogenetics*, 1974 (*in press*).

Forman, J., and Möller, G.: Generation of cytotoxic lymphocytes in mixed lymphocyte reactions: II. Importance of private and public *H-2* alloantigens on the expression of cytotoxicity. *Immunogenetics 1*:211–225, 1974.

Foschi, G. V., and Manson, L. A.: Radioimmune assay for histocompatibility antigens. *Nature 225*:583, 1970.

Foster, M., Petras, M. L., and Gasser, D. L.: The *Ea-1* blood group locus of the house mouse: Inheritance, linkage, polymorphism and control of antibody synthesis. In *Proc. International Congress of Genetics*, p. 245, Science Council of Japan, Tokyo, 1968. (*Abstract*).

Freed, J. H., Bechtol, K. B., Herzenberg, L. A., Herzenberg, L. A., and McDevitt, H. O.: Analysis of anti-(T,G)-A--L antibody in tetraparental mice. *Transplant. Proc. 5*:167–171, 1973.

Freiesleben-Sørensen, S., and Hawkes, S. P.: The genetic basis for cell-mediated lympholysis in mice. *Transplant. Proc. 5*:1361–1366, 1973.

Frelinger, J. A., Niederhuber, J. E., David, C. S., and Shreffler, D. C.: Evidence for the expression of Ia (H-2 associated) antigens on thymus derived lymphocytes. *J. Exp. Med. 140*: 1273–1284, 1974.

Friend, C.: Cell-free transmission in adult Swiss mice of a disease having the character of a leukemia. *J. Exp. Med. 105*:307–318, 1957.

Frye, L. D., and Edidin, M.: The rapid intermixing of cell surface antigens after formation of mouse-human heterokaryons. *J. Cell. Sci. 7*:319–335, 1970.

Fuji, H., Zaleski, M., and Milgrom, F.: Plaque-forming cell response to H-2 antigens of mice. *Proc. Soc. Exp. Biol. Med. 136*:239–241, 1971a.

Fuji, H., Zaleski, M., and Milgrom, F.: Allogenic nucleated cells as immunogen and target for plaque-forming cells in mice. *Transplant. Proc. 3*:852–855, 1971b.

Fuji, H., Zaleski, M., and Milgrom, F.: Immune response to alloantigens of thymus studied in mice with plaque assay. *J. Immunol. 106*:56–64, 1971c.

Fuji, H., Zaleski, M., and Milgrom, F.: Genetic control of immune response to θ-AKR alloantigen. *J. Immunol. 108*:223–230, 1972.

Gangal, S. G., Merchant, D. J., and Shreffler, D. C.: Characterization of the H-2 antigens of L-M mouse cells grown in culture. *J. Nat. Cancer Inst. 36*:1151–1159, 1966.

Gasser, D. L.: Genetic control of the immune response in mice. I. Segregation data and localization to the fifth linkage group of a gene affecting antibody production. *J. Immunol. 103*:66–70, 1969.

Gasser, D. L., and Shreffler, D. C.: Involvement of H-2 locus in a multigenically determined immune response. *Nature New Biol. 235*:155–156, 1972.

Gasser, D. L., and Silvers, W. K.: The genetic basis of male skin rejection in mice. *Transplantation 12*:412–414, 1971a.

Gasser, D. L., and Silvers, W. K.: Genetic control of the immune response in mice. III. An association between H-2 type and reaction to H-Y. *J. Immunol. 106*:875–876, 1971b.

Gates, W. H.: Linkage of short ear and density in the house mouse. *Proc. Nat. Acad. Sci. USA 13*:575–578, 1927.

Gelfand, M. C., Sachs, D. H., Lieberman, R., and Paul, W. E.: Ontogeny of B lymphocytes. III. H-2 linkage of a gene controlling the rate of appearance of complement receptor lymphocytes. *J. Exp. Med. 139*:1142–1153, 1974.

Gervais, A. G.: Detection of mouse histocompatibility antigens by immunofluorescence. *Transplantation 6*:261–276, 1968.

Gervais, A. G.: Transplantation antigens in the central nervous system. *Nature 225*: 647, 1970.

Gervais, A. G.: Localization of transplantation antigens in tissue sections: Effects of various fixatives and use of tissue preparations other than frozen sections. *Experientia 28*:342–343, 1972a.

Gervais, A. G.: Failure to detect H-2 antigens in mouse testis and heart by immunofluorescence. *Folia Biol. (Praha) 18*:50–52, 1972b.

Geyer-Duszynska, I.: Cytological investigations on the T locus in *Mus musculus* L. *Chromosoma 15*:478–502, 1964.

Gibson, T., and Medawar, P. B.: The fate of skin homografts in man. *J. Anat. 77*: 299–310, 1943.

Ginsburg, H.: Graft versus host reaction in tissue culture. I. Lysis of monolayers of embryo mouse cells from strains differing in the H-2 histocompatibility locus by rat lymphocytes sensitized *in vitro*. *Immunology 14*:621–635, 1968.

Ginsburg, H., and Sachs, L.: Destruction of mouse and rat embryo cells in tissue culture by lymph node cells from unsensitized rats. *J. Cell. Comp. Physiol. 66*: 199–220, 1965.

Gleichmann, E., and Gleichmann, H.: Differential immunogenicity of D- and K-end antigens and its possible significance for HL-A. *Transplantation 13*:180–183, 1972.

Gluecksohn-Schoenheimer, S.: The effect of an early lethal (t⁰) in the house mouse. *Genetics 25*:391–400, 1940.

Gluecksohn-Schoenheimer, S.: The effects of a lethal mutation responsible for duplications and twinning in mouse embryos. *J. Exp. Zool. 110*:47–76, 1949.

Gluecksohn-Waelsch, S., and Erickson, R. P.: The T locus of the mouse: Implications for mechanisms of development. *Curr. Topics Devel. Biol. 5*:281–316, 1970.

Goldberg, E. H., Aoki, T., Boyse, E. J., and Bennett, D.: Detection of H-2 antigens on mouse spermatozoa by the cytotoxicity tests. *Nature 228*:570–572, 1970.

Goldberg, E. H., Boyse, E. A., Bennett, D., Scheid, M., and Carswell, E. A.: Serological demonstration of H-Y (male) antigen on mouse sperm. *Nature 232*:478–480, 1971.

Goldman, M. B.: Immunogenetic factors in the survival of ovarian transplants. *Transplantation 17*:518–523, 1974.

Goldstein, P., Svedmyr, E. A. J., and Wigzell, H.: Cells mediating specific *in vitro* cytotoxicity. I. Detection of receptor-bearing lymphocytes. *J. Exp. Med. 134*: 1385–1401, 1971a.

Goldstein, P., Svedmyr, E. A. J., and Wigzell, H.: Cells mediating specific *in vitro* cytotoxicity. II. Detection of receptor-bearing lymphocytes. *J. Exp. Med. 134*: 1402–1415, 1971b.

Goodman, S. B., and Block, M. H.: The histogenesis of Gross viral induced leukemia. *Cancer Res. 23*:1634–1640, 1963.

Gorer, P. A.: The detection of a hereditary antigenic difference in the blood of mice by means of human group A serum. *J. Genetics 32*:17–31, 1936a.

Gorer, P. A.: The detection of antigenic differences in mouse erythrocytes by the employment of immune sera. *Brit. J. Exp. Pathol. 17*:42–50, 1936b.

Gorer, P. A.: The genetic and antigenic basis of tumour transplantation. *J. Pathol. Bacteriol. 44*:691–697, 1937a.

Gorer, P. A.: Further studies on antigenic differences in mouse erythrocytes. *Brit. J. Exp. Pathol. 18*:31–36, 1937b.

Gorer, P. A.: The antigenic basis of tumour transplantation. *J. Pathol. Bacteriol. 47*:231–252, 1938.

Gorer, P. A.: Antibody response to tumor inoculation in mice with special reference to partial antibodies. *Cancer Res. 7*:634–641, 1947.

Gorer, P. A.: The significance of studies with transplanted tumours. *Brit. J. Cancer 2*:103–107, 1948.

Gorer, P. A.: Studies in antibody response of mice to tumour inoculation. *Brit. J. Cancer 4*:372–379, 1950.

Gorer, P. A.: Some recent work on tumor immunity. *Adv. Cancer Res. 4*:149–186, 1956.

Gorer, P. A.: Some recent data on the H-2 system of mice. In *Biological Problems of Grafting*, F. Albert and P. Medawar (eds.), pp. 25–30, Blackwell, Oxford, 1959.

Gorer, P. A.: Interactions between sessile and humoral antibodies in homograft reactions. In *Symposium on Cellular Aspects of Immunity*, G. E. W. Wolstenholme and M. O'Connor (eds.), pp. 330–347, Little, Brown, Boston, 1960.

Gorer, P. A.: The antigenic structure of tumors. *Adv. Immunol. 1*:345–393, 1961.

Gorer, P. A., and Boyse, E. A.: Pathological changes in F_1 hybrid mice following transplantation of spleen cells from donors of the parental strains. *Immunology* 2:182–193, 1959.

Gorer, P. A., and Kaliss, N.: The effect of isoantibodies *in vivo* on three different transplantable neoplasms in mice. *Cancer Res.* 19:824–830, 1959.

Gorer, P. A., and Mikulska, Z. B.: The antibody response to tumor inoculation. Improved methods of antibody detection. *Cancer Res.* 14:651–655, 1954.

Gorer, P. A., and Mikulska, Z. B.: Some further data on the H-2 system of antigens. *Proc. Roy. Soc. (London) B 151*:57–69, 1959.

Gorer, P. A., and O'Gorman, P.: The cytotoxic activity of isoantibodies in mice. *Transplant. Bull.* 3:142–143, 1956.

Gorer, P. A., Lyman, S., and Snell, G. D.: Studies on the genetic and antigenic basis of tumour transplantation; linkage between a histocompatibility gene and 'fused' in mice. *Proc. Roy. Soc. (London) B 135*:499–505, 1948.

Gorer, P. A., Mikulska, Z. B., and O'Gorman, P.: The time of appearance of iso-antibodies during the homograft response to mouse tumours. *Immunology 2*:211–218, 1959.

Götze, D.: T(Iat)- and B(Iab)-cell alloantigens determined by the *H-2* linked *I* region in mice. *Immunogenetics*, 1974 (*in press*).

Götze, D., and Reisfeld, R. A.: Immunogenecity and partial purification of soluble H-2 antigens extracted with hypertonic salt. *J. Immunol. 112*:1643–1651, 1974.

Götze, D., Ferrone, S., and Reisfeld, R. A.: Serologic cross-reactivity between H-2 and HL-A antigens. I. Specific reactivity of rabbit anti-HL-A sera against murine cells. *J. Immunol. 109*:439–450, 1972.

Götze, D., Lee, S., Ferrone, S., Pellegrino, M. A., and Reisfeld, R. A.: Cross-reactivity between HL-A and H-2 antigens. II. Allogenic sensitization by xenogeneic soluble lymphocyte antigens (HL-A). *Transplant. Proc. 5*:467–470, 1973a.

Götze, D., Reisfeld, R. A., and Klein, J.: Serologic evidence for antigens controlled by the *Ir* region in mice. *J. Exp. Med. 138*:1003–1008, 1973b.

Govaerts, A.: Cellular antibodies in kidney homotransplantation. *J. Immunol. 85*:516–522, 1960.

Graff, R. J., and Bailey, D. W.: The non-H-2 histocompatibility loci and their antigens. *Transplant. Rev. 115*:26–49, 1973.

Graff, R. J., and Kandutsch, A. A.: Immunogenic properties of purified antigen preparations from a mouse sarcoma. *Transplantation 4*:465–473, 1966.

Graff, R. J., and Kandutsch, A. A.: An attempt to produce low-zone tolerance to tissue alloantigens. *Transplantation 8*:162–166, 1969.

Graff, R. J., Hildemann, W. H., and Snell, G. D.: Histocompatibility genes of mice. VI. Allografts in mice congenic at various non-H-2 histocompatibility loci. *Transplantation 4*:425–437, 1966a.

Graff, R. J., Silvers, W. K., Billingham, R. E., Hildemann, W. H., and Snell, G. D.: The cumulative effect of histocompatibility antigens. *Transplantation 4*:605–617, 1966b.

Graff, R. J., Mann, D. L., and Nathenson, S. G.: Immunogenic properties of papain-solubilized H-2 alloantigens. *Transplantation 10*:59–65, 1970.

Granger, G. A., and Weiser, R. S.: Homograft target cells: Specific destruction *in vitro* by contact interaction with immune macrophages. *Science 145*:1427–1429, 1964.

Grant, J. A., and Hood, L.: N-terminal analysis of normal immunoglobulin light chains. I. A study of thirteen individual humans. *Immunochemistry 8*:63–79, 1971.

Graziano, K. D., and Edidin, M.: Serological quantitation of histocompatibility-2 antigens and the determination of H-2 in adult and fetal organs. In, *Proc. Symp. Immunogenetics of the H-2 System*, A. Lengerová, and M. Vojtíšková (eds.), pp. 251–256, Karger, Basel, 1971.

Green, E. L.: Breeding systems. In *Biology of the Laboratory Mouse*, E. L. Green (ed.), pp. 11–22, McGraw-Hill, New York, 1966.

Green, E. L., and Doolittle, D. P.: Systems of mating used in mammalian genetics. In *Methodology in Mammalian Genetics*, W. J. Burdette (ed.), pp. 3–55, Holden-Day, San Francisco, 1963.

Green, M. C.: Methods for testing linkage. In *Methodology in Mammalian Genetics*, W. J. Burdette (ed.), pp. 56–82, Holden-Day, San Francisco, 1963.

Green, M. C.: Standard karyotype of the mouse, *Mus musculus. J. Hered. 63*:69–72, 1972.

Green, M. C., and Kaufer, K. A.: A test for histocompatibility between sublines of the CBA strain of mice. *Transplantation 3*:766–768, 1965.

Gregorová, S., and Iványi, P.: H-2-associated genetic differences in androgen dependent traits. The effect of castration and testosterone injections. *Folia Biol. (Praha) 19*:337–349, 1973.

Gropp, A., Tettenborn, U., and von Lehmann, E.: Chromosomenvariation vom Robertson'schen Typus bei der Tabakmaus, *M. poschiavinus*, und ihren Hybriden mit der Laboratoriumsmaus. *Cytogenetics 9*:9–23, 1970.

Gropp, A., Olert, J., and Maurizio, R.: Robertsonian chromosomal polymorphism in the mouse (*M. musculus domesticus*). *Experientia 27*:1226–1227, 1971.

Gross, L.: *Oncogenic Viruses*. 2nd ed., Pergamon Press, Oxford, 1970.

Grumet, F. C.: Genetic control of the immune response. A selective defect in immunologic (IgG) memory in nonresponder mice. *J. Exp. Med. 135*:110–125, 1972.

Grumet, F. C., and McDevitt, H. O.: Genetic control of the immune response. Relationship between the immune response-1 gene(s) and individual H-2 antigenic specificities. *Transplantation 13*:171–173, 1972.

Grumet, F. C., Mitchell, G. F., and McDevitt, H. O.: Genetic control of specific immune responses in inbred mice. *Ann. N.Y. Acad. Sci. 190*:170–177, 1971a.

Grumet, F. C., Mitchell, G. F., and McDevitt, H. O.: Selective effect of thymectomy on memory in a genetically controlled immune response. *Clin. Res. 19*:442, 1971b. (*Abstract*).

Grüneberg, H.: *The Genetics of the Mouse*. 2nd ed., Nijhoff, The Hague, 1952.

Grüneberg, H.: Genetical studies on the skeleton of the mouse. XXIII. The development of brachyury and anury. *J. Exp. Morphol. 6*:424–443, 1958.

Günther, E., Rüde, E., and Štark, O.: Antibody response in rats to the synthetic polypeptide (T,G)-A--L genetically linked to the major histocompatibility system. *Eur. J. Immunol. 2*:151–155, 1972.

Haenen-Severyns, A. M., Degiovani, G., Castermans, A., and Lejeune, G.: Improved method for preparing soluble transplantation antigens from normal mouse tissues. In *Advance in Transplantation*, J. Dausset, J. Hamburger, and G. Mathé (eds.), pp. 289–293, Williams & Wilkins, Baltimore, 1968.

Haldane, J. B. S.: The genetics of cancer. *Nature 132*:265–267, 1933.

Haldane, J. B. S., Sprunt, A. D., and Haldane, N. M.: Reduplication in mice. *J. Genetics 5*:133–135, 1915.

Halle-Pannenko, O., Florentine, I., Kiger, N., and Jolles, P.: Chromatographic purification of soluble graft antigens. In *Advance in Transplantation*, J. Dausset,

J. Hamburger, and G. Mathé (eds.), pp. 283–287, Williams & Wilkins, Baltimore, 1968.

Halle-Pannenko, O., Martyré, M. and Jollés, P.: Contribution to the study of the solubilization and purification of H-2 antigens obtained from BP-8 murine cell membranes. *Eur. J. Clin. Biol. Res.* 15:687–691, 1970.

Hamaoka, T., Osborne, D. P., Jr., and Katz, D. H.: Cell interactions between histoincompatible T and B lymphocytes. *J. Exp. Med.* 137:1393–1404, 1973.

Hämmerling, G. J., and McDevitt, H. O.: Frequency and characteristics of antigen binding cells in genetic high and low responder mice. *Transplant. Proc.* 5:179–182, 1973.

Hämmerling, G. J., and McDevitt, H. O.: Antigen binding T and B lymphocytes. I. Difference in cellular specificity and influence of metabolic activity on interaction of antigen with T and B cells. *J. Immunol.* 113:1726–1733, 1974a.

Hämmerling, G. J., and McDevitt, H. O.: Antigen binding T and B lymphocytes. II. Studies on the inhibition of antigen binding to T and B cells by anti-immunoglobulin and anti-H-2 sera. *J. Immunol.* 112:1734–1740, 1974b.

Hämmerling, G. J., Deak, B. D., Mauve, G., Hämmerling, U., and McDevitt, H. O.: B lymphocyte alloantigens controlled by the *I* region of the major histocompatibility complex in mice. *Immunogenetics* 1:68–81, 1974a.

Hämmerling, G. J., Mauve, G., Goldberg, E., and McDevitt, H. O.: Tissue distribution of Ia antigens. Ia on spermatozoa, macrophages, and epidermal cells. *Immunogenetics* 1974b (*in press*).

Hämmerling, U., and Eggers, H. J.: Quantitative measurement of uptake of alloantibody on mouse lymphocytes. *Eur. J. Biochem.* 17:95–99, 1970.

Hämmerling, U., Aoki, T., de Harven, E., Boyse, E. A., and Old, L. J.: Use of hybrid antibody with anti-γG and anti-ferritin specificities in locating cell surface antigens by electron microscopy. *J. Exp. Med.* 128:1461–1473, 1968.

Hämmerling, U., Aoki, T., Wood, H. A., Old, L. J., Boyse, E. A., and de Harven, E.: New visual markers of antibody for electron microscopy. *Nature* 223:1158–1159, 1969a.

Hämmerling, U., Shigeno, N., Old, L. J., and Boyse, E. A.: Labelling of mouse alloantibody with tritiated DL-alanine. *Immunology* 17:999–1006, 1969b.

Hämmerling, U., Davies, D. A. L., and Manstone, A. J.: Transplantation antigens in a high molecular weight form. I. Mouse H-2 antigens. *Immunochemistry* 8:7–16, 1971.

Hampl, R., Iványi, P., and Stárka, L.: Testosterone and testosterone binding in murine plasma. *Steroidologia* 2:113–120, 1971.

Hansen, T. H., Krasteff, T. N., and Shreffler, D. C.: Quantitative variations in the expression of the house serum antigen SS and its sex-limited allotype Slp. *Bioch. Genetics* 1974 (*in press*).

Harder, F. H., and McKhann, C. F.: Demonstration of cellular antigens on sarcoma cells by an indirect ^{125}I-labeled antibody technique. *J. Nat. Cancer. Inst.* 40:231–241, 1968.

Hardy, D. A., Ling, N. R., and Wallin, J.: Destruction of lymphoid cells by activated human lymphocytes. *Nature* 227:723–725, 1970.

Harris, T. N., Harris, S., and Ogburn, C. A.: Solubilization of H-2 histocompatibility antigens of the mouse by Triton X-100 and butanol. *Transplantation* 12:448–458, 1971a.

Harris, T. N., Harris, S., Ogburn, C. A., Bocchieri, M. H., and Farber, M. B.:

Accelerated rejection of allogeneic skin grafts in the mouse after injections of histocompatibility antigens solubilized by Triton, butanol and papain. *Transplantation 12*:459–463, 1971b.

Hartley, J. W., Rowe, W. P., and Huebner, R. J.: Host range restrictions of murine leukemia viruses in mouse embryo cell cultures. *J. Virol. 5*:221–225, 1970.

Hašková, V.: Transplantation immunity and immunological tolerance and the study of antigeniticy of tissues and their derivatives. In *Biological Problems of Grafting*, F. Albert and G. Lejeune-Ledant (eds.), pp. 95–106, Thomas, Springfield, Ill., 1959.

Hašková, V.: Differences in the antigenic effectiveness of the foetal part of mouse placenta depending on the strain combination employed. *Folia Biol. (Praha) 9*:99–103, 1963.

Hašková, V., and Hilgert, I.: Transplantation antigens in tumors, tumor extract and cell-free ascitic fluid. *Folia Biol. (Praha) 7*:81–86, 1961.

Hašková, V., and Hrubešová, M.: Part played by deoxyribonucleic acid in transplantation immunity. *Nature 182*:61–62, 1958.

Haughton, G.: Extraction of H-2 antigen from mouse tumour cells. *Transplantation 2*:251–260, 1964.

Haughton, G.: Naturally occurring soluble H-2 specificity in mouse tissues. *Immunology 9*:193–199, 1965.

Haughton, G.: Transplantation antigen of mice: Cellular localization of antigen determined by the H-2 locus. *Transplantation 4*:238–244, 1966.

Haughton, G., and Davies, D. A. L.: Tissue cell antigens: Antigens of mouse tumour cell ghosts. *Brit. J. Exp. Pathol. 43*:488–495, 1962.

Haughton, G., and McGhee, M. P.: Cytolysis of mouse lymph node cells by allo-antibody: A comparison of guinea-pig and rabbit complements. *Immunology 16*:447–461, 1969.

Hauptfeld, V., Klein, D., and Klein, J.: Serological identification of an Ir-region product. *Science 181*:167–169, 1973a.

Hauptfeld, V., Klein, D., and Klein, J.: Serological detection of antigens controlled by the Ir-region of the H-2 complex in the mouse. *Transplant. Proc. 5*:1811–1813, 1973b.

Hauptfeld, V., Hauptfeld, M., and Klein, J.: Tissue distribution of I region associated antigens in the mouse. *J. Immunol. 113*:181–188, 1974.

Hauschka, T. S.: Immunologic aspects of cancer: A review. *Cancer Res. 12*:615–633, 1952.

Hauschka, T. S.: Tissue genetics of neoplastic cell populations. *Proc. 2nd Canad. Cancer Res. Conf. 2*:305–345, 1957.

Hauschka, T. S., and Amos, D. B.: Cytogenetic aspects of compatibility. *Ann. N.Y. Acad. Sci. 69*:561–579, 1957.

Hauschka, T. S., and Levan, A.: Inverse relationship between chromosome ploidy and host-specificity in sixteen transplantable tumors. *Exp. Cell Res. 4*:457–467, 1953.

Hauschka, T. S., and Schultz, J.: Cytologic aspects of immunogenetic specificity. *Transplant. Bull. 1*:203–206, 1954.

Hauschka, T. S., Kvedar, B. J., Grinnell, S. T., and Amos, D. B.: Immunoselection of polyploids from predominantly diploid cell populations. *Ann. N.Y. Acad. Sci. 63*:683–705, 1956.

Häyry, P., and Andersson, L. C.: T-cells in mixed-lymphocyte-culture-induced cytolysis (MLC-CML). *Transplant. Proc. 5*:1697–1703, 1973.

Häyry, P., and Defendi, V.: Mixed lymphocyte cultures produce effector cells: Model *in vitro* for allograft rejection. *Science 168*:133–135, 1970.

Häyry, P., Andersson, L. C., Nordling, S., and Virolainen, M.: Allograft response *in vitro. Transplant. Rev. 12*:91–140, 1972.

Haywood, G. R., and McKhann, C. F.: Antigen specificities on murine sarcoma cells. Reciprocal relationship between normal transplantation antigens (H-2) and tumor-specific immunogenicity. *J. Exp. Med. 133*:1171–1187, 1971.

Hellström, I., and Sjögren, H. O.: Demonstration of H-2 isoantigens and polyoma specific tumor antigens by measuring colony formation *in vitro. Exp. Cell Res. 40*:212–215, 1965.

Hellström, K. E.: Studies on isoantigenic variation in mouse lymphomas. *J. Nat. Cancer Inst. 25*:237–269, 1960.

Hellström, K. E.: Studies on the mechanism of isoantigenic variant formation in heterozygous mouse tumors. II. Behavior of H-2 antigens D and K: Cytotoxic tests on mouse lymphomas. *J. Nat. Cancer Inst. 27*:1095–1105, 1961.

Hellström, K. E., and Bjaring, B.: Studies on the mechanism of isoantigenic variant formation in heterozygous mouse tumors. V. Quantitative studies of residual H-2 antigens in isoantigenic variant sublines isolated from a mouse lymphoma of F_1 hybrid origin. *J. Nat. Cancer Inst. 36*:947–952, 1966.

Hellström, K. E., and Hellström, I.: Syngeneic preference and allogeneic inhibition. In *Isoantigens and Cell Interactions*, J. Palm (ed.), pp. 79–93, Wistar Institute Press, Philadelphia, 1965.

Hellström, K. E., and Hellström, I.: Allogeneic inhibition of transplanted tumor cells. *Progr. Exp. Tumor Res. 9*:40–76, 1967.

Hellström, K. E., Hellström, I., and Haughton, G.: Demonstration of syngeneic preference *in vitro. Nature 204*:661–664, 1964.

Herberman, R., and Stetson, C. A.: The expression of histocompatibility antigens on cellular and subcellular membranes. *J. Exp. Med. 121*:533–549, 1965.

Herzenberg, L. A.: Chemical and serological characterization of purified H-2 antigens. In *Mechanisms of Immunological Tolerance*, Proc. Symp. Liblice-Prague, 1961, M. Hašek, A. Lengerová, and M. Vojtíšková (eds.), pp. 495–499, Publishing House of the Czechoslovak Academy of Sciences, Prague, 1962.

Herzenberg, L. A., and Herzenberg, L. A.: Association of H-2 antigens with the cell membrane fraction of mouse liver. *Proc. Nat. Acad. Sci. USA 47*:762–767, 1961.

Herzenberg, L. A., Tachibana, D. K., Herzenberg, L. A., and Rosenberg, L. T.: A gene locus concerned with hemolytic complement in *Mus musculus. Genetics 48*:711–715, 1963.

Herzenberg, L. A., Herzenberg, L. A., Goodlin, R. C., and Rivera, E. C.: Immunoglobulin synthesis in mice. Suppression by anti-allotype antibody. *J. Exp. Med. 126*:701–713, 1967.

Herzenberg, L. A., McDevitt, H. O., and Herzenberg, L. A.: Genetics of antibodies. *Ann. Rev. Genetics 2*:209–244, 1968.

Hess, M., and Davies, D. A. L.: Basic structure of mouse histocompatibility antigens. *Eur. J. Biochem. 41*:1–13, 1974.

Heston, W. E.: Development of inbred strains in the mouse and their use in cancer research. In *Lectures on Genetics, Cancer, Growth, and Social Behavior*, pp. 9–31, Roscoe B. Jackson Memorial Laboratory, Bar Harbor, Maine, 1949.

Hetherington, C. M.: The absence of any effect of maternal/fetal incompatibility at the H-2 and H-3 loci on pregnancy in the mouse. *J. Reprod. Fert. 33*:135–139, 1973.

Heyner, S., Brinster, R. L., and Palm, J.: Effect of alloantibody on pre-implantation mouse embryos. *Nature 222*:783–784, 1969.

Hicken, P., and Krohn, P. L.: The histocompatibility requirements of ovarian grafts in mice. *Proc. Roy. Soc. (London) B. 151*:419–433, 1960.

Hildemann, W. H.: A method for detecting hemolysins in mouse isoimmune serums. *Transplant. Bull. 4*:148–149, 1957.

Hildemann, W. H.: Early antibody production in relation to skin allograft reactions in mice. *Transplantation 5*:1001–1007, 1967.

Hildemann, W. H.: Components and concepts of antigenic strength. *Transplant. Rev. 3*:5–21, 1970.

Hildemann, W. H., and Pinkerton, W.: Alloantibody production measured by plaque assay in relation to strong and weak histocompatibility. *J. Exp. Med. 124*:885–900, 1966.

Hildemann, W. H., Morgan, M., and Grautnick, L.: Immunogenetic components of weaker histoincompatibility systems in mice. *Transplant. Proc. 2*:24–31, 1970.

Hilgert, I., and Krištofová, H.: Tolerance-inducing capacity of cell free spleen and liver extracts of various immunogenicity. In *Genetic Variations in Somatic Cells*, J. Klein, M. Vojtíšková, and V. Zelený (eds.), pp. 417–424, Publishing House of the Czechoslovak Academy of Sciences, Prague, 1966.

Hilgert, I., Castermans, A., and Lejeune, G.: Reversible association of histone with transplantation antigens. *Folia Biol. (Praha) 10*:206–211, 1964.

Hilgert, I., Kandutsch, A. A., Cherry, M., and Snell, G. D.: Fractionation of murine H-2 antigens with the use of detergents. *Transplantation 8*:451–461, 1969.

Hilgert, I., Koubek, K., and Krištofová, H.: Purification and immunogenicity of H-2 antigens. In *Immunogenetics of the H-2 System*, A. Lengerová and M.Vojtíšková (eds.), pp. 211–223, Karger, Basel, 1971.

Hillman, N.: The effect of spatial arrangement on cell determination during mouse development. *J. Embryol. Exp. Morphol. 28*:263–278, 1972.

Hillman, N., Hillman, R., and Wileman, G.: Ultrastructural studies of cleavage stage t^{12}/t^{12} mouse embryos. *Amer. J. Anat. 128*:311–340, 1970.

Hinzová, E., Démant, P., and Iványi, P.: Genetic control of haemolytic complement in mice: Association with H-2. *Folia Biol. (Praha) 18*:237–243, 1972.

Hirschberg, H., Kaakinen, A., and Thorsby, E.: The T-cell receptor: Does it stimulate allogeneic lymphocytes in MLC? *Transplant Proc. 5*:1615–1616, 1973.

Hirschfeld, J.: Serologic codes: Interpretation of immunogenetic system. *Science 148*:968–970, 1965.

Hirschfeld, J.: Immunogenetic model. *Nature 239*:385–386, 1972.

Hodes, R. J., and Svedmyr, E. A. J.: Specific cytotoxicity of H-2-incompatible mouse lymphocytes following mixed culture *in vitro. Transplantation 9*:470–477, 1970.

Hoecker, G., and Hauschka, T. S.: Apparent loss of specific isoantigens in heteroploid transplanted tumor cells. *Transplant. Bull. 3*:134–136, 1956.

Hoecker, G., and Pizarro, O.: The histocompatibility antigens. In *Proceedings of the International Symposium on Tissue Transplantation*, A. P. Cristoffanini and G. Hoecker (eds.) pp. 54–71, University of Chile, Santiago, Chile, 1962.

Hoecker, G., Counce, S., and Smith, P.: The antigens determined by the H-2 locus: A rhesus-like system in the mouse. *Proc. Nat. Acad. Sci. USA 40*:1040–1051, 1954.

Hoecker, G., Pizarro, O., and Ramos, A.: Some new antigens and histocompatibility factors in the mouse. *Transplant. Bull. 6*:407–411, 1959.

Howard, J. C.: On the relationship between initiator and effector cells in the response to major transplantation antigens. *Transplant. Proc. 5*:1451–1456, 1973a.

Howard, J. C.: On cell-mediated cytoxicity as an effector-cell assay in transplantation immunity. *Transplant. Proc. 5*:1647–1649, 1973b.

Howe, M., Berman, L., and Cohen, L.: Relationship between proliferative and effector phases of the mixed lymphocyte reaction and graft-vs-host reaction. *J. Immunol. 111*:1243–2349, 1973.

Huber, B., Penz-Martinez, J., and Festenstein, H.: Spleen cell transplantation in mice: Influence of non-H-2 M locus on graft-vs.-host and host-vs.-graft reactions. *Transplant. Proc. 5*:1373–1375, 1973a.

Huber, B., Démant, P., and Festenstein, H.: Influence of M-locus (non-H-2) and K-end and D-end (H-2 region) incompatibility on heart muscle allograft survival time. *Transplant. Proc. 5*:1377–1383, 1973b.

Huemer, R. P., Keller, L. S., and Lee, K. D.: Thymidine incorporation in mixed cultures of spleen cells from mice of differing H-2 types. *Transplantation 6*:706–715, 1968.

Hull, P.: Partial incompatibility not affecting total litter size in the mouse. *Genetics 50*:563–570, 1964a.

Hull, P.: Equilibrium of gene frequency produced by partial incompatibility of offspring with dam. *Proc. Nat. Acad. Sci. USA 51*:461–464, 1964b.

Hull, P.: Possible stability of polymorphism in a multiallele incompatibility system in the mouse. *Genetics 54*:1049–1053, 1966.

Hull, P.: Maternal-foetal incompatibility associated with the *H-3* locus in the mouse. *Heredity 24*:203–209, 1969.

Hull, P.: Notes on Dr. Snell's observations concerning the *H-2* locus polymorphism. *Heredity 25*:461–465, 1970.

Hull, P.: The fifth chromosome histocompatibility types of mouse strains Hg/Hu and C3Hf/A. *Heredity 26*:140–145, 1971.

Hull, P.: Maternal foetal interactions and gene frequency changes in populations of mice. *Heredity 28*:201–208, 1972.

Humphrey, J. H., and Dourmashkin, R. R.: Electron microscope studies of immune cell lysis. In *Ciba Foundation Symposium on Complement*, G. E. W. Wolstenholme and J. Knight (eds.), pp. 175–186, Little, Brown, Boston, 1965.

Ikeda, H., Stockert, E., Rowe, W. P., Boyse, E. A., Lilly, F., Sato, H., Jacobs, S., and Old, L. J.: Relation of chromosome 4 (linkage group VIII) to murine leukemia virus-associated antigens of AKR mice. *J. Exp. Med. 137*:1103–1107, 1973.

Irvin, G. L., Eustace, J. C., and Fahey, J. L.: Enhancement activity of mouse immunoglobulin classes. *J. Immunol. 99*:1085–1091, 1967.

Itakura, K., Hutton, J. J., Boyse, E. A., and Old, L. J.: Linkage groups of the θ and Ly-A loci. *Nature New Biol. 230*:126, 1971.

Itakura, K., Hutton, J., Boyse, E. A., and Old, L. J.: Genetic linkage relationships of loci specifying differentiation alloantigens in the mouse. *Transplantation 13*: 239–243, 1972.

Iványi, P.: The major histocompatibility antigens in various species. *Cur. Topics Microbiol. Immunol. 53*:1–90, 1970.

Iványi, P., and Démant, P.: Preliminary studies on histocompatibility antigens in wild mice (*Mus musculus*). In *Proc. 11th European Conf. on Animal Blood Groups and Biochem. Polymorphism*, W. Junk (ed.), pp. 547–550, N.V. Publishers, The Hague, 1970.

Iványi, P., and Micková, M.: Antigenic strength of non-H-2 systems in mice. *Folia Biol. (Praha) 15*:395–396, 1969.

Iványi, P., and Micková, M.: Further studies on genetic factors in the ninth linkage group influencing reproductive performance in male mice. In *Immunogenetics of the H-2 System*, A. Lengerová and M. Vojtíšková (eds.), pp. 104–119, Karger, Basel, 1971.

Iványi, P., and Micková, M.: Testing of wild mice for "private" H-2 antigens. Cross reactions or nonspecific reactions? *Transplantation 14*:802–804, 1972.

Iványi, P., Démant, P., Vojtíšková, M., and Iványi, D.: Histocompatibility antigens in wild mice (*Mus musculus*). *Transplant. Proc. 1*:365–367, 1969.

Iványi, P., Hampl, R., Stárka, L., and Micková, M.: Genetic association between H-2 gene and testosterone metabolism in mice. *Nature New Biol. 238*:280–281, 1972a.

Iványi, P., Gregorová, S., and Micková, M.: Genetic differences in thymus, lymph node, testes and vesicular gland weights among inbred mouse strains. Association with major histocompatibility (H-2) system. *Folia Biol. (Praha) 18*:81–97, 1972b.

Iványi, P. Gregorová, S., Micková, M., Hampl, R., and Stárka, L.: Genetic association between a histocompatibility gene (H-2) and androgen metabolism in mice. *Transplant. Proc. 5*:189–191, 1973.

Ivašková, E., Dausset, J., and Iványi, P.: Cytotoxic reactions of anti-H-2 sera with human lymphocytes. *Folia Biol. (Praha) 18*:194–197, 1972.

James, D. A.: Effects of antigenic dissimilarity between mother and foetus on placental size in mice. *Nature 205*:613–614, 1965.

James, D. A.: Some effects of immunological factors on gestation in mice. *J. Reprod. Fert. 14*:265–271, 1967.

James, D. A.: Antigenicity of the blastocyst masked by the zona pellucida. *Transplantation 8*:846–851, 1969.

Jeekel, J. J., McKenzie, I. F. C., and Winn, H. J.: Immunological enhancement of skin grafts in the mouse. *J. Immunol. 108*:1017–1024, 1972.

Jensen, C. O.: Experimentelle Untersuchungen über Krebs bei Mäusen. *Centralbl. Bakteriol. Parasitenk. Infektionskrankh. 34*:28–34, 122–143, 1903.

Jensen, E., and Stetson, C. A.: Humoral aspects of the immune response to homografts. II. Relationship between the hemagglutinating and cytotoxic activities of certain isoimmune sera. *J. Exp. Med. 113*:785–794, 1961.

Jerne, N. K.: The somatic generation of immune recognition. *Eur. J. Immunol. 1*:1–9, 1971.

Johannsen, W., *Elemente der exakten Erblichkeitslehre*. Gustav Fisher, Jena, 1909.

John, M., Carswell, E., Boyse, E. A., and Alexander, G.: Production of θ antibody by mice that fail to reject θ incompatible skin grafts. *Nature New Biol. 238*:57–58, 1972.

Johnson, D. R.: Private communication. *Mouse News Letter 47*:52, 1972.

Johnson, M. H., and Edidin, M.: H-2 antigens on mouse spermatozoa. *Transplantation 14*:781–786, 1972.

Johnson, P. G.: Male sterility in mice homozygous for the t^{w2} allele. *Austral. J. Biol. Sci. 21*:947–951, 1968.

Johnston, J. M., and Wilson, D. B.: Origin of immunoreactive lymphocytes in rats. *Cell. Immunol. 1*:430–444, 1970.

Jones, G.: The number of reactive cells in mouse lymphocyte cultures stimulated by phytohemagglutinin, concanavalin A or histocompatibility antigen. *J. Immunol.* *111*:914–920, 1973.

Kaczmarzyk, K.: Alimentary activity of a free house mouse population (*Mus musculus* L.) *Bull. Acad. Polon. Sci. 12*:201–205, 1964.

Kahan, B. D.: Isolation of a soluble transplantation antigen. *Proc. Nat. Acad. Sci. USA 53*:153–161, 1965.

Kahan, B. D.: The *in vivo* immunogenicity assay of transplantation antigens. In *Transplantation Antigens*, B. D. Kahan and R. A. Reisfeld (eds.), pp. 311–338, Academic Press, New York, 1972.

Kahan, B. D., Zajtchuk, R., Dawson, D., and Adams, W. E.: The kinetics of sensitization with whole and fractionated mouse spleen cells. A preliminary report. *Dis. Chest 46*:452–456, 1964.

Kaliss, N.: Regression or survival of tumor homoiografts in mice pretreated with injections of lyophilized tissues. *Cancer Res. 12*:379–382, 1952.

Kaliss, N.: Immunological enhancement of tumor homografts in mice. A review. *Cancer Res. 18*:992–1003, 1958.

Kaliss, N.: The transplanted tumor as a research tool in cancer immunology. *Cancer Res. 21*:1203–1208, 1961.

Kaliss, N.: Transplanted tumors. In *Biology of the Laboratory Mouse*, E. L. Green (ed.), pp. 563–570, McGraw-Hill, New York, 1966.

Kaliss, N.: Transfer from mother to offspring of antifetal antibody induced in the mouse by multiparity. *Proc. Soc. Exp. Biol. Med. 129*:83–85, 1968.

Kaliss, N.: Micromethod for assaying immune cytolysis by the release of ^{51}Cr. *Transplantation 8*:526–530, 1969.

Kaliss, N., and Robertson, T.: Spleen transplantation relationships among two inbred lines of mice and their F_1 hybrid. *Genetics 28*:78, 1943. (*Abstract*).

Kandutsch, A. A.: Intracellular distribution and extraction of tumor homograft-enhancing antigens. *Cancer Res. 20*:264–268, 1960.

Kandutsch, A. A.: The chemistry of transplantation antigens. *Transplant. Bull. 27*:135–140, 1961.

Kandutsch, A. A.: Isolation of transplantation isoantigens of mice. *Meth. Med. Res. 10*:70–75, 1964.

Kandutsch, A. A., and Stimpfling, J. H.: An isoantigen lipoprotein from sarcoma I. In *Ciba Foundation Symposium on Transplantation*, pp. 72–86, Little, Brown, Boston, 1962.

Kandutsch, A. A.: The enhancement assay for prolongation of graft survival. In *Transplantation Antigens*, B. D. Kahan and R. A. Reisfeld (eds.), pp. 383–390, Academic Press, New York, 1972.

Kandutsch, A. A., and Reinert-Wenck, U.: Studies on a substance that promotes tumor homograft survival (the "enhancing substance"). *J. Exp. Med. 105*:125–138, 1957.

Kandutsch, A. A., and Stimpfling, J. H.: Partial purification of tissue isoantigens from a mouse sarcoma. *Transplantation 1*:201–216, 1963.

Kandutsch, A. A., and Stimpfling, J. H.: Properties of purified isoantigenic preparations from a mouse sarcoma. In *Immunopathology*, 4th Int. Symp., P. Grabar and P. Miescher (eds.), pp. 134–144, Schwabe, Basel, 1965.

Kandutsch, A. A., Jurgeleit, H. C., and Stimpfling, J. H.: The action of snake venom on an isoantigenic lipoprotein from a mouse sarcoma. *Transplantation 3*:748–761, 1965.

Kantor, F. S., Ojeda, A., and Benacerraf, B.: Studies on artificial antigens. I. Antigenicity of DNP-polylysine and DNP copolymer of lysine and glutamic acid in guinea pigs. *J. Exp. Med. 55*:55–69, 1963.

Kaplan, H. S.: On the natural history of the murine leukemias: Presidential address. *Cancer Res. 27*:1325–1340, 1967.

Karnovsky, J., and Unanue, E. R.: Mapping and migration of lymphocyte surface macromolecules. *Fed. Proc. 32*:55–59, 1973.

Katz, D. H.: The allogeneic effect on immune responses: Model for regulatory influences of T lymphocytes on the immune system. *Transplant Rev. 12*: 141–179, 1972.

Katz, D. H., and Benacerraf, B.: The regulatory influence of activated T cells on B cell responses to antigen. *Adv. Immunol. 15*:1–94, 1972.

Katz, D. H., Paul, W. E., Goidl, E. A., and Benacerraf, B.: Carrier function in anti-hapten immune responses. I. Enhancement of primary and secondary anti-hapten antibody responses by carrier preimmunization. *J. Exper. Med. 132*:261–282, 1970.

Katz, D. H., Hamaoka, T., and Benacerraf, B.: Cell interactions between histo-incompatible T and B lymphocytes. II. Failure of physiologic cooperative inter-actions between T and B lymphocytes from allogeneic donor strains in humoral response to hapten-protein conjugates. *J. Exp. Med. 137*:1405–1418, 1973a.

Katz, D. H., Hamaoka, T., Dorf, M. E., and Benacerraf, B.: Cell interactions between histoincompatible T and B lymphocytes. The H-2 gene complex determines successful physiologic lymphocyte interactions. *Proc. Nat. Acad. Sci. USA 70*: 2624–2628, 1973b.

Katz, D. H., Hamaoka, T., Dorf, E. D., Maurer, P. H., and Benacerraf, B.: Cell interactions between histoincompatible T and B lymphocytes. IV. Involvement of the immune response (Ir) gene in the control of lymphocyte interactions in responses controlled by the gene. *J. Exp. Med. 138*:734–739, 1973c.

Kerman, R. H., and Harris, T. N.: Resistance to denaturation by periodate of a dialyzable form of BALB/c histocompatibility antigen. *Proc. Soc. Exp. Biol. Med. 141*:179–183, 1972.

Kerman, R. H., Harris, T. N., and Harris, S.: Preparation of dialyzable histo-compatibility antigen from BALB/c mice. *Proc. Nat. Acad. Sci. USA 69*:223–227, 1972.

Key, M., and Hollander, W. F.: *Thin fur*, a recessive mutant on chromosome 17 of the mouse. *J. Hered. 63*:97–98, 1972.

Kimura, A. K.: Inhibition of specific cell-mediated cytotoxicity by anti-T-cell receptor antibody. *J. Exp. Med. 139*:888–901, 1974.

Kindred, B.: Skin grafting between sub-lines of inbred strains of mice. *Austral. J. Biol. Sci. 16*:863–868, 1963.

Kindred, B., and Shreffler, D. C.: H-2 dependence of co-operation between T and B cells *in vivo. J. Immunol. 109*:940–943, 1972.

Kirby, D. R. S.: The immunological consequences of extrauterine development of allogeneic mouse blastocysts. *Transplantation 6*:1005–1009, 1968.

Kirby, D. R. S.: On the immunologic function of the zona pellucida. *Fertil. Steril. 20*:933–937, 1969.

Kirby, D. R. S., Billington, W. D., and James, D. A.: Transplantation of eggs to the kidney and uterus of immunized mice. *Transplantation 4*:713–718, 1966.

Kissmeyer-Nielsen, F., and Thorsby, E.: Human transplantation antigens. *Transplant. Rev. 4*:1–176, 1970.

Klein, D., Merchant, D. J., Klein, J., and Shreffler, D. C.: Persistence of H-2 and some non-H-2 antigens on long-term-cultured mouse cell lines. *J. Nat. Cancer Inst. 44*:1149–1160, 1970.

Klein, E.: Isoantigenicity of X-ray-inactivated implants of a homotransplantable and non-homotransplantable mouse sarcoma. *Transplant. Bull. 23*:420–424, 1959.

Klein, E.: Studies on the mechanism of isoantigenic variant formation in heterozygous mouse tumors. I. Behavior of H-2 antigens D and K: Quantitative absorption tests on mouse sarcomas. *J. Nat. Cancer Inst. 27*:1069–1093, 1961.

Klein, E., and Klein, G.: Studies on the mechanism of isoantigenic variant formation in heterozygous mouse tumors. III. Behavior of H-2 antigens D and K when located in the trans position. *J. Nat. Cancer Inst. 32*:569–578, 1964.

Klein, E., and Möller, E.: Relationship between host range and isoantigenic properties in different sublines of the same sarcoma. *J. Nat. Cancer Inst. 31*:347–364, 1963.

Klein, E., Klein, G., and Révész, L.: Permanent modification (mutation?) of a histocompatibility gene in a heterozygous tumor. *J. Nat. Cancer Inst. 19*:95–144, 1957.

Klein, E., Klein, G., and Hellström, K. E.: Further studies on isoantigenic variation in mouse carcinomas and sarcomas. *J. Nat. Cancer Inst. 25*:271–294, 1960.

Klein, G.: The usefulness and limitations of tumor transplantation in cancer research: A review. *Cancer Res. 19*:343–358, 1959.

Klein, G., and Hellström, K. E.: Transplantation studies on estrogen-induced interstitial-cell tumors of testis in mice. *J. Nat. Cancer Inst. 28*:99–113, 1962.

Klein, G., and Klein, E.: Detection of an allelic difference at a single gene locus in a small fraction of a large tumor-cell population. *Nature 178*:1389–1391, 1956.

Klein, G., and Klein, E.: Histocompatibility changes in tumors. *J. Cell. Comp. Physiol. 52* (suppl. 1):125–168, 1958.

Klein, G., and Klein, E.: Nuclear and cytoplasmic changes in tumors. In *Developmental Cytology*, 6th Symp. Soc. Study Devel. Growth, D. Rudnick (ed.), pp. 63–82, Ronald Press, New York, 1959.

Klein, G., and Perlmann, P.: *In vitro* cytotoxic effect of isoantibody measured as isotope release from labelled target cell DNA. *Nature 199*:451–453, 1963.

Klein, J.: Changes of transplantation characteristics in methylcholanthrene-induced tumors. Isolation of specific isoantigenic variants. *Neoplasma 12*:125–130, 1965a.

Klein, J.: Changes in the host range of the tumour cell. Immunological characteristics of specific isoantigenic variants. *Folia Biol. (Praha) 11*:34–40, 1965b.

Klein, J.: Transplantation immunity to antigens of the *H-1* and *H-3* locus: strength, the effect of dosage, the additive effect and the development of H-3 antigens. *Folia Biol. (Praha) 11*:169–176, 1965c.

Klein, J.: The ontogenetic development of H-2 antigens *in vivo* and *in vitro*. In *Blood Groups of Animals*, J. Matoušek (ed.), pp. 405–414, Junk, The Hague, 1965d.

Klein, J.: Strength of some H-2 antigens in mice. *Folia Biol. (Praha) 12*:168–175, 1966a.

Klein, J.: Further evidence on the origin of alloantigenic variants of F_1 tumours grown in semiisogenic F_1 hosts. In *Genetic Variations in Somatic Cells*, J. Klein, M. Vojtíšková, and V. Zelený (eds.), pp. 385–392, Academia, Prague, 1966b.

Klein, J.: Strength of histocompatibility genes in mice. In *Histocompatibility Testing 1967*, E. S. Curtoni, P. L. Mattiuz, and R. M. Tosi (eds.), pp. 21–29, Munksgaard, Copenhagen, 1967.

Klein, J.: Histocompatibility-2 (H-2) polymorphism in wild mice. *Science 168*:1362–1364, 1970a.

Klein, J.: Order of loci in the 2nd linkage group of the mouse with respect to the centromere. *Genetics 64*:s35, 1970b. (*Abstract*).

Klein, J.: Private and public antigens of the mouse H-2 system. *Nature 229*:635–637, 1971a.

Klein, J.: Cytological identification of the chromosome carrying the IXth linkage group (including *H-2*) in the house mouse. *Proc. Nat. Acad. Sci. USA 68*:1594–1597, 1971b.

Klein, J.: Histocompatibility-2 system in wild mice. I. Identification of five new H-2 chromosomes. *Transplantation 13*:291–299, 1972a.

Klein, J.: Is the H-2K locus of the mouse stronger than the H-2D locus? *Tissue Antigens 2*:262–266, 1972b.

Klein, J.: Polymorphism of the H-2 loci in wild mice. In *International Symposium on HL-A Reagents*, R. H. Regamey and J. V. Spärck (eds.), pp. 251–256, S. Karger, Basel, 1973a.

Klein, J.: List of congenic lines of mice. I. Lines with differences at alloantigen loci. *Transplantation 15*:137–153, 1973b.

Klein, J., and Bailey, D. W.: Histocompatibility differences in wild mice: Further evidence for the existence of deme structure in natural populations of the house mouse. *Genetics 68*:287–297, 1971.

Klein, J., and Egorov, I. K.: Graft-vs-host reaction with an H-2 mutant. *J. Immunol. 111*:976–979, 1973.

Klein, J., and Iványi, P.: Contributions to the detection of incomplete isoimmune antibodies in mice by means of the Coombs test. *Folia Biol. (Praha) 9*:305–308, 1963.

Klein, J., and Klein, D.: Position of the translocation break T(2;9)138Ca in linkage group IX of the mouse. *Genet. Res. (Camb.) 19*:177–179, 1972.

Klein, J., and Martínková, J.: A new non-H-2 antigen of C57BL mice. *Folia Biol. (Praha) 14*:240–241, 1968.

Klein, J., and Murphy, D. B.: The role of "private" and "public" H-2 antigens in skin graft rejection. *Transplant. Proc. 5*:261–265, 1973.

Klein, J., and Park, J. M.: Graft-versus host reaction across different regions of the H-2 complex of the mouse. *J. Exp. Med. 137*:1213–1255, 1973.

Klein, J., and Raška, K., Jr.: Deficiency of "ribosomal" DNA in t[12] mutant mice. *Proc. XII Internat. Congress of Genetics*, Vol. 1, p. 149, Science Council of Japan, Tokyo, 1968. (*Abstract*).

Klein, J., and Secosky, W. R.: Tooth transplantation in the mouse. II. The role of the histocompatibility-2 (H-2) system in tooth germ transplantation. *Oral. Surg. 32*:513–521, 1971.

Klein, J., and Shreffler, D. C.: The H-2 model for major histocompatibility systems. *Transplant. Rev. 6*:3–29, 1971.

Klein, J., and Shreffler, D. C.: Evidence supporting a two-gene model for the H-2 histocompatibility system of the mouse. *J. Exp. Med. 135*:924–937, 1972a.

Klein, J., and Shreffler, D. C.: HL-A model of the H-2 system? *Tissue Antigens 2*:78–83, 1972b.

Klein, J., Klein, D., and Shreffler, D. C.: H-2 types of translocation stocks T(2;9)138Ca, T(9;13)190Ca and an H-2 recombinant. *Transplantation 10*:309–320, 1970.

Klein, J., Widmer, M. B., Segall, M., and Bach, F. H.: Mixed lymphocyte culture reactivity and H-2 histocompatibility loci differences. *Cell. Immunol. 4*:442–446, 1972.

Klein, J., Bach, F. H., Festenstein, H., McDevitt, H. O., Shreffler, D. C., Snell, G. D., and Stimpfling, J. H.: Genetic nomenclature for the H-2 complex of the mouse. *Immunogenetics 1*:184–188, 1974a.

Klein, J., Hauptfeld, M., and Hauptfeld, V.: Evidence for a third, *Ir*-associated histocompatibility region in the *H-2* complex of the mouse. *Immunogenetics 1*:45–56, 1974b.

Klein, J., Livnat, S., Hauptfeld, V., Jeřábek, L., and Weissman, I.: Production of H-2 antibodies in thymectomized mice. *Eur. J. Immunol. 4*:44–48, 1974c.

Klein, J., Hauptfeld, M., and Hauptfeld, V.: Serological distinction of mutants B6.C— H(zl) and B6.M505 from strain C57BL/6. *J. Exp. Med., 140*: 1127–1132, 1974d.

Klein, J., Hauptfeld, V., and Hauptfeld, M.: Involvement of H-2 regions in immune reactions. In *Progress in Immunology II*, L. Brent (ed.), Excerpta Medica Press, 1974e (*in press*).

Klein, J., Hauptfeld, V., and Hauptfeld, M.: Evidence for a fifth region (*G*) in the *H-2* complex of the mouse. *Immunogenetics* 1974f (*in press*).

Kobozieff, N.: Recherches morphologiques et génétiques sur ·l'anourie chez la souris. *Bull. Biol. 69*:265–405, 1935.

Koene, R., McKenzie, I. F. C., Painter, E., Sachs, D. H., Winn, H. J., and Russell, P. S.: Soluble mouse histocompatibility antigens. *Transplant. Proc. 3*:231–233, 1971.

Kohn, H. I.: H-gene (histocompatibility) mutations induced by triethylenemelamine in the mouse. *Mutation Res. 20*:235–242, 1973.

Kohn, H. I., and Melvold, R. W.: Spontaneous histocompatibility mutations detected by dermal grafts: Significant changes in rate over a 10-year period in the mouse H-system. *Mutation Res.*, 1974 (*in press*).

Komai, T.: Private communication. *Mouse News Letter 12*:44, 1955.

Komuro, K., Boyse, E. A., and Old, L. J.: Production of TL antibody by mice immunized with TL cell populations. *J. Exp. Med. 137*:533–536, 1973.

Komuro, K., Itakura, K., Boyse, E. A., and John, M.: Ly-5; A new T-lymphocyte antigen system. *Immunogenetics*, 1974 (*in press*).

Konda, S., Kakao, Y., and Smith, R. T.: Immunologic properties of mouse thymus cells. Identification of T cell functions within a minor, low-density subpopulation. *J. Exp. Med. 136*:1461–1477, 1972.

Konda, S., Stockert, E., and Smith, R. T.: Immunologic properties of mouse thymus cells: Membrane antigen patterns associated with various cell subpopulations. *Cell. Immunol. 7*:275–289, 1973.

Kreth, H. W., and Williamson, A. R.: Cell surveillance model for lymphocyte cooperation. *Nature 234*:454–456, 1971.

Krištofová, H., Lengerová, A., and Rejzková, J.: Indirect mapping of spatial distribution of some H-2 antigens on the cell membrane. *Folia Biol. (Praha) 16*:81–88, 1970.

Krohn, P. L.: Ovarian transplantation in mice. In *Biological Problems of Grafting*, F. Albert and P. B. Medawar (eds.), pp. 146–157, Blackwell, Oxford, 1959.

Kuminek, K.: Private communication. *Mouse News Letter 20*:31, 1959.

Kyslíková, L., and Forejt, J.: Chiasma frequency in three inbred strains of mice. *Folia Biol. (Praha) 18*:216–220, 1972.

Lafferty, K. J., and Jones, M. A. S.: Reactions of the graft-versus-host (GVH) type. *Austral. J. Exp. Biol. Med. Sci. 47*:17–54, 1969.

Lamm, M. E., Boyse, E. A., Old, L. J., Lisowska-Bernstein, B., and Stockert, E.:

Modulation of TL (Thymus-Leukemia) antigens by Fab-fragments of TL antibody. *J. Immunol. 101*:99–103, 1968.

Lamm, M. E., Koo, G. C., Stackpole, C. W., and Hämmerling, U.: Hapten-conjugated antibodies and visual markers used to label cell-surface antigens for electron microscopy: An approach to double labeling. *Proc. Nat. Acad. Sci. USA 69*: 3732–3736, 1972.

Landsteiner, K.: *The Specificity of Serological Reactions.* Harvard University Press, Cambridge, Mass., 1945.

Lapp, W. S., and Bliss, J. Q.: Skin graft size: Its effect on graft survival in mice incompatible at a weak locus. *Transplantation 4*:754–755, 1966.

Law, L. W.: Genetic studies in experimental cancer. *Adv. Cancer Res. 2*:281–352, 1954.

Law, L. W., Apella, E., Wright, P. W., and Strober, S.: Immunologic enhancement of allogeneic tumor growth with soluble histocompatibility-2 antigens. *Proc. Nat. Acad. Sci. USA 68*:3078–3082, 1971.

Law, L. W., Appella, E., Strober, S., Wright, P. E., and Fischetti, T.: Induction of immunological tolerance to soluble histocompatibility-2 antigens of mice. *Proc. Nat. Acad. Sci. USA 69*:1858–1862, 1972.

Lederberg, J.: Prospects for a genetics of somatic and tumor cells. *Ann. N.Y. Acad. Sci. 63*:662–665, 1956.

Lejeune, G., Castermans, A., Dieu, H. A., Haenen-Severyns, A. M., and Vranken-Paris, M.: Chemical assays of transplantation antigens. *Ann. N.Y. Acad. Sci. 99*:487–496, 1962.

Lengerová, A.: *Immunogenetics of Tissue Transplantation.* North-Holland, Amsterdam, 1969.

Lengerová, A., and Viklický, V.: Relative "strength" of histocompatibility barriers as compared on the basis of different criteria. *Folia Biol. (Praha) 15*:333–339, 1969.

Lengerová, A., Matoušek, V., Poláčková, M., Viklický, V., and Vojtíšková, M.: "Strength" of H-2 and non-H-2 antigens. In *Immunogenetics of the H-2 System*, A. Lengerová and M. Vojtíšková (eds.), pp. 300–304, Karger, Basel, 1971.

Lengerová, A., Pokorná, Z., Viklický, V., and Zelený, V.: Phenotypic suppression of H-2 antigens and topography of the cell surface. *Tissue Antigens 2*:332–340, 1972.

Lerner, R. A., Oldstone, M. B. A., and Cooper, N. R.: Cell cycle-dependent immune lysis of Moloney virus-transformed lymphocytes: Presence of viral antigen, accessibility to antibody, and complement activation. *Proc. Nat. Acad. Sci. USA 68*:2584–2588, 1971.

Levan, A., Hsu, T. C., and Stich, H. F.: The idogram of the mouse. *Hereditas 48*:677–687, 1962.

Levin, B. R., Petras, M. L., and Rasmussen, D. I.: The effect of migration on the maintenance of a lethal polymorphism in the house mouse. *Amer. Nat. 103*:647–661, 1969.

Lewontin, R. C.: Interdeme selection controlling a polymorphism in the house mouse. *Amer. Nat. 94*:65–78, 1962.

Lewontin, R. C., and Dunn, L. C.: The evolutionary dynamics of a polymorphism in the house mouse. *Genetics 45*:705–722, 1960.

Lieberman, M., and Kaplan, H. S.: Leukemogenic activity of filtrates from radiation-induced lymphoid tumors of mice. *Science 130*:387–388, 1959.

Lieberman, R., and Humphrey, W., Jr.: Association of H-2 types with genetic control of immune responsiveness to IgA allotypes in the mouse. *Proc. Nat. Acad. Sci. USA 68*:2510–2513, 1971.

Lieberman, R., and Humphrey, W., Jr.: Association of H-2 types with genetic control of immune responsiveness to IgG (γ2a) allotypes in the mouse. *J. Exp. Med.* *136*:1222–1230, 1972.

Lieberman, R., and Paul, W. E.: Genetic control of antibody responses to myeloma proteins of mice. *Contemp. Topics Immunobiol.* *3*:117–139, 1974.

Lieberman, R., Paul, W. E., Humphrey, W., Jr., and Stimpfling, J. H.: H-2-linked immune reponse (Ir) genes. Independent loci for Ir-IgG and Ir-IgA genes. *J. Exp. Med.* *136*:1231–1240, 1972.

Lilly, F.: The inheritance of susceptibility to the Gross leukemia virus in mice. *Genetics 53*:529–539, 1966a.

Lilly, F.: The histocompatibility-2 locus and suceptibility to tumor induction. *Nat. Cancer Inst. Monographs 22*:631–641, 1966b.

Lilly, F.: Susceptibility to two strains of Friend leukemia virus in mice. *Science 155*: 461–462, 1967a.

Lilly, F.: The location of histocompatibility-6 in the mouse genome. *Transplantation 5*:83–85, 1967b.

Lilly, F.: The effect of histocompatibility-2 type on response to the Friend leukemia virus in mice. *J. Exp. Med. 127*:465–473, 1968.

Lilly, F.: The role of genetics in Gross virus leukemogenesis. *Bibl. Haemat. 36*:213–220, 1970.

Lilly, F.: The influence of H-2 type on Gross virus leukemogenesis in mice. *Transplant. Proc. 3*:1239–1242, 1971a.

Lilly, F.: H-2 membranes and viral leukemogenesis. In *Cellular Interactions in the Immune Response*, S. Cohen, G. Cudkowicz, and R. T. McCluskey (eds.), pp. 103–108, Karger, Basel, 1971b.

Lilly, F.: Genetic regulation of the expression of antigen specificity H-2K.31 on mouse erythrocytes. *Immunogenetics 1*:22–32, 1974.

Lilly, F., and Duran-Reynals, M. L.: Combined neoplastic effects of vaccinia virus and 3-methylcholanthrene. II. Genetic factors. *J. Nat. Cancer Inst. 48*:105–112, 1972.

Lilly, F., and Klein, J.: An H-2^g like recombinant in the mouse. *Transplantation 16*: 530–532, 1973.

Lilly, F., and Pincus, T.: Genetic control of murine viral leukemogenesis. *Adv. Cancer Res. 17*:231–277, 1973.

Lilly, F., Boyse, E. A., and Old, L. J.: Genetic basis of susceptibility to viral leukaemo-genesis. *Lancet 2*:1207–1209, 1964.

Lilly, F., Jacoby, J. S., and Coley, R. C.: Immunologic unresponsiveness to the H-2.2 antigen. In *Immunogenetics of the H-2 System*, A. Lengerová and M. Vojtíšková (eds.), pp. 197–199, Karger, Basel, 1971.

Lilly, F., Graham, H., and Coley, R.: Genetic control of the antibody response to the H-2.2 alloantigen in mice. *Transplant. Proc. 5*:193–196, 1973.

Lind, P. E., and Szenberg, A.: Quantitative aspects of the Simonsen phenomenon III. The effects of immunization of the donor fowl. *Austral. J. Exp. Biol. Med. Sci. 39*:507–514, 1961.

Lindahl, K. F.: Antisera against recognition sites. Lack of effect on the mixed leuko-cyte culture interaction. *Eur. J. Immunol. 2*:501–504, 1972.

Linder, O. E. A.: Comparisons between survival of grafted skin, ovaries, and tumors in mice across histocompatibility barriers of different strength. *J. Nat. Cancer Inst. 27*:351–373, 1961.

Linder, O. E. A.: Skin compatibility of different CBA sublines separated from each other in the course of a varying number of generations. *Transplantation 1*:58–60, 1963.

Linder, O., and Klein, E.: Skin and tumor grafting in coisogenic resistant lines of mice and their hybrids. *J. Nat. Cancer Inst. 24*:707–720, 1960.

Little, C. C.: A possible Mendelian explanation for a type of inheritance apparently non-Mendelian in nature. *Science 40*:904–906, 1914.

Little, C. C., and Johnson, W. B.: The inheritance of susceptibility to implants of splenic tissue in mice. I. Japanese waltzing mice, albinos, and their F_1 generation hybrids. *Proc. Soc. Exp. Biol. 19*:163–167, 1922.

Little, C. C., and Tyzzer, E. E.: Further experimental studies on the inheritance of susceptibility to a transplantable tumor, carcinoma (J.W.A.) of the Japanese waltzing mouse. *J. Med. Res. 33*:393–453, 1916.

Livnat, S., Klein, J., and Bach, F. H.: Graft versus host reaction in strains of mice identical for H-2K and H-2D antigens. *Nature New Biol. 243*:42–49, 1973.

Loeb, L.: Über Entstehung eines Sarkoms nach Transplantation eines Adenocarcinoms einer japanischen Maus. *Zeitschr. f. Krebsforschung 7*:80–110, 1908.

Lonai, P., Wekerle, H., and Feldman, M.: Fractionation of specific antigen-reactive cells in an *in vitro* system of cell-mediated immunity. *Nature New Biol. 235*:235–237, 1972.

Lotzová, E., and Cudkowicz, G.: Hybrid resistance to parental NZW bone marrow grafts. *Transplantation 12*:130–138, 1971.

Lotzová, E., and Cudkowicz, G.: Hybrid resistance to parental WB/Re bone marrow grafts. *Transplantation 13*:256–264, 1972.

Lotzová, E., and Cudkowicz, G.: Resistance of irradiated F_1 hybrid and allogeneic mice to bone marrow grafts of NZB donors. *J. Immunol. 110*:791–800, 1973.

Lotzová, E., and Cudkowicz, G.: Abrogation of resistance to bone marrow grafts by silica particles. Prevention of the silica effect by the macrophage stabilizer poly-2-vinylpyridine N-oxide. *J. Immunol. 113*:798–803, 1974.

Lozner, E. C., Sachs, D. H., Shearer, G. M., and Terry, W. D.: B-cell alloantigens determined by the H-2 linked Ir region are associated with mixed lymphocyte culture stimulation. *Science 183*:757–759, 1974a.

Lozner, E. C., Sachs, D. H., and Shearer, G. M.: Genetic control of the immune response to staphylococcal nuclease. I. Ir-Nase: Control of the antibody response to nuclease by the Ir region of the mouse H-2 complex. *J. Exp. Med. 139*:1204–1214, 1974b.

Lumsden, T.: Tumour immunity: II. Antiserum treatment of spontaneous mouse carcinoma. *J. Pathol. Bacteriol. 35*:441–450, 1932.

Lyon, M. F.: Hereditary hair loss in the tufted mutant of the house mouse. *J. Hered. 47*:101–103, 1956.

Lyon, M. F.: A new dominant T-allele in the house mouse. *J. Hered. 50*:140–142, 1959.

Lyon, M. F.: Private communication. *Mouse News Letter 36*:34–35, 1967.

Lyon, M. F., and Hawker, S.: Private communication. *Mouse News Letter 42*:27, 1970.

Lyon, M. F., and Meredith, R.: Investigations of the nature of t-alleles in the mouse. I. Genetic analysis of a series of mutants derived from a lethal allele. *Heredity 19*:301–312, 1964a.

Lyon, M. F., and Meredith, R.: Investigations of the nature of t-alleles in the mouse.

II. Genetic analysis of an unusual mutant allele and its derivatives. *Heredity* *19*:313–325, 1964b.

Lyon, M. F., and Meredith, R.: Investigations of the nature of t-alleles in the mouse. III. Short tests of some further mutant alleles. *Heredity 19*:327–330, 1964c.

Lyon, M. F., and Phillips, R. J. S.: Crossing-over in mice heterozygous for t-alleles. *Heredity 13*:23–32, 1959.

Lyon, M. F., Butler, J. M., and Kemp, R.: The positions of the centromeres in linkage groups II and IX of the mouse. *Genet. Res. (Camb.) 11*:193–199, 1968.

Lyon, M. F., Glenister, P. H., and Hawker, S. G.: Do the H-2 and T-loci of the mouse have a function in the haploid phase of sperm? *Nature 240*:152–153, 1972.

MacLaurin, B. P.: Thymus origin of lymphocytes reacting and stimulating reaction in mixed lymphocyte cultures—studies in the rat. *Clin. Exp. Immunol. 10*:649–659, 1972.

Mandel, M. A., Monaco, A. P., and Russell, D. S.: Destruction of splenic transplantation antigens by a factor present in liver. *J. Immunol. 95*:673–682, 1965.

Mangi, R. J., and Mardiney, M. R.: Transformation of mouse lymphocytes to allogeneic lymphocytes and phytohemagglutinin. *J. Immunol. 105*:90–97, 1970.

Mann, D. L.: The effect of enzyme inhibitors on the solubilization of HL-A antigens with 3 M KCL. *Transplantation 14*:398–401, 1972.

Mann, D. L., and Nathenson, S. G.: Comparison of soluble human and mouse transplantation antigens. *Proc. Nat. Acad. Sci. USA 64*:1380–1387, 1969.

Mann, L. T., Jr., Corson, J. M., and Dammin, G. J.: Homo transplant antigens: Preparation of active cellular fractions by a modified method; properties and attempted dose response. *Nature 193*:168–169, 1962.

Manson, L. A., and Palm, J.: The solubilization of mouse transplantation antigens. In *Advance in Transplantation*, J. Dausset, J. Hamburger, and G. Mathé (eds.), pp. 301–304, Williams & Wilkins, Baltimore, 1968.

Manson, L. A., and Simmons, T.: Induction of the alloimmune response in mouse lymphocytes by cell-free transplantation antigens *in vitro*. Enhancement of DNA synthesis and specific sensitization. *Transplant. Proc. 1*:498–501, 1969.

Manson, L. A., and Simmons, T.: An *in vitro* model for study of the development of the alloimmune response. In *Cellular Interactions in the Immune Response*, S. Cohen, G. Cudkowicz, and R. T. McCluskey (eds.), pp. 235–240, Karger, Basel, 1971.

Manson, L. A., Foschi, G. V., and Duplan, J. F.: Isolation and characterization of transplantation antigens. II. Isolation procedures. *Transplant. Bull. 27*:145–147, 1960a.

Manson, L. A., Foschi, G. V., and Duplan, J. F.: Isolation of transplantation antigens from a cultured lymphoblast L-5178Y. *Nature 188*:598–599, 1960b.

Manson, L. A., Foschi, G. V., and Palm, J.: *In vivo* and *in vitro* studies of histocompatibility antigens isolated from a cultured mouse cell line. *Proc. Nat. Acad. Sci. USA 48*:1816–1822, 1962.

Manson, L. A., Foschi, G. V., and Palm, J.: An association of transplantation antigens with microsomal lipoproteins of normal and malignant mouse tissues. *J. Cell. Comp. Physiol. 61*:109–118, 1963.

Manson, L. A., Foschi, G. V., Dougherty, T., and Palm J.: Microsomal lipoproteins as transplantation antigens. *Ann. N.Y. Acad. Sci. 120*:251–260, 1964.

Manson, L. A., Hickey, C. A., and Palm, J.: H-2-alloantigen content of surface membrane of mouse cells. In *Biological Properties of the Mammalian Surface Membrane*, L. A. Manson (ed.), pp. 93–112, Wistar Institute Press, Philadelphia, 1968.

Manson, L. A., Simmons, T., Mills, L., and Friedman, H.: *In vitro* induction of immunity. Detection by an antibody plaque-reduction assay. In *Proc. 4th Leukocyte Culture Conf.*, O. R. McIntyre (ed.), pp. 193–205, Appleton-Century-Crofts, New York, 1970.

Marchalonis, J. J., Cone, R. E., and Atwell, J. L.: Isolation and partial characterization of lymphocyte surface immunoglobulins. *J. Exp. Med. 135*:956–971, 1972.

Mariani, T., Damhof, J., and Good, R. A.: Germinal center formation in response to skin grafted across weak and strong histocompatibility (H_2) barriers. *Adv. Exp. Med. Biol. 29*:597–602, 1973.

Martin, W. J., Maurer, P. H., and Benacerraf, B.: Genetic control of immune responsiveness to a glutamic acid, alanine, tyrosine copolymer in mice. I. Linkage of responsiveness to H-2 genotype. *J. Immunol. 107*:715–718, 1971.

Mauel, J., Rudolf, H., Chapius, B., and Brunner, K. T.: Studies of allograft immunity in mice. II. Mechanism of target cell inactivation *in vitro* by sensitized lymphocytes. *Immunology 18*:517–535, 1970.

Maurer, P. H., and Merryman, C.: Genetic control of immune responses of inbred mice against the terpolymers poly($glu^{57}lys^{38}ala^5$) and poly($glu^{54}lys^{36}ala^{10}$). *Immunogenetics 1*:174–183, 1974.

McDevitt, H. O.: Genetic control of the antibody response. III. Qualitative and quantitative characterization of the antibody response to (T,G)-A--L in CBA and C57 mice. *J. Immunol. 100*:485–492, 1968.

McDevitt, H. O., and Benacerraf, B.: Genetic control of specific immune responses. *Adv. Immunol. 11*:31–74, 1969.

McDevitt, H. O., and Chinitz, A.: Genetic control of the antibody response: Relationship between immune response and histocompatibility (H-2) type. *Science 163*: 1207–1208, 1969.

McDevitt, H. O., and Sela, M.: Genetic control of the antibody response. I. Demonstration of determinant-specific differences in response to synthetic polypeptide antigens in two strains of inbred mice. *J. Exp. Med. 122*:517–531, 1965.

McDevitt, H. O., and Sela, M.: Genetic control of the antibody response. II. Further analysis of the specificity of determinant-specific control, and genetic analysis of the response to (H,G)-A--L in CBA and C57 mice. *J. Exp. Med. 126*:969–978, 1967.

McDevitt, H. O., and Tyan, M. L.: Genetic control of the antibody response in inbred mice. Transfer of response by spleen cells and linkage to the major histocompatibility (H-2) locus. *J. Exp. Med. 128*:1–11, 1968.

McDevitt, H. O., Shreffler, D. C., Snell, G. D., and Stimpfling, J. H.: Genetic control of the antibody response: Genetic mapping studies of the linkage between the H-2 and Ir-1 loci. In *Immunogenetics of the H-2 System*, A. Lengerová and M. Vojtíšková (eds.), pp. 69–75, Karger, Basel, 1971.

McDevitt, H. O., Deak, B. D., Shreffler, D. C., Klein, J., Stimpfling, J. H., and Snell, G. D.: Genetic control of the immune response. Mapping of the Ir-1 locus. *J. Exp. Med. 135*:1259–1278, 1972.

McDevitt, H. O., Oldstone, M. B. A., and Pincus, T.: Genetic control of specific immune responses to viral infection. In *Proc. Soc. Gen. Physiol.*, Raven Press, New York, 1974a (*in press*).

McDevitt, H. O., Bechtol, K. B., Hämmerling, G. J., Lonai, P., and Delovitch, T. L.:
Ir genes and antigen recognition. In *The Immune System. Genes, Receptors, Signals*, E. E. Sercarz, A. R. Williamson, and C. F. Fox (eds.), pp. 597–632, Academic Press, New York, 1974b.

McKenzie, I. F. C.: The effect of the H-2 gene dose on the rejection of skin grafts. *Transplantation 15*:555–563, 1973.

McKenzie, I. F. C., and Snell, G. D.: Comparative immunogenicity and enhanceability of individual *H-2K* and *H-2D* specificities of the murine histocompatibility-2 complex. *J. Exp. Med. 138*:259–277, 1973.

McKenzie, I. F. C., Koene, R. A., Painter, E., Sachs, D., Winn, H. J., and Russell, P. S.: Mouse soluble transplantation antigens. In *Immunogenetics of the H-2 System*, A. Lengerová and M. Vojtíšková (eds.), pp. 231–237, Karger, Basel, 1971.

McKhann, D. F.: Additive effect of multiple weak incompatibilities in transplantation immunity. *Nature 201*:937–938, 1964.

McLaren, A.: Genetic and environmental effects on foetal and placental growth in mice. *J. Reprod. Fert. 9*:79–98, 1965.

McPherson, J. C., Clamp, J. R., and Manstone, A. J.: Carbohydrate analysis of membrane derived glycoproteins carrying some cell surface expressed antigens. *Immunochemistry 8*:225–234, 1971.

Medawar, P. B.: The behaviour and fate of skin autografts and skin homografts in rabbits. *J. Anat. 78*:176–199, 1944.

Medawar, P. B.: Communication. *Nature 182*:62, 1958.

Medawar, P. B.: Iso-antigens. In *Biological Problems of Grafting*, F. Albert and G. Lejeune-Ledant (eds.), pp. 6–19, Thomas, Springfield, Ill., 1959.

Medawar, P. B.: The use of antigenic tissue extracts to weaken the immunological reaction against skin homografts in mice. *Transplantation 1*:21–38, 1963.

Melchers, I., Rajewsky, K., and Shreffler, D. C.: Ir-LDH$_B$: Map position and functional analysis. *Eur. J. Immunol. 3*:754–761, 1973.

Melvold, R. W., and Kohn, H. I.: Histocompatibility mutations: *H-2* and *non-H-2*. *Mutat. Res.* 1974 (submitted).

Meo, T., Vives, J., Miggiano, V., and Shreffler, D.: A major role for the Ir-1 region of the mouse H-2 complex in the mixed leukocyte reaction. *Transplant. Proc. 5*: 377–381, 1973a.

Meo, T., David, C. S., Nabholz, M., Miggiano, V., and Shreffler, D. C.: Demonstration by MLR test of a previously unsuspected intra-H-2 crossover in the B10.HTT strain: Implications concerning location of MLR determinants in the Ir region. *Transplant. Proc. 5*:1507–1510, 1973b.

Meo, T., Vives, G., Rijnbeck, A. M., Miggiano, V. C., Nabholz, M., and Shreffler, D. C.: A bipartite interpretation and tentative mapping of H-2-associated MLR determinants in the mouse. *Transplant. Proc. 5*:1339–1350, 1973c.

Merryman, C. F., and Maurer, P. H.: Genetic control of immune response to glutamic acid, alanine, tyrosine copolymers in mice. I. Association of responsiveness to H-2 genotype and specificity of the response. *J. Immunol. 108*:135–141, 1972.

Merryman, C. F., and Maurer, P. H.: Characterization of a new *Ir-GLT* gene and its location in the *I* region of the *H-2* complex. *Immunogenetics*, 1974 (*in press*).

Merryman, C. F., Maurer, P. H., and Bailey, D. W.: Genetic control of immune response in mice to a glutamic acid, lysine, phenylalanine copolymer. III. Use of recombinant inbred strains of mice to establish association of immune response genes with H-2 genotype. *J. Immunol. 108*:937–940, 1972.

Micklem, H. S., and Loutit, J. F.: *Tissue Grafting and Radiation*, Academic Press, New York, 1966.

Micklem, H. S., and Staines, N. A.: Alloantibody-forming cells in skin allografted mice detected by immunocytoadherence. *Adv. Exper. Med. Biol. 5*:333–340, 1969.

Micková, M., and Iványi, P.: Antigenic strength of non-H-2 systems in mice. *Folia Biol. (Praha) 15*:395–396, 1969.

Micková, M., and Iványi, P.: Histocompatibility antigens in the wild house mouse (*Mus musculus*). In *Immunogenetics of the H-2 System*, A. Lengerová and M. Vojtíšková (eds.), pp. 20–34, Karger, Basel, 1971.

Micková, M., and Iványi, P.: An estimate of the degree of heterozygosity at histocompatibility loci in wild populations of house mouse (*Mus musculus*). *Folia Biol. (Praha) 18*:350–359, 1972.

Miggiano, V. C., Bernoco, D., Lightbody, J., Trinchieri, G., and Ceppellini, R.: Cell-mediated lympholysis *in vitro* with normal lymphocytes as target: Specificity and cross-reactivity of the test. *Transplant. Proc. 4*:231–237, 1972.

Miller, D. A., and Miller, O. J.: Chromosome mapping in the mouse. *Science 178*: 949–955, 1972.

Miller, D. A., Kouri, R. E., Dev, V. G., Grewal, M. S., Hutton, J. J., and Miller, O. J.: Assignment of four linkage groups to chromosomes in *Mus musculus* and a cytogenic method for locating their centromeric ends. *Proc. Nat. Acad. Sci. USA 68*:2699–2702, 1971.

Miller, J. F. A. P., and Mitchell, G. F.: The thymus and the precursors of antigen reactive cells. *Nature 216*:659–663, 1957.

Miller, O. J., Miller, D. A., Kouri, R. E., Allderdice, P. W., Dev, V. G., Grewal, M. S., and Hutton, J. J.: Identification of the mouse karyotype by quinacrine fluorescence, and tentative assignment of seven linkage groups. *Proc. Nat. Acad. Sci. USA 68*:1530–1533, 1971.

Mintz, B.: Formation of genetically mosaic mouse embryos and early development of "lethal (t^{12}/t^{12})-normal" mosaics. *J. Exp. Zool. 157*:273–292, 1964.

Mishell, R.: Leukocyte agglutination in mice. *Meth. Med. Res. 10*:35–38, 1964.

Mishell, R. I., Herzenberg, L. A., and Herzenberg, L. A.: Leukocyte agglutination in mice: Detection of H-2 and non-H-2 isoantigens. *J. Immunol. 90*:628–633, 1963.

Mitchell, G. F., Grumet, F. C., and McDevitt, H. O.: Genetic control of the immune response. The effect of thymectomy on the primary and secondary antibody response of mice to poly-L(Tyr,Glu)-poly-D,L-Ala-poly-L-Lys. *J. Exp. Med. 135*: 126–135, 1972.

Mitchell, M. S., Bove, J. R., and Calabresi, P.: Simplified estimation of mouse iso-hemagglutinins by microassay. *Transplantation 7*:294–296, 1969.

Mitchison, N. A.: The effect on the offspring of maternal immunization in mice. *J. Genetics 51*:406–420, 1953.

Mitchison, N. A.: Passive transfer of transplantation immunity. *Proc. Roy. Soc. (London) B 142*:72–87, 1954.

Mitchison, N. A.: Antigens of heterozygous tumors as material for the study of cell heredity. *Proc. Roy. Phys. Soc. 250*:45–48, 1956.

Mitchison, N. A.: The carrier effect in the secondary response to hapten protein conjugates. I. Measurement of the effect with transferred cells and objections to the local environment hypothesis. *Eur. J. Immunol. 1*:10–17, 1971a.

Mitchison, N. A.: The carrier effect in the secondary response to hapten protein conjugates. II. Cellular cooperation. *Eur. J. Immunol. 1*:18–27, 1971b.

Mitchison, N. A., and Dube, O. L.: Studies on the immunological response to foreign tumor transplants in the mouse. II. The relation between hemagglutinating antibody and graft resistance in the normal mouse and mice pretreated with tissue preparations. *J. Exp. Med. 102*:179–197, 1955.

Mobraaten, L. E., and Bailey, D. W.: Private communication. *Mouse News Letter 48*:17, 1973.

Möller, E.: Quantitative studies on the differentiation of isoantigens in newborn mice. *Transplantation 1*:165–173, 1963.

Möller, E.: Isoantigenic properties of tumors transgressing histocompatibility barriers of the H-2 system. *J. Nat. Cancer Inst. 33*:979–989, 1964.

Möller, E.: Interaction between tumor and host during progressive neoplastic growth in histoincompatible recipients. *J. Nat. Cancer Inst. 35*:1053–1059, 1965.

Möller, G.: Demonstration of mouse isoantigens at the cellular level by the fluorescent antibody technique. *J. Exp. Med. 114*:415–434, 1961a.

Möller, G.: Studies on the development of the isoantigens of the H-2 system in newborn mice. *J. Immunol. 86*:56–68, 1961b.

Möller, G.: Phenotypic expression of isoantigens of the H-2 system in embryonic and newborn mice. *J. Immunol. 90*:271–279, 1963.

Möller, G.: Fluorescent antibody technique for demonstration of isoantigens in mice. *Meth. Med. Res. 10*:58–75, 1964.

Möller, G.: Survival of H-2 incompatible mouse erythrocytes in untreated and isoimmune recipients. *Immunology 8*:360–374, 1965.

Möller, G.: Biologic properties of 19S and 7S mouse isoantibodies directed against isoantigens of the H-2 system. *J. Immunol. 96*:430–439, 1966.

Möller, G. (ed.), *Strong and Weak Histocompatibility Antigens. Transplant Rev.*, vol. 3, pp. 5–102, Munksgaard, Copenhagen, 1970.

Möller, G., and Möller, E.: Reactions of various normal and neoplastic cells with humoral isoantibodies. In *Mechanisms of Immunological Tolerance*, M. Hašek, A. Lengerová, and M. Vojtíšková (eds.), pp. 459–487, Publishing House of Czechoslovak Academy of Sciences, Prague, 1962a.

Möller, G., and Möller, E.: Phenotypic expression of mouse isoantigens. *J. Cell. Comp. Physiol. 60 (Suppl.)*:107–128, 1962b.

Möller, G., and Möller, E.: Plaque-formation by non-immune and X-irradiated lymphoid cells on monolayers of mouse embryo cells. *Nature 208*:260–263, 1965.

Monaco, A. P., Wood, M. L., and Russell, P. S.: Preparation of murine transplantation antigens: Ultracentrifugal distribution, physical properties and biological activity. *Transplantation 3*:542–556, 1965.

Moreno, C.: Fractionation of H-2 antigenic specificities in A/Sn mice. *Proc. Soc. Exp. Biol. Med. 122*:368–373, 1966.

Morgado, F., Pizarro, O., and Ramos, A.: The mortality of lethally irradiated mice given marrow of varying degrees of histocompatibility. *Transplantation 3*:517–523, 1965.

Moser, G. C., and Gluecksohn-Waelsch, S.: Developmental genetics of a recessive allele at the complex T-locus in the mouse. *Devel. Biol. 16*:564–576, 1967.

Mosier, D., and Cantor, H.: Functional maturation of mouse thymic lymphocytes. *Eur. J. Immunol. 1*:459–461, 1971.

Mozes, E., Shearer, G. M., and Sela, M.: Cellular basis of the genetic control of immune responses to synthetic polypeptides. I. Differences in frequency of splenic precursor cells specific for a synthetic polypeptide derived from multichain polyproline (T,G)-Pro--L) in high and low responder inbred mouse strains. *J. Exp. Med. 132*:613–622, 1970.

Mühlbock, O., and Dux, A.: Histocompatibility genes and susceptibility to mammary tumor virus (MTV) in mice. *Transplant. Proc. 3*:1247–1250, 1971a.

Mühlbock, O., and Dux, A.: Histocompatibility genes and mammary cancer in mice. In *Immunogenetics of the H-2 System*, A. Lengerová and M. Vojtíšková (eds.), pp. 123–128, Karger, Basel, 1971b.

Muramatsu, T., and Nathenson, S. G.: Studies on the carbohydrate portion of membrane-located mouse H-2 alloantigens. *Biochemistry 9*:4875–4883, 1970a.

Muramatsu, T., and Nathenson, S. G.: Isolation of a chromatographically unique glycopeptide from murine histocompatibility-2 (H-2) membrane alloantigens labelled with H^3-fucose or H^3-glucosamine. *Biochem. Biophys. Res. Comm. 38*: 1–8, 1970b.

Muramatsu, T., and Nathenson, S. G.: Comparison of the carbohydrate portion of membrane H-2 alloantigens isolated from spleen cells and tumor cells. *Biochem. Biophys. Acta 241*:195–199, 1971.

Muramatsu, T., Nathenson, S. G., Boyse, E. A., and Old, L. J.: Some biochemical properties of thymus leukemia antigens solubilized from cell membranes by papain digestion. *J. Exp. Med. 137*:1256–1262, 1973.

Nabholz, M., Vives, J., Young, H. M., Meo, T., Miggiano, V., Rijnbeck, A., and Shreffler, D. C.: Cell mediated cell lysis *in vitro*: Genetic control of killer cell production and target specificities in the mouse. *Eur. J. Immunol. 4*:378–387, 1974a.

Nabholz, M., Young, H., Meo, T., Miggiano, V., Rijnbeek, A., and Shreffler, D.: Genetic analysis of an *H-2* mutant, B6.C-*H-2^{ba}*, using cell-mediated lympholysis: T- and B-cell dictionaries for histocompatibility determinants are different. *Immunogenetics*, 1974b (*in press*).

Nakamuro, K., Tanigaki, N., and Pressman, D.: Multiple common properties of human β_2-microglobulin and the common portion fragment derived from HL-A antigen molecules. *Proc. Nat. Acad. Sci. USA 70*:2863–2865, 1973.

Nandi, S.: The histocompatibility-2 locus and suceptibility to Bittner virus borne by red blood cells in mice. *Proc. Nat. Acad. Sci. USA 58*:485–492, 1967.

Nandi, S., Haslam, S., and Helmich, C.: Inheritance of susceptibility to erythrocyte-borne Bittner virus in mice. *Transplant. Proc. 3*:1251–1257, 1971.

Nathenson, S. G., and Davies, D. A. L.: Solubilization and partial purification of mouse histocompatibility antigens from a membranous lipoprotein fraction. *Proc. Nat. Acad. Sci. USA 56*:476–483, 1966a.

Nathenson, S. G., and Davies, D. A. L.: Transplantation antigens: Studies of the mouse model system, solubilization and partial purification of H-2 isoantigens. *Ann. N.Y. Acad. Sci. 129*:6–13, 1966b.

Nathenson, S. G., and Muramatsu, T.: Properties of the carbohydrate portion of mouse H-2 alloantigen glycoproteins. In *Glycoproteins of Blood Cells and Plasma*, G. A. Jamieson and T. J. Greenwalt (eds.), pp. 245–262, Lippincott, Philadelphia, 1971.

Nathenson, S. G., and Shimada, A.: Papain-solubilization of mouse H-2 isoantigens: An improved method of wide applicability. *Transplantation 6*:662–663, 1968.

Neauport-Sautes, C., Lilly, F., Silvestre, D., and Kourilsky, F. M.: Independence of H-2K and H-2D antigenic determinants on the surface of mouse lymphocytes. *J. Exp. Med. 137*:511–526, 1973.

Neauport-Sautes, C., Bismuth, A., Kourilsky, F. M., and Manuel, Y.: Relationship between HL-A antigens and β_2-microglobulin as studied by immunofluorescence on the lymphocyte membrane. *J. Exp. Med. 139*:957–968, 1974.

Němec, M., Nouza, K., and Démant, P.: Factors influencing different reactivity against H-2K and H-2D antigens in normal and ALS-suppressed mice. *Transplant. Proc. 5*:275–279, 1973.

Nesbitt, M. N., and Francke, U.: A system of nomenclature for band patterns of mouse chromosomes. *Chromosoma 41*:145–158, 1973.

Nicolson, G. L., Hyman, R., and Singer, S. J.: The two dimensional topographic distribution of H-2 histocompatibility alloantigens on mouse red blood cell membranes. *J. Cell Biol. 50*:905–910, 1971.

Nielson, H. E.: Reactivity of lymphocytes from germ-free rats in mixed leukocyte culture and in graft-versus-host reaction. *J. Exp. Med. 136*:417–424, 1972.

Nisbet, N. W., and Edwards, J.: The H-2D and H-2K regions of the major histocompatibility system and the M locus of the mouse investigated by parabiosis. *Transplant. Proc. 5*:1411–1415, 1973.

Nombela, J. J. A., and Murcia, C. R.: Identification of mouse chromosomes, in myeloid cells, by means of secondary constrictions. *Chromosoma 37*:63–73, 1972.

Nossal, G. J. V., and Ada, G. L.: *Antigens, Lymphoid Cells, and the Immune Response.* Academic Press, New York, 1971.

Nowell, P. C.: Phytohaemagglutinin: An initiator of mitosis in cultures of normal human leukocytes. *Cancer Res. 20*:462–466, 1960.

Odaka, T., and Yamamoto, T.: Inheritance of susceptibility to Friend mouse leukemia virus. *Jap. J. Exp. Med. 32*:405–413, 1962.

Old, L. J., and Boyse, E. A.: Antigens of tumors and leukemias induced by viruses. *Fed. Proc. 24*:1009–1017, 1965.

Old, L. J., Boyse, E. A., and Stockert, E.: Antigenic properties of experimental leukemias. I. Serological studies *in vitro* with spontaneous and radiation-induced leukemias. *J. Nat. Cancer Inst. 31*:977–986, 1963.

Old, L. J., Stockert, E., Boyse, E. A., and Kim, J. H.: Antigenic modulation. Loss of TL antigen from cells exposed to TL antibody. Study of the phenomenon *in vitro*. *J. Exp. Med. 127*:523–539, 1968.

Olds, P. J.: An attempt to detect H-2 antigens on mouse eggs. *Transplantation 6*:478–479, 1968.

Olds, P. J.: Effect of the T locus on sperm distribution in the house mouse. *Biol. Reprod. 2*:91–97, 1970.

Olds, P. J.: Effect of the T locus on fertilization in the house mouse. *J. Exp. Zool. 177*:417–434, 1971a.

Olds, P. J.: Effect of the T locus on sperm ultrastructure in the house mouse. *J. Anat. 109*:31–37, 1971b.

Oldstone, M. B. A., Dixon, F. J., Mitchell, G. F., and McDevitt, H. O.: Histocompatibility-linked genetic control of disease susceptibility. Murine lymphocytic choriomeningitis virus infection. *J. Exp. Med. 137*:1201–1212, 1973.

O'Neill, G. J., and Davies, D. A. L.: Behaviour of mouse H-2 specificities on polyacrylamide gel electrophoresis and polyacrylamide gel electrofocusing. *Biochim. Biophys. Acta 243*:337–342, 1971.

Oppltová, L., and Démant, P.: Genetic determinants for the graft-vs.-host reaction in the H-2 complex. *Transplant. Proc. 5*:1367, 1973.

Ordal, J. C., and Grumet, F. C.: Suppression of anti-(T,G)-A--L antibody production in nonresponder mice. *Transplant. Proc.* 5:175–178, 1973.

Oth, A., and Castermans, A.: Study of transplantation antigens from isolated nuclei. *Transplant. Bull.* 6:418–424, 1959.

Owen, R. D.: Immunogenetics. *Proc. Xth Internat. Congress Genetics*, pp. 364–374, University of Toronto Press, Toronto, Ont., 1959.

Owen, R. D.: Immunogenetic basis of transplant tolerance and rejection. In *Mechanisms of Immunological Tolerance*, M. Hašek, A. Lengerová and M. Vojtíšková (eds.), pp. 133–142, Publishing House of the Czechoslovak Academy of Sciences, Prague, 1962.

Ozer, H. L., and Herzenberg, L. A.: H-2 immunogenicity of liver cell membranes in the mouse. *Transplant. Bull.* 30:164–166, 1962.

Ozer, H. L., Klein, G., and Ozer, J. H.: Studies on the mechanism of isoantigenic variant formation in heterozygous mouse tumors. IV. H-2 component analysis of an (A/Sn × A.SW)F₁ lymphoma. *J. Nat. Cancer Inst.* 36:233–247, 1966.

Ozer, J. H., and Wallach, D. F. H.: H-2 components and cellular membranes: Distinctions between plasma membrane and endoplasmic reticulum governed by the H-2 region in the mouse. *Transplantation* 5:652–667, 1967.

Palm, J.: Serological detection of histocompatibility antigens in two strains of rats. *Transplantation* 3:603–612, 1964.

Palm, J., and Manson, L. A.: Tissue distribution and intracellular sites of some mouse isoantigens. In *Isoantigens and Cell Interactions*, J. Palm (ed.), pp. 21–36, Wistar Institute Press, Philadelphia, 1965.

Palm, J., Heyner, S., and Brinster, R. L.: Differential immunofluorescence of fertilized mouse eggs with H-2 and non-H-2 antibody. *J. Exp. Med.* 133:1282–1293, 1971.

Pancake, S. J., and Nathenson, S. G.: Selective loss of H-2 antigenic reactivity after chemical modification. *J. Immunol.* 111:1086–1092, 1973.

Pantelouris, E. M.: Absence of thymus in a mouse mutant. *Nature* 217:370–371, 1968.

Papermaster, B. W., and Herzenberg, L. A.: Isolation and characterization of an isoantigenic variant from a heterozygous mouse lymphoma in culture. *J. Cell. Physiol.* 67:407–420, 1966.

Parr, E. L., and Oei, J. S.: Immobilization of membrane H-2 antigens by paraformaldehyde fixation. *J. Cell Biol.* 59:537–548, 1973.

Passmore, H. C.: *Genetic and Hormonal Control of a Serum Protein Variant Associated with the H-2 Region of the Mouse.* Ph.D. Thesis, University of Michigan, Ann Arbor, 1970.

Passmore, H. C., and Shreffler, D. C.: A sex-limited serum protein variant in the mouse: Inheritance and association with the H-2 region. *Bioch. Genetics* 4:351–365, 1970.

Passmore, H. C., and Shreffler, D. C.: A sex-limited serum protein variant in the mouse: Hormonal control of phenotypic expression. *Bioch. Genetics* 5:201–209, 1971.

Pasternak, C. A., Warmsley, A. M. H., and Thomas, D. B.: Structural alterations in the surface membrane during the cell cycle. *J. Cell Biol.* 50:562–564, 1971.

Peacock, W. J., and Miklos, G. L. G.: Meiotic drive in *Drosophila*: New interpretations of the segregation distorter and sex chromosome system. *Adv. Genetics* 17:361–409, 1973.

Peck, A. B., and Click, R. E.: Immune responses *in vitro*. VII. Differentiation of H-2 and non-H-2 alloantigens of the mouse by a dual mixed leukocyte culture. *Transplantation 16*:331–338, 1973a.

Peck, A. B., and Click, R. E.: Immune responses *in vitro*. VIII. Mixed leukocyte culture reactivity induced by θ antigen. *Transplantation 16*:339–342, 1973b.

Peck, A. B., Bach, F. H., and Boyse, E. A.: Cellular reactivities associated with theta-antigen disparity. *Transplant. Proc. 5*:1611–1613, 1973.

Pellegrino, M. A., Ferrone, S., and Pellegrino, A.: Serologic detection of soluble HL-A antigens. In *Transplantation Antigens*, B. D. Kahan and R. A. Reisfeld (eds.), pp. 433–452, Academic Press, New York, 1972.

Peña-Martinez, J., Huber, B., and Festenstein, H.: The influence of H-2 and non-H-2 M locus on spleen colony formation after allogeneic bone marrow transplantation in irradiated mice, assayed by ^{59}Fe uptake and colony counting. *Transplant. Proc. 5*:1393–1397, 1973.

Perlmann, P., and Holm, G.: Studies on the mechanism of lymphocyte cytotoxicity. In *Mechanisms of Inflammation Induced by Immune Reactions* (Internat. Symp. Immunopathol. V), P. Miescher and P. Grabar (eds.), p. 325–341, Schwabe, Basel, 1968.

Peterson, P. A., Cunningham, B. A., Berggard, I., and Edelman, G. M.: β_2-microglobulin—A free immunoglobulin domain. *Proc. Nat. Acad. Sci. USA 69*:1697–1701, 1972.

Peterson, P. A., Rask, L., and Lindblom, J. B.: Highly purified papain-solubilized HL-A antigens contain β_2-microglobulin. *Proc. Nat. Acad. Sci. USA 71*:35–39, 1974.

Petras, M. L.: Studies of natural populations of *Mus*. I. Biochemical polymorphisms and their bearing on breeding structure. *Evolution 21*:259–274, 1967a.

Petras, M. L.: Studies of natural populations of *Mus*. II. Polymorphism at the T locus. *Evolution 21*:466–467, 1967b.

Petras, M. L.: Studies of natural populations of *Mus*. III. Coat color polymorphisms. *Canad. J. Genet. Cytol. 9*:287–296, 1967c.

Petras, M. L.: Studies of natural populations of *Mus*. IV. Skeletal variations. *Canad. J. Genet. Cytol. 9*:575–588, 1967d.

Petrusewicz, K.: Further investigation of the influence exerted by the presence of their home cages and own populations on the results of fights between male mice. *Bull. Acad. Polon. Sci. 7*:319–326, 1959.

Phillips, S. M., Carpenter, C. B., and Strom, T. B.: Cellular immunity in the mouse. III. *In vitro* kinetic studies on the relationship between recognition and effector phases. *Transplant. Proc. 5*:1669–1673, 1973.

Pincus, T., Hartley, J. W., and Rowe, W. P.: A major genetic locus affecting resistance to infection with murine leukemia viruses. I. Tissue culture studies of naturally occurring viruses. *J. Exp. Med. 133*:1219–1233, 1971a.

Pincus, T., Rowe, W. P., and Lilly, F.: A major genetic locus affecting resistance to infection with murine leukemia viruses. II. Apparent identity to a major locus described for resistance to Friend murine leukemia virus. *J. Exp. Med. 133*:1234–1242, 1971b.

Pizarro, O., and Dunn, L. C.: A study of recombination between the H-2 (histocompatibility) locus and loci closely linked with it in the house mouse. *Transplantation 9*:207–218, 1970.

Pizarro, O., and Vergara, U.: Relationship between locus R (Ea-2) and the other loci of the ninth linkage group of the house mouse. *Folia Biol. (Praha) 19*:89–94, 1973.

Pizarro, O., Hoecker, G., Rubinstein, P., and Ramos, A.: The distribution in the tissues and development of H-2 antigens of the mouse. *Proc. Nat. Acad. Sci. USA* 47:1900–1906, 1961.

Pizarro, O., Rubinstein, P., and Hoecker, G.: Properties of histocompatibility-2 antigens from different tissues. *Guy's Hosp. Rep. 112*:392–401, 1963.

Plate, J. M. D.: Mixed lymphocyte culture responses of mice: An analysis of the contribution of allelic differences at the various loci known to exist within the H-2 complex. *Transplant. Proc. 5*:1351–1359, 1973.

Plate, J. M. D.: Mixed lymphocyte culture responses of mice. Genetic analysis of the responses to H-2D^d specificities. *J. Exp. Med. 139*:851–860, 1974.

Plate, J. M. D., and McKenzie, I. F. C.: "B"-cell stimulation of allogeneic T-cell proliferation in mixed lymphocyte cultures. *Nature New Biol. 245*:247–249, 1973.

Popp, D. M.: A description of rho: A non-H-2 isoantigen in RFM mice. *Transplantation 5*:290–299, 1967.

Popp, D. M.: Histocompatibility-14: Correlation of the isoantigen rho and R-Z locus. *Transplantation 7*:233–241, 1969.

Popp, D. M.: *In vivo* lymphocyte transformation induced by H-2D and H-2K components of the H-2 locus. *Transplant. Proc. 5*:281–285, 1973.

Popp, D. M., and Davies, M. L.: *In vivo* lymphocyte transformation. In *Immunogenetics of the H-2 System*, A. Lengerová and M. Vojtíšková (eds.), pp. 182–187, Karger, Basel, 1971.

Potter, M., and Lieberman, R.: Genetics of immunoglobulins in the mouse. *Adv. Immunol. 7*:91–145, 1967.

Prehn, R. T., and Main, J. M.: Number of mouse histocompatibility genes involved in skin grafting from strain BALB/cAn to strain DBA/2. *J. Nat. Cancer Inst. 20*:207–209, 1958.

Premkamur, E., Shoyab, M., and Williamson, A. R.: Germ line basis for antibody diversity: Immunoglobulin V_H- and C_H-gene frequencies measured by DNA-RNA hybridization. *Proc. Nat. Acad. Sci. USA 71*:99–103, 1974.

Pressman, D., and Grossberg, A. L.: *The Structural Basis of Antibody Specificity.* W. A. Benjamin, Menlo Park, Calif., 1968.

Prout, T.: Some effects of variations in the segregation ratio and of selection on the frequency of alleles under random mating. *Acta Genet. Statist. Med. 4*:148–151, 1953.

Race, R. R., and Sanger, R.: *Blood Groups in Man.* Davis, Philadelphia, 1968.

Raff, M. C., and dePetris, S.: Movement of lymphocyte surface antigens and receptors: The fluid nature of the lymphocyte plasma membrane and its immunological significance. *Fed. Proc. 32*:48–54, 1973.

Ramseier, H.: Antibodies to receptors recognizing histocompatibility antigens. *Cur. Topics Microbiol. Immunol. 60*:31–78, 1973.

Ramseier, H., and Lindenmann, J.: Aliotypic antibodies. *Transplant. Rev. 10*:57–96, 1972.

Ranney, D. F., Gordon, R. O., Pincus, J. H., and Oppenheim, J. J.: Biological effects of murine histompatibility antigen solubilized with 3M potassium chloride. *Transplantation 16*:558–564, 1973.

Rapaport, F. T.: The biological significance of cross-reactions between histocompatibility antigens and antigens of bacterial and/or heterologous mammalian origin. In *Transplantation Antigens*, B. D. Kahan and R. A. Reisfeld (eds.), pp. 181–208, Academic Press, New York, 1972.

Rathbun, W. E., and Hildemann, W. H.: Genetic control of the antibody response to simple haptens in congenic strains of mice. *J. Immunol. 105*:98–107, 1970.

Reed, S. C.: The inheritance and expression of Fused, a new mutation in the house mouse. *Genetics 22*:1–13, 1937.

Reif, A. E., and Allen, J. M. V.: Specificity of isoantisera against leukemic and thymic lymphocytes. *Nature 200*:1332, 1963.

Reif, A. E., and Allen, J. M.: The AKR thymic antigen and its distribution in leukemias and nervous tissues. *J. Exp. Med. 120*:413–433, 1964.

Reimer, J. D., and Petras, M. L.: Breeding structure of the house mouse, *Mus musculus*, in a population cage. *J. Mammal. 48*:88–99, 1967.

Reimer, J. D., and Petras, M. L.: Some aspects of commensal populations of *Mus musculus* in Southwestern Ontario. *Canad. Field Nat. 82*:32–42, 1968.

Richards, F. F., and Konigsberg, W. H.: How specific are antibodies? *Immunochemistry 10*:545–563, 1973.

Robinson, R.: *Gene Mapping in Laboratory Mammals*. Part A, Plenum Press, New York, 1971.

Rosenau, W., and Moon, H. D.: Lysis of homologous cells by sensitized lymphocytes in tissue culture. *J. Nat. Cancer Inst. 27*:471–483, 1961.

Rosenfield, R. E., Allen, F. H., Jr., Swisher, S. N., and Kochwa, S.: A review of Rh serology and presentation of a new terminology. *Transfusion 2*:187–312, 1962.

Rowe, F. P., Taylor, E. J., and Chudley, A. H. J.: The numbers and movements of house-mice (*Mus musculus L.*) in the vicinity of four corn-ricks. *J. Anim. Ecol. 32*:87–97, 1963.

Rowe, W. P.: Studies of genetic transmission of murine leukemia virus by AKR mice. I. Crosses with Fv-1ⁿ strains of mice. *J. Exp. Med. 136*:1272–1285, 1972.

Rowe, W. P., and Brodsky, I.: A graded-response assay for the Friend leukemia virus. *J. Nat. Cancer Inst. 23*:1239–1248, 1959.

Rowe, W. P., and Hartley, J. W.: Studies of genetic transmission of murine leukemia virus by AKR mice. II. Crosses with Fv-1ᵇ strains of mice. *J. Exp. Med. 136*: 1286–1301, 1972.

Rowe, W. P., and Sato, H.: Genetic mapping of the Fv-1 locus of the mouse. *Science 180*:640–641, 1973.

Rowe, W. P., Humphrey, J. B., and Lilly, F.: A major genetic locus affecting resistance to infection with murine leukemia viruses. III. Assignment of the Fv-1 locus to linkage group VIII of the mouse. *J. Exp. Med. 137*:850–853, 1973.

Rubinstein, P.: Different immunogenicity of the H-2 antigens of liver and spleen in mice. *Transplantation 2*:695–706, 1964.

Rubinstein, P., and Ferrebee, J. W.: The H-2 phenotypes of random-bred Swiss-Webster mice. *Transplantation 6*:715–721, 1964.

Rugh, R.: *The Mouse: Its Reproduction and Development*. Burgess, Minneapolis, 1968.

Rychlíková, M., and Iványi, P.: Mixed lymphocyte cultures and histocompatibility antigens in mice. *Folia Biol. (Praha) 15*:126–135, 1969.

Rychlíková, M., Démant, P., and Iványi, P.: The predominant role of the K-end of the H-2 locus in lymphocyte transformation in mixed cultures. *Folia Biol. (Praha) 16*:218–221, 1970.

Rychlíková, M., Démant, P., and Iványi, P.: Histocompatibility gene organization and mixed lymphocyte reaction. *Nature New Biol. 230*:271–272, 1971.

Rychlíková, M., Démant, O., and Egorov, I. K.: Mixed lymphocyte reaction caused by an H-2D mutation. *Folia Biol. (Praha) 18*:360–363, 1972.

Rychlíková, M., Démant, P., and Iványi, P.: The mixed lymphocyte reaction in H-2K, H-2D and non-H-2 incompatibility. *Biomedicine 18*:401–407, 1973.

Rygaard, J., and Povlsen, C. O.: Is immunological surveillance not a cell-mediated immune function? *Transplantation 17*:135–136, 1974.

Sachs, D. H., and Cone, J. L.: A mouse B-cell alloantigen determined by gene(s) linked to the major histocompatibility complex. *J. Exp. Med. 138*:1289–1304, 1973.

Sachs, J. A., Huber, B., Peña-Martinez, J., and Festenstein, H.: Genetic studies and effect on skin allograft survival of DBA/2 DAG, Ly, and M-locus antigens. *Transplant. Proc. 5*:1385–1387, 1973.

Salmon, S. E., Krakauer, R. S., and Whitmore, W. F.: Lymphocyte stimulation: Selective destruction of cells during blastogenic response to transplantation antigens. *Science 172*:490–492, 1971.

Sanderson, A. R.: Applications of iso-immune cytolysis using radiolabelled target cells. *Nature 204*:250–253, 1964a.

Sanderson, A. R.: Cytotoxic reactions of mouse isoantisera: Preliminary considerations. *Brit. J. Exp. Pathol. 45*:398–408, 1964b.

Sanderson, A. R.: Quantitative titration, kinetic behaviour, and inhibition of cytotoxic mouse isoantisera. *Immunology 9*:287–300, 1965a.

Sanderson, A. R.: Cytotoxic reactions of mouse isoantisera: The scope of an assay using radiolabelled target cells. *Transplantation 3*:557–562, 1965b.

Sanderson, A. R., and Davies, A. L.: Enzymatic activity of mouse histocompatibility antigen preparations. *Nature 200*:32–33, 1963.

Sankowski, A., and Nouza, K.: The dynamics of graft-versus-host reaction across a strong and weak histocompatibility barrier. *Folia Biol. (Praha) 14*:372–382, 1968.

Sato, H., Boyse, E. A., Aoki, T., Iritani, C., and Old, L. J.: Leukemia-associated transplantation antigens related to murine leukemia virus. *J. Exp. Med. 138*:593–606, 1973.

Saunders, D., and Edidin, M.: Sites of localization and synthesis of Ss protein in mice. *J. Immunol. 112*:2210–2218, 1974.

Scheid, M., Boyse, E. A., Carswell, E., and Old, L. J.: Serologically demonstrable alloantigens of mouse epidermal cells. *J. Exp. Med. 135*:938–955, 1972.

Schendel, D. J., Alter, B. J., and Bach, F. J.: The involvement of LD- and SD-region differences in MLC and CML: A three-cell experiment. *Transplant. Proc. 5*:1651–1655, 1973.

Schierman, L. W., and Nordskog, A. W.: Relationship of blood type to histocompatibility in chickens. *Science 134*:1008–1009, 1961.

Schlesinger, M.: Serologic studies of embryonic and trophoblastic tissues of the mouse. *J. Immunol. 93*:255–263, 1964.

Schlesinger, M.: How cells acquire antigens. *Progr. Exp. Tumor Res. 13*: 28–83, 1970.

Schlesinger, M., and Chaouat, M.: Modulation of the H-2 antigenicity on the surface of murine peritoneal cells. *Tissue Antigens 2*:427–435, 1972.

Schlesinger, M., and Chaouat, M.: Antibody-induced alteration in the expression of the H-2 antigenicity on murine peritoneal cells: The effect of metabolic inhibitors on antigenic modulation and antigen recovery. *Transplant. Proc. 5*:105–110, 1973.

Schlesinger, M., Boyse, E. A., and Old, L. J.: Thymus cells of radiation-chimeras: TL phenotype, sensitivity to guinea-pig serum, and origin from donor cells. *Nature 206*:1119–1121, 1965.

Schlesinger, M., Cohen, A., and Hurvitz, D.: Characterization of cytotoxic isoantisera produced in RIII mice. II. Serological properties of antiserum fractions. In *Topics in Basic Immunology*, M. Sela and M. Prywes (eds.), pp. 101–110, Academic Press, New York, 1969.

Schlossman, S. F., and Williamson, A. R.: Discussion. In *Genetic Control of Immune Responsiveness*, H. O. McDevitt and M. Landy (eds.), pp. 54–60, Academic Press, New York, 1972.

Schrek, R., and Donelly, W. J.: Differences between lymphocytes of leukemic and non-leukemic patients with respect to morphologic features, motility, and sensitivity to guinea pig serum. *Blood 18*:561–571, 1961.

Schultz, J. S., and Shreffler, D. C.: Studies on the serum fraction containing soluble inhibitors of anti-HL-A. *Transplantation 13*:186–188, 1972.

Schwartz, B. D., and Nathenson, S. G.: Isolation of H-2 alloantigens solubilized by the detergent NP-40. *J. Immunol. 107*:1363–1367, 1971a.

Schwartz, B. D., and Nathenson, S. G.: Regeneration of transplantation antigens on mouse cells. *Transplant. Proc. 3*:180–182, 1971b.

Schwartz, B. D., Kato, K., Cullen, S. E., and Nathenson, S. G.: H-2 histocompatibility alloantigens. Some biochemical properties of the molecules solubilized by NP-40 detergent. *Biochemistry 12*:2157–2164, 1973a.

Schwartz, B. D., Wickner, S., Rajan, T. V., and Nathenson, S. G.: Biosynthetic properties of H-2 alloantigens: Turnover rate in H-2^d tumor cells. *Transplant. Proc. 5*:439–442, 1973b.

Schwarz, E.: On North American house mice. *J. Mammal. 26*:315–316, 1945.

Schwarz, E., and Schwarz, H. K.: The wild and commensal stocks of the house mouse, *Mus musculus Linnaeus. J. Mammal. 24*:59–72, 1943.

Searle, A. G.: Curtailed, a new dominant T-allele in the house mouse. *Genet. Res. (Camb.) 7*:86–95, 1966.

Searle, A. G.: Spontaneous frequencies of point mutations in mice. *Humangenetik 16*:33–38, 1972.

Searle, A. G.: Mutation induction in mice. *Adv. Rad. Biol. 4*:131–149, 1974.

Sela, M.: Antigenicity: Some molecular aspects. *Science 166*:1365–1374, 1969.

Selander, R. K.: Biochemical polymorphism in populations of the house mouse and old-field mouse. In *Variation in Mammalian Populations*, Symp. Zool. Soc. London No. 26, R. J. Berry and H. N. Southern (eds.), pp. 73–91, Academic Press, New York, 1970.

Selander, R. K., and Yang, S. Y.: Protein polymorphism and genic heterozygosity in a wild population of the house mouse (*Mus musculus*). *Genetics 63*:653–667, 1969.

Selander, R. K., Hunt, W. G., and Yang, S. Y.: Protein polymorphism and genic heterozygosity in two European subspecies of the house mouse. *Evolution 23*: 379–390, 1969a.

Selander, R. K., Yang, S. Y., and Hunt, W. G.: Polymorphism in esterases and hemoglobin in wild populations of the house mouse (*Mus musculus*). *Studies in Genetics 5*:271–338, 1969b.

Severson, C. D., and Thompson, J. S.: Quantitative semi-micro leuko- and hemagglutination with mouse cells. *Transplantation 6*:549–553, 1968.

Shearer, G. M., Mozes, E., and Sela, M.: Cellular basis of the genetic control of immune responses to synthetic polypeptides. II. Frequency of immunocompetent precursors specific for two distinct regions within (Phe,G)-Pro--L, a synthetic polypeptide derived from multichain polyproline, in inbred mouse strains. *J. Exp. Med. 133*:216–230, 1971.

Shimada, A., and Nathenson, S. G.: Solubilization of membrane H-2 isoantigens: Chromatographic separation of specificities determined by a single H-2 genotype. *Biochem. Biophys. Res. Comm. 29*:828–833, 1967.

Shimada, A., and Nathenson, S. G.: Murine histocompatibility-2 (H-2) alloantigens. Purification and some chemical properties of soluble products from H-2^b and H-2^d genotypes released by papain digestion of membrane fractions. *Biochemistry 8*:4048–4062, 1969.

Shimada, A., and Nathenson, S. G.: Removal of neuraminic acid from H-2 allo-antigens without effect on antigenic reactivity. *J. Immunol. 107*:1197–1199, 1971.

Shimada, A., Yamane, K., and Nathenson, S. G.: Comparison of the peptide composition of two histocompatibility-2 alloantigens. *Proc. Nat. Acad. Sci. USA 65*: 691–696, 1970.

Shinoi, K.: Study of skin homotransplantation (2nd report): Especially from the standpoint of immunological considerations and acid-base balance in the skin graft. *Tokyo J. Med. Sci. 46*:11, 1932.

Shons, A. R., Kromrey, C., and Najarian, J. S.: Xenogenic mixed lymphocyte response. *Cell. Immunol. 6*:420–428, 1973.

Shorter, R. G., Nava, C., Titus, J. L., and Hallenbeck, G. A.: Mixed leukocyte cultures as a measure of histocompatibility in inbred mice. *J. Surg. Res. 8*:555–557, 1968.

Shortman, K., Brunner, K. T., and Cerottini, J. C.: Separation of stages in the development of the "T" cells involved in cell-mediated immunity. *J. Exp. Med. 135*: 1375–1391, 1972.

Shreffler, D. C.: Serum protein types in X-irradiated mice treated with homologous hematopoietic tissues. *Transplant. Bull. 30*:146–151, 1962.

Shreffler, D. C.: A serologically detected variant in mouse serum: Further evidence for genetic control by the histocompatibility-2 locus. *Genetics 49*:973–978, 1964.

Shreffler, D. C.: The Ss system of the mouse—a quantitative serum protein difference genetically controlled by the H-2 region. In *Isoantigens and Cell Interactions*, J. Palm (ed.), pp. 11–19, Wistar Institute Press, Philadelphia, 1965.

Shreffler, D. C.: A new erythrocytic antigen in the house mouse. *Genetics 54*:362, 1966. (*Abstract*).

Shreffler, D. C.: Immunogenetics of the mouse *H-2* system. In *Blood and Tissue Antigens*, D. Aminoff (ed.), pp. 85–99, Academic Press, New York, 1970.

Shreffler, D. C.: Studies on genetic fine structure of the H-2 region. In *Immunogenetics of the H-2 System*, A. Lengerová and M. Vojtíšková (eds.), pp. 138–147, Karger, Basel, 1971.

Shreffler, D. C., and David, C. S.: Studies on recombination within the mouse *H-2* complex. I. Three recombinants which position the *Ss* locus within the complex. *Tissue Antigens 2*:232–240, 1972.

Shreffler, D. C., and David, C. S.: The H-2 major histocompatibility complex and the I immune response region: Genetic variation, function and organization. *Adv. Immunol.* 1974 (*in press*).

Shreffler, D. C., and Owen, R. D.: A serologically detected variant in mouse serum: Inheritance and association with the histocompatibility-2 locus. *Genetics 48*:9–25, 1963.

Shreffler, D. C., and Passmore, H. C.: Genetics of the H-2 associated Ss-Slp trait. In *Immunogenetics of the H-2 System*, A. Lengerová and M. Vojtíšková (eds.), pp. 58–68, Karger, Basel, 1971.

Shreffler, D. C., and Snell, G. D.: The distribution of thirteen H-2 alloantigenic specificities among the products of eighteen H-2 alleles. *Transplantation 8*:435–450, 1969.

Shreffler, D. C., Amos, D. B., and Mark, R.: Serological analysis of a recombination in the H-2 region of the mouse. *Transplantation 4*:300–322, 1966.

Shreffler, D. C., David, C. S., Passmore, H. C., and Klein, J.: Genetic organization and evolution of the mouse H-2 region: a duplication model. *Transplant. Proc. 3*:176–179, 1971.

Shreffler, D., David, C., Götze, D., Klein, J., McDevitt, H., and Sachs, D.: Genetic nomenclature for new lymphocyte antigens controlled by the *I* region of the *H-2* complex. *Immunogenetics 1*:189–190, 1974.

Shumova, T. E., Kryshkina, V. P., and Egorov, I. K.: Study of H-2 mutations in mice. I. Analysis of the mutation M504 by the F_1 hybrid method. *Genetika (Moscow) 8*:171–173, 1972. (*In Russian*).

Sidman, R. L., Dickie, M. M., and Appel, S. H.: Mutant mice (quaking and jimpy) with deficient myelination in the central nervous system. *Science 144*:309–311, 1964.

Silvers, W. K., Wilson, D. B., and Palm, J.: Typing and immunosuppression in rats. *Transplantation 5*:1053–1056, 1967.

Simmons, R. L., and Ozerkis, A. J.: The immunologic problem of pregnancy. IV. Histocompatibility antigens of aging mouse trophoblast. *Amer. J. Obst. Gyn. 99*:271–273, 1967.

Simmons, R. L., and Russell, P. S.: The antigenicity of mouse trophoblast. *Ann. N.Y. Acad. Sci. 99*:717–732, 1962.

Simmons, R. L., and Russell, P. S.: Histocompatibility antigens in transplanted mouse eggs. *Nature 208*:698–699, 1965.

Simmons, R. L., and Russell, P. S.: The histocompatibility antigens of fertilized mouse eggs and trophoblast. *Ann. N.Y. Acad. Sci. 129*:35–45, 1966.

Simonsen, M.: Graft-versus-host reactions. Their natural history and applicability as tools of research. *Progr. Allergy 6*:349–467, 1962a.

Simonsen, M.: The factor of immunization: Clonal selection theory investigated by spleen assays of graft-versus-host reaction. In *Ciba Foundation Symposium on Transplantation*, G. E. W. Wolstenholme and M. D. Cameron (eds.), pp. 185–209, Churchill, London, 1962b.

Simonsen, M.: The clonal selection hypothesis evaluated by grafted cells reacting against their hosts. *Cold Spring Harbor Symp. Quant. Biol. 32*:517–523, 1967.

Simonsen, M., and Jensen, E.: The graft versus host assay in transplantation chimaeras. In *Biological Problems of Grafting*, F. Albert and G. Lejeune-Ledant (eds.), pp. 214–236, Thomas, Springfield, Ill., 1959.

Simpson, G. G.: The principles of classification and a classification of mammals. *Bull. Amer. Museum Nat. Hist. 85*:88–90, 1945.

Singer, M., Foster, F. M., Petras, M. L., Tomlin, P., and Sloane, R. W.: A new case of blood group inheritance in the house mouse. *Genetics 50*:285–286, 1964. (*Abstract*).

Singer, S. J., and Nicolson, G. L.: The fluid mosaic model of the structure of cell membranes. *Science 175*:720–731, 1972.

Skoskiewicz, M., Case, C., Winn, H. J., and Russell, P. S.: Kidney transplants between mice of graded immunogenetic diversity. *Transplant. Proc. 5*:721–725, 1973.

Smith, L. J.: A morphological and histochemical investigation of a preimplantation lethal (t^{12}) in the house mouse. *J. Exp. Zool. 132*:51–83, 1956.

Smith, R. T., and Landy, M. (eds.): *Immune Surveillance*. Academic Press, New York, 1970.

Snell, G. D.: Antigenic differences between the sperm of different inbred strains of mice. *Science 100*:272–273, 1944.

Snell, G. D.: Methods for the study of histocompatibility genes. *J. Genetics 49*:87–108, 1948.

Snell, G. D.: A fifth allele at the histocompatibility-2 locus of the mouse as determined by tumor transplantation. *J. Nat. Cancer Inst. 11*:299–1305, 1951.

Snell, G. D.: Enhancement and inhibition of the growth of tumor homoiotransplants by pretreatment of the hosts with various preparations of normal and tumor tissue. *J. Nat. Cancer Inst. 13*:719–729, 1952.

Snell, G. D.: The genetics of transplantation. *J. Nat. Cancer Inst. 14*:691–700, 1953.

Snell, G. D.: Histocompatibility genes of the mouse. I. Demonstration of weak histocompatibility differences by immunization and controlled tumor dosage. *J. Nat. Cancer Inst. 20*:787–824, 1958a.

Snell, G. D.: Histocompatibility genes of the mouse. II. Production and analysis of isogenic resistant lines. *J. Nat. Cancer Inst. 21*:843–877, 1958b.

Snell, G. D.: Transplantable tumors. In *The Physiopathology of Cancer*, 2nd ed., F. Homburger (ed.), pp. 293–345, Hoeber-Harper, New York, 1958c.

Snell, G. D.: The H-2 locus of the mouse: Observations and speculations concerning its comparative genetics and its polymorphism. *Folia Biol. (Praha) 14*:335–358, 1968.

Snell, G. D.: The histocompatibility systems. *Transplant. Proc. 3*:1133–1138, 1971.

Snell, G. D., and Borges, P. R. F.: Determination of the histocompatibility locus involved in the resistance of mice of strains C57BL/10-*x*, C57BL/6-*x*, and C57BL/6Ks to C57BL tumors. *J. Nat. Cancer Inst. 14*:481–484, 1953.

Snell, G. D., and Bunker, H. P.: Histocompatibility genes of mice. V. Five new histocompatibility loci identified by congenic resistant lines on a C57BL/10 background. *Transplantation 3*:235–252, 1965.

Snell, G. D., and Cherry, M.: Genetic factors in leukemia. Loci determining cell surface alloantigens. In *RNA Viruses and Host Genome in Oncogenesis*, P. Emmelot and P. Bentvelzen (eds.), pp. 221–228, North-Holland, Amsterdam, 1972.

Snell, G. D., and Cherry, M.: Hemagglutination and cytotoxic studies of H-2. IV. Evidence that there are 3-like antigenic sites determined by both the K and the D crossover regions. *Folia Biol. (Praha) 20*:81–100, 1974.

Snell, G. D., and Higgins, G. F.: Alleles at the histocompatibility-2 locus in the mouse as determined by tumor transplantation. *Genetics 36*:306–310, 1951.

Snell, G. D., and Stevens, L. C.: Histocompatibility genes of mice. III. *H-1* and *H-4*, two histocompatibility loci in the first linkage group. *Immunology 4*:366–379, 1961.

Snell, G. D., and Stevens, L. C.: Early Embryology. In *Biology of the Laboratory Mouse*, 2nd ed., E. L. Green (ed.), pp. 205–245, McGraw-Hill, New York, 1966.

Snell, G. D., and Stimpfling, J. F.: Genetics of tissue transplantation. In *Biology of the Laboratory Mouse*, 2nd ed., E. L. Green (ed.), pp. 457–491, McGraw-Hill, New York, 1966.

Snell, G. D., Cloudman, A. M., and Woodworth, E.: Tumor immunity in mice induced with lyophilized tissue, as influenced by tumor strain, host strain, source of tissue and dosage. *Cancer Res. 8*:429–437, 1948.

Snell, G. D., Smith, P., and Gabrielson, F.: Analysis of the histocompatibility-2 locus in the mouse. *J. Nat. Cancer Inst. 14*:457–480, 1953a.

Snell, G. D., Russell, E., Fekete, E., and Smith, P.: Resistance of various inbred strains of mice to tumor homoiotransplants, and its relation to the H-2 allele which each carries. *J. Nat. Cancer Inst. 14*:485–491, 1953b.

Snell, G. D., Staats, J., Lyon, M. F., Dunn, L. C., Grüneberg, H., Hertwig, P., and Heston, W. E.: Standardized nomenclature for inbred strains of mice, second listing. *Cancer Res. 20*:145–169, 1960.

Snell, G. D., Hoecker, G., Amos, D. B., and Stimpfling, J. H.: A revised nomenclature for the histocompatibility-2 locus of the mouse. *Transplantation 2*:777–784, 1964.

Snell, G. D., Cudkowicz, G., and Bunker, H. P.: Histocompatibility genes of mice. VII. H-13, a new histocompatibility locus in the fifth linkage group. *Transplantation 5*:492–503, 1967a.

Snell, G. D., Hoecker, G., and Stimpfling, J. H.: Evidence that the "R" and "Z" blood group specificities of mice are allelic and distinct from H-2. *Transplantation 5*:481–491, 1967b.

Snell, G. D., Démant, P., and Cherry, M.: Hemagglutination and cytotoxic studies of H-2. I. H-2.1 and related specificities in the EK crossover regions. *Transplantation 11*:210–237, 1971a.

Snell, G. D., Cherry, M., and Démant, P.: Evidence that H-2 private specificities can be arranged in two mutually exclusive systems possibly homologous with two subsystems of HL-A. *Transplant. Proc. 3*:183–186, 1971b.

Snell, G. D., Démant, P., and Cherry, M.: An H-2 chart arranged to show postulated structural features of H-2. In *Immunogenetics of the H-2 System*, A. Lengerová and M. Vojtíšková (eds.), pp. 2–9, Karger, Basel, 1971c.

Snell, G. D., Graff, R. J., and Cherry, M.: Histocompatibility genes of mice. XI. Evidence establishing a new histocompatibility locus, H-12, and new H-2 allele, H-2^{bc}. *Transplantation 11*:525–530, 1971d.

Snell, G. D., Cherry, M., and Démant, P.: H-2: Its structure and similarity to HL-A. *Transplant. Rev. 15*:3–25, 1973a.

Snell, G. D., Cherry, M., McKenzie, I. F. C., and Bailey, D. W.: Ly-4, a new locus determining a lymphocyte cell-surface alloantigen in mice. *Proc. Nat. Acad. Sci. USA 70*:1108–1111, 1973b.

Snell, G. D., Démant, P., and Cherry, M.: Hemagglutination and cytotoxic studies of H-2. V. The anti-27,28,29 family of antibodies. *Folia Biol. (Praha) 20*:145–160, 1974.

Solliday, S., and Bach, F. H.: Cytotoxicity: Specificity after *in vitro* sensitization. *Science 170*:1406–1409, 1970.

Sørenson, S. F.: The mixed lymphocyte culture interaction. Techniques and immunogenetics. *Acta Path. Microbiol. Scand.* Suppl. *230*:1–82, 1972.

Southwick, C. H.: The population dynamics of confined house mice supplied with unlimited food. *Ecology 36*:212–225, 1955a.

Southwick, C. H.: Regulatory mechanisms of house mouse populations: Social behavior affecting litter survival. *Ecology 36*:627–634, 1955b.

Southwick, C. H.: Population characteristics of house mice living in English corn ricks: Density relationships. *Proc. Zool. Soc. London 131*:163–175, 1958.

Sparks, F. C., Ting, C. C., Hammond, W. G., and Herberman, R. B.: An isotopic antiglobulin technique for measuring antibodies to cell-surface antigens. *J. Immunol. 102*:842–847, 1969.

Sparks, F. C., Canty, T. G., Ting, C. C., Hammond, W. G., and Herberman, R. B.: Antibody response to skin allografts in mice. *Proc. Soc. Exp. Biol. Med. 133*: 1392–1396, 1970.

Spencer, R. A., Hauschka, T. S., Amos, D., and Ephrussi, B.: Co-dominance of iso-antigens in somatic hybrids of murine cells grown *in vitro. J. Nat. Cancer Inst. 33*:893–903, 1964.

Spooner, R. L., Bowden, F. W., and Carpenter, R. G.: Description and analysis of a simple micro-titration immune cytolytic test. *J. Hyg. (Camb.) 63*:369–381, 1965.

Sprent, J.: The proliferative response of T lymphocytes to alloantigens in irradiated mice: A mixed lymphocyte reaction *in vivo. Transplant. Proc. 5*:1725–1729, 1973.

Sprent, J., and Miller, J. F. A. P.: Interaction of thymus lymphocytes with histo-incompatible cells. I. Quantitation of the proliferative response of thymus cells. *Cell. Immunol. 3*:361–384, 1972a.

Sprent, J., and Miller, J. F. A. P.: Interaction of thymus lymphocytes with histo-incompatible cells. II. Recirculating lymphocytes derived from antigen-activated thymus cells. *Cell. Immunol. 3*:385–404, 1972b.

Sprent, J., and Miller, J. F. A. P.: Interaction of thymus lymphocytes with histo-incompatible cells. III. Immunological characteristics of recirculating lymphocytes derived from activated thymus cells. *Cell. Immunol. 3*:213–230, 1972c.

Staats, J.: The laboratory mouse. In *Biology of the Laboratory Mouse*, 2nd ed., E. L. Green (ed.), pp. 1–9, McGraw-Hill, New York, 1966.

Staats, J.: Standardized nomenclature for inbred strains of mice: Fifth listing. *Cancer Res. 32*:1609–1946, 1972.

Stackpole, C. W.: Topography of cell surface antigens. *Transplant. Proc. 3*:1199–1201, 1971.

Stackpole, C. W., Aoki, T., Boyse, E. A., Old, L. J., Lumley-Frank, J., and De Harven, E.: Cell surface antigens: Serial sectioning of single cells as an approach to topographical analysis. *Science 172*:472–474, 1971.

Štark, O., Křen, V., and Frenzl, B.: Erythrocyte and transplantation antigens in four inbred rat strains. Serological analysis of strain-specific antigens. *Folia Biol. (Praha) 13*:85–92, 1967.

Steeves, R. A., Bennett, M., Mirand, E. A., and Cudkowicz, G.: Genetic control by the *W* locus of susceptibility to (Friend) spleen focus forming virus. *Nature 218*: 372–374, 1968.

Stephenson, E. M., and Stephenson, N. G.: Karyotype analysis of the B16 mouse melanoma with reassessment of the normal mouse idiogram. *J. Nat. Cancer Inst. 45*:789–800, 1970.

Stetson, C. A., and Esko, B.: Reactions between some antimicrobial sera and mouse erythrocytes. In *Cross-reacting Antigens and Neoantigens* (with Implications for Autoimmunity and Cancer Immunity), J. J. Trentin (ed.), pp. 61–68, Williams & Wilkins, Baltimore, 1967.

Stimpfling, J. H.: The use of PVP as a developing agent in mouse hemagglutination test. *Transplant. Bull. 27*:109–111, 1961.

Stimpfling, J. H.: Immunogenetics of mouse cellular isoantigens. In *Isoantigens and Cell Interactions*, J. Palm (ed.), pp. 5–10, Wistar Institute Press, Philadelphia, 1965.

Stimpfling, J. H.: Recombination within a histocompatibility locus. *Ann. Rev. Genetics* 5:121–142, 1971.

Stimpfling, J. H.: Presentation at the H-2 workshop, Bar Harbor, Maine, 1973.

Stimpfling, J. H., and Durham, T.: Genetic control by the H-2 gene complex of the alloantibody response to an H-2 antigen. *J. Immunol.* 108:947–951, 1972.

Stimpfling, J. H., and McBroom, C. R.: The effect of H-2 on the humoral antibody response to a non-H-2 blood group antigen. *Transplantation 11*: 87–89, 1971.

Stimpfling, J. H., and Pandis, D. E.: The effect of heterozygosity on the humoral antibody response in mice. *Folia Biol. (Praha)* 15:233–238, 1969.

Stimpfling, J. H., and Pizarro, O.: On the antigenic products of the H-2^m allele in the laboratory mouse. *Transplant. Bull.* 28:102–106, 1961.

Stimpfling, J. H., and Reichert, A. E.: Strain C57BL/10ScSn and its congenic resistant sublines. *Transplant. Proc.* 2:39–47, 1970.

Stimpfling, J. H., and Reichert, A. E.: Male-specific graft rejection and the H-2 locus. *Transplantation* 12:527–531, 1971.

Stimpfling, J. H., and Reichert McBroom, C.: The effect of H-2 on the humoral antibody response to a non-H-2 blood group antigen. *Transplantation 11*:87–89, 1971.

Stimpfling, J. H., and Richardson, A.: Recombination within the histocompatibility-2 locus of the mouse. *Genetics 51*:831–846, 1965.

Stimpfling, J. H., and Richardson, A.: Periodic variations of the hemagglutinin response in mice following immunization against sheep red blood cells and allo-antigens. *Transplantation 5*:1496–1503, 1967.

Stimpfling, J. H., and Snell, G. D.: Detection of a non-H-2 blood group system with the aid of B10.129(5M) mice. *Transplantation 6*:468–475, 1968.

Stimpfling, J. H., Reichert, A. E., and Hudson, P.: The serological properties of some H-2 recombinant alleles. In *Immunogenetics of the H-2 System*, A. Lengerová and M. Vojtíšková (eds.), pp. 10–17, Karger, Basel, 1971.

Stockert, E., Old, L. J., and Boyse, E. A.: The G_{IX} system. A cell surface allo-antigen associated with murine leukemia virus; implications regarding chromosomal integration of the viral genome. *J. Exp. Med. 133*:1334–1335, 1971.

Stockert, E., Sato, H., Itakura, K., Boyse, E. A., and Old, L. J.: Location of the second gene required for expression of the leukemia-associated mouse antigen G_{IX}. *Science 178*:862–863, 1972.

Strecker, R. L., and Emlen, J. T.: Regulatory mechanisms in house mouse popula-tions: The effect of limited food supply on a confined population. *Ecology 34*: 375–385, 1953.

Strom, R., and Klein, E.: Fluorometric quantitation of fluorescein-coupled antibodies attached to the cell membrane. *Proc. Nat. Acad. Sci. USA 63*:1157–1163, 1969.

Strong, L. C.: The establishment of the "A" strain of inbred mice. *J. Hered. 27*: 21–24, 1936.

Strong, L. C.: The origin of some inbred mice. *Cancer Res. 2*:531–539, 1942.

Stutman, O.: Tumor development after 3-methylcholanthrene in immunologically deficient athymic-nude mice. *Science 183*:534–536, 1974.

Summerell, J. M., and Davies, D. A. L.: Further characterization of soluble mouse and human transplantation antigens. *Transplant. Proc. 1*:479–482, 1969.

Summerell, J. M., and Davies, D. A. L.: Physical properties of mouse H-2 trans-plantation alloantigens. *Biochim. Biophys. Acta. 207*:92–104, 1970.

Svehag, S. E., and Schilling, W.: Solubilization of species-specific antigens and murine alloantigens by pulsed high frequency sonic energy. *Scand. J. Immunol. 2*:115–123, 1973.

Tachibana, T., and Klein, E.: Detection of cell surface antigens on monolayer cells. I. The application of immune adherence on a micro scale. *Immunology 19*:771–782, 1970.

Tachibana, T., Worst, P., and Klein, E.: Detection of cell surface antigens on mono-layer cells. II. The application of mixed haemadsorption on a micro scale. *Immunology 19*:809–816, 1970.

Takahaski, T.: Possible examples of antigenic modulation affecting H-2 antigens and cell surface immunoglobulins. *Transplant. Proc. 3*:1217–1220, 1971.

Takahashi, T., Old, J., and Boyse, E. A.: Surface alloantigens of plasma cells. *J. Exp. Med. 131*:1325–1341, 1970.

Takasugi, M., and Hildemann, W. H.: Regulation of immunity toward allogeneic tumors in mice. I. Effect of antiserum fractions on tumor growth. *J. Nat. Cancer Inst. 43*:843–856, 1969.

Tanigaki, N., Nakamuro, K., Apella, E., Poulik, M. D., and Pressman, D.: Identity of the HL-A common portion fragment and human β_2-microglobulin. *Biochem. Biophys. Res. Com. 55*: 1234–1239, 1973.

Taylor, B. A., Meier, H., and Huebner, R. J.: Genetic control of the group-specific antigen of murine leukemia virus. *Nature New Biol. 241*:184–186. 1973.

Taylor, G. M., and Bennet, J.: A modified plaque test for the detection of cells forming antibody to alloantigens. *J. Immunol. Methods 2*:213–219, 1973.

Taylor, R. B., Duffus, P. H., Raff, M. C., and DePetris, S.: Redistribution and pino-cytosis of lymphocyte surface immunoglobulin molecules induced by anti-immunoglobulin antibody. *Nature New Biol. 233*:225–229, 1971.

Tennant, J. R.: Derivation of a murine lymphoid leukemia virus. *J. Nat. Cancer Inst. 28*:1291–1303, 1962.

Tennant, J. R.: Susceptibility and resistance to viral leukemogenesis in the mouse. II. Response to the virus relative to histocompatibility factors carried by the prospective host. *J. Nat. Cancer Inst. 34*:633–641, 1965.

Tennant, J. R.: Additional evidence for implication of histocompatibility factors in resistance to viral leukemogenesis in the mouse. In *Advance in Transplantation*, J. Dausset, J. Hamburger, and G. Mathé (eds.), pp. 507–514, Williams & Wilkins, Baltimore, 1968.

Tennant, J. R., and Snell, G. D.: Some experimental evidence for the influence of genetic factors on viral leukemogenesis. *Nat. Cancer Inst. Monogr. 22*:61–72, 1966.

Tennant, J. R., and Snell, G. D.: The H-2 locus and viral leukemogenesis as studied in congenic strains of mice. *J. Nat. Cancer Inst. 41*:597–604, 1968.

Terasaki, P. I., and Rich, N. E.: Quantitative determination of antibody and com-plement directed against lymphocytes. *J. Immunol. 92*:128–138, 1964.

Theiler, K.: *The House Mouse*, Springer-Verlag, New York, 1972.

Theiler, K., and Gluecksohn-Waelsch, S.: The morphological effects and the develop-ment of the Fused mutation in the mouse. *Anat. Rec. 125*:83–103, 1956.

Thomas, L.: Discussion. In *Cellular and Humoral Aspects of the Hypersensitive States*, H. S. Lawrence (ed.), pp. 529–532, Cassell, London, 1959.

Thorsby, E.: A tentative new model for the organization of the mouse H-2 histo-compatibility system. Two segregant series of antigens. *Eur. J. Immunol. 1*:57–59, 1971.

Ting, C-C., and Herberman, R. B.: Inverse relationship of polyoma tumour specific cell surface antigen to H-2 histocompatibility antigens. *Nature New Biol. 232*: 118–120, 1971.

Tissot, R. G., and Cohen, C.: Histocompatibility in the rabbit. *Tissue Antigens 2*:267–279, 1972.

Tomazic, V., Rose, N. R., and Shreffler, D. C.: Autoimmune murine thyroiditis. IV. Localization of genetic control of the immune response. *J. Immunol. 112*:965–969, 1974.

Tridente, G., Cappuzzo, G. M., and Chieco-Cianchi, L.: Lymphocyte interaction in mixed mouse leukocyte cultures (a preliminary report). In *Histocompatibility Testing 1967*, E. S. Curtoni, P. L. Mattiuz, and R. M. Rosi (eds.), pp. 67–73, Munksgaard, Copenhagen, 1967.

Tyan, M. L.: Rejection of allogeneic skin grafts by sublethally irradiated and non-irradiated mice sensitized with spleen cells and Freund's adjuvant. *Transplantation 3*:54–61, 1965.

Tyan, M. L.: Genetically determined immune responses: *In vitro* studies. *J. Immunol. 108*:65–72, 1972.

Tyan, M. L., and Cole, L. J.: Development of transplantation isoantigens in the mouse embryo plus trophoblast. *Transplant. Bull. 30*:526–530, 1962.

Tyan, M. L., and McDevitt, H. O.: Antibody responses to two synthetic polypeptides: The role of the thymic epithelial reticulum. *J. Immunol. 105*:1190–1193, 1970.

Tyan, M. L., and Ness, D. B.: Mouse blood leukocytes: *In vitro* primary and secondary responses to two synthetic polypeptides. *J. Immunol. 106*:289–291, 1971.

Tyan, M. L., and Ness, D. B.: Modification of the mixed leukocyte reaction with various antisera. *Transplantation 13*:198–201, 1972.

Tyan, M. L., McDevitt, H. O., and Herzenberg, L. A.: Genetic control of the antibody response to a synthetic polypeptide: Transfer of response with spleen cells or lymphoid precursors. *Transplant. Proc. 1*:548–550, 1969.

Tyzzer, E. E.: A study of inheritance in mice with reference to their susceptibility to transplantable tumors. *J. Med. Res. 21*:519–573, 1909.

Uhr, J. W., and Anderson, S. G.: The placenta as a homotransplant. *Nature 194*:1292–1293, 1962.

Uphoff, D. E.: Drug-induced immunological "tolerance" for homotransplantation. *Transplant. Bull. 28*:110–114, 1961.

Vaiman, M., Renard, C., LaFage, P., Ameteau, J., and Nizza, P.: Evidence for a histocompatibility system in swine (SL-A). *Transplantation 10*:155–164, 1970.

Vaz, N. M., and Levine, B. B.: Immune responses of inbred mice to repeated low doses of antigen: Relationship to histocompatibility (H-2) type. *Science 168*: 852–854, 1970.

Vaz, N. M., Vaz, E. M., and Levine, B. B.: Relationship between histocompatibility (H-2) genotype and immune responsiveness to low doses of ovalbumin in the mouse. *J. Immunol. 104*:1572–1574, 1970.

Vaz, N. M., Phillips-Quagliata, J. M., Levine, B. B., and Vaz, E. M.: H-2-linked genetic control of immune responsiveness to ovalbumin and ovomucoid. *J. Exp. Med. 134*:1335–1348, 1971.

v.Boehmer, H.: Separation of T and B lymphocytes and their role in the mixed lymphocyte reaction. *J. Immunol. 112*:70–77, 1974.

Vedernikov, A. A., and Egorov, I. K.: Study of H-2 mutations in mice. II. Recombination analysis of the mutation 504. *Genetika* (Moskva) *9*:60–66, 1973. (In Russian).

Virolainen, M., Häyry, P., and Defendi, V.: Effect of presensitization on the mixed lymphocyte reaction of rat spleen cell cultures. *Transplantation 8*:179–188, 1969.

Vitetta, E. S., Bianco, C., Nussenzweig, V., and Uhr, J. W.: Cell surface Ig. IV. Distribution among thymocytes, bone marrow cells, and their derived populations. *J. Exp. Med. 136*:81–93, 1972a.

Vitetta, E. S., Uhr, J. W., and Boyse, E. A.: Isolation and characterization of H-2 and TL alloantigens from the surface of mouse lymphocytes. *Cell. Immunol. 4*: 187–191, 1972b.

Vitetta, E. S., Klein, J., and Uhr, J. W.: Partial characterization of Ia antigens from murine lymphoid cells. *Immunogenetics 1*:82–90, 1974a.

Vitetta, E. S., Uhr, J. W., and Boyse, E. A.: Metabolism of H-2 and Thy-1 (θ) allo-antigens in murine thymocytes. *Eur. J. Immunol. 4*:276–282, 1974b.

Vladutiu, A. O., and Rose, N. R.: Autoimmune murine thyroiditis. Relation to histo-compatibility (H-2) type. *Science 174*:1137–1139, 1971.

Voisin, G. A., Kinsky, R. G., and Jansen, F. K.: Transplantation immunity: Localization in mouse serum of antibodies responsible for haemagglutination, cytotoxicity and enhancement. *Nature 210*:138–139, 1966.

Voisin, G. A., Kinsky, R., Jansen, F., and Bernard, C.: Biological properties of anti-body classes in transplantation immune sera. *Transplantation 8*:618–632, 1969.

Vojtíšková, M.: H-2^d antigens on mouse spermatozoa. *Nature 222*:1293–1294, 1969.

Vojtíšková, M., and Pokorná, Z.: H-2 antigens on diploid spermatogenic cells. In *Immunogenetics of the H-2 System*, A. Lengerová and M. Vojtíšková (eds.), pp. 261–266, Karger, Basel, 1971.

Vojtíšková, M., and Pokorná, Z.: Cellular antigens of mouse spermatozoa as possible markers of gene action. In *The Genetics of the Spermatozoon*, R. A. Beatty and S. Gluecksohn-Waelsch (eds.), pp. 160–176, Edinburgh, 1972a.

Vojtíšková, M., and Pokorná, Z.: Developmental expression of H-2 antigens in the spermatogenic cell series: Possible bearing on haploid gene action. *Folia Biol. (Praha) 18*:1–9, 1972b.

Vojtíšková, M., Poláčková, M., and Pokorná, Z.: Histocompatibility antigens on mouse spermatozoa. *Folia Biol. (Praha) 15*:322–332, 1969.

Vranken-Paris, M., Lejeune, G., Castermans, A., Dieu, H. A., and Haenen-Severyns, A. M.: Essais de séparation et d'identification des antigènes de transplantation. *Bull. Soc. Chim. Biol. 44*:365–377, 1962.

Vriesendorp, H. M., Rothengatter, C., Box, E., Westbroek, D. L., and van Rood, J. J.: The production and evaluation of dog allolymphocytotoxins for donor selection in transplantation experiments. *Transplantation 11*:440–445, 1971.

Wallach, D. F. H.: *The Plasma Membrane: Dynamic Perspectives, Genetics and Pathology*. Springer-Verlag, New York, 1972.

Warburton, F. E.: Maintenance of histocompatibility polymorphisms. *Heredity 23*: 151–152, 1968.

Weber, W.: Genetical studies on the skeleton of the mouse. III. Skeletal variation in wild populations. *J. Genetics 50*:174–178, 1950.

Weinrach, R. S., Lai, M., and Talmage, D. W.: The relation between hemolysin concentration and hemolytic rate as measured with chromium[51] labeled cells. *J. Inf. Dis. 102*:60–73, 1958.

Wekerle, H., Lonai, P., and Feldman, M.: Fractionation of antigen reactive cells on a cellular immunoadsorbent: Factors determining recognition of antigens by T-lymphocytes. *Proc. Nat. Acad. Sci. USA 69*:1620–1624, 1972.

Wernet, D., Vitetta, E. S., Uhr, J. W., and Boyse, E. A.: Synthesis, intracellular distribution, and secretion of immunoglobulin and H-2 antigen in murine splenocytes. *J. Exp. Med. 138*:847–857, 1973.

Wheeler, L. L.: XVI. Inheritance of allozymes in subspecific F_1 hybrids of *Mus musculus* from Denmark. *Studies in Genetics 7*:319–325, 1972.

Wheeler, L. L., and Selander, R. K.: XIII. Genetic variation in populations of the house mouse, *Mus musculus*, in the Hawaiian Islands. *Studies in Genetics 7*:269–296, 1972.

Widmer, M. B., and Bach, F. H.: Allogeneic and xenogeneic response in mixed leukocyte cultures. *J. Exp. Med. 135*:1204–1208, 1972.

Widmer, M. B., Alter, B. J., Bach, F. H., and Bach, M. L.: Lymphocyte reactivity to serologically undetected components of the major histocompatibility complex. *Nature New Biol. 242*:239–241, 1973a.

Widmer, M. B., Omodei-Zorini, C., Bach, M. L., Bach, F. H., and Klein, J.: Importance of different regions of H-2 for MLC stimulation. *Tissue Antigens 3*:309–315, 1973b.

Widmer, M. B., Peck, A. B., and Bach, F. H.: Genetic mapping of H-2 LD loci. *Transplant. Proc. 5*:1501–1505, 1973c.

Widmer, M. B., Schendel, D. J., Bach, F. J., and Boyse, E. A.: The H(Tla) histocompatibility locus: A study of *in vitro* lymphocyte reactivity. *Transplant Proc. 5*:1663–1666, 1973d.

Wigzell, H.: Quantitative titrations of mouse H-2 antibodies using Cr^{51}-labelled target cells. *Transplantation 3*:423–431, 1965.

Wilson, D. B., and Fox, D. H.: Quantitative studies on the mixed lymphocyte interaction in rats. VI. Reactivity of lymphocytes from conventional and germfree rats to allogeneic and xenogeneic cell surface antigens. *J. Exp. Med. 134*:857–870, 1971.

Wilson, D. B., and Nowell, P. C.: Quantitative studies on the mixed lymphocyte interaction in rats. IV. Immunologic potentiality of the responding cells. *J. Exp. Med. 131*:391–407, 1970.

Wilson, D. B., and Nowell, P. C.: Quantitative studies on the mixed lymphocyte interaction in rats. V. Tempo and specificity of the proliferative response and the number of reactive cells from immunized donors. *J. Exp. Med. 133*:442–453, 1971.

Wilson, D. B., Silvers, W. K., and Nowell, P. C.: Quantitative studies on the mixed lymphocyte interaction in rats. II. Relationship of the proliferative response to the immunologic status of the donors. *J. Exp. Med. 126*:655–665, 1967.

Wilson, D. B., Blyth, J. L., and Nowell, P. C.: Quantitative studies on the mixed lymphocyte interaction in rats. *J. Exp. Med. 128*:1157–1181, 1968.

Wilson, D. B., Howard, J. C., and Nowell, P. C.: Some biological aspects of lymphocytes reactive to strong histocompatibility alloantigens. *Transplant. Rev. 12*:3–29, 1972.

Winn, H. J.: The participation of complement in isoimmune reactions. *Ann. N.Y. Acad. Sci. 101*:23–44, 1962.

Winn, H. J.: Hemolysis and complement fixation. *Meth. Med. Res. 10*:48–57, 1964.

Winn, H. J.: Effects of complement on sensitized nucleated cells. In *Ciba Foundation Symposium on Complement*, G. E. W. Wolstenholme and J. Knight (eds.), pp. 133–148, Little, Brown, Boston, 1965a.

Winn, H. J.: Complement fixation in typing histocompatibility systems. In *Histocompatibility Testing*, pp. 61–69, Nat. Acad. Sci., Washington, 1965b.

Yamane, K., and Nathenson, S. G.: Murine histocompatibility-2 (H-2) alloantigens. Purification and some chemical properties of a second class of fragments (class II) solubilized by papain from cell membranes of H-2^b and H-2^d mice. *Biochemistry* 9:1336–1341, 1970a.

Yamane, K., and Nathenson, S. G.: Biochemical similarity of papain-solubilized H-2^d alloantigens from tumor cells and from normal cells. *Biochemistry* 9:4743–4750, 1970b.

Yamane, K., Shimada, A., and Nathenson, S. G.: Peptide comparison of two histocompatibility-2 (H-2^b and H-2^d) alloantigens. *Biochemistry* 11:2398–2401, 1972.

Yanagisawa, K.: Studies on the mechanism of abnormal transmission ratios at the T-locus in the house mouse. II. Test for physiological differences between t- and T-bearing sperm manifested *in vitro. Jap. J. Genetics* 10:87–92, 1965a.

Yanagisawa, K.: Studies on the mechanism of abnormal transmission ratios at the T-locus in the house mouse. III. Test for physiological differences between t^1- and T-sperm manifested during storage period in the epididymis and vas deferens. *Jap. J. Genetics* 40:93–96, 1965b.

Yanagisawa, K.: Studies on the mechanism of abnormal transmission ratios at the T-locus in the house mouse. IV. Some morphological studies on the mature sperm in males heterozygous for t-alleles. *Jap J. Genetics* 40:97–104, 1965c.

Yanagisawa, K., Dunn, L. C., and Bennett, D.: On the mechanism of abnormal transmission ratios at T-locus in the house mouse. *Genetics* 46:1635–1644, 1961.

Yanagisawa, K., Bennett, D., Boyse, E. A., Dunn, L. C., and Dimeo, A.: Serological identification of sperm antigens specified by lethal t-alleles in the mouse. *Immunogenetics* 1:57–67, 1974a.

Yanagisawa, K., Pollard, D. R., Bennett, D., Dunn, L. C., and Boyse, E. A.: Transmission ratio distortion at the T-locus: Serological identification of two sperm populations in t-heterozygotes. *Immunogenetics* 1:91–96, 1974b.

Young, H., Strecker, R. L., and Emlen, J. T., Jr.: Localization of activity in two indoor populations of house mice, *Mus musculus. J. Mammal.* 31:403–410, 1950.

Young, J. M., and Gyenes, L.: The induction of cellular immunity with soluble murine histocompatibility antigens. *Cell. Immunol.* 6:231–242, 1973.

Yu, A., and Cohen, E. P.: Studies on the effect of specific antisera on the metabolism of cellular antigens. I. Isolation of Thymus Leukemia antigens. *J. Immunol.* 112:1285–1295, 1974a.

Yu, A., and Cohen, E. P.: Studies on the effect of specific antisera on the metabolism of cellular antigens. II. The synthesis and degradation of TL antigens of mouse cells in the presence of TL antiserum. *J. Immunol.* 112:1296–1307, 1974b.

Yunis, E. J., and Amos, D. B.: Three closely linked genetic systems relevant to transplantation. *Proc. Nat. Acad. Sci. USA* 68:3031–3035, 1971.

Zajtchuk, R., Kahan. B. D., and Adams, W. E.: The tissue distribution of a water soluble antigen. *Dis. Chest* 50:368–371, 1966.

Zaleski, M.: Immune response of mice to Thy-1.1 antigen: Studies on congenic lines. *Immunogenetics* 1:226–238, 1974.

Zaleski, M., and Klein, J.: Immune response of mice to Thy-1.1 antigen: Genetic control by alleles at the *Ir-5* locus loosely linked to the H-2 complex. *J. Immunol.* 113:1170–1177, 1974.

Zaleski, M., and Milgrom, F.: Complementary genes controlling immune response to θ-AKR antigen in mice. *J. Immunol.* 110:1238–1244, 1973.

Zaleski, M., Fuji, H., and Milgrom, F.: Evidence for multigenic control of immune response to theta-AKR antigen in mice. *Transplant. Proc. 5*:201–204, 1973.

Zmijewski, C. M.: *Immunohematology*. Appleton-Century-Crofts, New York, 1968.

Zoschke, D. C., and Bach, F. H.: Specificity of allogeneic cell recognition by human lymphocytes *in vitro. Science 172*:1350–1352, 1971.

Author Index

Subject Index

Many entries occur repeatedly throughout the text; for these only reference to the page is given where they are defined or described in detail.